Naturopathic Medicine

Fraser Smith

Naturopathic Medicine

A Comprehensive Guide

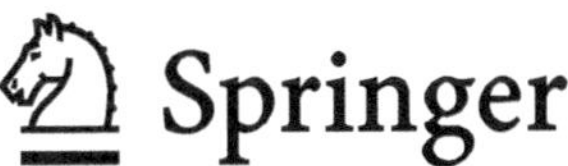

Fraser Smith, MATD, ND
National University of Health Sciences
Lombard, IL, USA

ISBN 978-3-031-13390-9 ISBN 978-3-031-13388-6 (eBook)
https://doi.org/10.1007/978-3-031-13388-6

This Springer imprint is published by the registered company Springer Nature Switzerland AG
The registered company address is: Gewerbestrasse 11, 6330 Cham, Switzerland

I dedicate this book to my wife Debra. You encouraged me to dream it, go for it, and to get the writing done! Love always, Fraser

Preface

Naturopathic Medicine: A Comprehensive Guide was written to exposit the principles, processes, and application of this approach to medicine. Naturopathic medicine, being both first contact health care and a particular approach to creating conditions for healing, needs to be understood as a dynamic system. Therefore, this textbook builds from the premise that the body can often heal itself, but not always, and that it often needs assistance, in some cases the kind of immediate and forceful assistance that is best delivered by conventional medical approaches. The book also explains why even clearly indicated medical interventions can yield diminishing returns, if the physiology, biochemical, and genetic reserves of a patient are perpetually imbalanced and unstable.

The dynamic approach of this book is based on the premise that there are two major types of responses to injury, or disruptions to determining factors of health, that we can observe. There are adaptive responses which can maintain homeostasis and often repair damaged tissues or organs. There are maladaptive responses that might have started out as helpful, or are simply byproducts of a very strong pathogenic or traumatic force. The maladaptive responses can frustrate our efforts to heal—sometimes reducing them allows healing to proceed, provided that other conditions are met. Undergirding this all is the fact that basic physiological requirements for health and function must be met in order to heal, and their inadequacy is often behind many chronic problems.

The book, by necessity, explores the progression of disease. The factors that can injure the body are numerous, and they often work in unison across multiple systems. They can be ignored for a long time in some cases, but their bill eventually comes due. These injurious factors can lead to compensatory responses, as well as directly interfering with homeostasis. Over time, this process leads to certain states that are the ground from which various clinically recognizable diseases emerge, for instance, disruption to the microbiome and the immune system, or fundamental imbalances in the bioregulatory systems that create homeostasis. The process of unwinding the resilient and healthy state to one where multiple breakdowns occur is one that is understandable in biological terms.

With this in mind, the book examines various organ systems, and treatments, in light of various levels of dysfunction. These range from the serious but superficial, to structural, to exhibiting decline of function based on disruption to tissues. Understanding the nature of this dysfunction is important in creating a treatment plan, and in anticipating what improvements and exacerbations may be on the way. The book proposes a model of healing that is dynamic, just as living systems are. Since disturbed or inadequate determining factors of health are often found in ill patients, therapy should at least start with addressing these. On the side of enhancing adaptive responses, the use of natural means to provide biochemical support, to give whole person support (broadly impacting health or nutritional status), and using treatments that have a hormetic mode of action can all be done in a coherent way. Dampening maladaptive responses is also important, and both natural and pharmaceutical ways to do this are discussed. Finally, for a number of reasons, some creation of homeostasis through external means is unavoidable for some patients. Naturopathic medicine is very helpful in a wide array of outpatient situations and many examples are provided in this book. The approach to these conditions, and the way that various therapies are useful within the aforementioned model of healing, is an overarching theme.

The manner in which scientifically derived knowledge can be applied to naturopathic medical practice is discussed, as well as the best ways to create more of that knowledge. It is true that a system such as naturopathic medicine that addresses causative factors of disease is partially supported by the simple study of the structure and function of the body. But this is an inadequate knowledge base. As a practice, applied research is needed. The sort of knowledge that derives from randomized controlled trials is important and certainly accurate if done well, but it is not wholly relevant to all aspects of naturopathic medicine. This is because of the individualization and the process-oriented approach that defies extreme generalizations arising from attempts to randomize. Such studies and aggregations of them can tell us a lot, but not everything about what to do for a patient.

Finally, the role of naturopathic medicine in primary care settings and in society is a final note of this book. It is very easy for allosteric systems of practice such as naturopathic medicine to drift into anomie and a lack of rootedness in the phenomenological approach that helped it gain traction in the first place. Or, it can assimilate into standard medical care out of a desire for acceptance and access to resources, becoming almost indistinguishable from conventional practice. It might also become so iconoclastic that it places itself outside of healthcare, which can lead to unfortunate outcomes should patients be given false dilemmas about which approach to choose. Or it can become pseudo-professional, with more of a consulting or retail presence. None of these fates have befallen naturopathic medicine yet, but there is much work to do in articulating and expanding the knowledge basis of this field. There are many excellent resources in publication that address diagnosis and therapy. This book is intended to guide the reader through the process of analysis of problems and synthesis of solutions, in a way that incorporates scientific discovery and traditional knowledge. When this is done well, it is naturopathic medicine at its best—an approach to medicine that can help many people.

Lombard, IL, USA
July 5, 2022

Fraser Smith

Acknowledgments

I wish to express my thanks to those in naturopathic medicine whose work and leadership have been so instrumental in my own learning. Dr. Jared Zeff and Dr. Pamela Snider, both in their published works and in conversation, have helped me to understand healing as a process. My colleague and friend Dr. Louise Edwards has over the years helped me to appreciate how fundamental the determining factors of health are in setting the stage for health, or for disease if those determinants are insufficient or disturbed. Dr. Edwards also helped me to appreciate, on a deeper level, just how capable and ready we are to heal, if the conditions for health are met and the right support and guidance is provided.

But I am particularly indebted to my long-term teacher, mentor, colleague, and friend, Dr. Paul Saunders. Through the many, many times he has imparted his knowledge, and always through his example, I've come to appreciate how scientific discoveries, carefully curated clinical observations, and sound reasoning can come together to create a naturopathic treatment plan. I first met Dr. Saunders when I was a soon to be naturopathic medical student and was simply coming to the teaching clinic at Canadian College of Naturopathic Medicine (CCNM), to see what it was all about. His sharp mind and calm but energized demeanor made an impression on me. As a naturopathic medical student, I took many classes with him, and upon graduating I had the opportunity to do my residency under his auspices. It was a time where I wanted to keep learning and be very much a part of the explosive growth of CCNM in the late 1990s. He has been a source of encouragement since I came to National University of Health Sciences (NUHS) in 2005 to work with the University to start the Doctor of Naturopathic Medicine degree program. Since 2018 Dr. Saunders has been part-time faculty at NUHS, teaching principles of intravenous therapy and lately botanical medicine. Not only am I exceedingly happy for our students, but it is a thrill to see a new generation learn from someone who is so well read, with so many publications, so experienced in patient care, and who can synthesize knowledge from so many sources and bring it to the clinic. I urge any student of healthcare, including naturopathic medicine, to follow this example of constantly seeking knowledge and better ways to help patients.

I thank my associates here at NUHS, and our amazing students whose quest to become outstanding naturopathic physicians inspires me.

Finally, my thanks to my editor Ms. Margaret Moore, Mr. Vinodh Thomas, the production coordinator for this book, and the team at Springer-Nature. It's a pleasure to get to work with a world-class scientific publishing house, which is a fitting home for books about my field, naturopathic medicine.

Fraser Smith, MATD, ND
Lombard, Illinois
June 2022

Contents

Chapter 1
The Nature of Health, Homeostasis, Adaptation, Biological Plasticity, Repair

Definitions of Health

Health is a state of being that practically everyone wants to enjoy. Living according to good habits helps to preserve it. The absence of the determinants of health will erode it. The judicious use of standard medical therapies can preserve it, by negating, for a time, the breakdown processes that occur when a state of health is not sustainable.

Health does not just happen, and it is more than the absence of disease as the World Health Organization (WHO) once pointed out. It is also much more than just a state of wholeness of high function. The ground of the experience we know as health is the result of millions of concurrent processes that sustain these very complex entities we know as our bodies. The amount of synchronicity and organization that this involves is staggering. It is, in fact, beyond what we can grasp in its totality. But we can study its components, and we can create very useful and research-supported models that can guide our decisions about prevention and treatment.

It is useful to describe health in terms of physiological processes, keeping in mind that the subjective experience of health matters. That is, a person may seem fine on a routine physical examination, bloodwork, and imaging studies. But they might have a sense of despair or futility in their life and suffer from lassitude and a sense of emptiness. Or at a different level, latent processes such as expression of oncogenes and failure of their cancer suppression genes have put them on track for developing cancer in the next 5–10 years even though at the moment, they are in a state of high function.

A relevant, but limited, concept used in defining health is that of homeostasis. This is the proper functioning of bioregulatory systems in the body that keep the conditions for life within certain normal limits (Fig. 1.1). For example, our cells need a certain concentration of the cation potassium (K+) inside themselves, within their cell membranes. They need a certain concentration of sodium on the outside,

F. Smith, *Naturopathic Medicine*, https://doi.org/10.1007/978-3-031-13388-6_1

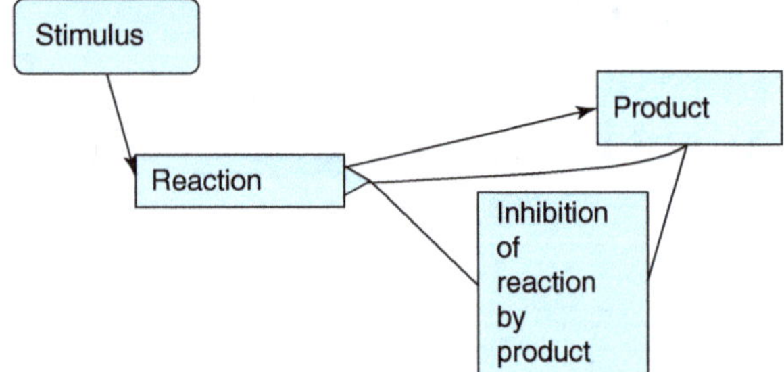

Fig. 1.1 Homeostasis: The classical model of homeostasis involves various negative feedback loops. Processes needed for function are inhibited by the accumulation of their own product/effect and sometimes by other processes

in the extracellular compartment between cells. This is maintained by the integrity of the cell membrane, but more actively by a specific ion pump that establishes a gradient of more K+ within the cell than without. This sodium-potassium ATPase requires energy, but it is energy well spent. Body temperature is important as temperatures that are too high begin to impact the central nervous system and then the organs. Temperatures that are too low disrupt metabolism and damage cells. While there are limits to what our bodies can do to maintain temperature homeostasis, the increased use of the circulatory system, shivering, sweating, and adjustment of the basal metabolic rate, can all impact our body temperature. There are hundreds of bioregulatory events happening at all times in our bodies.

Our bodies have additional layers of adaptation and responsiveness. Our homeostatic mechanisms are absolutely necessary, but they are just part of the story. Our bodies can coordinate several actions at once to preserve life. And our bodies respond to stress, damage, and work by remodeling themselves in order to adapt to current conditions. Even more, our bodies can receive information about the environment and react proactively via preconditioning responses.

An example of coordination can be seen in patients with lung damage that has led to chronic obstructive pulmonary disease (COPD). If the variant of COPD is emphysema, then a destructive process has led to dissolution of the alveolar membrane in many locations in the lung. This results in much larger alveolar sacs that simply cannot have the same contact with oxygen bringing (and carbon dioxide removing) blood vessels as normal, grapelike clusters of alveoli that are each wrapped in their own cluster of vasculature. This means that the ratio of ventilation (air in and out) to perfusion (circulation of blood to pick up and drop off gasses into the lung spaces) is now disturbed. In areas of the lung where big empty spaces have displaced normal smaller breathing or alveolar sacs, the ratio of ventilation to perfusion is decreased, and this means oxygen deficits and carbon dioxide elevation. These are conditions that are dangerous to life. The body will address this by shunting the circulation of blood to those lung areas that are still healthy or at least not as degenerated. The trapping of air in the stiff, emphysemic lung that has lost its normal recoil due to dissolution of elastin tissue creates other problems—the obstruction aspect. The body will recruit muscle power from intercostal muscles or clavicle elevating scalene muscles in order to expand the chest and then push air out. This eventually can remodel the chest to be more barrel-like with an increased

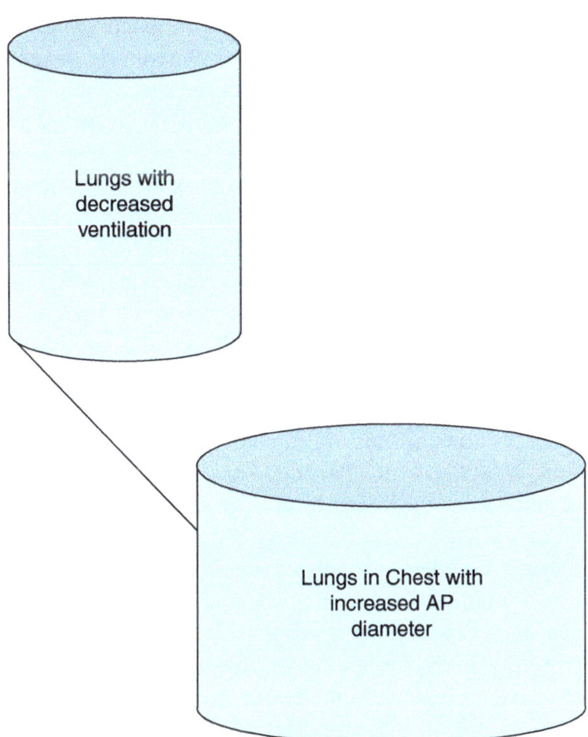

Fig. 1.2 Remodeling: The increase in the anterior-posterior chest diameter in emphysema helps to compensate for stiff, poorly ventilated lungs. But it comes with a price—respiratory muscle function in the chest and the diaphragm becomes disadvantaged

anterior-posterior diameter (Fig. 1.2). The neurologic inputs into blood flow to the lung and the recruitment of accessory muscles of respiration are a basic, but illustrative example of coordination of adaptive processes to maintain homeostasis (and the eventual failure of such compensations is something well understood by all physicians).

Naturopathic Medicine and Health

Naturopathic medicine is rooted in a concept that goes back to the Greek physician Hippocrates. This principle is that of the *vis medicatrix naturae*. A rough translation of that term would be "the healing power of nature." This is an acceptable colloquial translation, but it is potentially misleading. It implies that nature is the healer, and while this *naturalistic* worldview has aspects that are correct and amenable to investigation (i.e., studies on the effects of exposure to nature and effects on stress and wellbeing), it is not an accurate summation of the *vis* concept. Hippocrates was describing the force of survival and adaptation in the body. In his writings, the nature of the disease, the constitutional state of the patient, the aspects of their surroundings (like the seasons), and their diet and finally the physician as actor are all factors in the matrix of the medical art. Hippocrates observed in a vast experience of his own and those of the fellow physicians in his guild that patients have an ability to overcome and recover from disease. Some diseases are too strong to overcome, and some diseases are mismanaged. Instead of allowing the body's self-repair systems to be ascendant, the wrong treatment at the worst possible time can actually inflict harm on the patient, even if it seems minor, such as feeding the patient a lot, or giving the patient a very restricted diet. Sometimes a simple treatment can extinguish a pathological process and allow the body to resume its normal functions. But chronic diseases are not so simple to alleviate, as their manifestations can easily be confused with the generative factors that give rise to them.

But the underlying force (or in Greek, the *physis*) that *physicians* are counting on is what Hippocrates predicated his treatments on. Aside from metaphysical beliefs, which have their own importance in the life of belief, faith, intuition, and transpersonal phenomena, there is an observable set of processes that are now exponentially better described then in Hippocrates' time. There is also a better contemporary description of the higher level of complexity of many of these processes working in harmony in a living person (Fig. 1.3). Emergent properties from complex systems are found everywhere in a living being, especially a human being. For instance, the 200,000 billion neurons in the human central nervous system can often sprout 10,000 connections with other neurons. This results in trillions of synaptic connections. The presence of relay systems among groups of synapse-linked neurons brings the number of signaling processes in a human brain to another exponential level. Even though a single neuron has microprocessor-like aspects, the aggregate of many neurons has many levels of complexity and function higher than this. The harmonization of many such systems (circulatory, nervous, endocrine, immune, extracellular matrix signaling, and more) in a human being creates a dynamic entity that is most certainly a vital partner in the processes of disease and healing. Moreover, the underlining genome and proteome create a ground for untapped resources and an intense responsiveness to

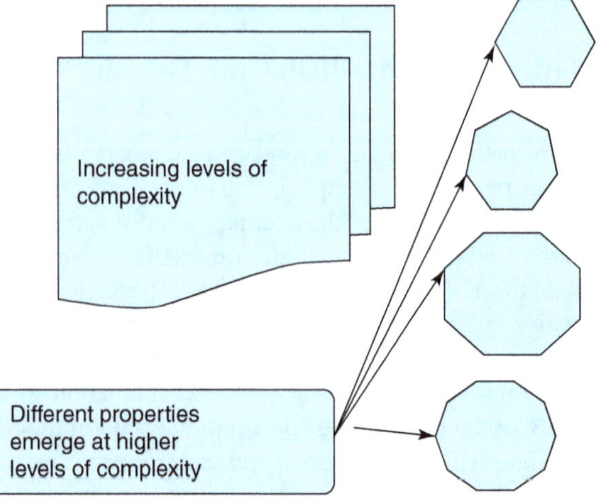

Fig. 1.3 Levels of complexity: As the complexity of a biological system increases, from molecule, to organelle, to cell, to community of cells/organ, and organism, emergent properties are seen at the higher complexity levels that are dormant or absent at lower levels

stimuli. This results in a consistently dynamic responsiveness in a human being in contact with their environment, or coping with some internal dysfunction leading to symptoms, or even the inputs from physicians and their remedies.

Healing as Process

Healing can be observed and described according to different criteria depending on which aspects are highlighted, such as structural or functional restoration. A simple and illuminating example is the healing of a wound. This is captivating, not only because the body fills in and often completely eliminates a defect with new tissue, but because the entire process is so carefully coordinated. Even the busiest construction site for an office tower cannot compare to what the human body does with a wound in terms of project management.

In early stages of injury and wound formation, lymph and blood flow into the area. Blood clotting is activated, and platelets create a fibrin mesh that will form scaffolding for regeneration. Fibroblasts lay down collagen, and over time a new extracellular matrix is formed. Granulation tissue is formed as the wound heals, and if the wound is on skin, then epithelial cells migrate from the margins of the wound toward the center. This thin coating of epithelium will thicken over time. Revascularization will see blood vessels sprout into the area, which is what will allow for more growth and the creation of a strong tissue bond.

Our bodies can replace damaged tissue, and the process has its own control. It is designed to terminate once healing is complete and tissues are remodeled to fit their environment (Fig. 1.4). More complex levels of healing can occur in more complicated tissue structures, such as the liver, kidney, heart muscle cell, and central nervous system tissues. An important question to ask is what defines healing. A consistent set of phenomena, played out in different ways, is observable:

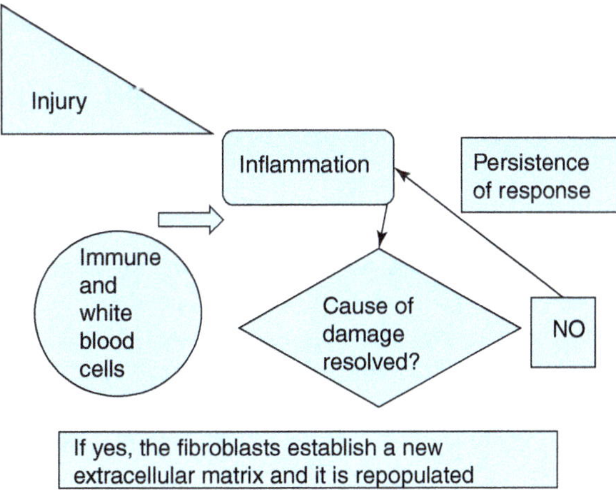

Fig. 1.4 Inflammation: The inflammatory process is meant to be self-terminating and to resolve. But it may fail to do so due to unrepaired injury, infection, or other prompts for inflammation

- Short-term damage is limited including hemorrhage.
- Scaffolding for tissue structure is laid down.
- Tissue replacement begins.
- Tissue differentiation starts.
- An extracellular matrix becomes identifiable.
- Organization returns.
- Blood supply becomes intrinsic to the new tissue.
- Inflammation subsides.
- Control systems return—the healed area behaves like its neighbors.
- Strength, function, and integration with surrounding tissues improve to its maximum potential.

A recreated structure always precedes an improvement in function, but this can proceed in steps and in levels of organization.

Some healing phenomena are easy to comprehend by observing structural changes. The example of the healing of a wound, as provided above, is useful for the purpose of studying a healing pathway. But functional phenomena can occur as well. For instance, a person might eat a diet very heavy in processed foods that are difficult to digest. It leads to excessive proteins in the colon that putrefy (the patient complains of foul-smelling stools). Should they take 2 days to eat fruits, vegetables, and broth and take a few botanical medicines that activate the liver, they suddenly have very loose stools. Their gut is clearing itself and undergoing a type of watery discharge. This is a kind of rebalancing that helps prevent chronic problems.

Bioregulatory systems have their own ways of setting a pace, of oscillating between highs and lows of activity. Cortisol secretion from the adrenal glands peaks at about dawn and winds down in the late evening. Healing can be a result of the stabilization and correction of bioregulatory systems that are out of balance. By this we mean they hypofunction, or hyperfunction, or behave erratically.

Or with an even more systemic example, a patient presents with fatigue, headaches, sore muscles in the shoulders (trapezius), and difficulty concentrating. Their bloodwork and physical exam are within normal limits. It turns out that they only sleep 5 h/night due to the demands of obtaining a degree, taking evening courses, and wanting to watch television past midnight in order to unwind. We know that chronic sleep deprivation leads to biochemical changes in the brain. As sleep is obtained, especially the deeper stages of sleep, the brain can make the growth factors, repair connections, and adjust neurotransmitters that lead to well-being. The symptoms the patient reported just fade away.

Some creatures can regenerate entire body parts, such as axolotls. The axolotls are a type of salamander that are being studied for their regenerative properties. They can regenerate a limb. This is dependent on, but not wholly attributable to, an intact nervous system input into the area. Moreover, sequential amputations of an axolotl limb will result in a less well-developed replacement limb by the fourth or fifth regrowth. It appears that axolotls stay in a juvenile or larval sort of body, even after sexual maturity. So they retain some pluripotency.

Healing as an Ordered Process

Many medical systems, in many cultures across time, have recognized that the healing process follows a certain order. This usually started with examining modes of living (good and bad habits), diet, and family relations and then considered the mind (mood, hope, faith, thought habits). This might lead to treatments with herbs, hands, or water that strengthened the person. Or if more action was required, specific herbal medicines were used for pain, fever, agitation, wounds, etc.

In modern naturopathic medicine, the idea of an order to healing was introduced by Dr. Jared Zeff, in a 1997 article entitled A Hierarchy of Healing. With his collaborator Dr. Pamela Snider, this was expanded to the Therapeutic Order, a seven-level model of steps to healing.

The central concept behind the order is that healing follows an order that is biologically intrinsic. Influencing the body and mind to help the patient return to health means following that order. That is to say, a certain isomorphism between therapy and the normal progression of healing is most productive. In the Textbook of Natural Medicine, Zeff, Snider, Myers, and DeGrandpre outline these steps of the therapeutic order, which are paraphrased below:

1. Create the conditions for health (address determining factors of health that might be deficient or disturbed, such as lack of sleep or hydration; address inborn/congenital and legacy medical issues).
2. Stimulate the vis medicatrix naturae—specifically with therapies that are chosen based on very specific patient attributes, such as acupuncture or homeopathy. Or use nonspecific methods such as hydrotherapy.
3. Support weakened organ systems—provide nutritional, catalytic, and biochemical support to organs and tissues that are under duress.
4. Address structural integrity, such as the skeletal and myofascial system.
5. Address pathology using natural pharmacology, such as botanicals that provide symptom relief or which downregulate dangerously overactive symptoms.
6. Address pathology with synthetic pharmacology, such as pharmaceuticals designed to bind to a receptor and induce a different physiological state.
7. Suppress pathology using high-force interventions such as surgery, gamma rays, transplants, etc.

Students of naturopathic medicine, in addition to this volume, are encouraged to read the works of Zeff, Snider, and their collaborative colleagues.

Some interesting points come to light in this concept. One is that different situations call for different starting points. A patient having a myocardial infarction does not need a diet analysis; they need a rapid trip to a cardiac catheterization lab. It is also apparent that many natural therapies can be used in different ways, but the dose, or the frequency of use, can shift them from being supportive and nutritional to more interventional and higher force. For instance, a small amount, such as 2 mL of a tincture of the herb *Passiflora incarnata*, will help a typical adult relax near bedtime and be better able to get into sleep mode. But 6 mL of the same herb will have a mild sedative effect that might lessen acute anxiety. While individual responses and actual preparations of natural medicines may make it seem that a dose or amount is more art than science, practitioners tend to use a small amount—*when the patient is not having an urgent or emergency situation*—and perhaps work their way up in dose. But overall, many treatments are not only supportive, or only addressing pathology. They can be, depending on the therapy, much more versatile.

The Approach of This Textbook

The work of Zeff, Snider, and their associates has been seminal and foundational to works such as this, as the discipline of naturopathic medicine has moved forward due to the codification of fundamental principles and models. In this current text, the intent is to examine the process of dysfunction in the body and how choices can be made about how to address the symptoms and consequences of the dysfunction. Patients are typically in some mode of adaptive or maladaptive responses (Fig. 1.5). The fundamental choice is this: to what degree does a patient, at this moment in time, need help to:

1. Correct deficiencies or disturbances to the factors that are necessary for normal function
2. Bring out the best in their various pro-survival or adaptive responses at the cell, tissue, and organism level
3. Reduce the intensity and severity of maladaptive responses, such as excessive inflammation or overly exuberant healing by fibrosis
4. Enforce a state of homeostasis through artificial means because the body simply cannot, such as providing insulin to a type I diabetic who cannot produce their own

To arrive at some of the answers to this question, it is necessary to examine the following questions, in addition to the nature of healing:

What is disease?

When is combating a disease versus supporting intrinsic healing the more important priority (beyond obvious examples such as massive trauma or extreme congenital defects)?

What precisely are the factors that injure and cause dysregulation to the body?

What are naturopathic therapeutics and where do they come into play in terms of the four needs that a patient might have (listed above)?

What are some of the states of being that give rise to diseases—what unifying chronic declines in health or function lead to the breakdown states that we know as diagnosable diseases?

How is a model of assessment and treatment that follows naturopathic concepts applied to the various organ systems of the body?

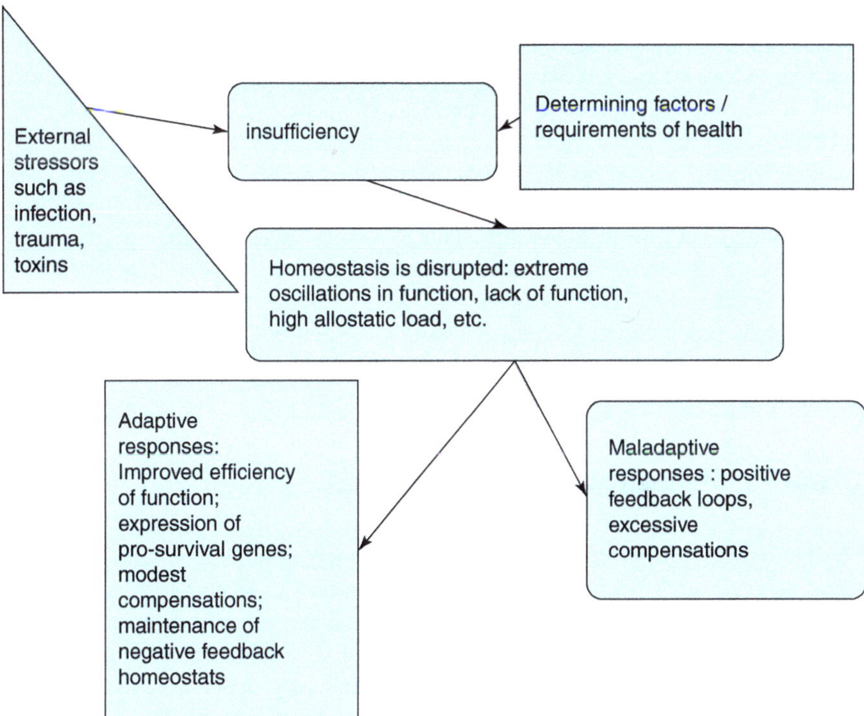

Fig. 1.5 Generation of body responses: Disruptions to homeostasis can occur from a basic lack of determining factors of health or due to some form of trauma or infection. This gives rise to adaptive responses from the body that increase resilience and lead to repair or at least better function. Disturbed homeostasis, especially when determining factors of health are very deficient, can also give rise to maladaptive responses, such as excessively intense inflammation, prolonged blood clotting, excessive scar tissue formation, etc.

What is the application of naturopathic medicine in primary care, across different age groups and populations?

What is the role of a naturopathic physician in primary care, specialty care, so-called integrative care?

In what way is naturopathic medicine scientific, where can it improve, and what limitations in medical science in general are inhibiting scientific progress in understanding the facilitation of healing?

What will be the roles of machine learning, advanced computing, and assisted decision-making in the future or naturopathic physicians?

What is the role of the naturopathic physician in the community, in society, and in global-level issues such as deforestation, water scarcity, loss of biodiversity, food insecurity, communicable diseases, and climate change?

Why do healing mechanisms fail?

This is a central question in naturopathic medicine and all health care. One key consideration is, of course, that our healing mechanisms almost never fail. No machine of any complexity has ever demonstrated reliability and resilience on so many levels like the human body possesses. Thousands of times a day, our body quenches unpaired electrons before they can damage our cells or our DNA. We break down innumerable toxins, human made or of natural origin. We replace tissues that only last for a few days. Our body repairs the damage of life, due to gravity, ultraviolet and cosmic radiation, mechanical stressors, and simple entropic decay.

Sooner or later, powerful stressors, random accidents, or some inherent weakness allows an imbalance to grow in our body. This can emerge, too, from simple lack of some precondition for normal function—a nutrient deficiency or a lack of a determining factor of health such as sleep are prime examples.

Disturbed Biologically Essential Factors

The biologically essential (for survival) factors such as water, sunlight, breathing, movement, etc. are sometimes referred to in naturopathic medicine as the "determinants of health." This term is used in public health and essentially refers to the same kinds of things. Due to the focus of naturopathic medicine on individual patients who suffer from distinct encumbrances and have very different histories, these determinants include more patient-oriented issues than perhaps looking at larger populations and the data about them. However, the research around these population effects is part of the scientific basis of studying what happens when these essential factors or determinants are disturbed. This is accompanied by research into pathophysiology. For example, the impact of dehydration on cognition is a physiological imbalance that is relevant to perceiving certain symptoms in a patient presentation and connecting them to a deficient essential factor.

But clearly all disease is not simply the result of a shortcoming in meeting some biological essentials, even if these unmet essentials are a major factor in disease genesis. Sometimes, there is a simple failure of the healing mechanisms to create a healing event. This is an unpleasant fact of life that human resilience can be overstretched and broken. Situations that can bring this about include the following:

- Toxins that are more potent than a human being can process
- Lasting pathological impressions from toxins and traumatic experiences
- Ultravirulent microbes and viruses
- Overly exuberant inflammatory reactions
- Loss of structural integrity—permanent disorganization
- Loss of innervation
- Limits to biological plasticity by age, nutritional status, or genetic potential
- Genetic predisposition
- Aging and loss of viability of the extracellular matrix
- Mutations and progression to neoplasia

Examining the above list, there is a distinction between these etiologic factors. Some of them are simply overwhelming—such that our physical and genetic resources are not capable of meeting them. For instance, exposure to enough ionizing radiation will break down our cells and radically damage our DNA. Other factors listed above become more difficult to control as they gain momentum. Mutations that then lead to cell anaplasia and then finally a cancer cell are easier to delete early on and eventually very difficult to defeat when they become full-blown cancer cells. Other factors are a type of collateral damage that occurs in response to stressors—the body's own reactions can be difficult to endure sometimes. Some pathogens excel at provoking those reactions to an extreme—such as gram-negative bacteria that can trigger disseminated intravascular coagulation by virtue of their endotoxins. Breakdown of the extracellular matrix is usually at the end of a long road of dysfunction.

Healing can become more challenging as degenerative changes set in and a loss of organization and structure become evident. This is not always irreversible—our organs can heal and sometimes the 60% function of an organ is enough for the body as a whole to manage (for example, someone who has had a lobe of their lung removed can, given time, adapt and live an active life). Nevertheless, disorganization of an organ creates a situation where normal healing mechanisms can fail in their purpose. A simple example is cirrhosis of the liver. The hepatic stellate cells release so much fibrous tissue that the liver becomes crosscut with a type of scar tissue. This massively disrupts the biliary system. The liver is not only the hepatocytes. The organization of the liver depends on infiltration of blood from the portal system for nutrient delivery and filtering, plus the arrival of arterial blood (which can also carry substances that require biotransformation or "detox") and the drainage of bile through many thousands of biliary canals. Once this distribution system is literally cut off by scar tissue, the liver cannot function properly. The remaining hepatocytes can continue to function and so some work, but the scar tissue cannot be removed. Have patients with cirrhosis recovered somewhat and gone on to lead healthy lives? Yes, provided that the inciting injuries ended (alcohol, other chemicals). Some cases are too advanced even for our very adaptive bodies. So the value of medical-based therapies for those who have lesions or damage to their body that blocks a return to function is beyond question.

A rather different set of conditions prevails when the determining factors of health, or biologically essential factors, as described above, are disturbed. In this case, baseline physiological function is disordered, because some essential component of health is missing or greatly reduced. That disorder will create its own symptoms. For example, those with mild dehydration experience decrease in cognitive performance and increase bronchial sensitivity. At the same time, our basic biology tends to respond to disordered physiology with various counterreactions. Some are right on time and apropos for the situation, and others are less specific, too late, or too forceful. As an example, in dehydration the kidneys will begin to reduce urinary output. A more hyperosmolar urine is created. This is a positive adaptation. But imagine a person who subsists on soft drinks and coffee and is usually running at mild dehydration. Their risk of renal lithiasis (kidney stones) goes up over the long haul because of that concentrated urine.

If our bodies were designed to only operate under ideal conditions, then all disturbed determinants would lead to disease in a short time, and this is not the observed effect. What is more likely is that a cluster of acute symptoms appears caused chiefly by a physiological disruption. The body's countermeasures (assuming the disturbance or deficiency continues) may also be perceptible. Left unchecked, the acute reactions become chronic ones, and over time, degenerative changes occur. The term "degenerative" is composed of a prefix "de," meaning to move downward, or descend, and it contains the root word generative, which means to create, grow, or spawn. A degeneration is where the body has moved away from regrowth, repair, and replacement and is now in the process of letting tissues exhaust themselves. The tissues in a degenerative situation are more like machine parts than living tissue. Parts of tools and machines are designed to be replaced—such as filters, blades, washers, etc. They do not self-heal. In a degenerative situation, the disorganization and the disturbed determinants (which engender a chronic reaction as described by Zeff and Snider) lead to a collapse of normal "generative" responses. The body does not have the conditions for health, and the instructions for healing are further stymied by physical or chemical blockages due to damage.

Again, in degenerative situations, a synthetic medicine can do for the body what it no longer can do for itself. A pharmaceutical medicine, in many cases, will create a compensation for a problem that the body can tolerate. In time that effect leading to a compensation (sodium depletion that lower's blood pressure, GABA receptor allosteric binding that lessens anxiety, etc.) might attenuate. Then a secondary drug, or a new drug, or a stronger dose, must be employed. The concept of adverse effects of drugs are well known, and outright drug toxicity is a reason in itself to first consider natural and noninvasive methods to ameliorate or cure a disease state. Nevertheless, synthetic medicines are taken with great frequency—about half of all Americans used a prescription pharmaceutical in any 30-day period. Despite their risks, and their shortcomings, they can change a person's situation for the better.

Unfortunately, the ease with which this can be accomplished has led many patients to believe that a disease process is inevitable. This is a worldview where diseases just happen, and the only way to escape it is to be cured with pills or surgery. It also can lead to a blindness to the generative factors of the body and how potent those healing resources can be especially when the conditions for health are established. That is, someone who only knows medicine as pills and surgery can be quite unaware that their body has a vast capacity to reorganize itself, to heal, as it were. This naivete about the body's intrinsic healing, and the passivity it engenders, has several pernicious consequences. One is simply a type of learned helplessness. That leads to increased stress when illness develops. It also makes it more likely that a person will bypass, or scarcely realize that they have any capacity for physical and psychological renewal. An extension of this mindset is that health is something that is given to a person by a professional. While it is certainly true that *help* and sometimes lifesaving assistance is provided by health-care professionals, the belief that healing is a result of extrinsic forces that are out of the patient's control can turn the patient into a supplicant, one who must beg. Yet another is that even if the patient avails themselves of whatever help can be offered by allopathic medicine, if they are under the influence of the cultural belief that they themselves cannot really overcome any real disease state beyond a mild respiratory tract infection, then they will not take actions that could alter the outcome of their situation for the positive. Their situation is real, but they do not consider all of the options, because of a **bounded rationality** with which they have been enculturated. This is also a reliable feature of the stress response—a narrowing of perspective and a fleeing of awareness of options. And nothing can stress a human being as much as the intrusion of an illness they are neither prepared to experience nor to accept.

The Origins of the Naturopathic Approach

Naturopathic medicine traces its roots back to the Hippocratic school of medicine. Although Hippocratic medicine is a progenitor to Western medicine in general, due to the establishment of a method based on observation and clinical reasoning, the history of medicine is in fact more complex in this tradition. And there are other traditions that have deep roots and have influenced and contributed to both naturopathic and Western medicine in general.

The Hippocratic school was not without its rivals in the 400 BCE ferment of Greek civilization. Hippocrates emphasized the understanding of the patient and their environment and an observation of the development of a disease in a patient. Many conditions could be eliminated by the body, with the proper support and guidance. The role of the physician was to assist and remove obstacles to healing, so that this natural phenomena of healing, which Hippocrates termed the *vis medicatrix naturae*, was able to operate freely. Emphasis was on addressing determining factors of health and, in disease, on using herbs, diet, and water (plus warmth and cold), to help with the cooking off ("coction") of disease. Prognosis was important to these physicians as they believed that the healing reactions that the body went through were vital and often somewhat predictable.

A rival school of the time focused more on the establishment of disease categories. True, observable diseases could be known, and once it was determined what disease the patient had, the choice of remedy was rather obvious. The patient's reactions, their status relative to the determining factors of health, and tactics to enhance the self-healing systems were secondary at best.

The historian of medicine Harris Coulter described these two perpetual strings of medicine in his four volume work *Divided Legacy*. He contrasts the rationalist school (the rivals of Hippocrates who put emphasis on disease categories are an example) and the empirical school. Coulter notes that prevailing rationalist schools eventually stagnate, even as the information they accumulate becomes more impressive. They begin to have difficulty treating the diseases of the day and responding to the nature of health problems in their contemporary milieu. An empirical movement rises up and infuses the dominant school with new methods and fresh thinking. Over time, that particular empirical movement, for the most part, becomes rather brittle and behaves like the system it used to critique, or it is simply assimilated into the "conventional" profession. Precise biochemical or structural descriptions of disease processes do not seem to completely stop this pendulum from swinging, for reasons that range from economics to epistemology.

It should be clear which school became predominant over time. For many patients, a disease-centric model is the only one they have known their entire life. It may in fact appear to them that this is the only rational and scientific approach to patient care.

Clearly, it is not a matter of which approach was absolutely correct; rather, these two perspectives together allow a range of response to patient needs that cover a wide span of timing, evolution and causes, patient resilience, prevention, treatment, suppression, and simple palliation. Medicine became one sided truly when the perspective to use scientific information was only from this perspective. But this approach to therapy is not in itself a theory. It is a practice that puts the patient's self-healing abilities on the margin.

Legacies of Healing

The approach of naturopathic medicine is a unique fusion of European natural cures/hydrotherapy and North American healing modalities. The connection of understanding health-generating and health-deteriorating factors using a biomedical perspective is a step beyond those traditions. The career role preparation to practice primary care medicine is yet another advance.

Nevertheless, the edifice upon which naturopathic medicine rests (that is, if it is more than just a milder or therapeutically broadened version of standard medicine) is one that has been laid down for thousands of years. In many cultures across time, indigenous healers have used medicines from the earth to stimulate or support the body. They have helped those in disharmony with nature and with themselves find a way to resynchronize with the seasons, the laws of nature, and their own instincts for healthy behaviors. Traditional medicine systems, such as Ayurvedic medicine, have been used by millions and millions of people through time.

In the North American context, three great traditional systems intersect as naturopathy (later naturopathic medicine) takes off (to be joined by others later on). One is the European spa cure taught by Father Sebastian Kneipp and others. A second is a vast repository of medicines that come from various Indigenous bands, tribes, and nations. Many of these medicines, such as Echinacea species, found their way into the eclectic (herbally skilled MD) tradition where they were further researched and documented. A third pillar is a strong legacy of herbal and natural healing developed and taught by African-American healers. Some of these methods were created based on available herbs and substances. Some were learned from the Indigenous peoples and further developed. And some were brought over from Africa. These healers brought health care to Black Americans when access to conventional doctors was very limited and African-Americans in many states were not allowed to practice medicine. Over time, some of these herbs were incorporated into herbal medicine and even the allopathic medicines that came out of the US pharmacopeia (which had many, many plant medicines until the 1930s), but Black healers have not been properly credited for their contributions.

In this sense, naturopathic medicine remains a fusion of useful natural practices that support self-healing. It is more than the practices; however, it is an approach that seeks to establish the conditions of health and then assist the patient in regaining it. It is a record of observation of healing practices and a window into how the very latest discoveries also can support healing. The fact that it alone is not appropriate for all situations, or that technologically driven allopathic procedures can be stunningly successful, does not negate the need for a naturopathic approach. Because without it, in a one-sided approach to health care, the fight against pathology and the chase after disease symptoms are endless, with spiraling costs and a population that is chronically less healthy with each passing year.

Naturopathic medicine is a modern successor to that purely Hippocratic school which is focused on the patient's reactions, the patient's adaptations, and the prognosis that can be created by working with the vis medicatrix naturae. Should naturopathic medicine in its contemporary form simply merge and dissolve into mainstream practice, which is entirely possible, then some other organized force that flies the banner of the "empirical" school of medicine will wear the mantle of Hippocrates in the mid- to late twenty-first century.

In the chapters that follow, each of the above questions about health, and disease, will receive more in-depth discussion. This is followed by an examination of chronic states of ill health and how these manifest in various organ systems. We will examine the naturopathic therapies and the way in which these can work to ameliorate disease states and support health restoration. Applications of this knowledge to particular organ systems, patient populations, and practice contexts follow on this discussion.

Chapter 2
Theory of Disease

Feedback Loops and Bioregulation

The role of feedback systems in the body has been well understood for over a century. The human body has many systems that follow basic cybernetic principles. An example is thermoregulation. A certain set point exists for core body temperature. When it is beginning to drop, the hypothalamus commands the autonomic nervous system to commence shivering, and the metabolic rate may increase if the cold stimulus is prolonged.

The basic functions of homeostasis are well described [1]. For our purposes, it is important to note that the human body has hundreds of negative feedback loops in operation constantly. That is, the product of these reactions has an inhibitory effect on the reaction. Should the product drop too low, it allows the reaction to continue (Fig. 2.1) A few positive feedback loops exist in the body. One example is the role of oxytocin in childbirth; another is blood clotting (although some built in inhibition is also seen in clotting factors).

These feedback systems can function smoothly, or they can become untuned. What does that look like? It can appear as a slowness in creating a product as the levels of that product dissipate (lack of responsiveness to stimuli), or conversely it can appear as a tardiness in inhibiting the formation of a product even when it is piling up in the bloodstream (a failure of the "off-switch").

A feedback loop can become "stuck" in a higher output state, with the bottom of the loop still higher than it ideally ought to be [2]. Blood pressure that fluctuates from 150/90 to 160/99 mmHg over the course of a day is one example. Or it can become stuck in a lower output state with the top of the loop still lower than it ideally ought to be. Feedback loops can also begin to behave erratically, with an actual set point being difficult to discern due to so much variability.

F. Smith, *Naturopathic Medicine*, https://doi.org/10.1007/978-3-031-13388-6_2

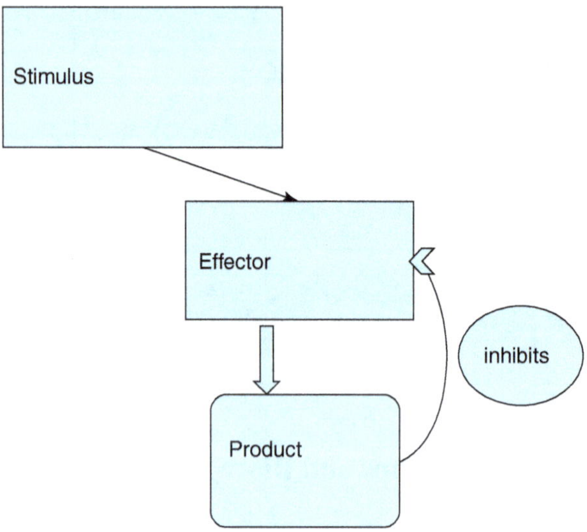

Fig. 2.1 Negative feedback: In a typical negative feedback loop, the effector is inhibited by the product. Increased stimulus on the effector may create more forward activity and production of a product, but that product has inhibitory effects. The set point for inhibition is an important aspect of this control system

We will explore contemporary science on this topic below. As a simple example, imagine the thermostat on a wall, if it is a digital thermostat, and for some reason its chipset is damaged; it may allow the temperature in a house to drop to a very uncomfortable 55 °C before kicking in to allow the heat to come and raise the temperature a point or two above the chosen set point of, say, 70 °F. Or imagine a thermostat on a wall, and a homeowner places a lamp with a halogen bulb too near to it. The heat of the lamp is detected by the thermostat, and furnace activation is suppressed, even as the room itself is chilly.

Feedback loops get even more interesting in a living being however. The basic concept in feedback loops in the body is the Goodwin oscillation [3]. These are based on the work of Brian Goodwin, whose seminal works on this topic described, in mathematical terms, the three-cycle oscillation. In this process, a gene is expressed by transcription, and transfer RNA leads to the creation of a protein. As the protein accumulates, it suppresses RNA formation from the gene. This is seen with many processes in the body, including NfKB production, p53 expression, calcium homeostasis, and more.

The oscillations of this type are also now known to be tied to mammalian circadian rhythms. Newer research shows how these can all be interconnected. Some products can impact *other* feedback loops. And it appears that a small number of oscillations can allow for *positive feedback* (where the product enhances the machinery of production instead of inhibiting it) so as to allow more impact from a small set of oscillators. This is the body's version of a snowball effect.

Aside from giving us even more appreciation of the awesome scope of self-regulation that the human body displays, this science can inform us about the causes of disease and how to improve health. Some of the scientific disciplines that can provide information are neurocybernetics and more broadly biocybernetics.

Circadian and Neurological Oscillations

A neuron undergoes oscillations in the generation of action potentials (Hodgkin-Huxley model) [4]. Depolarization (with exchange of ions across the cell membrane) and repolarization balance each other. Groups of neurons can coordinate their firing and oscillate as a whole. They wire together and fire together, simply put. Certain brain regions oscillate together and usually have a bidirectional communication. The cerebral cortex and the thalamus have various radiations that connect.

In oscillations [5, 6], there are:

- Variations in amplitude but not frequency. For example, the frequency of the adrenocorticotropic hormone (ACTH) from the pituitary is stable, but the amount of secretion, the amplitude, can vary (and thus the amount of cortisol secretion from the adrenal glands can vary) [7] (Fig. 2.2).
- Variations in frequency but not amplitude. For example, heart rate can be variable depending on someone's activity level, or emotional state, but the actual amount of blood ejected from the left ventricle, per beat, remains more or less the same.

An example of a disturbed oscillatory cycle in health would be Parkinson's disease (Fig. 2.3). The patient suffers from rigidity and tremor, due to lack of dopamine input by various modulators along the corticospinal tract (i.e., the basal ganglia). Another oscillatory disturbance is where cortisol secretion rises to exaggerated

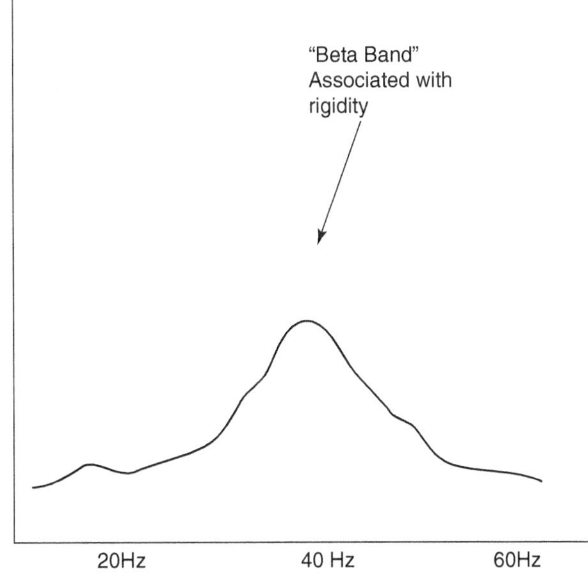

Fig. 2.2 Parkinson's disease: Neural oscillations in symptomatic Parkinson's disease patients show a characteristic band

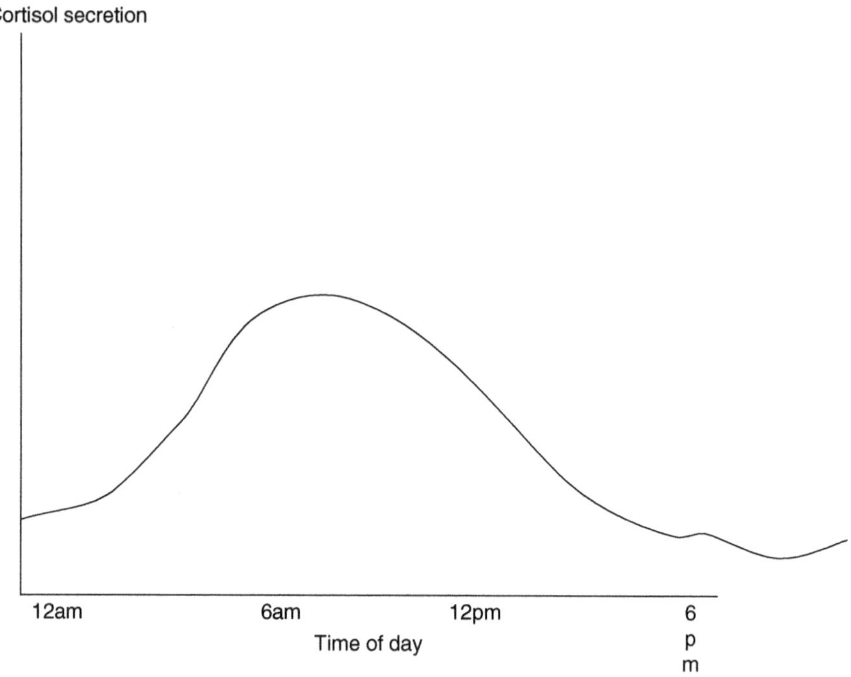

Fig. 2.3 Cortisol secretion: Humans have a daily oscillating cortisol secretion with an early morning/dawn peak and a trough in the night. This can become imbalanced or erratic, as seen in chronic stress responses

levels as noted above, which can happen in chronic stress, as in Dr. Hans Selye's general adaptation syndrome.

Circadian rhythms, protein transcription, cell migration, and glycolysis all follow oscillatory rhythms. As science progresses, we will have clearer insight into how the human body, as a dynamic system, becomes "untuned." This is relevant because of its connection with disease and aging [8, 9].

Degenerative Changes

Degenerative changes are typically the consequence of an imbalance that continues to the point that it causes a chronic inflammatory reaction. Normally, cell destruction and injury are balanced by replacement and repair [10]. A classic example of where this can go wrong is cirrhosis of the liver. This exuberant fibrotic reaction usually occurs after a long period of hepatitis due to alcohol consumption in excess, extreme steatohepatitis, or other causes of injury (viruses, toxins, autoimmune processes, etc.). The damage, and healing, and reinjury continued for a long time. Eventually, the "regeneration," the recreation of healthy tissue, is less than ideal. Architecture or structure might be intact, but not enough healthy cells are present.

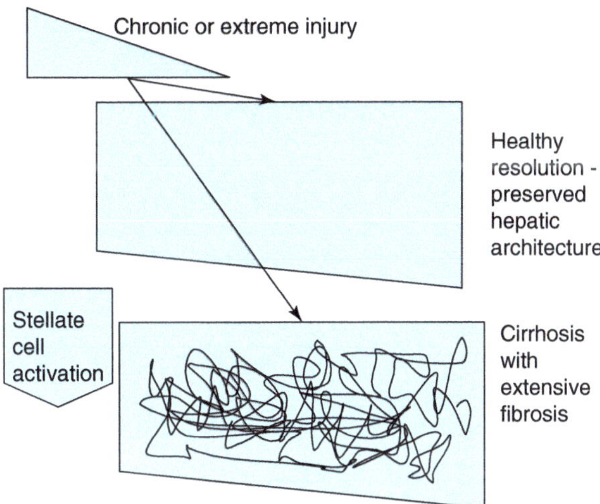

Fig. 2.4 Cirrhosis of the liver: An example of maladaptive responses, hepatic stellate cells are overstimulated and produce massive amounts of collagen. Rather than buttressing the liver structure, this abundance of collagen distorts hepatic architecture and impairs function

Or cellular mitosis can proceed, but the structure of a tissue is compromised. In the case of cirrhosis, this is attended by fibrotic tissue that disturbs the normal highly organized structure of the biliary system (Fig. 2.4).

Not all degenerative events take years to manifest. Sometimes a direct trauma leads to irreversible loss of healthy tissue. One example is sudden blood loss that leads to ischemia of the anterior pituitary and various endocrinopathies in the weeks and months that follow. Or in the more recent example of SARS CoV-2 infection, fibrosis of the lung or vascular damage throughout the body can manifest in a few weeks [11].

What is interesting about some of the degenerative processes is that they exhibit ongoing attempts by the body to try to heal, to reintegrate, or simply to stabilize. But it is not enough, and the inflammation, resolution, and scarring that occur can be deleterious. Somewhat like a car stuck in a snow drift or mud that is spinning its wheels, but gets nowhere except getting deep into the trap in spite of high RPMs, the body's usual tactics to heal become unhelpful in this situation.

This can be a chronic condition that fails to resolve, or it can become the dangerous positive feedback loop. In this case, a product of a reaction leads to more production of itself.

Neoplasms

This is the ultimate form of degeneration, in that a set of cells that were derived from the human body break away from normal controls on growth and behavior and act invasively. The scientific understanding of carcinogenesis is rather deep and yet continuously advancing. What seems to be the case is that the mutations to the DNA

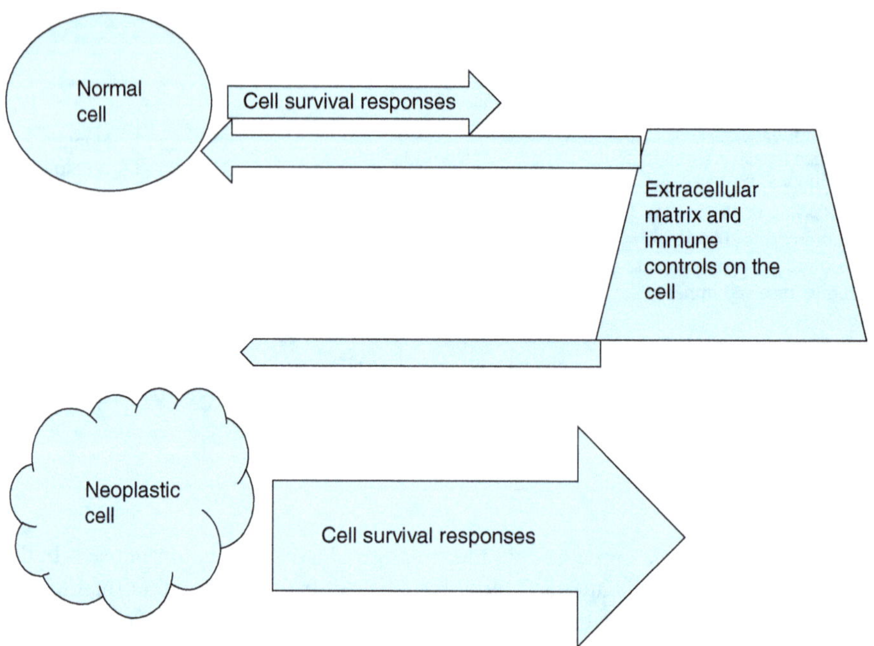

Fig. 2.5 Neoplastic cells: Normal cells express various survival responses, but they are controlled by immune, extracellular matrix, and other signaling mechanisms. Neoplastic (cancer) cells exhibit extreme expression of survival responses and unrestrained by the normal control systems

of a cell destined to become the first in a line of tumor cells in a patient, are *enabled* by a set of circumstances that are variable to some degree.

Perhaps cancer is the ultimate breakdown, because it unleashes pro-survival responses of the neoplastic cells that no longer connect with the rest of the body (Fig. 2.5). Like a drowning person who is panicking and will climb over or push down their rescuer (unless that rescuer knows lifesaving techniques in the water or has a big size differential), cancer cells simply express every gene transcription strategy they can to generate more cancer cells as an option to annihilation.

There are scientific findings that (a) cancer cells arose from mutation *and* distressed tissues and (b) the nutritional, oxygenated, and extracellular matrix environment or "milieu" of that cancer was somehow abnormal and functioned as a more fertile environment for neoplastic proliferation. Notably, this is important in a chemoprevention sense, but it should be stated that it does not negate the importance of targeted medical therapies against cancer. The oncology situation is a "disease crisis"—it tends toward a poor prognosis—because it is now operating outside the normal rules of the body.

The Extracellular Matrix

The unsung hero of the entire human physiology, the extracellular matrix, is what allows our cells to properly function. It has been said that the concept of a cell as such is an abstraction when considered separately from the extracellular matrix (ECM). It would be easy to overlook the truth of that statement, in that 140 years of cellular biology and a good 70 years of molecular cell biology have yielded a massive amount of information about cells including how they are constituted, regulated, injured, and repaired and the interactions between nucleus and cell membrane. And yet, cells in a living organism really do not function independently of the ECM, and it interacts with them. In fact, the ECM facilitates communication between cells and is most likely a preneural form of communication and reactivity going back to very ancient modes of life on our planet.

The extracellular matrix is the space where nutrients and oxygen flow to the cell. It is also a transit area where waste products and carbon dioxide can be collected and removed from the vicinity of a cell.

The ECM is composed of proteins and glycoproteins (Fig. 2.6). The most abundant are glycosaminoglycans (GAGs) [12, 13]. A special protein known as integrin

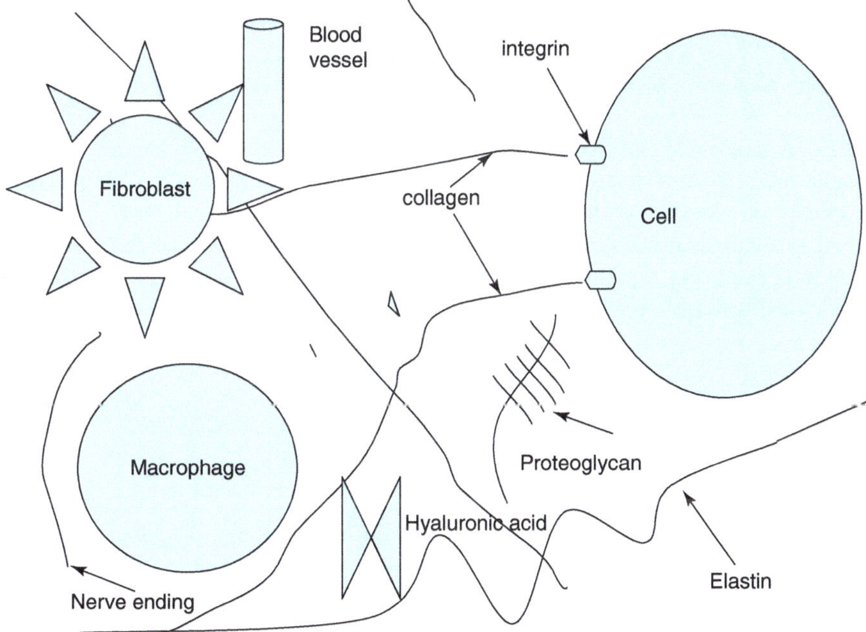

Fig. 2.6 The extracellular matrix (ECM): The ECM is the necessary milieu for cells. It contains proteins, proteoglycans, fibroblasts, immune cells, nerve endings, and certain hormones and signaling molecules. It is a transit zone for nutrients to the cell and toxins out. The protein scaffolding of the ECM connects to the microtubule assembly of cells via the transmembrane integrin protein

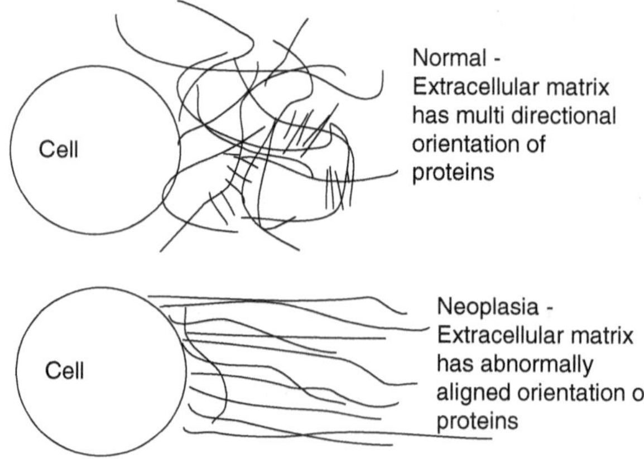

Fig. 2.7 Extracellular matrix and neoplasia: Neoplastic cells rearrange the extracellular matrix, forming an unnatural parallel array of protein fibers. This provides stimulation to the cancer cells, spurring more proliferation

connects the matrix to the cell by passing through the cell membrane. The physical nature of the ECM has an influence on the behavior of cells. For example, these interactions can promote cellular division, and they can provide inhibition of mitosis so that a healing or growth reaction knows when to stop. Cells in this way have a sensory or touch experience with their immediate environment. A healthy matrix precedes normal cellular function and tissue formation.

Conversely, unhealthy or abnormal ECM permits various types of cellular dysfunction. When the ECM becomes rigid, losing elasticity, it is not as effective a transit space for molecules to pass through. Newer research has described how, in the case of cancerous solid tumors, the ECM immediately adjacent to the tumor becomes thickened and stiff and has the odd characteristic of high degrees of alignment of collagen fibrils (they should be assorted randomly) [14–17]. This physical property provides a high level of overstimulation to the tumor cells, aiding them in their action of nonstop mitosis (Fig. 2.7). This hyperproliferation of cancer cells is partly genetic, but the tumor cells reorganize the ECM so as to conform to their biological activities, not that of normal tissue.

Mitochondrial Dysfunction

Mitochondrial dysfunction is another hallmark of a system that is corrupted and on its way to expressing pathology. The creation of ATP is the major function of this organelle and for anaerobic organisms is absolutely vital. An intact mitochondrial member system, a complement of specific enzyme, and a precisely controlled gradient of protons on either side of the inner mitochondrial membranes are some of the conditions for proper function [18, 19].

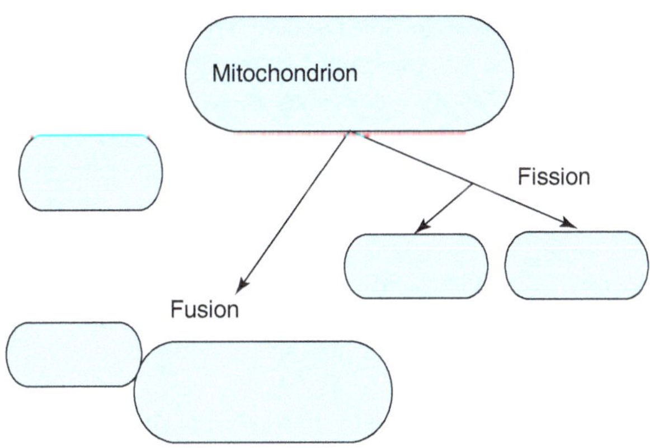

Fig. 2.8 Mitochondrial metamorphosis: Mitochondria can fuse with each other, and they can undergo fission, which leads to their dissolution. Both events are normal to a point, but excessive fusion or fission is associated with pathology

Under excessive stress, mitochondria are less able to fuse together to provide extra energy generation. They become overloaded with calcium. As aging and degeneration progresses, deletions in mitochondrial DNA occur [20–23]. It is hypothesized.that cellular transformation into neoplastic cells can be promoted by a loss of mitochondrial DNA. Some tumor cells can create energy by glycolysis (Warburg phenomenon), and perhaps this alternate pathway (for what is normally an aerobic cell) is an adaptation to loss of mitochondria and the normal way of conducting oxidative phosphorylation [24]. Even in health, mitochondria create reactive oxygen species (ROS) because they are using oxygen in a reactive form. ROS are rapidly neutralized by various antioxidant systems in the mitochondria. Degenerate tissues, such as diseased heart tissues, are well known to be lacking in mitochondria. Their mitochondria are also not as efficient as normal and display excessive mitochondrial fission (Fig. 2.8).

Stem Cell Depletion–Differentiation–Dedifferentiation

Stem cells are well known as the pluripotent undifferentiated cells in the center of the blastocyst that can become the many tissue types in the human body. This unfolding, in its scope and coordination, is a breathtaking phenomenon. Stem cells are integral to homeostasis, in postembryonic human. Depending on the tissue and its rate of turnover, stem cells may be involved in repair, or in regeneration. For instance, renal stem cells are mostly functioning on the repair side. The stem cells in the lining of the gut are used for regeneration [25, 26].

The rules of stem cell behavior in the mature human and how they are expressed in different contexts is an area of intense research. What is clear is that epigenetic phenomena drive the developmental pathways of stem cells. A situation of decreased reserves of health, the ground of true disease states, would be insufficient stem cell recruitment. Or stem cells may be available, but they cannot be transformed into differentiated cells that are needed. This failure can be due to the contextual breakdowns that have been referenced earlier in this chapter. An obvious one is the breakdown of the extracellular matrix. A disorganized matrix, with loss of "touch" functions provided by microtubule frameworks, might impair the unfolding of stem cell development. A stiff and disorganized matrix might make it difficult for stem cells to migrate to where they are needed. A linearly arranged matrix might allow stem cells to travel and may in fact provide a springboard of sorts for stem cell migration.

New investigations into stem cells are showing that in high-turnover tissues, such as the gut epithelium, stem cells can be created by "dedifferentiation" of more mature cells. Instead of calling upon a reservoir of stem cells, cells that are more specialized can be reverted back to stem cells, which themselves can be used to spawn various new specialty cells that are needed in different aspects of the gut epithelium.

Cellular Proteins

Protein balance in cells is in a state of constant turnover. Too little production leads to cellular failure [27–29]. MicroRNA has emerged as a mediator of actual translation of RNA into proteins [30]. Lack of breakdown and control leads to accumulation of misfolded protein, a term known as autophagy. This process has several pathways, but one involves the attachment of a protein called ubiquitin (not to be confused with ubiquinone or coenzyme Q10). When one or more ubiquitins are attached to a protein, it will be brought to the proteasome, an organelle that breaks proteins down (Fig. 2.9). Neurodegenerative diseases, but other organ systems, can have defective autophagy. Conversely, toxins such as mercury can interfere with protein synthesis.

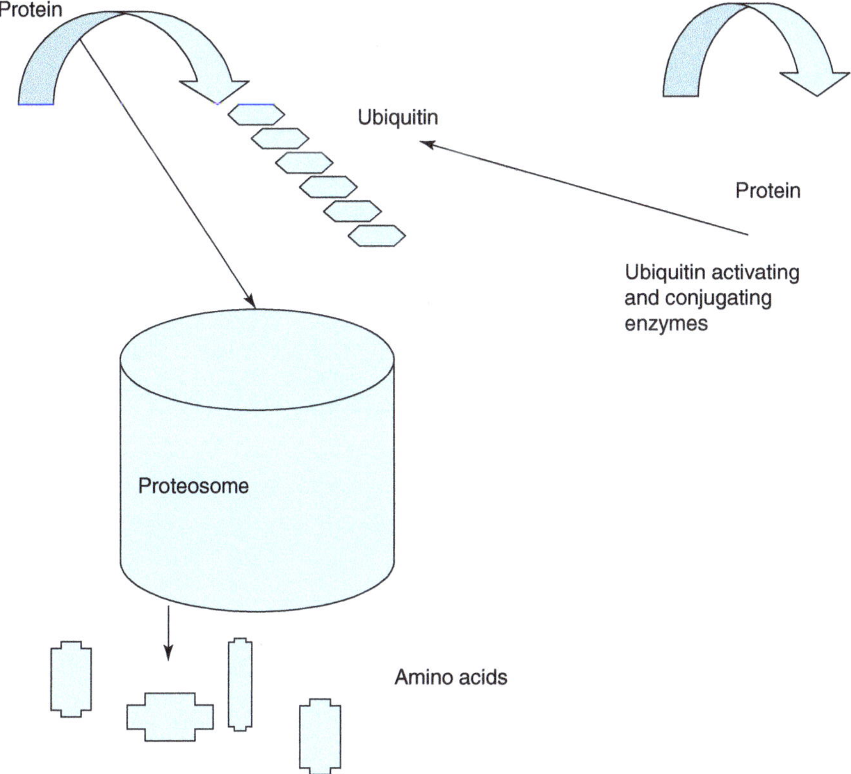

Fig. 2.9 The proteasome: Proteins in the cell are broken down when they are tagged with the protein ubiquitin, which leads to degradation in the proteasome

Long-Term Effects of Using Pharmaceutical Drugs

It is obvious and non-disputable that pharmaceutical interventions save and improve the quality of life for many people. They allow the system to operate "as if" the original disharmony did not exist. This can work well indefinitely in the best-case scenario. But it can also allow a more progressive problem that is intrinsically unstable, or one that arose from disturbances that will lead to degenerative changes, to continue to march on.

Conversely, the very act of creating a higher order of organization using a chemical compound introduced into the system can cause countering changes in the body that are adverse. For instance, an adapting or countering response from the body can lead to unwanted symptoms and the need to keep increasing the dose of the drug. Statins are an example, as they can lower LDL and stabilize plaques, but at the same time (mostly in intensive statin therapy) damage muscle cells (Fig. 2.10). Otherwise, the presence of that drug can cause other pathways and effects to occur that do not so much as oppose the drug as they lead to the appearance of a novel state of

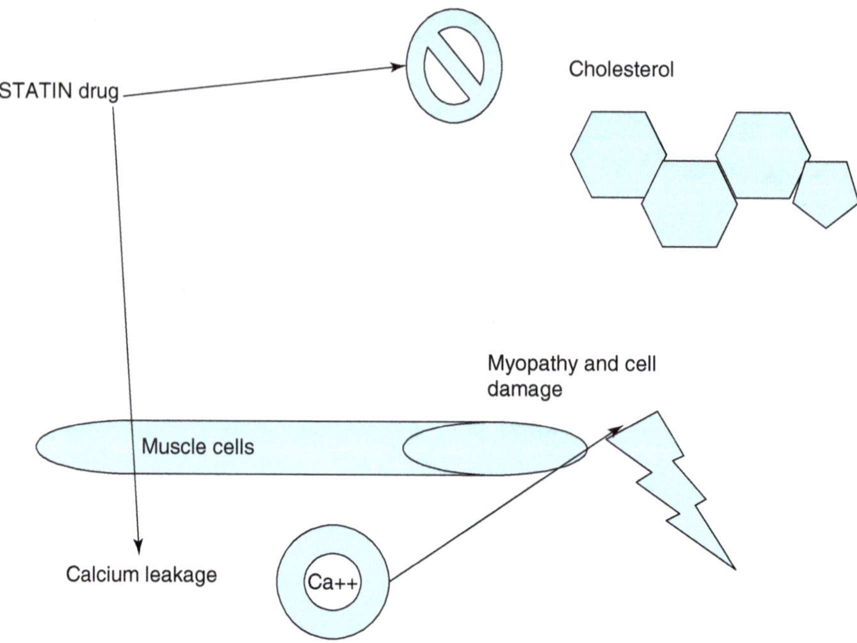

Fig. 2.10 Statins and muscle damage. Statins can cause calcium leakage from muscle cells, leading to necrosis

organization in the body. This is akin to what the physician Samuel Hahnemann referred to as an iatrogenic dissimilar disease. These states of being are not always that serious and can be rather tolerable. But they can also lead to benighted situations that are arguably worse than the initial problem that the drug was given to ameliorate.

Cause and Effect

Insofar as an existing disease can result in new damage and dysfunction, it is also natural that prior to the establishment of a disease, these states of dysfunction and dysregulation can lead to a disease state. A "disease" does not lead to these states of decay. It is these entropic states that allow diseases to emerge. Unfortunately, sometimes the efficacy of physiologically alternating medications has given the public a false sense of security. Many people allow themselves to settle into states which are in fact quite dangerous because they are the ground, or emerging field, of a number of consequences. Metabolic syndrome, and the inflammation that is pervasive in this state, is a common example.

We can also look at disease as a process, which is important to understand that dysfunction can proceed into a more profound disorder in the system. But it is also important to note that many of these disturbances can continue to act as a person becomes sicker and that sometimes, such as in infection or trauma, a person can jump from normal to very advanced pathology in an instant. Many other situations are more aptly described as chronic and progressive.

Disease as Process

Disease typically evolves in a process, with more irreversible changes occurring as one progresses further into it. Trauma, exposure to virulent pathogens, and toxins are events that can instantly cause a disease state. In many more cases it is gradual. This process can be understood in the following seven steps:

1. Hypofunction
2. Impaired communication and circulation
3. Inflammation
4. Deeper inflammation and immune involvement
5. Fibrosis and extracellular matrix degeneration
6. Decline of function
7. Neoplasm

Hypofunction

A gradual loss of function is what precedes more blatant pathological states. This hypofunction can occur for the simple reason that some factor that is essential for health is not being adequately met. The degree to which this disturbed determinant of health is impacted can make a difference on how long this stays as a subacute problem. For example, mild dehydration can impact cognition, lung function, urinary tract clearance of salts, etc. More severe dehydration can lead to confusion, agitation, and cardiac arrhythmias.

Not all states of hypofunction have a one-degree connection with a single disturbed detriment of health. Some are outcomes of several issues with meeting basic biological and psychological needs. A process can set in, where a chronic reaction involving multiple tissues and cells can set the stage for much more blatant breakdowns. An example would be insulin resistance, where the mechanisms of a process are all still operating, but one aspect is notably less efficient (Fig. 2.11).

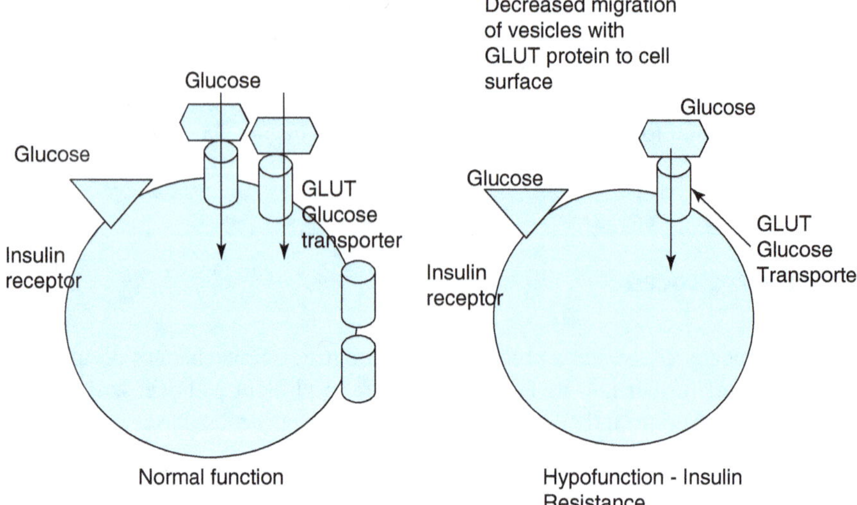

Fig. 2.11 Insulin resistance: The glucose transporter will malfunction in situations of insulin resistance, leading to impaired muscle glucose uptake, increased serum glucose levels, and, if possible, increased insulin secretion. This can become a self-reinforcing process

Impaired Communication and Circulation

Specific failure in a degree that becomes more acute is the progression from the impeded normal state to an abnormal, but still repairable state. For example, a person might have extensive triglyceride storage in their liver, a true steatosis, but carry on much like they always have (even though blood lipids and insulin resistance are silently setting in). But if the canaliculi of the liver become inflamed and swollen, this will impede the drainage of bile. That leads to cholestasis, which might be so extreme that it leads the patient to hyperbilirubinemia and hospitalization, or simply makes them very food adverse, tired, uncomfortable, and generally suffering from malaise.

This is a hallmark of a stage of disturbance that has progressed beyond hypofunction. At this point, communication with the rest of the body and circulation is impaired. All tissues must be in communication with their immediate environment and with the greater organism. For example, cells are connected to the extracellular matrix by connections such as integrins [31, 32]. Cells and tissues composed of them must have circulation. Waste products go out and nutrients and oxygen come in. Those gasses and other chemical compounds must transit through the matrix. Many tissues have a particular secretory or circulatory function. This can become impaired or erratic in some way as disturbance progresses. For example, as disturbances to determinants of health and hypofunction in the cardiovascular system begin to progress, the circulation of blood can become more difficult due to vascular

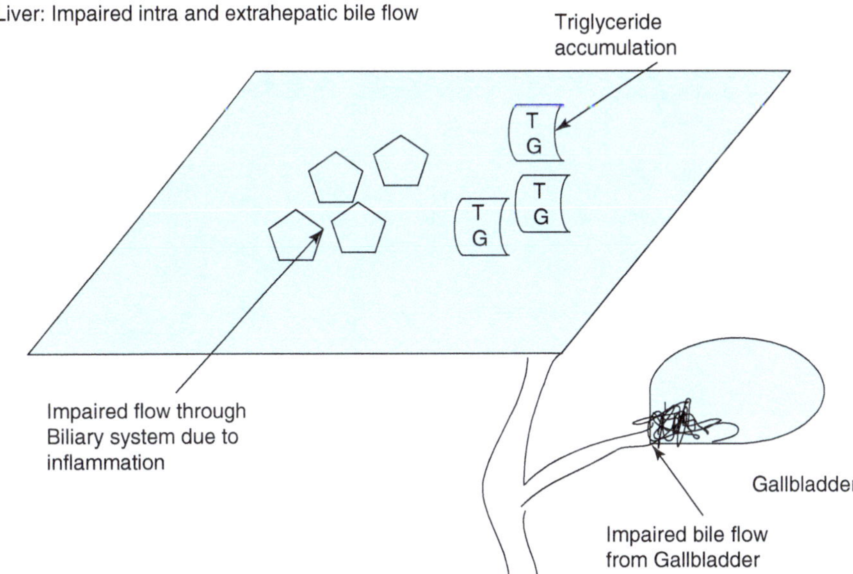

Fig. 2.12 Cholestasis: In liver conditions such as fatty liver disease, triglyceride accumulates in the hepatic cells. Biliary flow through the liver canaliculi can become impaired due to inflammation. Bile quality issues, such as lack of bile salts, can lead to poor biliary flow through the larger ducts and the gallbladder

resistance. Yet another example is intrahepatic cholestasis, often coupled with biliary stasis or "bile sludge" which can create a poor draining of bile and waste products from the liver (Fig. 2.12).

Inflammation

Tissues that have begun to form an abnormal relationship with their surrounding extracellular matrix and that have ceased having normal circulation of wastes and toxins out and nutrients and oxygen in will begin to show signs of inflammation. This is concurrent with overall decline of viability. Under these conditions, cellular damage begins to accrue. This is not necessarily from some outside source such as exogenous toxins or bacteria, although it can be. It can also be caused by loss of management of the normal oxidative and metabolic products within the cell. Once this begins to occur, some degree of inflammation in response to injury will occur.

For example, mitochondrial uncoupling can occur in cells that have poor enzymatic function, including the ability to make enough superoxide dismutase, and glutathione, for protection of cell and organelle membranes. Mitochondria create oxidative agents by virtue of their role in oxidative phosphorylation. If damaged or

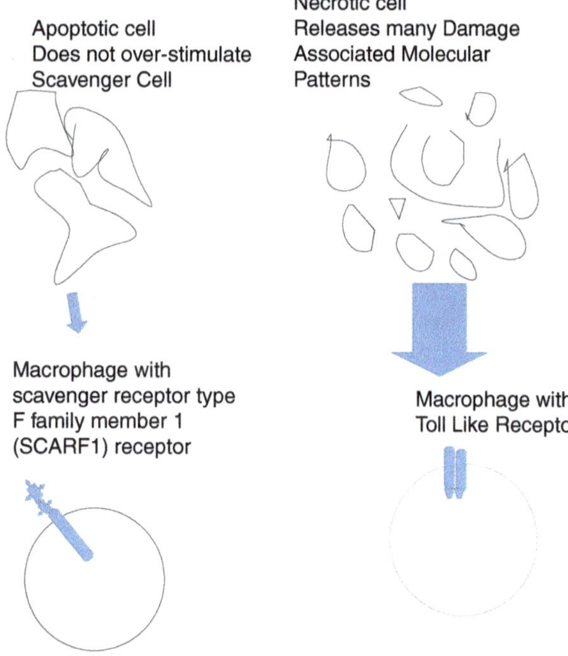

Fig. 2.13 Apoptosis versus necroptosis. Normal cell death via apoptosis does not trigger substantial inflammation. But cell fragments from necroptosis, by releasing damage-associated molecular patterns, gain the attention of the immune system

improperly supplied (with cofactors) mitochondria show uncoupling, then it can discharge excessive amounts of oxygen free radicals [33, 34]. This damages the mitochondrial membrane, which in turn leads to the rupture of this organelle. That, in turn, releases even more oxidative species into the cell. This can lead to cellular necrosis and an inflammation reaction. The damage-associated molecular patterns of necrotic cells will bind to toll-like receptors on antigen-presenting cells (Fig. 2.13).

Deeper Inflammation with Immune Involvement

As loss of function, and aggregate impairment, and unresolved inflammation progress, there will be greater damage and more intervention by the immune system.

For example, growth of an atheroma in an artery progresses initially from oxidative stress to inflammatory processing, evidenced by elevated C-reactive protein. As years go by, a new and more dangerous phase of inflammation arises (Fig. 2.14). White blood cells release substances such as myeloperoxidase and more white blood cells, and more oxidative stress leads to further damage to the artery. When initially inflammation cannot be resolved, and healing with remodeling cannot occur, a chronic inflammation sets in. White blood cells that under normal circumstances would create a natural event of cellular turnover and removal of foreign

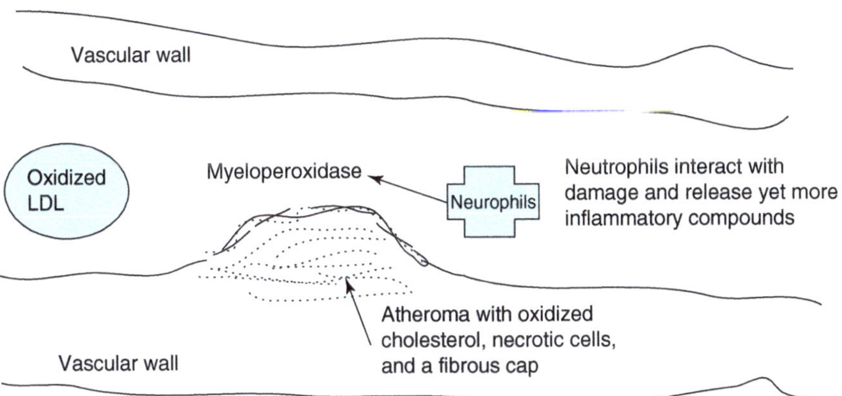

Fig. 2.14 Inflamed vascular wall. The initial damage done to the vascular endothelium and then the intima leads to a permanent deposition of oxidized cholesterol. This creates a circular phenomenon whereby white blood cells generate reactive oxygen species, accelerating the process of atherosclerotic plaque development

pathogens or cellular debris now begin to destroy local tissue. An open wound of sorts becomes a constant feature, which releases more signaling for further immune involvement.

Fibrosis and Extracellular Matrix Degeneration

With prolonged and unresolved inflammation and a disruption to normal communication and circulation, beleaguered tissues will undergo a fibrotic reaction. This is a secondary response and not often an adaptive one. Tissues that are stressed and which then have a normal resolution to inflammation and normal remodeling will eventually respond by fibrin deposition and a type of scarring (vide supra Fig. 2.7). This is concurrent with a dissolution of an extracellular matrix and is in a sense defined by that dissolution [35–37]. Without proper controls on this kind of collagen formation, which should be reasonably loose and anisotropic (multiple directions of orientation), a denser, clustered collagen assembly that chokes off normal communication even further can become elaborated. An example is the later stages of ongoing damage to the liver. When liver cells die because of toxins (alcohol, acetaldehyde, oxidized cholesterol, excessive free fatty acids), they release damage-associated patterns (DAMPs). These compounds, including high-mobility group box-1 (HMGB1), can directly activate the hepatic stellate cells, which are able to elicit a massive fibrotic reaction. There are antifibrotic mechanisms in the liver, but these are overmatched by a push to fibrosis. DAMPs can also activate macrophages and lymphocytes. This type of response is the undoing of the liver, because the fibrosis is irreversible, and the breakdown of normal architecture creates a myriad of new challenges. Although, with medical assistance and naturopathic assistance, there are people who have suffered hepatic fibrosis and have rehabilitated their body to the degree that remaining healthy patches of the liver can sustain life, for many patients this evolution is lethal.

Decline of Function

In organs that have remodeled themselves after a substantial amount of injury and no longer are structurally or physiologically the same, they can head toward a total breakdown of function [38]. In medical terms, this can be referred to as organ failure. What leads to a final breakdown? One factor is that the level of attrition of healthy cells is so high that there simply is not enough output from that organ to sustain life. This is accentuated in tissue breakdown that is concentrated in highly specialized functional units. For example, a loss of a broad swath of left ventricular muscle due to the aftereffects of a myocardial infarction might still permit the person to rehabilitate, or perhaps allow them to live with medical and naturopathic assistance for years with a very slowly progressive congestive heart failure. But if the brunt of the damage involves critical electrical junctures, such as the sinoatrial node, the patient might be headed for lethal cardiac events much sooner. Or a stroke, a cerebral vascular accident that impacts part of the temporal lobe will have very serious and debilitating effects, but the patient might rehabilitate to a high degree and it will be survivable. But if the damage from a stroke is in the brain stem, the vital functions of life might cease.

Another form of terminal breakdown is the aforementioned liver failure due to extensive fibrosis. The liver has an extensive filter structure, with precise locations of portal system vein dispersion, bile disposal, and arterial blood flow. When this is crosscut with collagen, the liver can no longer physically work, and the portal blood cannot access hepatocytes. Waste products cannot easily find their way through the rigid extracellular matrix and into the bile and efferent circulation.

A similar situation arises with emphysema, a form of chronic obstructive pulmonary disease. When the lung becomes less elastic and shot through with vacuoles and empty spaces, the ventilation (air dispersion) to perfusion (blood coming to the alveoli to pick up oxygen) ratio changes for the worse (Fig. 2.15).

The example of emphysema illustrates another dimension of breakdown. The lack of oxygen leads to a high-output cardiac state, as the heart attempts to speed up circulation to better supply organs (including the brain) with O_2. The right ventricle must push blood through a fibrotic lung matrix. These patients often die of *cor pulmonale* or right-sided heart failure. The knock on effects of the organ's breakdown leads to death, as there are so many interdependencies between specialized tissues of the body.

Sometimes, an event can occur in the severely damaged organ that simply leads to an acute and rapidly deteriorating situation. A patient with congestion of the

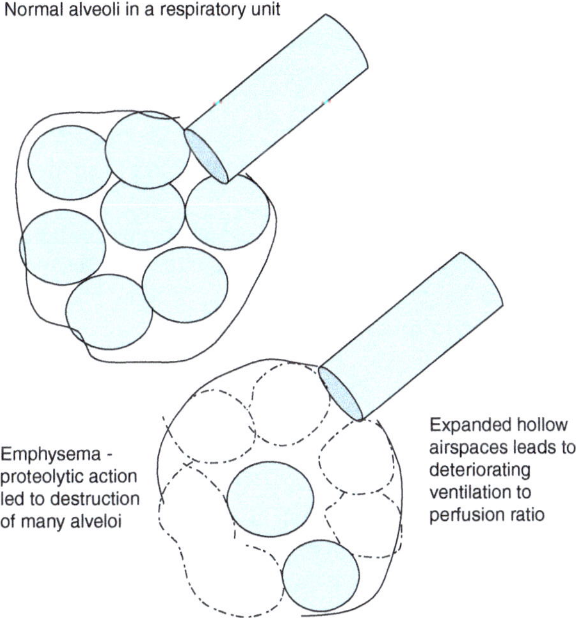

Fig. 2.15 Emphysema: The destruction of proteins such as elastin and collagen by proteolytic enzymes creates hollow spaces that are not efficiently ventilated nor perfused

portal circulation due to cirrhosis develops dilatation of the esophageal veins, begins to vomit up blood, and dies of a hemorrhage.

Neoplasm

In some cases, there is an ultimate consequence of breakdown in function, which is neoplasia. Entropic disorganization of tissues is not the primary cause of neoplasia. Mutations and various gene expression alterations are. However, this breakdown is a powerful facilitator of the oncogenic process. It could be described as literally paving the way for transformed cells to succeed. In 1889, surgeon Stephen Paget described cancer metastasis as an interplay between the migrating tumor cells (the "seed") and its microenvironment (the "soil"). The early naturopathic physicians thought the same way, which is abundantly clear in the works of Henry Lindlahr.

What has been clearly described in the twenty-first century is that as tumor cells begin to divide, the nearby extracellular matrix begins to change its structure [39]. There is a communication between tumor cells and the ECM. More fibronectin and collagens I, III, and IV create a different environment. Stromally derived lysyl oxidases begin to align the collagen, changing it from a normally diffuse and random configuration to a more lined up configuration. The "stiff" matrix has constant communication with the tumor cells and, via signaling mechanisms, begin to enable even more proliferation of tumor cells.

While healthy tissue can give rise to a neoplasm, it seems likely that degenerated tissues have a corrupted matrix that is more easily manipulated by neoplastic cells and easier to realign to suit the growth and the travel of tumor cells through migration tracks. Like a warlord exploiting a local situation of lawlessness for their own ends, a tumor cell is readily able to reconfigure cell signaling, homeostasis, and migration by co-opting the microenvironment primarily through the extracellular matrix.

For example, in Barrett's esophagus, ongoing damage from gastric acid and even bile acids will lead to a metaplasia of the distal esophagus. High levels of inflammation also can progress to neoplasia. In some breast cancers, stromal reorganization is key to their proliferation and spread.

Disease Is a Process

Disease is a process that follows predictable stages. Naturopathic medicine considers where a patient is in this progression. This allows for a therapeutic plan that can address the needs of the patient. In some cases, a simple correction of deficient biological essentials is all that is needed. In other cases, biochemical support through plant extracts and nutrients will help someone to exit an inflammatory or confused state and function normally again. In other situations, reducing symptoms is necessary for patient quality of life and often life-saving, because the symptoms in question are manifestations of a breakdown of function.

Seeing disease as a process is commensurate with recognizing disease entities as observable and measurable in cells and tissues (pathology reports, CT scans, bloodwork, physical examination, etc.). This process view, the backstory of a given patient's pathology (and in clinical practice, it always comes down to one patient, at one point in time), opens the door for therapeutic interventions that allow the adaptation responses of the body to assert themselves. These adaptations are not only biochemical fail-safes. The human body, and other lifeforms, can be reintegrated and reestablish coordinated function. They can be made whole again and, if not completely restored, then at least move toward health.

References

1. Franco E, Galloway KE. Feedback loops in biological networks. Methods Mol Biol. 2015;1244:193–214.
2. Smith A, Bianchi A, Kuestermann K, O'Byrne A, Van Brandt B. Introduction to bioregulatory medicine. Stuttgart: Thieme; 2009.
3. Gonze D, Ruoff P. The Goodwin oscillator and its legacy. Acta Biotheor. 2020;69:857.
4. Stiles PJ, Gray CG. Improved Hodgkin-Huxley type model for neural action potentials. Eur Biophys J. 2021;50(6):819–28.

5. Blanchini F, Cuba Samaniego C, Franco E, Giordano G. Homogeneous time constants promote oscillations in negative feedback loops. ACS Synth Biol. 2018;7(6):1481–7.
6. Ananthasubramaniam B, Herzel H. Positive feedback promotes oscillations in negative feedback loops. PLoS One. 2014;9(8):e104761.
7. Gjerstad JK, Lightman SL, Spiga F. Role of glucocorticoid negative feedback in the regulation of HPA axis pulsatility. Stress. 2018;21(5):403–16.
8. Pomatto LCD, Davies KJA. The role of declining adaptive homeostasis in ageing. J Physiol. 2017;595(24):7275–309.
9. Davies KJA. Adaptive homeostasis. Mol Asp Med. 2016;49:1–7. https://pubmed.ncbi.nlm.nih.gov/27112802.
10. Lauzon RJ, Ishizuka KJ, Weissman IL. Cyclical generation and degeneration of organs in a colonial urochordate involves crosstalk between old and new: a model for development and regeneration. Dev Biol. 2002;249(2):333–48.
11. Abedi F, Rezaee R, Hayes AW, Nasiripour S, Karimi G. MicroRNAs and SARS-CoV-2 life cycle, pathogenesis, and mutations: biomarkers or therapeutic agents? Cell Cycle. 2021;20(2):143–53.
12. Ac IAH, Histology M. Matrix Histol Physiol. 2007:1–55.
13. Yue B. Biology of the extracellular matrix: an overview. J Glaucoma. 2014;23(8 Suppl 1):S20–3. https://pubmed.ncbi.nlm.nih.gov/25275899.
14. Pickup MW, Mouw JK, Weaver VM. The extracellular matrix modulates the hallmarks of cancer. EMBO Rep. 2014;15(12):1243–53.
15. Moreira AM, Pereira J, Melo S, Fernandes MS, Carneiro P, Seruca R, et al. The extracellular matrix: an accomplice in gastric cancer development and progression. Cells. 2020;9(2):394.
16. Kai F, Drain AP, Weaver VM. The extracellular matrix modulates the metastatic journey. Dev Cell. 2019;49(3):332–46.
17. Filipe EC, Chitty JL, Cox TR. Charting the unexplored extracellular matrix in cancer. Int J Exp Pathol. 2018;99(2):58–76.
18. Mohanraj K, Nowicka U, Chacinska A. Mitochondrial control of cellular protein homeostasis. Biochem J. 2020;477(16):3033–54.
19. Bhatti JS, Bhatti GK, Reddy PH. Mitochondrial dysfunction and oxidative stress in metabolic disorders - a step towards mitochondria based therapeutic strategies. Biochim Biophys Acta Mol basis Dis. 2017;1863(5):1066–77.
20. Nunnari J, Suomalainen A. Mitochondria: in sickness and in health. Cell. 2012;148(6):1145–59.
21. Giorgi C, Marchi S, Simoes ICM, Ren Z, Morciano G, Perrone M, et al. Mitochondria and reactive oxygen species in aging and age-related diseases. Int Rev Cell Mol Biol. 2018;340:209–344. https://pubmed.ncbi.nlm.nih.gov/30072092.
22. Meyer JN, Leuthner TC, Luz AL. Mitochondrial fusion, fission, and mitochondrial toxicity. Toxicology. 2017;391:42–53.
23. Brand MD, Nicholls DG. Assessing mitochondrial dysfunction in cells. Biochem J. 2011;435(2):297–312. https://pubmed.ncbi.nlm.nih.gov/21726199.
24. Srinivasan S, Guha M, Kashina A, Avadhani NG. Mitochondrial dysfunction and mitochondrial dynamics-the cancer connection. Biochim Biophys Acta Bioenerg. 2017;1858(8):602–14.
25. Calabrese EJ. Hormesis and stem cells enhancing cell proliferation, differentiation and resilience to inflammatory stress in bone marrow stem cells and their therapeutic implications. Chem Biol Interact. 2021;351:109730. https://doi.org/10.1016/j.cbi.2021.109730.
26. Gehart H, Clevers H. Tales from the crypt: new insights into intestinal stem cells. Nat Rev Gastroenterol Hepatol. 2019;16(1):19–34.
27. Brundel BJJM. The role of proteostasis derailment in cardiac diseases. Cells. 2020;9(10):2317. https://pubmed.ncbi.nlm.nih.gov/33086474.
28. Roth DM, Balch WE. Modeling general proteostasis: proteome balance in health and disease. Curr Opin Cell Biol. 2011;23(2):126–34.
29. Morimoto RI, Cuervo AM. Proteostasis and the aging proteome in health and disease. J Gerontol A Biol Sci Med Sci. 2014;69(Suppl 1):S33–8.

30. Alvarez-Garcia I, Miska EA. MicroRNA functions in animal development and human disease. Development. 2005;132(21):4653–62.
31. Ge H, Tian M, Pei Q, Tan F, Pei H. Extracellular matrix stiffness: new areas affecting cell metabolism. Front Oncol. 2021;11:631991. https://pubmed.ncbi.nlm.nih.gov/33718214.
32. Theocharis AD, Manou D, Karamanos NK. The extracellular matrix as a multitasking player in disease. FEBS J. 2019;286(15):2830–69.
33. Faas MM, de Vos P. Mitochondrial function in immune cells in health and disease. Biochim Biophys Acta Mol basis Dis. 2020;1866(10):165845.
34. Verma SK, Garikipati VNS, Kishore R. Mitochondrial dysfunction and its impact on diabetic heart. Biochim Biophys Acta Mol basis Dis. 2017;1863(5):1098–105.
35. Lu P, Takai K, Weaver VM, Werb Z. Extracellular matrix degradation and remodeling in development and disease. Cold Spring Harb Perspect Biol. 2011;3(12):a005058. https://pubmed.ncbi.nlm.nih.gov/21917992.
36. Monnier VM, Sell DR, Nagaraj RH, Miyata S, Grandhee S, Odetti P, et al. Maillard reaction-mediated molecular damage to extracellular matrix and other tissue proteins in diabetes, aging, and uremia. Diabetes. 1992;41(Suppl 2):36–41.
37. Burgstaller G, Oehrle B, Gerckens M, White ES, Schiller HB, Eickelberg O. The instructive extracellular matrix of the lung: basic composition and alterations in chronic lung disease. Eur Respir J. 2017;50(1):1601805. http://erj.ersjournals.com/content/50/1/1601805.abstract.
38. Brunet A, Berger SL. Epigenetics of aging and aging-related disease. J Gerontol A Biol Sci Med Sci. 2014;69(Suppl 1):S17–20.
39. Walker C, Mojares E, Del Río Hernández A. Role of Extracellular Matrix in Development and Cancer Progression. Int J Mol Sci. 2018;19(10):3028.

Chapter 3
Where Does a Naturopathic Approach Apply?

Why Are Allopathic Therapies Sometimes Not Enough?

The advent of pharmaceutical-based medicine informed by advances in understanding of physiology, pharmacology, pathology, and other biomedical sciences has been undeniably successful. This has been to the great benefit of humanity. Anyone who has, or has had, a loved one in need of an allopathic approach can appreciate the precision and rapidity of this approach. There is a powerful combination of observable results that can be statistically validated and abstract logic derived from known biological processes. Followed to its conclusion, this approach would suggest that all breakdown of our bodies, all disease, can be fixed if we understand the point of breakdown and can find an agent that reverses it.

That quest for more and more agents that will patch up the myriad points of breakdown in the body has yielded both spectacular successes and diminishing returns. The useful and sometimes amazing results of drug therapy have shown the efficacy of targeted therapies. The persistent presence of chronic disease and the acceleration of health issues for individual patients and our society as a whole belies that notion that all that is needed in medicine are better drug treatments coupled with a few common sense lifestyle practices.

There are an incredible number of enzymatic processes, molecular movement, energy transfer, and communication (nervous, endocrine, immune, extracellular matrix—microtubule) events every second in the human body. A drug might have to only impact one of them to make a positive therapeutic difference. It would be logical to presume that any problem that comes along can be treated with a receptor-targeted therapy. But the complexity, velocity, and sheer number of events happening in an organized system of the human body preclude the power of an external agent to manage all possible dysfunctions that might arise.

That may seem to be begging the question—if the human system works well enough a lot of the time and sometimes simply breaks down, why is that a

F. Smith, *Naturopathic Medicine*, https://doi.org/10.1007/978-3-031-13388-6_3

shortcoming of pharmaceutical-based therapies that can reverse or at least reduce the consequences of that breakdown?

There are several reasons why this question of the limits of an allopathic paradigm are critically important:

1. Eliminating the "X factor" of the body's creative adaptations to stressors is to ignore an extremely important factor in the equation of healing. This adaptive and inherent responsiveness is not only a major force in the healing process (ask any surgeon who sees a carefully approximated wound heal). This adaptive response limits and alters the effects of therapies (Fig. 3.1). Pretending that human adaptations are low in relevance is useful for creating generalizable knowledge about drug effects, but it is incomplete. It is possible to temporarily bypass the self-healing mechanisms in emergency situations and practical to do so. In longer-term treatment and in the preservation of health, it is counterproductive. It is no wiser than building a bridge without considering the prevailing winds, or shearing stresses from turbulent water, or effects of acidic rain on structural integrity. Thinking about how to purposefully stimulate these healing mechanisms, instead of presuming that they are inert, would be more productive.
2. Cause and effect. A "disease" does not lead to these states of decay. It is these entropic states that allow diseases to emerge (Fig. 3.2). Treating only late process effects of underlying dysfunction can be effective to a point, but eventually becomes a game of endless blockades of breakdown symptoms. Disease states

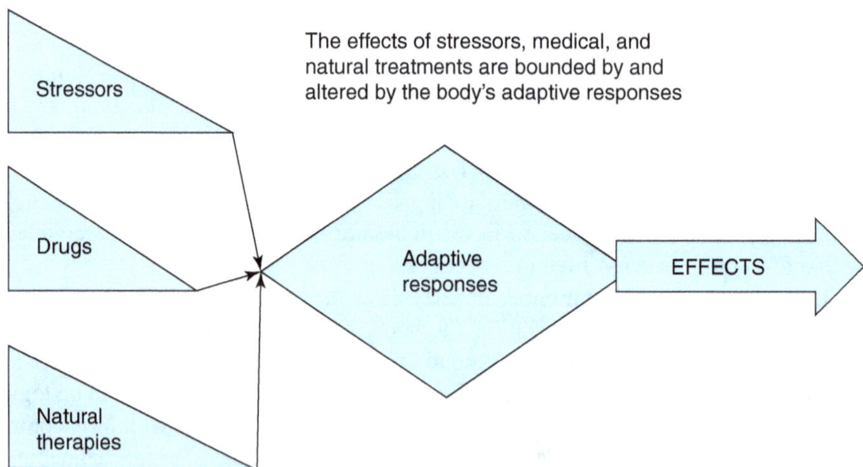

Fig. 3.1 Central role of adaptive responses: The body's adaptive responses set a limit to what stressors, pharmaceutical treatments, and natural therapies can achieve. Any input to the body, including vigorous receptor binding by a drug, must rely on downstream biological activity to create an observable effect. Adaptive responses also alter the effects of these inputs. For example, when alpha blocking agents were experimented with in the 1950s, they dropped blood pressure dramatically, but it came back up as the baroreceptors activated an increase in heart rate

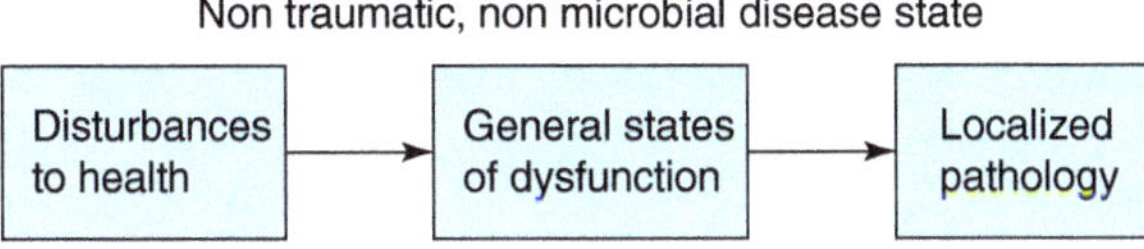

Fig. 3.2 Sequence of disease generation: Premorbid, degenerative states give rise to clinical pathologies. If the disturbances to health are not too great, and if most body systems remain intact, then treating the resultant localized pathology can alleviate symptoms (although this may lead to simply a slower breakdown). Diseases—localized pathologies—certainly create their own ramifying consequences that must be managed medically. But their generative ground are the states of dysfunction that arise from disturbances to health

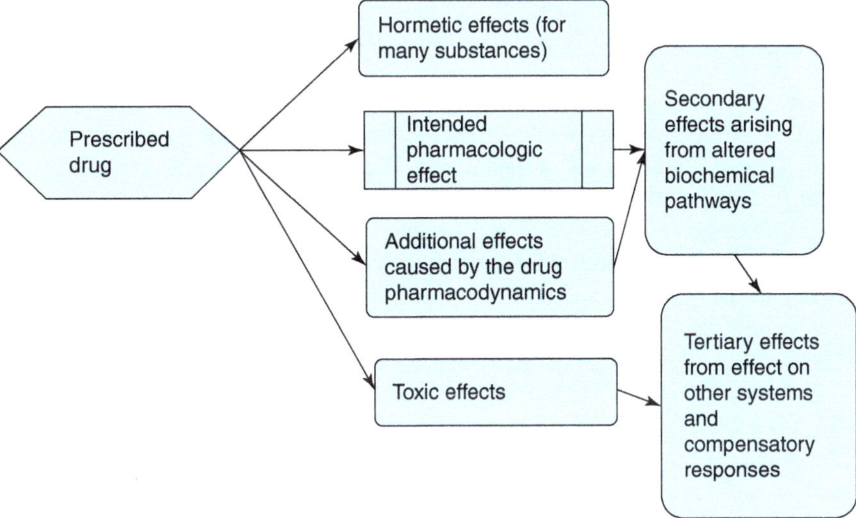

Fig. 3.3 Drug treatment has broad effects: Pharmaceutical treatments, including some herbal extracts at higher doses, lead to a manifold of effects. Secondary effects arise both as an effect of the primary receptor-binding purpose of the drug (effects are not always totally specific to just the therapeutic benefit), but also from allosteric binding sites and knock-on effects of the drug. Other organ systems may respond to these actions, which can also occur with toxicity. Hormetic effects are unique, in that they are from doses below any dose at which any observable adverse effect is noted and the magnitude of the hormetic effect is modest. This leads to adaptive responses, but in a different manner than the compensatory responses to a drug

will eventually self-propagate but, aside from trauma or infection, are usually preceded by premorbid changes.

3. These adaptive responses referred to in [1] above are a major determinant on the results and course of allopathic therapies (Fig. 3.3). The ability of allopathic medicine to ignore the obvious biphasic dose response nature of many, many drugs and to incuriously write down many biological effects as "side effects" is an astounding example of bounded rationality. It is possible to prescribe these medications based on a truncated, linear, dose-response curve, but this fails to

make use of the predictive power of a full spectrum of dose-response relationships. That would be responses at lower doses than typically thought of as a threshold for inhibitory activity.

4. In some cases, the consequence of blocking an enzyme, or strongly stimulating a receptor beyond what the body would normally do, can become a knock-on effect of significance. Aside from the effects noted in [2] above, this is a question of magnitude and clinical significance. For instance, antidepressant medications can help children and adolescents but can also lead to suicidal ideation. Conversely, a less dramatic but more common example would be the benefits of blocking the COX-1 enzyme from taking NSAID drugs such as aspirin (Fig. 3.4). This can inhibit the proactive mucosal lining of the stomach. The higher-risk effects of drugs, understandably, get more attention as they can impact clinical decision-making. But it is important to recognize that most pharmaceuticals using therapeutic levels will have ramifying consequences in a complex system such as the human body. Testing medications versus a null hypothesis has been a very productive (and with the right biostatistical controls) and accurate method to determine the efficacy of medications. But the many *other* effects of introducing a drug into the human system are not understood clearly. They are observed, and documented, during the process of preapproval studies for drugs, and in after-market surveillance. Sometimes these are beneficial effects and may even suggest new uses for a drug. For instance, aspirin will reduce pain and fever, but also has value in colon cancer prevention.

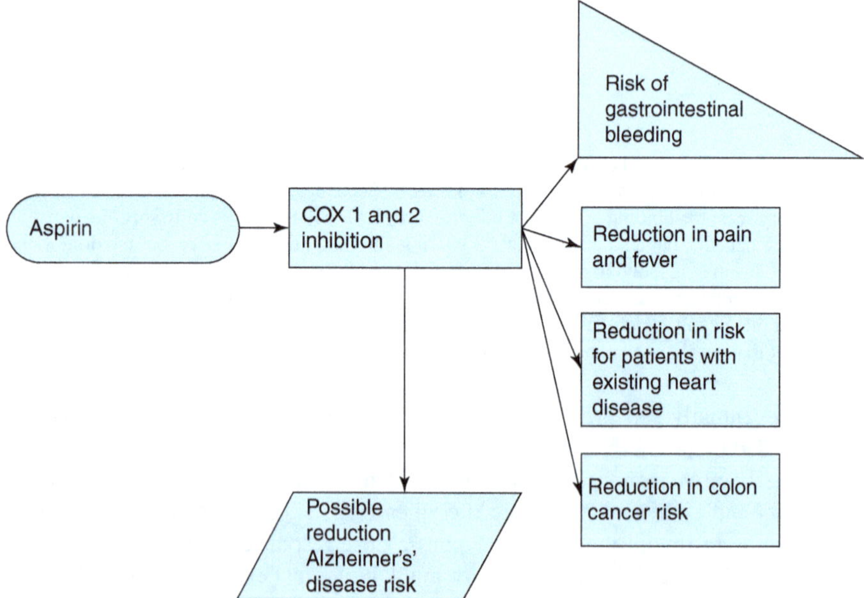

Fig. 3.4 Cyclooxygenase inhibition: Some of the consequences of cyclooxygenase inhibition, beyond pain and fever reduction, are clinically important

5. The knowledge base about genes, their activation or suppression, and how they work together continues to advance. The use of software to manage this manifold of knowledge makes it possible to model and predict effects in complex systems. Drug therapy that focuses on a single target and precludes larger system effects (provided they are not a nuisance) is a mode of thinking that dates back to the late nineteenth century. It was useful then, and it still is. But to become stuck at this level of therapeutic guidance is to miss out on a very promising, whole systems approach to healing that can make use of today's and tomorrow's technologies.

The question is not one of allopathic medicine being invalid because of these factors. It is demonstrably valid and indispensable. The problem is the belief in, and commitment to, the idea that targeted alterations to pathophysiology are the only form of treatment (aside from surgery and some physical therapies) that scientific information can be used to create. This is an unfortunate oversight, a *magna omissio*, that itself threatens to make the delivery of allopathic health care itself economically unsustainable.

Why Natural Approaches Are Sometimes Not Enough

There are many situations where natural approaches are not enough. Although a naturopathic approach, using all its modalities, can meet the challenges of many clinical situations, there are real limits to what treatment with tools apart from synthetic pharmacology, surgery, and radiation therapies can accomplish.

Timeframe and Speed of Events

The velocity at which some pathological events take place sometimes make a natural approach ideal. Although natural treatments tend to have longer term, and beneficial cumulative effects, they can also work quickly. But sometimes a superrapid and reproducible result is the appropriate standard of care, and the more natural approaches are insufficient (Fig. 3.5). There are treatments such as acupuncture, or higher-dose botanicals, that *can* work. An example is the use of intramuscular epinephrine to treat an allergic reaction that is closing the airway. Another would be nitroglycerine to relieve an acute angina pectoris episode. This kind of treatment is not about changing the biological terrain in the long term. It is about dealing with a situation in the contracted timeframe of seconds.

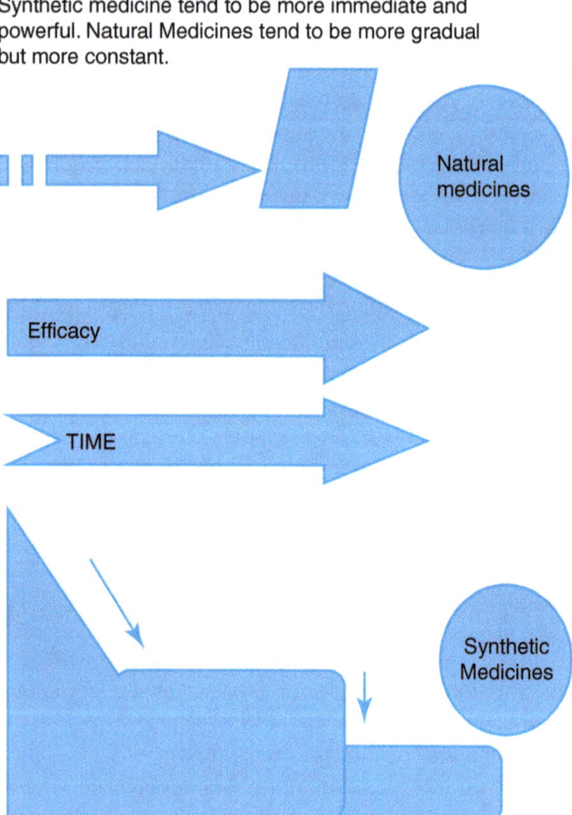

Fig. 3.5 Velocity of action versus duration of efficacy: Synthetic medicines can work immediately and forcefully, but after time often lose impact as the body adapts or underlying pathological processes progress. Natural approaches often take longer to build up effect, but can have persistent benefits. The choice of therapy in emergency situations is obvious

Overwhelming Severity of Pathology

Sometimes a pathological situation is so drastic that the only way to preserve life is the use of powerful synthetic treatments. An example would be toxic shock syndrome and disseminated intravascular coagulation, or an infection of the central nervous system (Fig. 3.6). A noninfectious example would be an acute inflammatory reaction that is rapidly destroying the kidneys. In these cases, the ability of systems in the body to reestablish homeostasis is not able to assert itself. The system cannot "reboot."

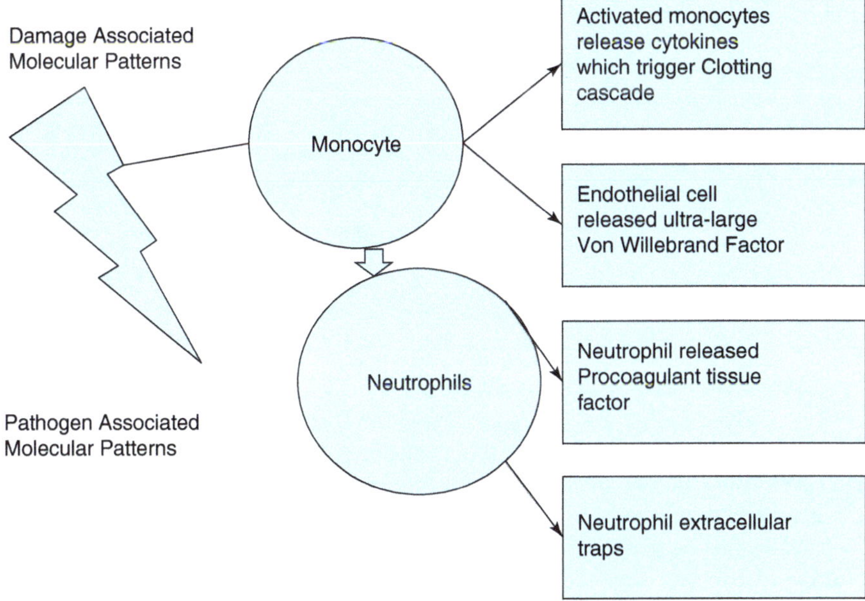

Fig. 3.6 Disseminated intravascular coagulation. A chain reaction of inflammatory events can be rapidly fatal. This is the type of situation where rapid activity pharmaceutical medications that create a clear-cut effect are the medically indicted treatment

Degree of Chronic System Breakdown

The ability of the human body to stay functional, to find a way to maintain homeostasis, is amazing. But as chronic disease progresses, there comes a point where outside help is needed to make it continue functioning. The tendency in contemporary health care is to assume that biological adaptation cannot occur, and many people are not even aware that they could improve function or even heal from certain diseases. They have been raised and enculturated to think that their options are pills and surgery, or death.

Nevertheless, patients can reach a point where this is true, and we can be exceedingly grateful that ways to prolong, and enhance life, are available. An example would be a patient with insulin-dependent diabetes mellitus—they simply cannot make enough insulin and need to inject it. A more chronic example would be a patient who lost so much cardiac function due to a myocardial infarction that they need some kind of allopathic therapy to offset this situation. Their dependence on

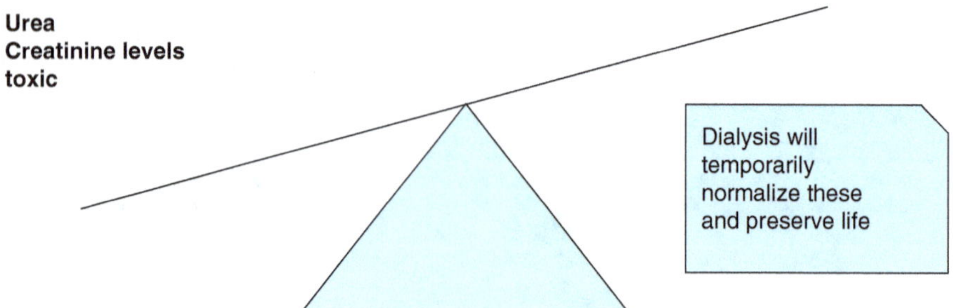

Fig. 3.7 Renal dialysis: Patients obtain the desired effect of removing uremic toxins from the blood and must obtain this treatment in order to stay alive

this therapy will be lessened if they use a naturopathic approach, in many situations. However, some diuretic, or some therapy aimed at reducing peripheral resistance to the heart's pumping of blood, is going to come into play. The question becomes: "what does this patient have to work with?" Sometimes, the answer is so very little that in order to stay alive they need a specific medical therapy. In the case of renal dialysis (Fig. 3.7), the absence of renal function makes the therapy effective and necessary.

Interaction of Comorbidities That Have Distinctive Causes

A patient can have several disease processes in motion at one time. By the time these breakdowns in homeostasis have become well established, they no longer yield to attempts to remove the original causative conditions. While addressing disturbances to the determinants of health is still a high priority, it will not be enough. An example is a patient with advanced diabetes mellitus (NIDDM), neuropathy, kidney disease, and heart disease (Fig. 3.8). Much like a country attempting to fight a war on three fronts, eventually the person cannot juggle all of the issues going on.

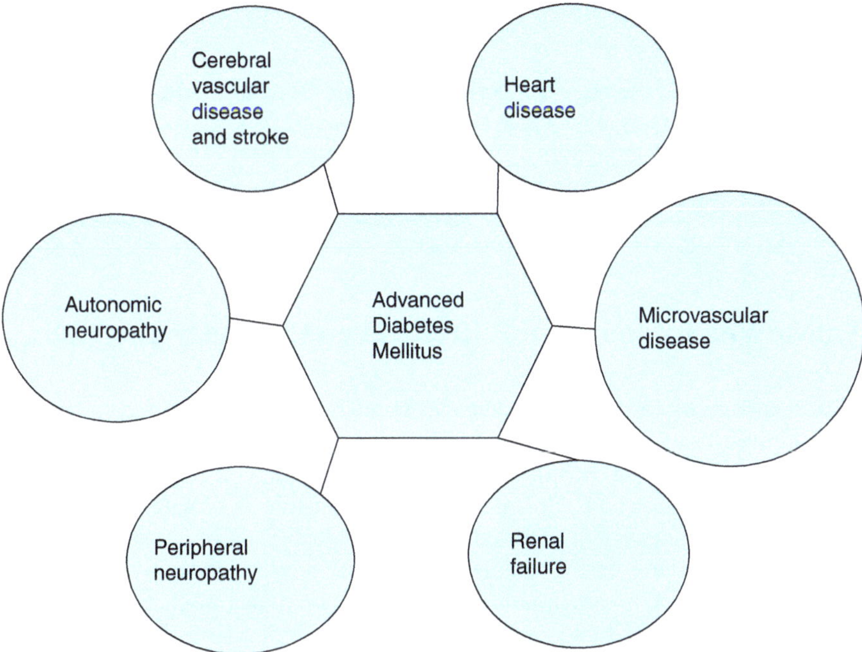

Fig. 3.8 Diabetes mellitus complications: Diabetes eventually becomes a multisystem disease

Genetic Predispositions or Causes That Have a Large-Magnitude Effect

All human beings have genetic predispositions, or a potential for various diseases. That does not mean that they will develop those illnesses, nor can we predict at this time, all of the multifarious ways that genes, environment, and behavior interact. But in some cases, a genetic tendency is so strong that it will be expressed and will have a negative impact. Beyond a vague "predisposition" or "tendency," there are well-established links between genes and certain maladies. Cystic fibrosis, Huntington's disease, and chronic myeloid leukemia are all examples of this type of linkage.

Trauma

Traumatic injury to the body can destroy or disable structures to the point that normal repair mechanisms are not able to restore it. Trauma itself can be so overwhelming that the patient's system is under extreme duress. Examples would be a motor vehicle accident, electrocution, gunshot wounds, and exposure to extreme cold or heat.

Patient Vitality and Overall Health at an Extremely Low Ebb

The compensatory responses to challenges or intentionally used stimuli can move a patient toward healing. But if the patient lacks sufficient resources to mount an effective response, then their dependence on an allopathic approach is going to be much greater. While good can still result from the methods of naturopathic medicine, the patient does not have the energy or biological plasticity to get all the way back to a homeostatic state. Examples include very advanced age, exhaustion after chronic viral or tick-borne disease, conclusion of a regimen of chemotherapy and radiation to eradicate a tumor, and chronic poor health in general (such as years of neglected NIDDM).

Patient Does Not Wish to Participate in The Process of Healing

Not all natural therapies require great effort from the patient. Some therapies, such as hydrotherapy, allow the patient to receive a physical treatment. Nevertheless, for healing to happen often requires some change of behavior, some willingness to address the disturbed determinants of health. If a patient is unable to, or unwilling to participate in their own healing process, then a more purely allopathic approach is needed. An example would be a patient with COPD, and heart disease, who does not wish to give up smoking, or make very extensive changes to their diet. In this case, that patient is going to need bronchodilating agents, statins, and probably a beta blocker just to continue to function. That does not mean that they cannot still benefit from other therapies, but they will have at least one foot on the pharmaceutical side of treatment.

Severe Psychological and Socioeconomic Constraints

Disease and healing are not always simple phenomena. In some situations, the patient has limited ability to change their circumstances. This can be due to poverty, or a common situation of having to work two jobs just to keep their head above water financially. They can barely find a few minutes a day to sit down and relax and must remain in a high functioning state most of the time. In this case, they might need the advantages of symptom control through the use of pharmaceuticals. There are downsides to this of course; the ultimate toll that this situation might take on them could be very high. Morbid obesity is another example. Simply knowing that energy expenditure and caloric intake must be balanced is not going to make a big dent in a multifactorial condition such as this. Psychological counseling, changes to decades-old habits, exploration of the role that food plays, slow introduction of exercise to tolerance, etc. are all going to be needed.

Virulent Pathogens

Pathogens can exceed the ability of the human organism to withstand them. In these cases, morbidity can be so rapid, and so extreme, that a natural approach alone cannot gain a foothold. The rabies virus is a clear example (Fig. 3.9). As stated in other examples, this does not preclude the use of natural approaches while using other approaches. The dichotomizing view that a patient *can only use X*, or *can only use Y*, is counterproductive. An example would be SARS CoV-2. Many people exposed to this agent developed flu-like symptoms and recovered. Some patients, including

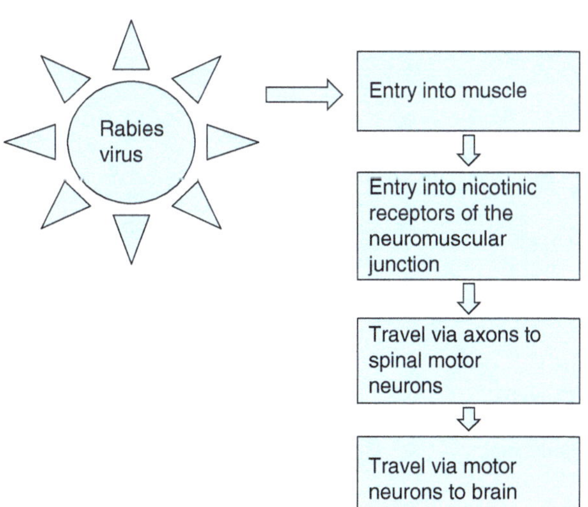

Fig. 3.9 Rabies virus: The relentless progression from the muscle to the nerves and to the spinal cord and brain makes infection with the rabies virus almost universally fatal, without medical treatment early on

those who were young and healthy, developed extreme reactions—vasculitis, cerebral inflammation, myocarditis, and much more. The way in which infectious agents can defeat the body's defenses, or provoke those defenses into an extreme overcompensation response, is a fact of living in the biological world. Technologies that can interrupt this process do save lives, which would be lost if the matter were left entirely up to nature.

Truly Structural or Surgical Situations

Bodies can break, and surgical interventions can be the appropriate therapies. Even in these surgical cases the healing mechanisms of the body are needed to not only mend the incisions, but to allow the surgical therapy to help the person to move back toward health. Examples include the decompression and ablation of osteophytes on the spine that are measurably obstructing nerve roots, congenital defects such as pulmonary hypertension, pulmonary embolism (Fig. 3.10), and infection of the large bowel secondary to infarction of the mesenteric artery.

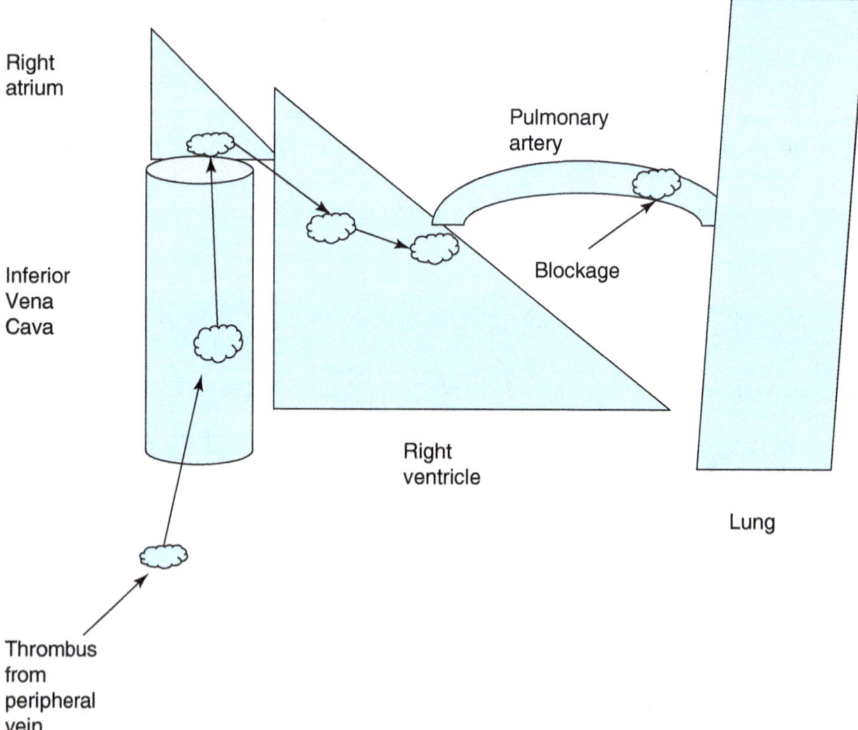

Fig. 3.10 Pulmonary embolism: The location of this embolus makes it fatal, but modern cardiology has found ways to dislodge and dissolve it

Threshold for Healing No Longer Being Intrinsic

It can be difficult to determine any measurable threshold beyond which naturopathic medicine approaches cannot help due to the fact that self-repair processes are not able to function. Certainly there are many situations where this is plainly obvious. The causes are discussed above. In practice, naturopathic physicians will use more interventional therapies in these cases—that is why in naturopathic medicine there is a widely accepted and studied therapeutic order, or hierarchy, that acknowledges that moving healing forward, or preserving life and limb [1], requires, at certain times, suppressive or high-force therapies.

If there is a threshold, it would fall into one of five categories (Fig. 3.11):

Structural integration is not possible—loss of organization, cohesion, and normal geometric structure cannot be attained. This can be at the organ level, or the extracellular matrix level. Excessive trauma, or fibrotic tissue, is one cause. But repeated insult can simply erase the fundamental structural guidance for replacement tissue and result in an amorphous, dysfunctional tissue.

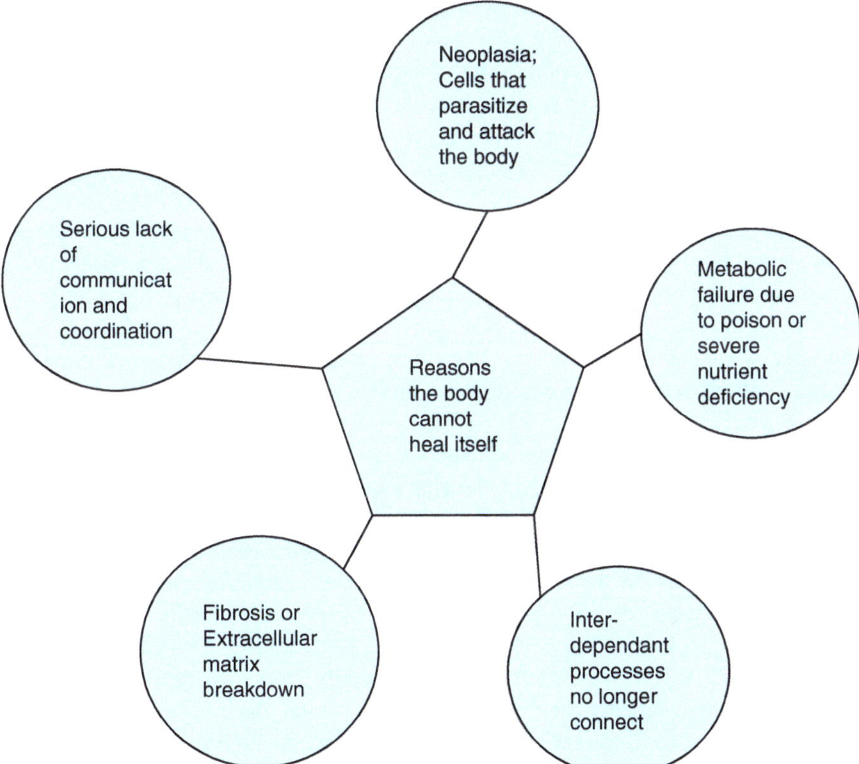

Fig. 3.11 Situations that defy self-healing: The states confound the normal adaptive responses of the body. They require medical intervention, although in nonemergency situations patients often exit these states with appropriate naturopathic treatment

The cellular turnover, genetic expression, or pluripotency of the source tissues is exhausted. This can be seen with aging, and while organisms have many cards to play in terms of finding ways to keep tissues functioning, there does come a time where it is not enough. In a different sense, loss of neural tissue in a young person can be catastrophic, but the potential for repair might be better than someone older. Some losses of tissue in any organ are so extensive that in organisms like humans that do not have the regenerative capability of an axolotl or salamander, the deficit cannot be filled.

The cells and tissue in question have dedifferentiated to the point where the cells no longer interact normally with surrounding cells—they are neoplastic. (This does not preclude the possibility of the host immune system, or any still functioning caspase enzymes, defeating the neoplasm, but this becomes rapidly unlikely at this threshold.)

The cellular machinery cannot carry out its functions. This can be due to the arresting effects of toxins (i.e., mercury, cyanide, etc.). Or it can be due to excessive oxidative stress. It can also occur due to macro- or micronutrient deficiencies.

The synchronization of events necessary for healing cannot be achieved. Like a machine that cannot time its own events and stalls, this can happen locally in various disorders. This can be due to some of the above factors. Or it can be due to systematic issues. Poor circulation in an area of the body due to vascular disease might sabotage healing of a wound, even though the other requirements for repair are being met. Some blood flow and oxygen are present, but at some critical stage: inflammation, or tissue replacement, or remodeling. Events cannot proceed quickly enough.

It is worth mentioning that patients can be brought back below this threshold with natural therapies in many instances. For example, the breakdown of metabolic functions due to extreme nutrient deficiency can be remedied by supplying the nutrients if intake is the problem. But many other issues, such as the lack of communication in the body resulting from a spinal cord injury due to a vertebral fracture, simply require external intervention that is conventional medical or surgical in nature.

Biological plasticity depends on these factors such as inflammation, resolution, and tissue repair and remodeling (and it also requires nutritional inputs and a reserve supply of stem cells). They function successfully every moment of our lives. It is the rare times that they break down that get our attention as disease states. In many instances, we examine the causes and deficiencies in the determining factors of health, and when we address these disturbances, the system rights itself. Conversely, more tailored approaches are needed to support self-healing mechanisms, such as the use of nutritional, herbal, or structural therapies. In the case of the five conditions under which intrinsic healing is not likely to take place (vide supra), we can impact these to some degree. For instance, lack of biochemical substrates for proper healing functions can be corrected by improving nutritional status and providing those substrates if needed.

The fact that in situations where natural approaches, used in isolation, cannot *solely* be enough can still contribute to overall healing is one we will explore next.

The usefulness of natural approaches beyond this point of "natural therapy only" is one of a number of false dichotomies that currently beset medicine. Abandoning helpful measures simply because they cannot unilaterally repair lesions is an undermining practice. The medical model of seeing all diseases as a lesion or biochemical imbalance that works along one axis and that can be altered with one therapy is a model that precludes the understanding and management of whole systems. It is a good model for testing pharmaceutical therapies. As an organizing principle for primary care in general, it is very limited.

Importance of Naturopathic Approaches Even When Complete Cure Is Not Possible

Quality of life is one important reason why it makes sense for patients to use naturopathic medicine when cure or total symptom remission is not possible. Adequate function rather than optimal function is still a worthy goal. There can also be additive effects of naturopathic effects and allopathic effects—there can be a degree of synergy between the two modes of treatment (Fig. 3.12).

Another reality that makes co-treatment with naturopathic medicine helpful is the spreading effect of organ dysfunction—and the knock-on effects stemming from failure of an organ. Decline of one organ can put pressure on other organs as well. Minimizing that decline is important. Naturopathic therapies can support organs and improve quality of life.

Some degree of disease burden may impact the patient's ability to meet the requirements for their determinants of health. This can be due to pain interfering with good movement and exercise. Additionally, excessive stress and inflammation from a chronic infection can lead to poor appetite and poor digestion. Sometimes patients who take diuretics for blood pressure treatment self-limit their water intake, so that they do not have as many trips to the bathroom, which can be onerous for those with arthritis and poor balance. Often, it is the chronically ill that might be reliant on conventional medicine, but really need a naturopathic doctor to help them examine their biological essentials. Not only are they quite possibility deficient, but this kind of patient can least afford the consequences.

Reducing dependence on medications means that there is room to ascend in dose, lower risk of toxicity, and possibly less risk of drug-drug or drug-herb interactions. This is important, as all drugs have efficacy limits and tolerance limits. Even if a naturopathic approach cannot set the stage for complete healing, the improvements that result can allow for other treating physicians to prescribe less of a drug, simply because for the time being, less is needed to reach the therapeutic goals.

Psychologically, if a patient has the experience that doing proactive things results in an improvement in their level of functioning, it is a strong motivation to continue to make good choices. It also teaches them that their body has self-healing abilities. Doing nothing except managing the worsening symptoms may simply allow a degenerating condition to proceed into disorganization and dysfunction much faster.

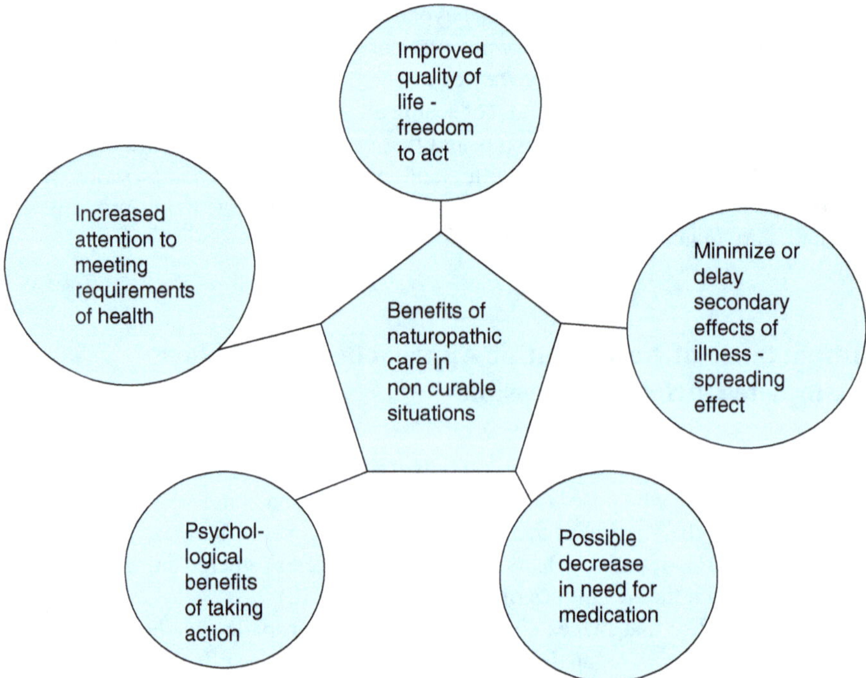

Fig. 3.12 Benefits of naturopathic treatment in noncurable situations: Better coping, improved response to other treatments, and improved quality of life can result from naturopathic care. The very act of taking steps to help oneself, even in the face of a situation that is chronic, can awaken some latent adaptive potential

If the patient has a chronic condition that is not completely curable, staying as healthy as possible may grant that patient time for newer allopathic therapies to come along.

The idea that improvement is not desirable just because a single drug (or nutrient, or herbal extract) has not been proven to completely ameliorate the patient's malady is a very benighted way of thinking. In naturopathic medicine, we attempt to help the patient do as much as possible with what they have to work with at the present time. That patient's situation, *their particular experience of disease, their idiosyncratic illness, and the benefits that they derive from proactive measures* are what is most relevant to that individual patient.

The Role of the Naturopathic Physician in Setting the Stage for Healing

The primary role of naturopathic medicine, beyond that very important task of helping patients stay in balance and falling into a disease state, is to maximize the homeostatic, pro-survival, and self-repair mechanisms.

Homeostatic refers to the ongoing, continuous, and self-regulating processes that keep our bodies functioning.

Pro-survival means the adaptive and stress-resisting responses that humans and all organisms exhibit. An example would be heat-shock proteins, or responses to oxidative stress.

Self-repair means the ability to call upon reserves of stem cells and to express developmental genes that create new tissue that is differentiated and suited to its intended purpose. An example would be restoration of the gastric mucosa after an ulceration, with intact tissue and a newly resilient mucous protection. A more functional (versus structural) example would be the adaptation of the heart and lungs to a lobectomy (where a lobe of the lung is removed). Perfusion of blood to high ventilations in this new configuration occurs, and the heart must adapt to the more difficult task of harvesting oxygen from the lungs.

The Model Used in This Book

The model of therapy used in this book takes the perspective that in order for healing to occur (Fig. 3.13), the body must be:

- Reasonably unencumbered (by nutritional deficiencies, toxins, overstimulating influences, and deficient biological essentials)
- Not held captive by maladaptive responses to degenerative processes and inflammation that simply perpetuate or intensify themselves (such as a cardiac muscle

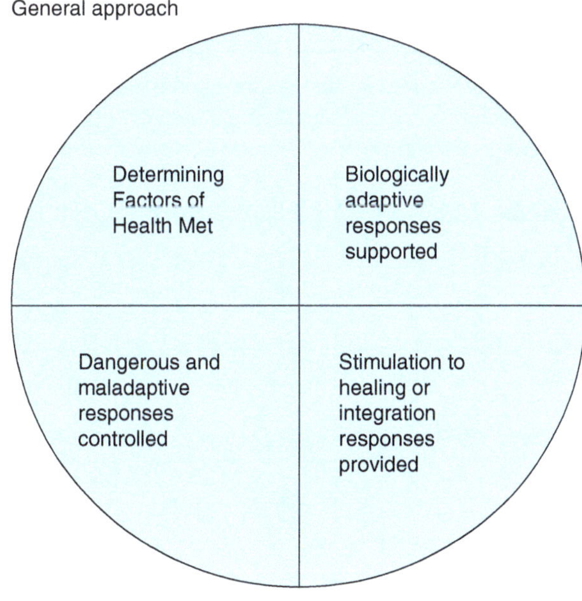

Fig. 3.13 The general approach in naturopathic medicine: Ensuring that patients meet requirements for health, that they receive stimulatory inputs for healing responses, that these responses are biochemically supported, and that dangerous or persistent maladaptive responses are lessened (those that do not disappear when other conditions are met) comprises the basis of the naturopathic approach

that has a blocked arterial inflow, or autoimmune flare-ups that create organ damage and yet more inflammation)

- Supported in its very critical adaptive responses, without which repair and a move toward integration and whole system harmony are not possible

There is also the acknowledgement that, sometimes, artificial means to establish homeostasis must be given. Providing insulin to a type 1 diabetic who no longer has insulin-secreting beta cells in their pancreas, or giving L-dopa to a patient who has lost most of their dopaminergic cells in the basal ganglia and has rigidity and tremor—Parkinson's disease—are examples of this.

Address Essential Biological Factors

These factors or "determinants of health" are going to have to be met, if healing is to occur. As has been well described by Zeff et al. [1], and others, such as Dr. Louise Edwards, one of the profession's foremost teachers in this area, it is not uncommon in naturopathic medicine to see patients revert back to a state of balance after finally addressing these disturbances [3]. They may have lived without the conditions for health being in place, and now that they are, their body can still execute its design plans so to speak, for health and wholeness.

Increase Adaptive Responses

All living things have adaptive responses to life. Change, stressors, growth, reproduction, and performance all make demands on the organism. All living things have various genetic factors that can be expressed to rise to the occasion.

Moreover, very complex beings, namely, humans, have adaptive responses that involve genes and proteins, but are cybernetic in nature. That is to say, various systems in the body influence each other, and there are multiple control systems.

There are three principal approaches to support these responses therapeutically (Fig. 3.14).

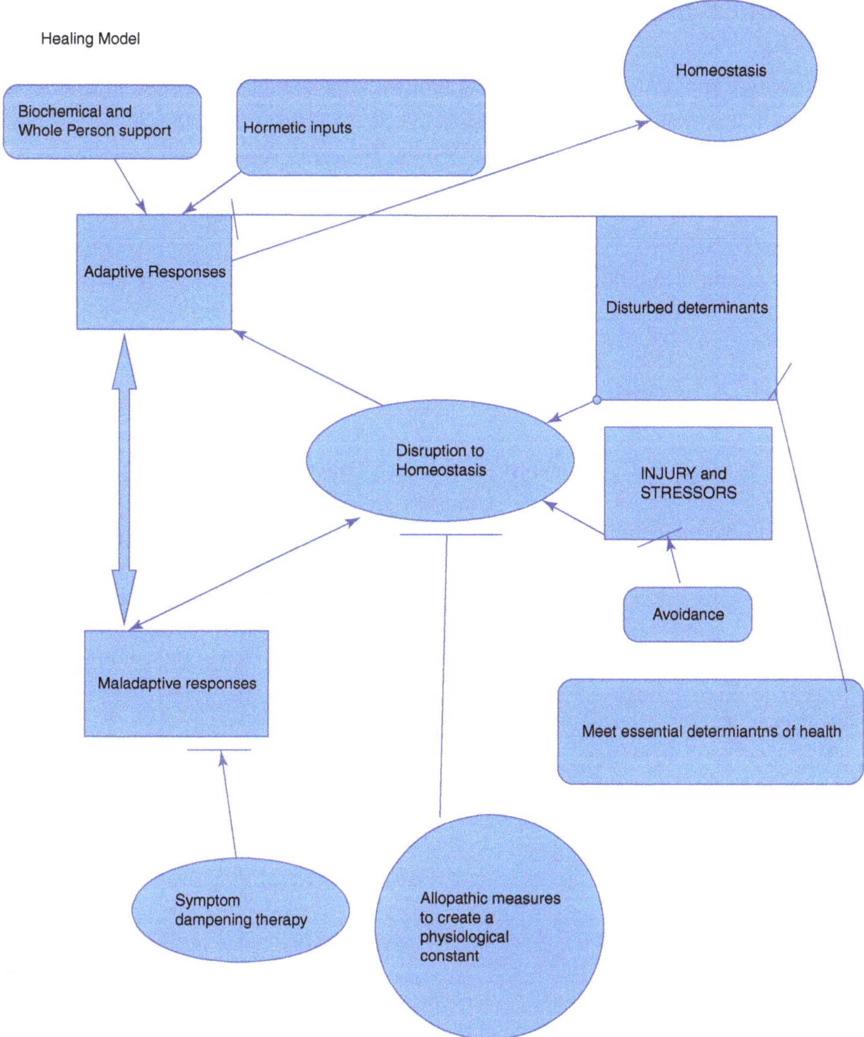

Fig. 3.14 Model of Healing: Homeostasis can be disrupted by a lack of the factors that are necessary requirements for health. It can also be disrupted by pathogens, trauma, genetic issues, and wear and tear effects of aging. The reestablishment of homeostasis must include ensuring that the requirements or "determining factors" of health are met. But it also needs to biochemically support and stimulate the adaptive responses of the body's cells and tissues

Biochemical Support

This involves providing molecules, as plant extracts, foods, or isolated nutrients, to support chemical/enzymatic processes. A simple example of biochemical support is to give additional alpha-lipoic acid and coenzyme Q10 to a patient who has mitochondrial dysfunction. Else, the support may be a gentle way of enhancing protective systems. When patients take silymarin, a group of flavonoids from *Silybum marianum* (milk thistle), their glutathione levels in liver (and other) cells rise. This might be an important boost to one of the body's major adaptations to stressors.

Hormetic Stimulation

Hormesis is from the Greek word "to excite." This concept as a pharmacological one has been studied for over 140 years. According to Edward Calabrese, hormesis is a modest stimulation in the low-dose zone [2, 4]. Often, this stimulation effect in the dose zone between zero dose and the dose we associated with a stronger drug effect (and where it is possible to have adverse effects) is opposite in nature to the high dose. For instance, alcohol sedates at larger doses, and at much smaller doses it can stimulate the CNS. Hormesis is a stimulatory effect that creates modest overcompensation responses. These include the expression of genes that code for enzymes that create antioxidant enzymes, heat-shock proteins, protein chaperones, and more. The forerunner to hormesis was the Ardnt Shultz principle that "low doses stimulate and large doses inhibit." In the twenty-first century, hormetic research is extensive. This type of low-dose stimulations elicit adaptive responses at basically no cost to the organism.

Whole Person Therapies

Naturopathic medicine has a number of therapies that work in a whole person manner, such as hydrotherapy. This is important because healing is a self-integration and rebalancing that our bodies can do. It can be blocked by lack of biological essentials, or stymied by overly exuberant inflammation and immune reactions. But healing is something we know how to do. Providing experiences and various therapies that encourage a healing response is important, even though it is more general. It is in fact the blanket nature of these therapies that makes them so valuable.

Decreasing Maladaptive Responses

It should be clear that a health-care approach that is mostly preoccupied with thwarting maladaptive resources, but neglects the biological essentials and does not tune up the adaptive responses, nor encourages healing, is incomplete. Merely decreasing maladaptive responses to an imbalance in the body cannot be counted on to lead to healing in many cases.

However, it can provide time, and resources, for the body to do what it can. An example would be a patient that had an extreme allergic reaction. It is so dangerous that they needed one infusion of intravenous prednisone, but once they broke down the escalation of the information, things began to return to normal. Another example would be someone who is in very good health, but encounters a strain of *Mycobacterium tuberculosis* that is simply very virulent. They get an infection, but treatment with antimicrobials causes so much attenuation of the Mycobacteria that their immune system does the rest, and they return to a rather robust state.

Both pharmaceutical drugs and some natural approaches can work *contra* maladaptive resources. What makes something maladaptive is when it is too prolonged, too forceful, and too costly and becomes a threat in its own way. Patients with heart failure will retain sodium as a result of renin release by the kidney which is in danger of shutting down due to poor perfusion. This is at first adaptive but becomes maladaptive when the renin and sympathetic nervous system responses no longer function in balance with other systems. The sodium retention, increase in blood osmolarity, and high blood pressure can cause fluid to leak into the alveolar spaces, waterlogging the lungs and suffocating the person.

Inducing Homeostasis

It is possible to create a homeostatic balance by extrinsic means. This might be necessary on a temporary basis, or a long-term one. The unique aspect of this therapy approach is that it goes beyond lowering dangerous compensations. It creates a balance and induces bioregulation, but only as far as it is possible through chemical manipulation. An example would be a patient with renal failure that has progressed to the point where many glomeruli are attenuated, and the extracellular matrix of the kidney has expanded. Filtration of blood is so decreased that the person will die due to toxin accumulation and electrolyte disturbance. This patient undergoes regular dialysis treatments, which temporarily puts the osmolarity and nitrogen levels of the blood back within a normal range. This might not be healing, but it creates the conditions for a level of health that would not be possible if an advanced pathology exerted its effects unhindered. This approach is more or less doing for the body what it cannot do for itself.

This stimulation can be hormetic, using low-dose stimuli to activate adaptation, or whole person, which includes these cell responses, but also the mind, immune system, and organ systems beyond that which is afflicted. Relieving or dampening maladaptive responses is often necessary as they can commandeer resources and keep the system in constant imbalance. Sometimes simply reducing these maladaptive responses brings about healing. In yet other situations, a tissue or organ is so damaged, or a pathogen so strong, that enforcing a state of temporary homeostasis through extrinsic means (surgery, drugs, dialysis, etc.) is necessary.

The level of dysfunction can indicate how initial emphasis might be placed on these different therapeutic approaches. Someone who is at risk of a number of compilations is probably going to receive some treatments that dampen maladaptive resources. But that does not mean that addressing the biological essentials and supporting adaptive resources are not done very early on in treatment.

Individuals differ in their physiological capacities, their mental and emotional state, and the various stressors and burdens on their body's regulation systems and tissues. For this reason, one sequence of treatments, or one golden proportion of each of these approaches, is not generalizable across all patients.

In the experience of naturopathic medicine, and as seen in many traditional medical systems, the starting point ought to include addressing biological essentials and then gentle, minimally disruptive treatments that support, stimulate, and help organize the inherent resources of the person.

References

1. Zeff J, Snider P, Myers S. Naturopathic model of healing-the process of healing revisited. Integr Med. 2019;18(4):26–30.
2. Calabrese EJ, Dhawan G, Kapoor R, Iavicoli I, Calabrese V. HORMESIS: a fundamental concept with widespread biological and biomedical applications. Gerontology. 2016;62(5):530–5.
3. Dr. Louise Edwards. Personal conversations. 2005–2021.
4. Calabrese EJ. Hormesis: path and progression to significance. Int J Mol Sci. 2018;19(10):2871.

Chapter 4
Causes of Ill Health

Naturopathic physicians make it a point to direct their efforts to treating the cause of the patient's problems. There are some preliminary thoughts about causes to consider. Causality of disease exists at different levels (Fig. 4.1). A proximate cause of disease is the more immediate, the easier to associate factors that led to an event. For example, a 38-year-old male patient needed to take large doses of prednisone in order to quell an autoimmune condition that would have destroyed his kidneys. The prednisone calmed the autoimmune flare-up and the kidney function tests and kidney imaging showed great improvement. But the patient had a compression fracture in his spinal vertebrae at L1. Radiographs reveal that the patient has osteopenia. It is ascribed to the prednisone, which can cause this. Another example would be a myocardial infarction in a patient that had coronary arterial plaques that were found, upon an angiogram the preceding year, to block 80% of the right coronary artery and circumflex artery. The atheromas were ascribed as the cause of a thrombus in those arteries (an atheroma had ruptured and a blood clot formed).

Causes that are removed in time can take much more investigation to attribute causality. For instance, the theory that high circulating LDL is a cause of atheromas is difficult to prove. It is certainly proven that high LDL is a major risk factor for atherosclerosis. It increases the probability that one will develop that disease. This is clinically actionable information. In a naturopathic model, we would also examine the mitigating factors in an LDL to atherosclerosis progression. For example, in patients with low oxidative stress in their arteries and whose blood sugar and insulin levels are normal throughout their life, a mildly elevated LDL is a true risk factor (being apparently healthy in this case is not the same as being truly healthy, in that "no obvious signs or symptoms" is not the same as "optimal nutritional status, no physiological perturbations, low inflammation level, etc.").

This raises the question of a third causal consideration, which are multifactorial causes. For example, a patient with age-related macular degeneration may have developed this because of borderline zinc status, poor plant food intake for many years including low serum levels of tocopherols and ascorbic acid, and a 20 packs/

F. Smith, *Naturopathic Medicine*, https://doi.org/10.1007/978-3-031-13388-6_4

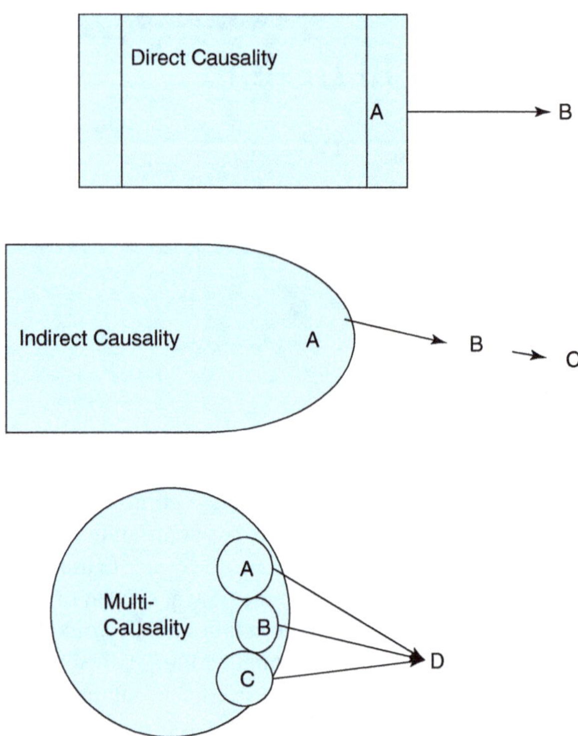

Fig. 4.1 Causality: The causes of an observable clinical state have direct, indirect, and sometimes multiple causes. Discerning what level of causality to direct efforts at treatment is an important question for all physicians

year history of smoking. In this case, there are several possible causes. Assuming that they also made this patient more vulnerable to degenerative retinal changes, these causes also interact with each other in some respects. For instance, cigarette smoking is such a drain on the body's antioxidant system that it depletes ascorbic acid and glutathione. Not eating many plant foods means that there are not a lot of polyphenolic molecules that can offset a low alpha tocopherol (vitamin E) status.

A clinical question is, if it is difficult to establish causality, is it a good use of time to attempt to eliminate the types of stressors and injurious agents discussed in this chapter? Perhaps they are not that relevant to what a patient is suffering from. The association between elevated LDL and atherosclerosis has been the subject of a massive amount of research, much of it done very well with large populations. If even that is on some level incomplete, should we worry about less clearly developed risk factors?

Part of the answer to this question lies in the fact that conditions that weaken the human body can work additively together. Attempting to limit and prevent these often injurious behaviors and environmental factors is prudent. Moving from the important concept of prevention to the management of patients who currently have a problem, the idea of causes takes on new meaning. If factors such as toxin exposure, lack of sleep, nutrient deficiency, etc., can lead to physiological disturbance, when we are confronted with a patient who has disturbed function, inflammation, or degeneration of some aspect of their body, it becomes even more important to reduce these damaging factors (Fig. 4.2). In some cases, these actions will improve quality of life and the patient may feel that they have more resources to summon to work toward recovery. In other cases, their symptoms will abate to some extent because the disturbing environmental or behavioral factor was generating the physiological imbalance that was behind the illness. In other cases, no immediate discernable change happens when addressing these factors, but doing so appears to help more specific interventions (biochemical support, hormetic stimulation, symptom-directed treatment, etc.) to actually work. Since in naturopathic medicine, we are trying to support and stimulate various whole systems to come back into balance and proper function, simply permitting dysregulating influences to persist runs counter to an efficient and effective approach. The notion of a very direct and linear causality has its place, especially in the actual science of diagnosis. But in working with patients to be able to exit a repetitive physiological loop that is dysfunctional and leading to symptoms, or degenerative and increases risk of mortality, we must go beyond linear causality and provide the body's systems of regulation with operating conditions that are conducive to balance and good function. This means the best function for a specific person, at a specific moment in time, such as they are, and not only creating conditions that are probabilistically health generative across a large population.

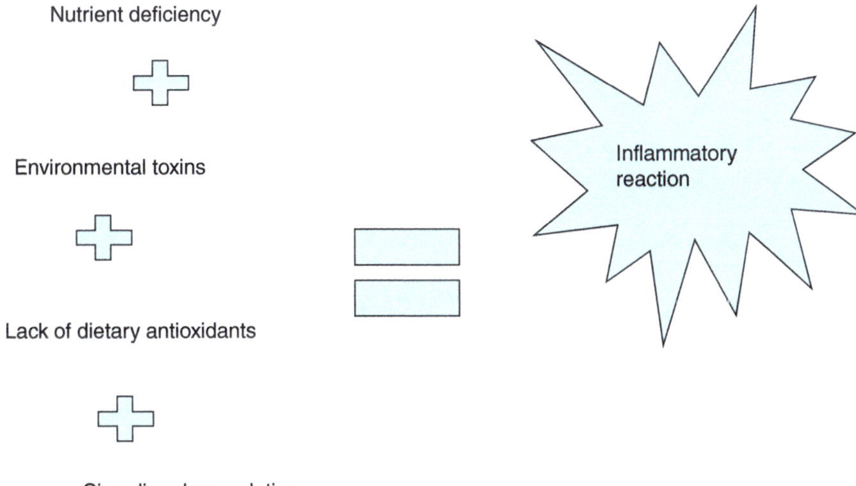

Fig. 4.2 Inflammation: Although there are various molecular pathways that can be described in the inflammatory process, various factors, aside from microbial infection, can trigger it. Often, several of these factors are present at the same time, lowering the threshold for activation of inflammation

Circadian Dysregulation

Humans have a sleep-wake cycle, which is set by so-called zeitgebers or time-givers. These include sunlight of course, as well as mealtimes, work schedule, and exercise. They program the suprachiasmatic nucleus (SCN), which is found in the hypothalamus [1]. This is supplemented by and synchronizes various peripheral clocks in the organs that are themselves directly influenced by activity, feeding, and temperature. Even cells appear to have their own oscillating clock, which is enhanced by the presence of the extracellular matrix and its fibroblasts (Fig. 4.3).

The circadian rhythm is on a 24-h clock (slightly longer in fact, at about 24.18 h). The functions that are chronologically synchronized with this cycle go far beyond sleep-wake cycles. Circadian rhythms are also connected with:

- Hunger and the drive to find food
- Neuroendocrine hormonal release
- Metabolic processes and body temperature
- Autonomic control of blood pressure

Decreased rhythmicity of the circadian rhythms has been found to be a risk factor or Parkinson's disease, in a 2020 analysis of 3135 males [2]. Although Alzheimer's disease and other dementia conditions have been associated with sleep disturbance

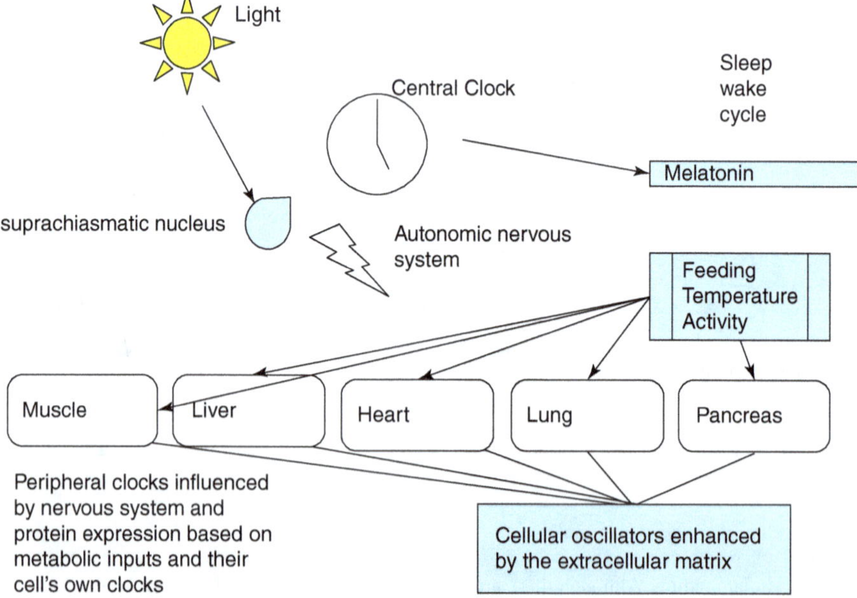

Fig. 4.3 Circadian clocks: A central clock in the suprachiasmatic nucleus, which is chronologically set by light exposure. Peripheral clocks, which synchronize with the central clock, also have their own "zeitgebers" or time-givers, such as feeding and activity. Even cells have oscillations that follow a 24-h cycle—this seems to be reinforced by the presence of the extracellular matrix

for many years, newer evidence demonstrates an increased risk of developing Alzheimer's disease in individuals with a chronic sleep disturbance [3].

Metabolic syndrome is characterized by hypertension, dyslipidemia, and obesity. Circadian disruption, that is, interruptions to the establishment of consistently programmed circadian rhythms, increases the risk of diabetes (NIDDM), cardiovascular disease, hypertension, sleep apnea, nonalcoholic fatty liver disease, and dyslipidemia [4].

Disrupted circadian clocks have been shown to be an inducer of certain cancer cell behaviors, such as angiogenesis and mitosis. While the sole or main cause of cancer, circadian disruption, and lack of synchrony seems to increase the risk of cancer promotion and progression [5].

These examples underlie that one bioregulatory system, which happens to be connected with a very prevalent disturbed determining factor of health (or essential biological requirement), can be an initiator or promoter of dysfunction and eventually observable pathologies in a number of different systems of the body.

Lack of Social Engagement and Loneliness

Human beings need each other, and although personal relationships can require effort and growth and at times are fraught, most people wither in their absence. Social isolation in some studies has increased the 5-year mortality by 50%. This might be due to poor eating habits, negative mindset, reluctance to get medical screening tests, etc. But it does seem that the human need for others must be met, or the mind and body will decline. Our society has issues with social isolation. The geography of living conditions for many people is very spread out, with the automobile being the only way to physically get in contact with others. Civic engagement and participation have declined, and membership in clubs and mutual interest organizations is not what it once was. Social media connects people in a way and can at least be a way to communicate. But much social media activity lacks authenticity and a real sense of connection. Hence, those who turn to social media for companionship find that they must post and reply frequently to remain relevant and part of the conversation or attention-grabbing object of the moment. Those who have proximity to family, who spend time with family, who have close friends (and friend head count is less important than quality and the attributes of honesty, true concern for friends, positive interactions, etc.), and who engage in civic or places of worship activities have a network of social support.

A 2018 review by Zia and Li [6] noted that chronic social isolation has been shown to increase the risks of morbidity and mortality similar to known factors, including high blood pressure, smoking, and obesity [7]. A 2016 systematic review and meta-analysis involving data from 16 longitudinal datasets, for a total of 4628 CHD and 3002 stroke events, showed the deficiencies in social relationship were associated with cardiovascular disease. The mechanisms are not clear. Immune function decreases and blood pressure rises in these lonely conditions. Behaviors that are higher risk may increase. It is generally noted that without the requirement for social engagement properly met, one is more likely to be unhealthy.

Screen Time

In a very technologically connected world, people spend more time looking into a computer screen than ever before. This can be a work-related screen, or the use of smartphones, computers, and tablets for personal entertainment, communication, and social media exploration. This activity has been associated with increased risk of depression, especially in adolescents and children. These cohorts are not only more likely to spend their socializing (or potential socializing) time there, but they may lack the psychological defenses an adult may have to insulate themselves against, or to avoid negative interactions, bullying, and the sheer power of suggestion that thousands of images and video clips can transmit. The problem with excessive screen time is that it displaces other forms of human interaction, or time that could be spent in more solitary but constructive pursuits, as simply as riding a bike or doing a hobby. According to the American Academy of Child and Adolescent Psychiatry, children aged 8–12 years spend an average of 4–6 h a day on screened devices and adolescents, up to 9 [8]. Not all of this time is negative, and some of it certainly replaces broadcast television or recorded movies. But this is a large amount (25% or 33% of one's day) spent in feeds and interactions that are rapidly cycling, non-authentic, manipulative, orchestrated by companies that acquire personal data for sale, and sometimes threatening.

Deficiencies of Exercise and Movement

Humans are meant to move. While it is possible to live with little movement, and the types of movement available to those with certain physical limitations can be of a smaller range, in general, the human organism responds to movement and exercise (Fig. 4.4). The benefits of exercise are well documented. The cardiovascular system gets stronger. Vascular networks enlarge. The brain responds favorably to the sensory input and increased blood flow of exercise. Bone density can improve. Overall stress levels can decrease. Movement in general keeps the myofascial system from becoming tight and restrictive. It helps the lymph system pump. Exercise also can induce protective responses such as the expression of genes to make sirtuins.

One-third of the global population aged 15 years and older engages in insufficient physical activities, which affects health [9]. The lack of exercise and movement has detrimental effects. High levels of cognitive activity and no movement can increase stress. If sleep duration or quality is low because of literally sitting all day,

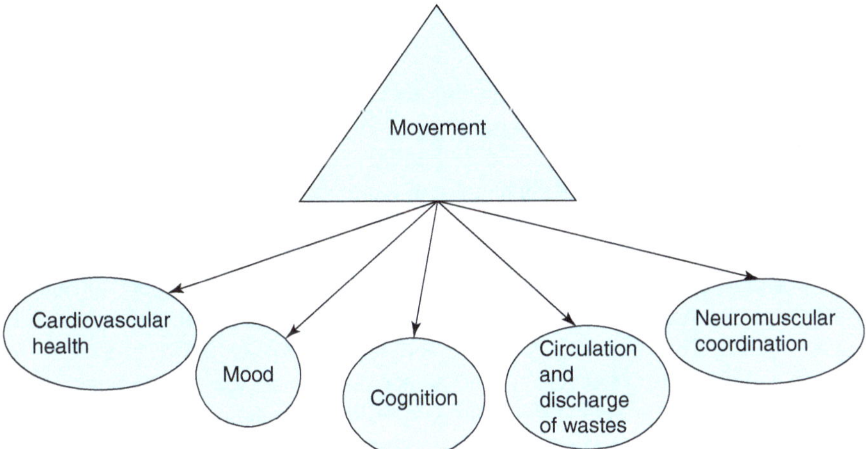

Fig. 4.4 Exercise benefits: The effects of movement and exercise are far ranging and go beyond strength, but as examples, nervous, cardiovascular, and metabolic systems all respond to and are dependent on movement and exercise. It is a determining factor of health

leptin levels will decrease and the person may want to eat more. If the diet is higher carbohydrate, glycemic levels can rise. And depending on the sedentary person's caloric intake, there may be in an imbalance with regards to energy, which can lead to obesity.

Children need movement, and a lack of it can be a threat to children and adolescent's health. Body mass index, motor coordination, and mental health are all adversely affected by a sedentary way of living. Clinical studies about pediatric nonalcoholic fatty liver disease indicate that 10% of children have it. According to the CDC, about 1 in 2 adults do not get enough aerobic physical activity, and the figure for high school students is worse, at 77% [10]. With 20% of the US adolescent population now considered prediabetic, which has strong dietary causes as well, this is another underscoring of the need to move. Many excellent public health initiatives have worked to turn this tide. The social isolation of 2020–2021 did not help matters.

The WHO guidelines for physical activity stress that some physical activity is better than none [11]. The correlations between lack of exercise and various disease outcomes are still being established. Obesity has much evidence of a correlation, and many cancers do not have as strong a correlation. The amount of minutes of aerobic activity needed to avoid disease is a topic of debate.

This clinical epidemiology is of course interesting to naturopathic physicians. But what is more relevant is that a lack of movement and exercise creates a deviation from normal function. This disordered function may be directly causal of later occurring diseases, or indirectly. But to starve oneself of movement is to allow the body to drift into a state that it is not optimized for.

Electromagnetic Fields

Humans are exposed to electromagnetic fields (EMFs) far more than in the past. Electricity creates EMFs, and of course electricity, with all of its benefits, is everywhere. Additionally, there are about 270 million mobile phone users in the United States, who have a strong EMF generator at their side or their head for much of the day. The research into how any of these EMF might cause cancer or neurodegenerative disease is unclear. What we have to consider is the cumulative effect and length of exposure to these forces. One clue to this is that those with ongoing substantial EMF exposure increases oxidative stress (Fig. 4.5). This is well demonstrated in rodents and neurons in vitro. This is yet another source of oxidative stress that can sap the body's redox systems [12]. Researchers have found that real damage occurs if the body's redox systems (which are controlled by genetic expression, endogenous antioxidants, immune reactions, dietary components) are disturbed over a long period of time, either *permanently or repeatedly*. In the case of repeated disturbances, brain repair and brain cell differentiation and development can be impacted. Likewise, oxidative stress, while an important signal in the immune system, can damage that system if it is excessive or induced in an artificial way for too long.

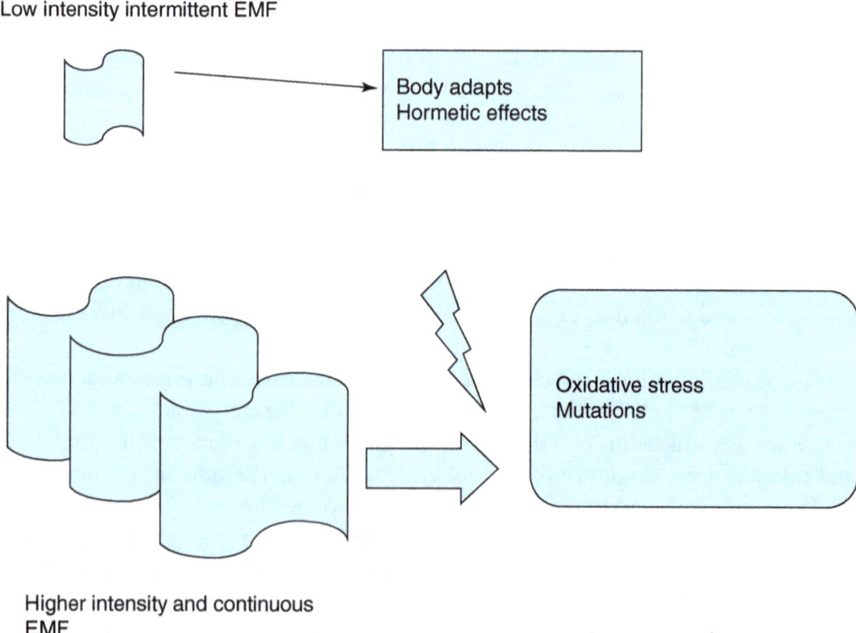

Fig. 4.5 Electromagnetic fields: EMF can be tolerated at lower doses and shorter exposures, but as the total load and cumulative effect hits a certain threshold, damaging oxidative stress is generated

Societal and Economic Forces

It is increasingly recognized that disparities in health care can be frequent and significant [13]. These disparities, from even a cursory read of data at the website of the CDC, often break down across races. They can also be across income strata and, of course, gender. LGBTQ persons, including adolescents, suffer from health disparities [14].

People move through their life starting from their earlier influences and circumstances. Opportunities, influences, and obstacles, in some way, form the person (including their growth as they take the opportunities or overcome the obstacles). But these external factors also change a person's trajectory. And while a person might adapt to them, they can also frustrate that person's efforts to improve their own life. So it is that in the United States, millions of people, African-American, Indigenous, and others, begin their life with legacy and transgenerational effects of racism. The effects of trauma, or cumulative effects of socioeconomic disadvantages, work against them. This is to not say that all of these very real factors are so deterministic that a person's health cannot be good because of their racial heritage or identity. But if we practice a system of medicine that addresses disturbances to the determining factors of health, then the facts and current situation for many: lack of access to health care, lack of equal treatment in some health-care settings, lack of access to healthy food, patterns of eating and living that replaced over generations what was in fact traditions with many wise healing practices, and the effects of violence and trauma.

Health statistics are useful to help point out what the facts are. It is important to also apply the principle of finding the cause [15]. Diabetes might be more common in some populations, but that does not mean that it is deterministically so, or that it is by choice. Public health education measures addressed to a certain city, community, or even neighborhood might fail to have an impact, but that does not mean that there is no need for them. Perhaps such a program in healthy eating, or breastfeeding, or cooking, is simply written for someone else, and the people who could most benefit should be given the opportunity to help create it. Health literacy improvements are needed as much as merely providing more information [16].

General Nutrition

Nutrient Deficiencies

Lack of a truly required nutrient can have multiple effects on health. This ranges from failure of a metabolic pathway to stress on other pathways and multiple tissues due to the allostatic load on those systems that occurs when a biochemical pathway is partially blocked. The following nutrients serve as examples:

Vitamin A

Vitamin A deficiency can manifest in inadequate diets, but also for those who suffer from malabsorption. This fat-soluble vitamin will not find its way into the lymphatics if fats cannot be absorbed. All *trans* retinal (Fig. 4.6) is converted into retinaldehyde and retinoic acid (RA), which can exist as all-*trans* or several *cis* isomers. In addition to its well-known function in the visual cycle, vitamin A controls a wide array of gene expression. Deficiency is far more common in the developing world. According to Timoneda et al., vitamin A deficiency has been associated with histopathological changes in the pulmonary epithelial lining and lung parenchyma which lead to disruption of the normal lung physiology and predispose to severe tissue dysfunction and respiratory diseases [17]. This impacts the extracellular matrix (ECM) and basement membrane (BM) protein content and distribution. As we have seen, ECM degradation has a major effect on disease development. About a third of US adults get less than the recommended daily allowance of vitamin A. Groups at risk include young females, African-Americans, smokers, people with pancreatic insufficiency due to cystic fibrosis or other causes due to fat malabsorption, and those with fat malabsorption due to gastrointestinal illness [18].

Vitamin A is used to help "home" T and B cells to travel to the gut. Moreover, vitamin A is used to differentiate IgA antibody in the gut-associated mucosal tissue. Vitamin A has an overall immune-supporting effect and an antiatherogenic effects.

We can expect those with poor vitamin A status to be less immune competent. It is also likely that due to difficulties with epithelial function and particularly with impairment of defenses in the gut, higher inflammation and antigen penetration in the gut are likely. This can potentially exacerbate inflammation, allergy, and some autoimmune conditions.

Vitamin D

Vitamin D is a fat-soluble vitamin derived from the diet and from the action of ultraviolet light (from sunlight) on vitamin D precursor ergosterols in the skin. It is really a hormone, but one that requires an extrinsic input (sunlight) or dietary supply. There are receptors for vitamin D throughout the body, and it is important for growth, regulation of epithelial surfaces, inflammation, immune function, and

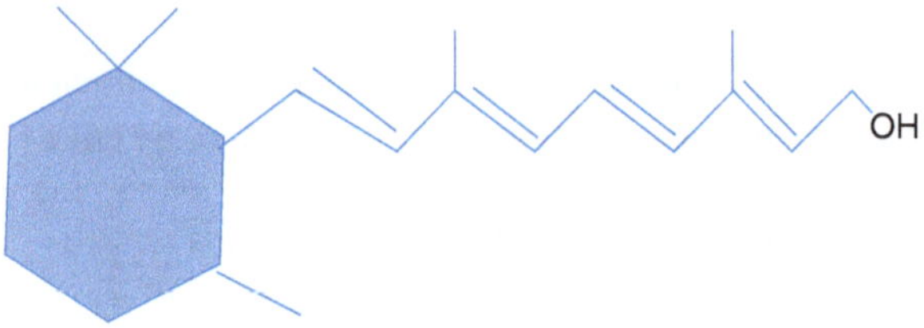

Fig. 4.6 All trans retinol: A common form of vitamin A

OH

nervous system function. People with poor sun exposure and with fat malabsorption (or simply poor vitamin D intake) are at risk. Vitamin D deficiency is characterized as serum levels of <20 ng/mL and vitamin D insufficiency as <20–30 ng/mL. This is the case for almost one billion people worldwide, many of them in North America [19].

The line between low status and some inevitable pathology is not always clear (beyond the classic extreme deficiency picture of osteomalacia and rickets). The evidence that poor vitamin D status *exacerbates* numerous problems in the body is very strong. Inflammatory conditions can be more intense [20], bone density lowers, and cancer risk increases. Moreover, the individual requirement for vitamin D can be increased due to certain genetic polymorphisms that render someone in need of much more vitamin D than the contemporary typical diet or sun-sheltered lifestyle might provide.

Vitamin E

Vitamin E, alpha tocopherol, is a key antioxidant in the body. It protects lipids from oxidation, particularly the propagating reactions that happen in clusters of fatty acids. Foods such as wheat germ or natural, unprocessed oils contain vitamin E. It is present in nature to protect the fats. We need it to protect our nervous system, and in general it is part of a system that regenerates the major antioxidant glutathione [21]. What should be a source of vitamin E—fats—is often low in it. The rather extensive processing of edible oils in contemporary diets will simply strip tocopherols (and polyphenols—a separate but also powerful antioxidant class of molecules). Moreover, the presumption of seed oils such as canola, soy, cottonseed, sunflower, etc. puts stress on the body. But the lack of accompanying antioxidants with those oils creates an even bigger burden of fatty acids that are potentially oxidized. It is analogous to the consumption of refined grains and sugars that do not come with their own supply of B complex vitamins as they would in nature.

Vitamin C

Some people have actual vitamin C deficiency because they do not consume enough foods that are rich in it [22]. This includes citrus, potatoes, bell pepper, and berries. There is a basic level of vitamin C that is necessary for the body to function properly, particularly in the sense of making the protein collagen. Vitamin C (ascorbic acid) is important in the hydroxylation of the amino acid proline, which is part of collagen's fiber-based structure. When this hydroxylation is lacking, the fibers can unravel, much like a worn shoelace. This wreaks havoc on blood vessels, skin, and gum tissue, as well as the gut. But there are many more functions of ascorbic acid in the body (Fig. 4.7). It is integral to the recharging of one of our primary

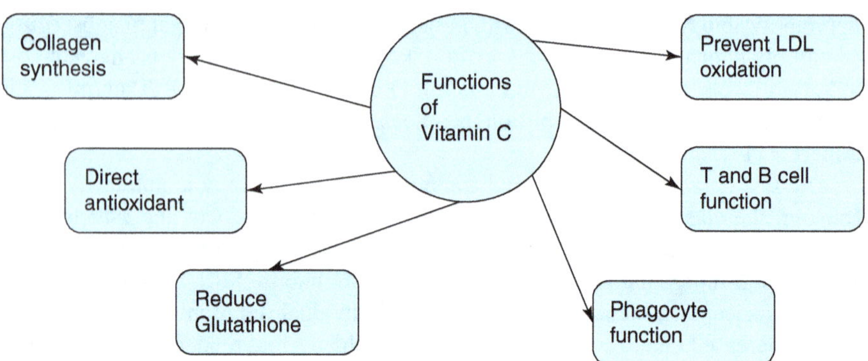

Fig. 4.7 Some functions of vitamin C: Ascorbic acid has multiple roles in the body, supporting structure, immune function, and antioxidant systems

antioxidant systems—glutathione. When this major antioxidant is spent absorbing some reactive oxygen-containing compound, it can be "deoxidized" or reduced, by an enzyme known as glutathione reductase. Vitamin C (and E) and the mineral selenium are needed for that chemical reaction.

Ascorbic acid also shows up in the thyroid, to make thyroid hormone, and in the adrenal gland medulla, to make epinephrine. Ascorbic acid is a free-floating, water-soluble antioxidant that can act as a free radical trap in the cytosol and in the plasma of our circulatory system. It is also important to keep our extracellular matrix from aging too quickly due to oxidation. Vitamin C is important for our immune function, as it is found in phagocytic cells [23]. It can support primary white blood cell defensive functions such as chemotaxis (moving to an area of bacterial invasion), phagocytosis (engulfing bacteria), and generation of reactive oxygen species (which destroy bacteria). Vitamin C is also important in sweeping away cellular debris which accumulates during inflammation. Vitamin C might support proliferation of B and T cells, and deficiency of C can impair our immune function. Infection and inflammation not only require C, but also use it up, underscoring the need for increased amounts of this vitamin when the body is under attack.

Mineral: Selenium

Selenium is a required cofactor in many enzymes, including many aspects of the immune system. Selenoproteins are crucial there, and there are about 25 types that connect with immune function. Needs for selenium vary between individuals [24]. In deficiency there is more risk of overly exuberant inflammatory responses, chronic infection, and succumbing to diseases that are fought off by a fully operational cell-mediated immune response (infections by *Mycobacterium tuberculosis* are an example). T cell proliferation and natural killer cell activity are enhanced when selenium status is optimal. Too much selenium can lead to alopecia, dermatitis, and even an increased risk of some cancer.

Dietary: Excessive Sugars and Carbohydrates

In our culture of food preoccupation (and food overconsumption), it is not that helpful to single out one macronutrient as harmful. But in the case of sugars and very refined carbohydrate, the excesses in the contemporary diet ensure that carbohydrates have to be considered as a problem area. In lesser amounts, they are simply a good source of energy that are already precursors of the glucose that the human brain and heart like to feed on. The United States has the highest per capita daily consumption of sugar in the world, at 126.40 g/day [25]. While the average American in 1915 consumed about 17.5 lb of sugar per year, that has grown to 150 lb/year by 2011. Even allowing for inaccuracy with the 1915 survey data, there has been a substantial increase (Fig. 4.8). A connection between sugary drinks and all-cause mortality has been established. A far amount of time has been spent attempting to prove that table sugar (sucrose) or high-fructose corn syrup causes or does not cause non-insulin-dependent diabetes mellitus. This makes for an interesting scientific debate. What is more relevant is to examine what the metabolic state is for someone who consumes 150 lb of sugar annually and also eats a fair amount of very refined grains. What happens to the insulin-glucagon system, and what happens to the levels of inflammation in the body? The fact that this behavior may or may not "give" someone type 2 diabetes is less consequential than the fact that this massive sugar intake will undermine health. In a dysregulated, inflamed, and nutrient-depleted state, this creates a ground out of which many pathological situations are more likely to arise.

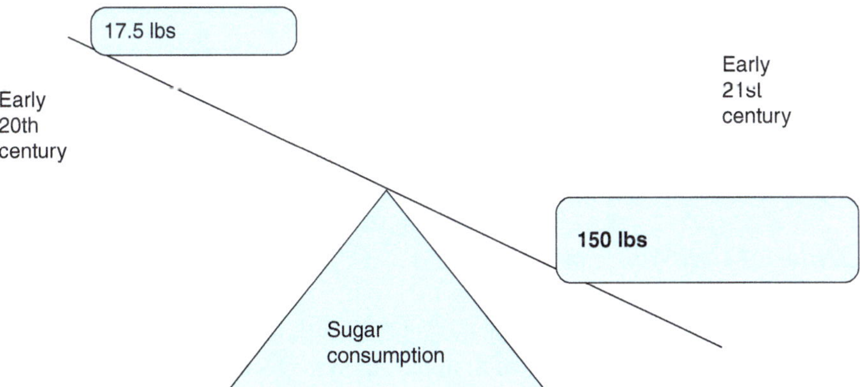

Fig. 4.8 Sugar consumption in the United States: Sugar consumption has increased dramatically in the last century

In excessive sugar intake, there are changes to brain chemistry which lead to short-term dopamine releases as a reward response. Over time, this becomes a tolerance-dependent phenomena, with larger and more frequent amounts of sugars needed to avert a downturn in mood and pleasure. Extreme sugar intake causes sustained insulin release, which not only can exhaust the pancreas endocrine function after years of overstimulation, but will also increase the risk of insulin resistance. Some people avert insulin resistance by offsetting sugar intake with high nutrient-dense foods also consumed, supplementation, intense exercise, and lucky genetics (a normally high-functioning GLUT4 receptor). But many more will eventually develop peripheral insulin resistance. This is a hallmark of the metabolic syndrome, which has the concomitants of hypertension and hyperlipidemia. These factors are major risks for cardiovascular disease, cancer, and progression to diabetes mellitus.

Sugar in excess can disrupt the gut microbiome, for although much of the sugar is absorbed, some is not, and this causes excess fermentation and a shift in species of gut microorganisms. It is in the opposite direction of foods such as high-fiber complex carbohydrates and vegetables that provide a fermentation substrate that creates butyrate and other short-chain fatty acids. These are tonic to the intestine. The impact of disturbing the microbiota on the brain is an area of investigation. But it is clear that the gut influences the brain via the vagus nerve and the immune system, as well as neuroactive compounds that are produced locally in the gut and find their way to the circulation and eventually the brain.

The liver is a major target for excessive sugar. When that much carbohydrate is consumed, it cannot possibly be burned off. Much of it will become stored as triglyceride. The acetate units formed by processing monosaccharides will be used to create free fatty acids, which themselves will be attached to a glycerol backbone and then stored. The liver will absorb much of this, and nonalcoholic fatty liver disease (NAFLD) has become far more common. NAFLD has overtaken alcohol fatty liver disease as the main cause of this phenomena. The liver will turn bright yellow as it becomes saturated with triglyceride. Some patients will develop inflammation, and in some (fortunately not all) the inflammation will progress to be a form of serious hepatitis. A few will even progress to cirrhosis. The presence of fatty acids in the storage form of triglycerides in other body compartments, including intra-abdominal fat, has its own risks, as this is associated with increased mortality.

Microbiome

Bacterial Cell Wall Components

Lipopolysaccharide (LPS) is a toxin found in the cell walls of gram-negative bacteria. Some LPS can be translocated from the gut to the bloodstream. LPS can enter along with fats and chylomicrons, or through defects in the cell junctions of the intestine. Normally, they are removed by the Kupffer cells (phagocytes) of the liver.

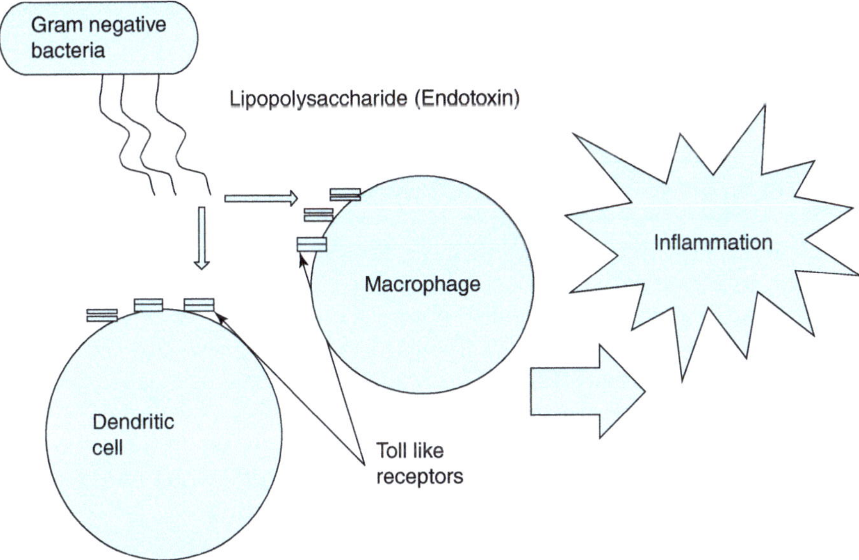

Fig. 4.9 Lipopolysaccharide and inflammation: LPS can enter the bloodstream from the gut or from foci of infection in the body. It is picked up by specialized receptors and is a strong activator of the inflammatory responses, including innate defenses such as complement

Those that get into the general circulation can provoke systemic inflammation and can increase the inflammatory response to any other cause (Fig. 4.9). Interestingly, LPS can bind to the spike protein of SARS CoV-2 [26]. LPS has been linked to obesity and metabolic syndrome [27]. The risk factors that make someone more susceptible to LPS are chronic gut inflammation, excessive fats in the diet (which are not a sole cause), and disruptions to the normal microbiota of the gut leading to more gram-negative bacteria and fewer productive species.

Persistent Biofilms

Bacteria can create a home for themselves, where they can attach to a surface, spawn more bacteria, and even communicate with each other. This proteoglycan matrix is called a biofilm [28]. A typical place for this to happen is in the lining of the bladder, which leads to bacteria resisting the antibiotic treatments for recurring bladder infections. A biofilm that most people are familiar with is that of plaque on the teeth. Plaque is formed by bacteria in the mouth, and while regular brushing and flossing can keep it in check, having it literally scraped off by a dental hygienist is eventually necessary (and it will be worse for those who consume a lot of sugar or do not have good oral hygiene). Just as our own cells need an extracellular matrix to survive, many bacteria oxidized fatty acids.

Mind and Body

Disharmonies

Physicians and healers in most, if not all, of the world's traditional medical systems have recognized the connection between mind and body. Systems such as Traditional Chinese Medicine see mind and body as perhaps distinct but inseparable. Traditional systems seem to come back to the idea that a disturbance in the mind or soul eventually finds its way to the body. These systems also consider the connection between the individual and the family and their immediate community—with healing ceremonies that have group involvement. There is more of an emphasis on establishing harmony between the individual and their family, community and nature, and less preoccupation with exercising power over disease.

In our own way, in twenty-first century health care, we are coming around to truly recognizing this once again. Observational studies that look at stress or trauma and their effects on health outcomes make it clear that these things are connected [29]. At the physiological and cellular level, the nature of these connections are being more understood [30]. For example, a state of trauma and fear can compromise the immune system. The effects of chronic stress include increased risk of cancer [31] and cardiovascular disease [32].

In addition to the direct effects of prolonged depression of mood, inner conflicts, unresolved suffering, etc., there are behavioral implications. One impact of note is that in a highly stressed or disturbed state, people tend to see fewer options. Their mental field of vision becomes like tunnel vision. This is important in illness, as at precisely the moment when someone ought to realize that they can access hitherto unused resources for healing in themselves and to seek out help beyond their typical health-care regimen, they may be struck with a sense of helpfulness that leads to inaction. Furthermore, in prolonged negative states of mind (with high levels of anger, guilt, resentment, fear, etc.), many people turn to self-destructive behaviors such as compulsive eating, drinking, drug use, and revenge behaviors such as self-abuse or staying up extremely late every night to retreat into alcohol, television, unfulfilling sexual encounters, etc. Revenge in this case is a type of anger directed at self but it can certainly affect those around them at home and in the community and those for whom they work.

Toxins

A toxin is something that disrupts homeostasis, damages tissues, or disrupts normal cellular and biochemical activity. A substance can be toxic at a certain threshold and tolerable below that threshold. There are a few toxins which have a threshold that is so low that they are considered toxic in any amount. Some toxic substances can damage our DNA, thus creating mutations of the kind that can lead to cancer.

Toxins fall into categories such as:

- Pesticides (can impact the human nervous system)
- Herbicides (can be carcinogenic)
- Mycotoxins (fungus-produced toxins)
- Industrial solvents (not naturally occurring but used in many ways)
- Heavy metals
- Halogens
- Dichlorophenols
- Cigarette-borne toxins
- Adulterants of and direct effects of drugs of abuse
- Alcohol (a threshold effect and an addiction effect)
- Pharmaceutical drugs
- Dietary supplements
- Damaged fatty acids
- Burnt food
- Endocrine disruptors
- Internal at mucous membranes
- Biofilms
- Protein putrefactive products
- Microbial imbalances

Pesticides

Pesticides are everywhere. They are used to protect crops from insects, and they are sprayed widely in homes and businesses. Hotels, warehouses, restaurants, and hospitals are heavy sprayers of pesticides.

These compounds kill insects usually through some mechanism that destroys nerve tissues [33]. Some may also destroy cell architecture or mitochondrial function [34].

Herbicides

Although these were designed to increase crop yields, their ubiquitous presence in the food system presents health risks [35]. Glyphosate is a very commonly used weed killer. Crops are designed to resist it, so that they do not succumb to its toxic effects. That allows farmers to use more glyphosate. It has been linked to insulin dysregulation, infertility, immune system dysfunction, gut inflammation, and cancer. American diets have several times more glyphosate than European ones. There is a small amount of it in European diets due to the use of some US corn and soy for animal feed in Europe.

Mycotoxins (Fungus-Produced Toxins)

Mycotoxins are produced by fungi. Low levels of these from normal ecological processes, such as the degradation of leaves in a backyard, or rotting of a log in a nearby wooded area, do not pose a problem for most people. But when these toxins accumulate in a home or public space, especially one that people spend prolonged time in, then they can result in serious morbidity. The opportunities for fungal growth are the conditions one would expect: moisture, lack of sunlight, and some kind of material that acts as a substrate for fungal digestion. They can be carcinogenic, harmful to the nervous system, alter the microbiome, and suppress the immune system [36, 37]. Poisoning is more dangerous in conditions such as vitamin deficiency, low-calorie intake, alcohol abuse, or the presence of an infectious disease (Omotayo). Aflatoxins are some of the better known and can be hepatotoxic and carcinogenic. There are many other types, such as fumonisins and trichothecenes, which are immunosuppressive. Infections of the lung and brain in patients with compromised immune systems by Aspergillus species is well known. What is striking about the toxins produced by fungi is that exposure is widely spread, and this presents another burden on the detoxification systems, as well as direct health impacts depending on the length and intensity of exposure.

Damaged Polyunsaturated Fatty Acids

Heating dietary oils creates toxic substances. This is of importance because of the large amount of frying that occurs in many modern diets. Vegetable oils are added to many foods, which then go on to be cooked. The oversimplification of the nature of fatty acid requirements and metabolism has overemphasized the downsides of saturated fats and often ignores the problems with polyunsaturated fats [38]. In the oil of a deep fryer, or a pan, the action of heat at first hydrolysis triglycerides, freeing the fatty acids from glycerol. As the heat continues and in the presence of oxygen, initial free radicals are formed (Fig. 4.10). First, peroxyl radicals are formed, and these then further propage the free radical reaction, forming hydroperoxyls [39]. Over time, polymerized molecules form, as oxidation runs its course. These products, when consumed in the diet, can induce more oxidative stress and cause increases in inflammation. They may be carcinogenic. They are damaging to the arteries. Antioxidants in the diet can offset this damage. There are antioxidants in oils—tocopherols and polyphenols (in the case of virgin olive oil)—but these are usually consumed in the early stages of oil heating. When large quantities of these heat-damaged oils are consumed, as in the North American diet and many other diets globally, this adds a toxic burden to the person eating it.

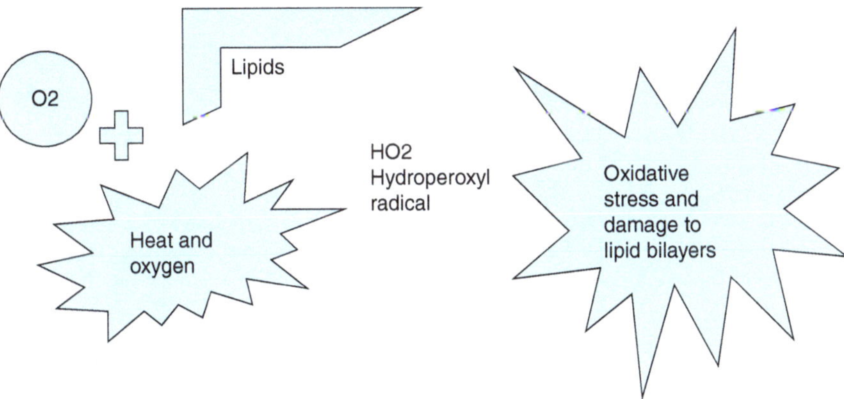

Fig. 4.10 Formation of hydroperoxyl radical (HO_2): During heating of food oils, oxygen and heat create a number of reactive oxygen species including the HO_2 radical. These free radical reactions easily propagate

Heavy Metals

Arsenic

Arsenic is found in soil, water, and various foods that humans consume. It is number 33 on the periodic table. It is found throughout the earth's crust, sometimes in combination with other minerals such as sulfur and sometimes as an arsenic crystal. Worldwide, arsenic toxicity and exposure is a serious problem that causes morbidity and mortality [40]. It is found in much of the world's ground water, and those who drink well water are at particular risk. Rice, a major world food staple that grows in high water conditions, is particularly good at concentrating arsenic, but other foods such as apples and apple juice can be high in it. Chronic overexposure leads to skin lesions, organ damage, and increased risk of cancer. Arsenic uncouples the electronic transport chain, thus disrupting the oxidative phosphorylation process in the mitochondria.

Tiny exposures are tolerable, and interestingly, micro-exposures probably have a hormetic effect in increasing mitochondrial coupling (Fig. 4.11). But for many people exposed to arsenic, there is a health risk. In the United States, about half of all well water has arsenic, and about 7% of well water sources exceed the limit of 10 μg/L that the USEPA has set. This is a more prevalent problem in the southwest, but examples are found in other regions [41].

One particular organ system that can be damaged by arsenic is the cardiovascular system. The ability of toxic (but not immediately lethal) chronic arsenic exposure to increase the risk of cardiac death and progression of atherosclerosis is well documented.

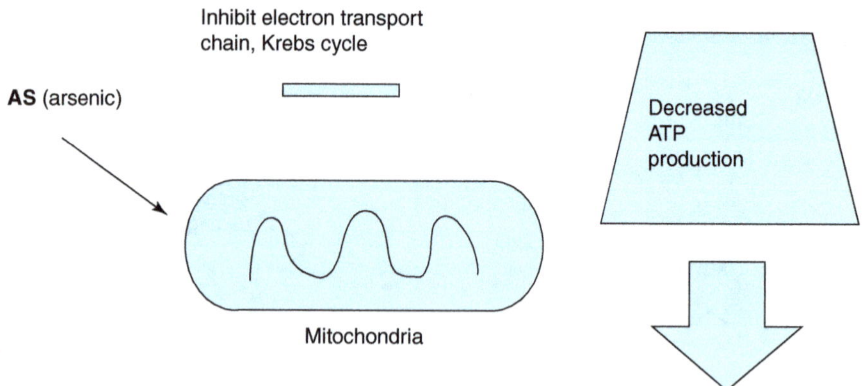

Fig. 4.11 Arsenic and mitochondria: Arsenic reduces the ability of the mitochondria to produce ATP via a decoupling mechanism

Mercury

Mercury is found throughout the world, often in conjunction with sulfur. Alchemists were fascinated with the properties of "quicksilver" and it had some early industrial uses. It later became incorporated into human infrastructure as part of electrical systems, as part of switches, batteries, and semiconductors. Mercury was incorporated into the "amalgam" of metals that made dental fillings. In medicine, Theophrastus Von Hohenheim (Paracelsus), who had traveled widely and studied ancient texts, saw the relation of mercury as an agent of transformation. He experimented with microdoses of it. While at first ridiculed, the use of minerals in medicine, including mercury but soon joined by antinomy, gold, zinc, and others, became the norm. Mercury was a desperate treatment for a tsunami of syphilis that sixteenth-century physicians had no guidance to treat from the writers of Galen they had studied in medical college. This was taken to toxic levels which became the normal for two centuries. By the early twentieth century, mercury use had been reduced to the use of purgatives with "calomel" (as opposed to vapors of mercury in sweat rooms) and fell out of use by the time scientifically informed allopathic medicine swept the scene.

Mercury is unfortunately found throughout the oceans, and creatures that are at certain high predator places in the food web, like sharks, tuna, and swordfish, will aggregate mercury. Daily fish eaters, depending on the species, can develop mercury toxicity. Pregnant females are advised to limit their intake of those fishes that are highest in mercury.

Mercury can inhibit methylation enzymes, which broadly interferes with DNA synthesis, neurotransmitter synthesis, and detoxification (Fig. 4.12). Mercury is toxic to the nervous system. Chronic exposure can cause neurotoxicity and permanent deficits. Mercury may also increase inflammation and autoimmune issues [42].

A source of exposure for mercury is thimerosal, which is used as a preservative in some medicines. In the past, some nasal sprays for allergy contained it, and

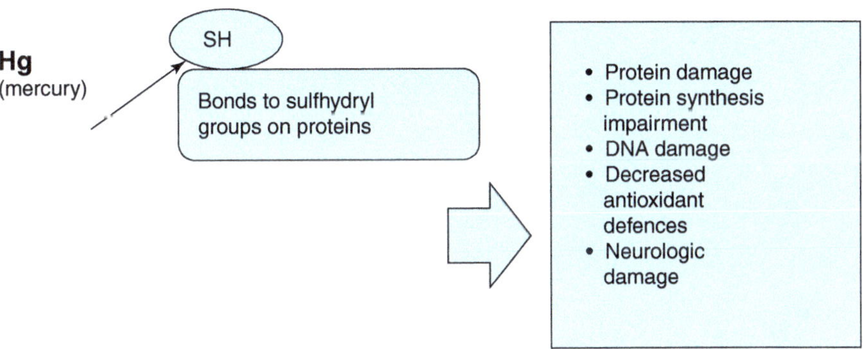

Fig. 4.12 Mercury toxicity: By binding to sulfhydryl groups on proteins, mercury can damage multiple systems including protein and DNA synthesis, and antioxidant defenses. The nervous system is particularly vulnerable to this toxicity

heavy, chronic users of those sprays developed toxicity. It is added to some vaccinations, with the Centers for Disease Control and Prevention stating that the intake is subtoxic. This is most likely the case for most children. However, those children with impaired detoxification systems due to poor nutritional status or simply genetic predisposition are likely to be sensitive to any additional intake of heavy metals. Moreover, those who have a genetic polymorphism that results in a sharp reduction in methylation enzymes (including the sometimes over-attributed yet very real MTHFR polymorphism) are going to have difficulty with any toxin that requires methylation to clean it up [43]. Those patients with strong methylation systems and good nutritional status are more likely to tolerate the small amounts of thimerosal in contemporary medicines.

Another source are ultraprocessed foods in general that contain corn syrup, bleached flours, and food coloring. These are processed with mercury alkali and deliver a cumulative dose of inorganic mercury [44]. This can damage enzyme systems. It also damages glycemic regulation—GLUT 4 gene expression is suppressed directly by inorganic mercury. The fact that the ultraprocessed diet is a rapid road to metabolic syndrome and diabetes is clearly more than simply caloric intake [45].

Lead

Lead has a long history in human usage. The term "plumber" is derived from the Latin term for lead, "plumbum," which is the basis for the symbol for lead in the periodic table—Pb. Lead has been used for glazing earthenware and the Romans even went so far as to sweeten some wine with lead acetate. Gasoline was treated with lead as an anti-knocking agent into the 1970s. Lead binds to sulfhydryl groups in sulfur-containing antioxidant proteins, such as glutathione synthase and superoxide dismutase (Fig. 4.13). Lead is neurotoxic, and it causes a type of anemia, which has some distinct features, particularly the stippled appearance of basophils in a

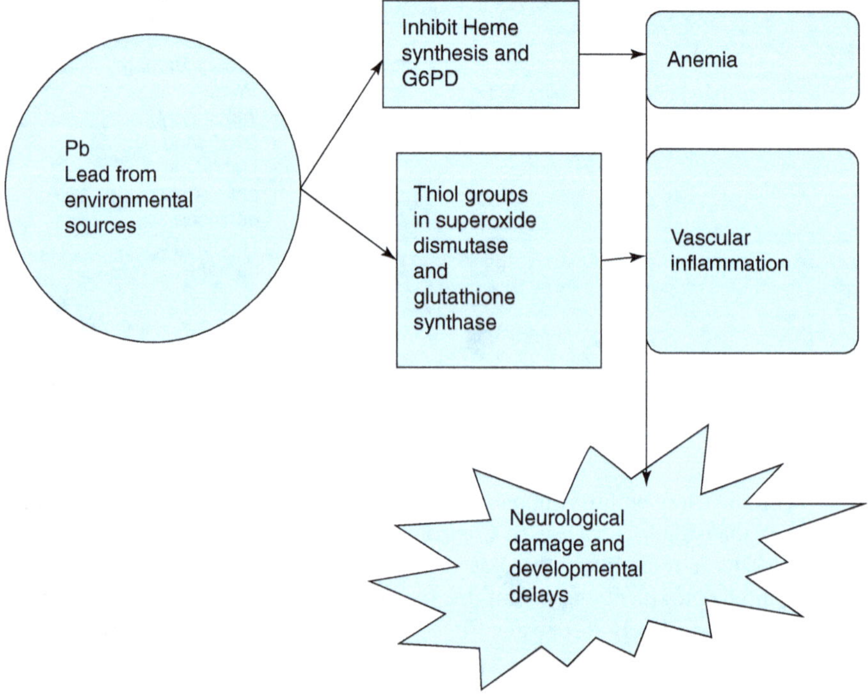

Fig. 4.13 Lead toxicity: Lead inhibits enzymes that are key to antioxidant functions and has direct actions against red blood cells. Poisoning with lead leads to anemia, vascular inflammation, neurological damage, and, in children, developmental delays

blood smear [46]. Lead causes developmental delays when children are exposed, and this harm can be profound. One of the greatest threats to children has traditionally been the legacy of leaded house paint. In many older homes, underneath the more contemporary layers of paint on the wall are older layers going back to the mid-twentieth century and earlier that contain lead [47]. Dust from renovations or simply ingesting paint chips can contaminate the home's residents. More recently, the great risks of those "plumbum" pipes in the water supply has been brought into stark focus. The water crisis in Flint, Michigan, dramatically illustrated this. When Flint went off of the Detroit water supply, the poor quality control of local water sources, and the treatment of very old pipes, led to toxic levels of lead in the water supply. Many residents developed symptoms and became ill [48]. This is not confined to Flint—and other municipalities have similar issues.

Lead, like mercury, has an ability to accumulate in the body. Early life exposures can have long-term and profound effects. There are associations, but not pure causation, between mercury and lead exposure and dementia.

If we consider the total metabolic and genetic reserve potential of a human being, clearly heavy metal intoxication reduces the available resources. Lead inhibits vitamin D synthesis, cell membrane integrity, and DNA synthesis. It is hard to imagine a more disruptive toxin especially for the young.

Pharmaceutical Drugs

Pharmaceutical products provide an enormous amount of good. They relieve suffering, prolong life, and in many cases can almost completely nullify the symptoms of a disease. Sometimes they are completely curative. Nevertheless, given the massive amount of pharmaceuticals that are consumed, there are bound to be toxic effects. Some of this toxicity is inherent in the nature of these substances, they create a benefit at a cost, and some people are more susceptible to the adverse effects. In other cases, the drug is used at too high a dose or for too long a period of time. Drugs can interact with each other at different levels of the body: in the detoxification systems of the body, in the bloodstream, at the target receptor on whatever tissue is the destination for the drug, or even through simply opposing or additive effects at the physiological level [49, 50].

According to the Food and Drug Administration, one set of estimates (the less conservative set than those of the Institute of Medicine) would mean that there are more than 2,216,000 serious Adverse Drug Reactions (ADR) in hospitalized patients, causing over 106,000 deaths annually [51]. If true, then ADRs are the fourth leading cause of death—ahead of pulmonary disease, diabetes, AIDS, pneumonia, accidents, and automobile deaths. These statistics do not include the number of ADRs that occur in ambulatory settings. Also, it is estimated that over 350,000 ADRs occur in US nursing homes each year.

This is not to disparage or diminish the many lives improved or saved by medical interventions using pharmaceuticals. But we must look at the facts which indicate that adverse effects, both predictable based on the mode of action and known pharmacodynamics of the drug and completely surprising or unpredictable, are a major problem. Drugs in general do put a burden on the hepatic processing of compounds, although in many cases it is a minor stress. Drug interactions remain a major risk. Pharmacology has gotten more sophisticated in its ability to identify those who are most susceptible to ADRs for any given drug, and that bodes well for reducing the number of injuries due to drug therapy.

The relevance to this chapter is that these medicines are ubiquitous, and many people use a lot of them. It is estimated that in 2019, for instance, 4.39 billion retail prescriptions were filled [52]. Without disparaging the many accomplishments of this industry—neonatal infections cured, diseases prevented, adults with chronic illnesses extending their lifespan, and many other compelling examples—we have to list pharmaceuticals as a force to consider in causes of ill health, at least for some people.

Dietary Supplements

Many dietary supplements are safe to use, but there is a wide variation in quality. This is due to the nature of regulation and manufacture of dietary supplements. Manufacturers are required to follow good manufacturing practices brought in by the FDA in about the late 2000s [53]. The GMPs were created with industry input. The regulatory framework for dietary supplements, the DSHEA from the 1990s, gives manufacturers the ability to bring supplements to market without the kind of extremely expensive premarket testing that is required for pharmaceuticals. It allows for a dietary supplement industry that provides innovative products for consumers. But the FDA has a small pool of resources to monitor what has become a vast industry (over 40 billion dollars a year spent in the United States). The FDA can and does investigate, warn, and order removal from market products that pose a risk to the public's health. A manufacturer can bring to market a dietary supplement by claiming to follow certain practices, but this might not be true. Their globally sourced (very often the case) constituents might have contaminants. The Certificate of Analysis that attests to the contents being as stated, and being free from adulterants, might be false, or forged.

In fairness to this industry, there are excellent companies who follow the highest standards of quality control. They submit to review by third-party accreditation. There are resources for determining what level of quality a company adheres to including voluntary programs where manufacturers share their quality assurance accreditation information.

Many natural products are quite safe. But with over 70% of Americans using them, that allows for the adverse events even if just a small fraction of products are not safe [54]. That can be due to the compounds found in the products, such as pyrrolizidine alkaloids and hepatotoxicity, neurotoxic plant compounds, heavy metal contamination, solvent contamination, fungal or bacterial contamination, and herb-drug interactions, as just some examples.

Burnt Food

Polycyclic aromatic hydrocarbons (PAH) are produced by heating food and certainly by burning it. They can arise from fat dripping onto coals or a grill, from burnt food such as toast and very significantly within frying oil [55]. The intensity and the length of frying will increase these molecules. PAHs are strong inducers of phase 1 detoxification and can increase oxidative stress in the body. They are carcinogenic, although food antioxidants and cellular antioxidants can provide some defense. They are implicated in gastrointestinal cancers including cancers of the esophagus and stomach. For those who inhale PAH due to occupation, such as line cooks or those who are around burning wood or coal, there is an increased risk of lung cancer [56].

Endocrine Disruptors

Endocrine disruptors are compounds that bind to a hormonal receptor in the body. They might directly stimulate it—“as if” they were a bona fide hormone (Fig. 4.14). Or they may alter the behavior of the cell itself, including the way that the cell DNA behaves and therefore act as a receptor modifier. These compounds can act to enhance the proliferation of cancers that are sensitive to hormonal inputs, such as certain the types of breast cancer [57]. They disrupt microflora which can have immune and metabolic consequences [58]. They can also dysregulate normal hormonal function, by adding an uncontrollable stimulus that is not wired into the negative feedback systems of the body’s own hormonal system. This can make conditions such as endometriosis far more active and painful [59]. Aside from introducing confusion in what would normally be a balanced system, they can also cause untoward effects by overstimulating the receptors. An extreme example of this are the obesogens, which are endocrine disruptors that cause adipose tissue to proliferate [60, 61]. Unfortunately, many of the products and substances that our industrialized world is constructed from have compounds in them that can act as endocrine disruptors. Examples include food packaging, receipt paper, plastics in all manner of products, and industrial solvents. There have been laudable efforts to reduce these compounds in products such as water bottles in the lining of canned food. But they are still ubiquitous.

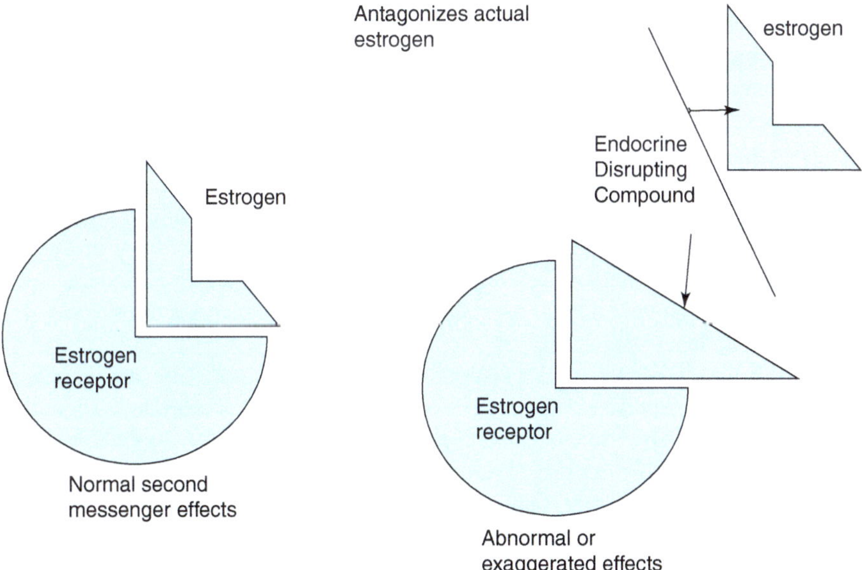

Fig. 4.14 Endocrine-disrupting compounds (EDC): Plasticizers and many industrial compounds can act as EDC. They occupy the same receptors as estrogen and other hormones. This can lead to dysregulation of function, or a strong endocrine effect that can increase the risk of the proliferation of cancer cells

Obesogens are a type of endocrine disruptor that cause adipocytes to multiply and to aggregate more fatty acids. In that process, the adipocytes also absorb more obesogens and further expand. Other pernicious effects include lower metabolic rate, increase in appetite, and increase in the storage of calories. While these compounds are not the sole cause of obesity, they have to be considered as an important driver of obesity, another negative force that has pushed the general population to unprecedented higher rates of obesity. Persistent organochlorines, bisphenol A, and parabens are examples. The effects of these obesogens appear to be multigenerational.

Another major concern about these substances are their impact on fertility and reproductive organ and tissue development. Exposure in utero, in childhood, and as an adult can impact reproductive tissues and function [62–64].

Drugs of Abuse

Many people use and are often addicted to an array of mind-altering chemicals. Heroin, methamphetamine, fentanyl, cocaine, synthetic cannabinoids, and others are illegal. They can be rife with impurities, adulterants, or toxins that are simply part of their synthesis (such as iodine used in the preparation of methamphetamine). Prescription drugs, particularly but not exclusively opioids, are an epidemic level of abuse. A common pathway to addiction is for a person to begin taking a prescription medication, such as Oxycontin (their prescription, relative's, or shared by a friend), and then this becomes an addiction. This can be very expensive, and they may transition to another nonprescription opioid.

Alcohol, while quite possible for many people to use in a moderate way, is as always a major drug of abuse. About 140,000 people die from excessive alcohol use in the United States each year [65]. There are still 29,000 alcohol-related liver disease deaths per year in the United States [66], which does not include many other causes of alcohol-related death such as seizures, motor vehicle accidents, and actual alcohol poisoning. Cannabis, while possible for people to use in a moderate way and despite its many medicinal uses, can also be used in excess and in a way that denotes dependency.

Opioids have become a major source of morbidity and mortality, and in spite of their long-standing presence as a drug of abuse, their use has accelerated. According to the Centers for Disease Control and Prevention [67], from 1999 to 2019, nearly 841,000 people died from a drug overdose, with about 70,000 perishing in 2019 and 92,000 in 2020. In that year, 68,630 people died of opioid overdose, meaning for 2020, 75% of overdose deaths involved an opioid, like prescription opioids, heroin, or synthetic opioids (like fentanyl).

These substances lead to other problems and to massive disruptions to the factors that make a person healthy. Infections due to routes of delivery (intravenous, skin popping, respiratory), sexually transmitted diseases particularly due to the exchange of sex for drugs, lack of nutrition, homelessness, despair, violence, and other damaging factors create a cloud of poor health around the abuse of these drugs. There are knock-on damages to the community but particularly to those who love, including the children of people who suffer with addiction.

People can recover from these addictions, with various treatment programs and especially, for many, the way of 12-step programs. This was initially Alcoholic Anonymous [68], but other groups such as Narcotics Anonymous follow the same principles and program of action.

There are long-term effects of these substances. Hepatitis C and B are a high risk from intravenous needle use, via needle sharing. There are direct toxicities such as vasoconstriction (which can even cause ischemia to internal organs) from amphetamines, and cocaine in particular has a long history of induced cardiac arrhythmias. As noted, alcohol can damage the liver and brain. Long-term and often delayed neurological consequences are still being found from many drugs of abuse.

A cursory look at methamphetamine reveals many toxins [69], which combined with the drug itself can damage many organs including the central nervous system. It is a substance that is synthesized from pseudoephedrine, using a series of chemical reactions to make a crystalline substance (Fig. 4.15). These chemical labs range from rather elaborate operations in rural areas to kitchen-based smaller operations and even to car trunk mobile operations [70]. They release many chemicals that not only harm the one who "cooks" the drugs, but any nearby neighbor or resident (including children) in the building.

Methamphetamine contains the following [71]:

Acetone—a powerful solvent found in nail polish remover and in construction and painting.

Lithium—a highly reactive alkali metal that is used in batteries; minute amounts are used cautiously in mood stabilization.

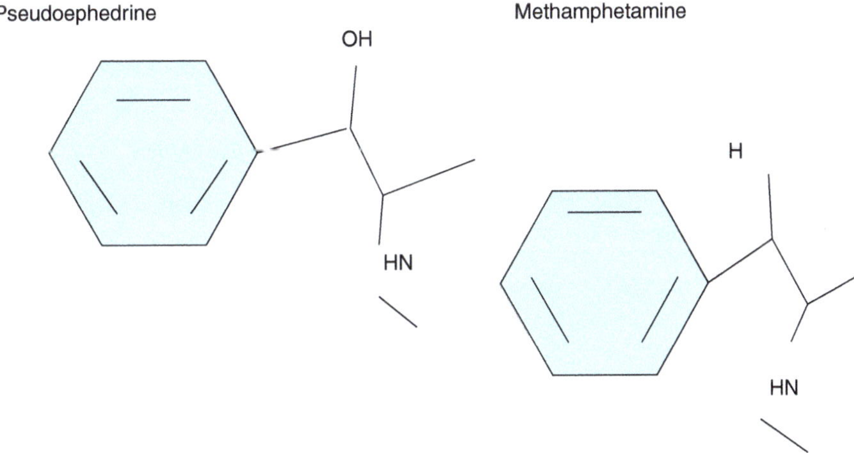

Fig. 4.15 Methamphetamine: In spite of the multitude of chemicals involved in the production of methamphetamine, it is structurally very similar to its parent compound, pseudoephedrine

Toluene—an industrial solvent that is carcinogenic.

Red phosphorus—a highly reactive form of phosphorus that can cause organ damage.

Hydrochloric acid, sulfuric acid, sodium hydroxide—strong acid and base that can damage mucus membranes.

Fentanyl, as noted above, is a leading cause of overdose death [72]. It is an incredibly potent opioid being 100 times more potent than morphine (Fig. 4.16). It is used with precision and care in anesthesia. Fentanyl is manufactured by criminal organizations and smuggled into the United States. It is sold directly and is also an adulterant in other drugs. It can cause immediate poisoning and even poison nearby people and first responders.

Prescription opioids can also be obtained illegally, through street traffic as well as "pill mills" that irresponsibly prescribe hundreds of prescriptions a week without any due medical process. These are not busy pain clinics; they are essentially walk-in operations for easy prescriptions. Many communities have been hit by a combination of these prescription drugs, heroin, and fentanyl.

Urban use of opioids is a major source of morbidity, in addition to cocaine and all other drugs. Medium-sized cities, smaller towns, and finally rural areas have been swept up in the opioid epidemic. A 2019 review outlined this problem, focusing on West Virginia with the highest rates of overdoses accounting for 41.5 deaths per 100,000 people among the 33,091 deaths in 2015 [73]. This state has had an accelerating trend of this problem. The number of people injecting drugs increased from 36% in 2005 to 54% in 2015. The authors attributed this to sociocultural factors, a depressed economy, lack of education, and a high rate of prescribing and dispensing of prescription opioids.

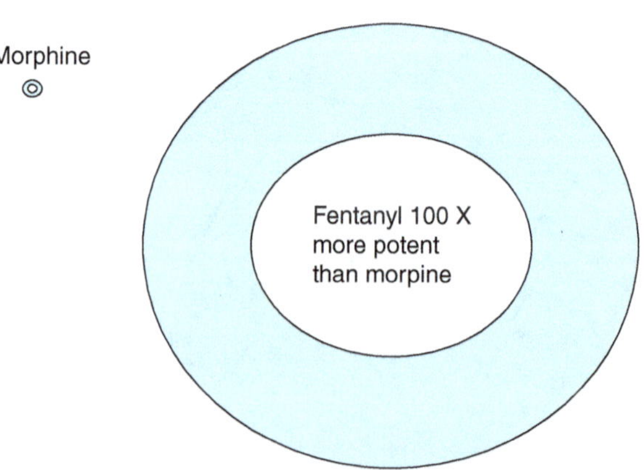

Fig. 4.16 Morphine versus fentanyl: Although morphine is a powerful anodyne, fentanyl, a drug which used to be only used with care and precision in clinical anesthesia, is vastly more potent, making it all that much more deadly as a drug of abuse

Smoking

According to the Centers for Disease Control and Prevention, about 40 million US adults still smoke cigarettes [74]. About 2.55 million middle and high school students use at least one tobacco product, including e-cigarettes. Annually, nearly half a million Americans die prematurely of smoking or exposure to secondhand smoke. At least 16 million live with a serious illness caused by smoking.

The health effects of smoking are well known. For some time, until the 1950s, it was thought to be a fairly tolerable activity until one got to be too old. Athletes who smoked tended to get winded more easily, and it seemed to be rough on the skin as one aged. In 1958, only 44% of Americans believed that smoking caused cancer. In spite of the fact that the generations that smoked those cigarettes and other tobacco forms did grow up eating more unprocessed food for the most part and less sugars and high-fructose corn syrup and had a lower toxin load in some cases (those who did not live in industrial cities at least), the tobacco was a pleasure that took a huge toll on their health. In fact, smoking adoption took decades for the full health implications, including cancer, to manifest, as carcinogenesis from induction to promotion to clinical progression can be a long process. It was obvious to thoracic surgeons that long-term smoking could devastate the lungs, and that most of their lung cancer patients were smokers. In spite of laboratory, epidemiological, and surgical evidence, up to the time that the Surgeon General Luther L. Terry issued his famous 1964 report, on June 7, 1962, the majority of Americans did not believe that smoking caused cancer. Dr. Terry's report came after a 2-year review of scientific literature by a committee of experts on the smoking question. It had an impact, and by 1968, 78% of Americans believed that smoking caused cancer [75]. Tobacco companies used a defense that the health authorities could not prove beyond a doubt that it was causative and that there were statistical reasoning flaws. This has a strange parallel today where a certain agnosticism about direct observation, pathology reports, physician experience, laboratory data, and basic common sense exists in the face of a deference to statistical computations of probability. This deep faith in statistical reasoning is found on subjects that lend themselves well to those statistical approaches and very often to those that do not.

Smoking has decreased, but is not gone. It has well-known effects of increasing cancer risk of the lung and other organs. This is due to the massive amount of carcinogenic compounds that cigarettes exude, including radioactive isotopes. Smoking increases the risk of stroke, heart disease, and peripheral vascular disease. It generates a lot of free radical stress, and it is a vasoconstrictor. The toxins in cigarettes harm the vascular lining. Smoking-derived toxins also activate the cytochrome P450 system, which generates a lot of free radical stress in the process, and this uses up the available antioxidant systems of glutathione, superoxide dismutase, ascorbic acid, etc. It is well known that chronic obstructive pulmonary disease, such as emphysema and chronic bronchitis, is most often caused by smoking. Damage to the lung parenchyma releases inflammatory compounds. For some that means over-activation of proteases that cause matrix disintegration which leads to fibrosis and dead air spaces in the lungs (emphysema). For others, excessive mucus, edema, coughing, and smooth muscle proliferation (chronic bronchitis) leads to obstruction.

Nicotine is a very addictive substance. Peripherally, it is a ganglionic blocker in the autonomic nervous system, which is a very profound action. Centrally, it can cause relaxation or stimulation. In withdrawal, there can be anxiety, irritability, and intense cravings. Nicotine and various carrier substances that are found in vaping are still being studied with respect to their level of risk [76]. In and of itself, a hypertensive agent like nicotine is not a safe daily agent for teens or any adult. The degree to which inhaled nicotine is causing injury is still being studied, but the CDC already has a term for it: vaping product use-associated lung injury (EVALI). One example noted is the use of vitamin E acetate as a carrier. At higher heats, it becomes a toxic ketone, diacetyl. In some patients it has caused a diffuse lung injury with alveolar damage and a condition called bronchiolitis obliterans, where the terminal airways become inflamed and damaged, thus depriving the respiratory units of actual oxygen. This condition was at first called "popcorn lung" due to the occupational health reports of workers in microwave popcorn factories who were applying diacetyl to popcorn to give it a "butter flavor" who developed bronchiolitis obliterans (this is a good reminder about what is meant for something to be an ultraprocessed food—that it is highly artificial and can contain all sorts of compounds that are not normally in a more unprocessed or "natural" food). Time will tell to what extent vaping is going to cause long-term lung damage in the millions who use it, including the young. Similarly to smoking in the past, pathology reports, laboratory studies, clinical observation, and common sense would indicate that it will not be a happy ending.

Infectious Disease: Chronic, Occult, and Sequelae

Infectious diseases create their own pathophysiology state, which requires accurate diagnosis and treatment. In this chapter, we are more concerned with long-term impacts. It is certainly a benefit to humanity that diseases such as tuberculosis, leprosy, staphylococcal infections, malaria, and many more infections have very reliable treatments. Although the human immune system and overall levels of health remain important to the overall question of infectious diseases, many lives are not cut short in these times thanks to the advances in medicine.

In those who recover from an infectious disease, aside from trivial and expected events, such as mild rotavirus infections or uncomplicated URI, there can be an aftermath of damaged organs. For example, the organism *Trypanosoma cruzi*, a parasite with a life cycle in humans, the triatomine bug (and animal reservoirs), is found in the United States [77]. It used to be confined to South America, but with rising temperatures, it has made its way well into the mid-continent of North America. The triatomine bug takes a blood meal from a human or animal infected with *T. cruzi* and passes the parasite on to other humans. The mature trypomastigotes burst out of cells and elaborate a toxin that can severely damage the heart leading to cardiomyopathy.

Many people have had tick-borne diseases, such as Lyme disease or Rocky Mountain spotted fever (Fig. 4.17). These conditions, such as RMSF, can be quite dangerous. There are patients with chronic Lyme disease due to *Borrelia burgdorferi* who develop chronic symptoms [78]. The acute phases of the disease can lead to skin, neurological, and cardiac inflammation. Posttreatment, there can be lack of eradication of the bacteria, and even after complete clearance, myalgia, fatigue, and cognitive changes can occur. This issue is illustrative of the challenges of contemporary medicine in addressing chronic dysfunction. Patients have found that their reports about ongoing symptoms were rebuffed by their doctor, on the basis of low-sensitivity testing. Higher-sensitivity testing can often uncover an occult persistent infection. As with many higher sensitivities, the number of false positives will increase. This can lead to a certain derisive skepticism about patients who have "never been well since" a Lyme diagnosis. Physicians have to make allowances for the fact that patients may be incorrect, or even misled about the nature of their diagnosis (or that an autoimmune disease is undiagnosed because an assumption has been made that the patient's symptoms are all due to Lyme disease). But in chronic

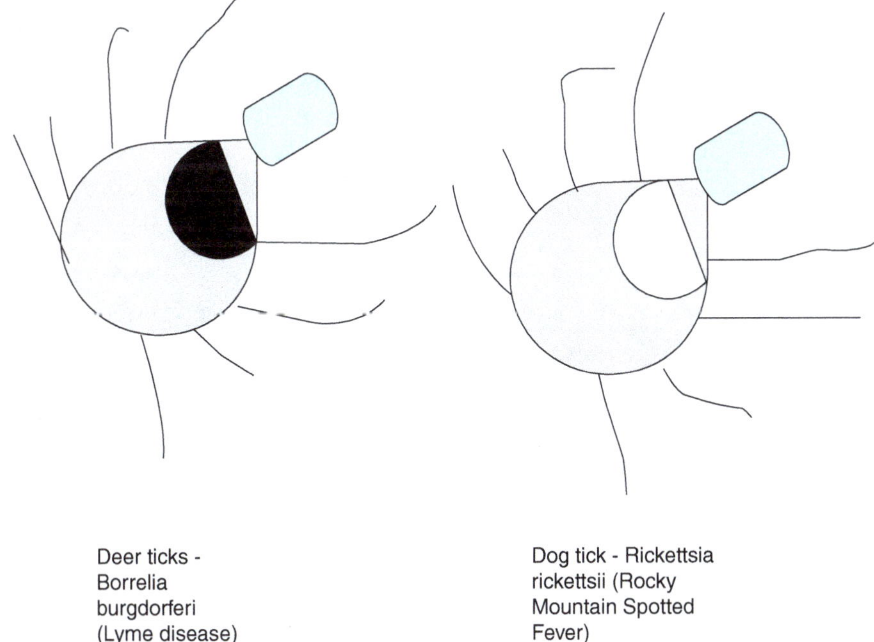

Fig. 4.17 Ticks: Different types of ticks serve as disease vectors for different bacteria

Lyme disease, to refuse to acknowledge that there is a spectrum of presentations, both acute and chronic, is a disservice to patients. This relates to the tendency to apply methods and reasoning that is appropriate to the acute diagnosis and treatment of disease to issues that are chronic and systemic in nature. The procedures in diagnosis and treating an acute infectious disease are different than those in a persistent or even an after-effect situation once the agent has been cleared. For instance, neuroinflammation during acute, or ongoing low-level, attacks by *B. burgdorferi* will lead to exposure of the brain to the immune system in ways that are not supposed to be. As an "immune-privilege" tissue, it has immune defenses, but it also has tight control over immune interaction with the central nervous system (the blood-brain barrier being an example). The breach of that barrier, and the loss of immune privilege, can lead to a chronic neuroinflammation. If a practitioner is only trained to address static states or has clinical reasoning that only allows for 1 degree of cause and effect relationships, then they will have difficulty in confronting this sort of situation. A naturopathic physician is trained to think of how function can gradually decrease, stay at a disturbed and chronically maladaptive level, and what to do to allow the self-repair mechanism to better reassert themselves.

HPV

Human papillomavirus is widely spread throughout the population, with different strains of varying virulence and potential for carcinogenesis [79]. HPV can be mutagenic and lead to cervical dysplasia, then carcinoma in situ, and invasive cervical cancer [80] (Fig. 4.18). It is also implicated in some throat cancers. New immunizations to prevent transmission will have an impact on the prevalence of this virus. Nevertheless, it is an example of a viral infection that in the short term can cause warts, but in the long term greatly increases the risk of developing cancer.

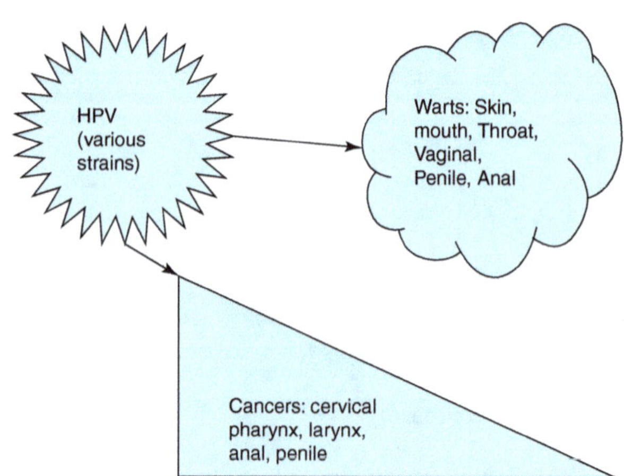

Fig. 4.18 HPV and cancer: The human papilloma virus is a powerful mutagen and is linked to, or proven to be causative of, many cancers

Bacteria and Atherosclerosis

There are many risk factors for atherosclerosis, and the inflammation and plaque deposition that leads to the atheroma is a multivariable process. The ability of oral bacteria to translocate to the bloodstream, raise inflammation, and even contribute to a biofilm matrix to the arterial lining is under investigation [81, 82]. The ability of some bacteria to produce the atherogenic metabolite trimethylamine-N-oxide from the amino acid choline is also under investigation [83].

Varicella Zoster

The virus that causes the disease chickenpox has the ability to become quiescent and remain in the ganglia of cranial and dorsal nerves [84]. When a person's immune surveillance wanes, it can begin to replicate, causing painful lesions that blister along the course of a nerve on the trunk or face typically. This condition is known as shingles and is an example of latency.

Treponema pallidum

This spirochete causes the disease known as syphilis [85]. It has been afflicting the human race for a long time, and its origins are unclear. It may have existed in the Americas in the pre-Columbian era or existed globally. Outbreaks in Europe in the early sixteenth century, especially contracted and spread by mercenaries during the 30 years' war, rapidly spread the disease. It was at first a virulent and rapidly fatal disease. It causes a rash and then muscle pains, fever, headaches, and other symptoms. Often the immune system can somewhat suppress it, and then in a decade or longer, a fatal progression of the infection leads to heart failure, neurologic damage, vasculitis, and organ failure (Fig. 4.19). These days the majority of people who have untreated syphilis do not develop tertiary presentations, but if they do, it can be devastating. Neurosyphilis is a feared complication with both nerve changes observable on physical exam and dementia. Congenital syphilis is where the spirochetes are transmitted in utero to the baby, and this can cause a number of anomalies and definite damage to the nervous system. There are still about 2000 cases of congenital syphilis in the United States each year. Syphilis reached a low in case counts in the year 2000 and has risen since—during 2020, there were 133,945 new cases of syphilis (all stages) [85]. In the 1950s, most cases of aortic aneurysm were associated with a positive test for syphilis.

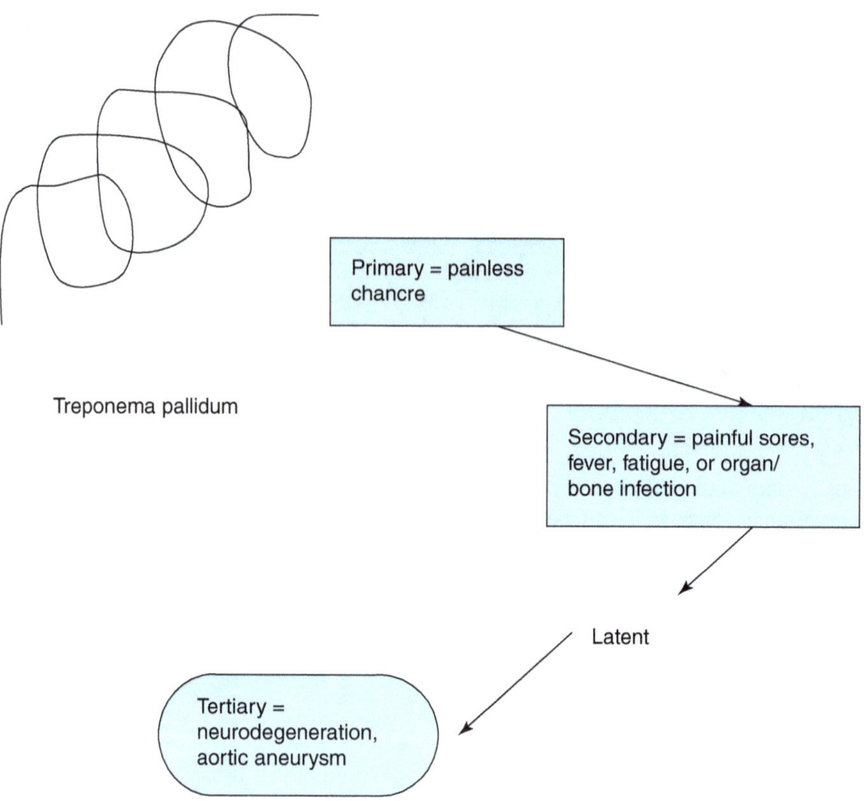

Fig. 4.19 Syphilis: Infection with *Treponema pallidum* has primary, secondary, and tertiary manifestations

This disease serves as a reminder that the relationship between pathogen and host is complex, and diseases continue to evolve. Mercury was used for many years to treat syphilis, resulting in massive mercury toxicity to those who did the treatment. If it worked at all, it was possibly due to the fact that mercury vapors were administered in a hot steam bath, and the spirochetes are heat labile (so it was a form of thermotherapy, albeit very dangerous). The antibiotic benzathine penicillin G is now given by injection. A single injection is usually curative in early syphilis and up to three injections are needed to eradicate *Treponema pallidum* in latent presentations. This has had a historic impact on public health in ways that are hard to appreciate now. Syphilis is an example of how an infection can be slow burning, and through its destruction and the involvement of the immune system—effective or not—create massive damage at a later time.

Dehydration and Water Quality

Water is essential to body chemistry, and when the various compartments of the body, vascular, extracellular, and intracellular, are not adequately filled, there are health risks. The kidneys will concentrate urine (increasing long term the risk of kidney stones) and the colon will reclaim as much water as it can (leading to constipation). Joint pain, mental concentration impairment, and bronchial sensitivity all get worse with dehydration. And of course it can be fatal if it progresses. Water quality is a global issue. Water scarcity is a direct threat for hundreds of millions of people and an incipient threat for billions [86]. In the United States, water management has improved, but many parts of the country have intense droughts and dropping reservoir levels. Contamination of groundwater with industrial by-products is always a concern, and contamination can occur in lakes, rivers, and streams. Groundwater in some parts of the country, such as well water in much of the southwest, can contain levels of arsenic far above the EPA limits [41]. Tap water in some communities with aging pipe systems can contain lead. This was illustrated by the tragedy of the Flint water crisis. In 2014, when Flint, Michigan, changed its water supply from the Detroit Water and Sewage Department (DWSD) to the Karegnondi Water Authority (KWA), the pipes started to rust from the inside, releasing toxic amounts of lead [48]. This has been repeated in other communities. Water conservation, management, and quality are bound to be major health issues across the world in the rest of the twenty-first century.

Summary

These factors that can dysregulate and damage the body are illustrative of a very large arsenal of challenges. If they are proven to directly cause an illness, this makes them of even higher relevance. A strong association with a disease end state is also valuable information.

But of importance to naturopathic medicine is that these factors lead to a biochemical and physiological malfunction. In this state, normal function is compromised. When multiple injurious factors additively impact the same process or system in the body, they can create an even more dramatic malfunction. When multiple processes and systems malfunction, they can have adverse effects together due to the intersystem reliance that is inherent in the body.

To not address these factors is to increase the risk of disease, but also to create conditions where normal function and structure become less likely. Any form of treatment may take longer to work, or fail, if the body's systems cannot reassert control and return to normal function. Although the human body can be incredibly adaptive, there are points at which dysregulating influences simply take their toll.

References

1. Steele TA, St Louis EK, Videnovic A, Auger RR. Circadian rhythm sleep-wake disorders: a contemporary review of neurobiology, treatment, and dysregulation in neurodegenerative disease. Neurother J Am Soc Exp Neurother. 2021;18(1):53–74.
2. Leng Y, Blackwell T, Cawthon PM, Ancoli-Israel S, Stone KL, Yaffe K. Association of Circadian Abnormalities in older adults with an increased risk of developing Parkinson disease. JAMA Neurol. 2020;77(10):1270–8.
3. Pase MP, Himali JJ, Grima NA, Beiser AS, Satizabal CL, Aparicio HJ, et al. Sleep architecture and the risk of incident dementia in the community. Neurology. 2017;89(12):1244–50.
4. Zimmet P, Alberti KGMM, Stern N, Bilu C, El-Osta A, Einat H, et al. The Circadian syndrome: is the metabolic syndrome and much more! J Intern Med. 2019;286(2):181–91.
5. Lee Y. Roles of circadian clocks in cancer pathogenesis and treatment. Exp Mol Med. 2021;53(10):1529–38.
6. Xia N, Li H. Loneliness, social isolation, and cardiovascular health. Antioxid Redox Signal. 2018;28(9):837–51.
7. Valtorta NK, Kanaan M, Gilbody S, Ronzi S, Hanratty B. Loneliness and social isolation as risk factors for coronary heart disease and stroke: systematic review and meta-analysis of longitudinal observational studies. Heart. 2016;102(13):1009–16.
8. Of AA of C and AP. Screen time and children. https://www.aacap.org/AACAP/Families_and_Youth/Facts_for_Families/FFF-Guide/Children-And-Watching-TV-054.aspx.
9. Park JH, Moon JH, Kim HJ, Kong MH, Oh YH. Sedentary lifestyle: overview of updated evidence of potential health risks. Korean J Fam Med. 2020;41(6):365–73.
10. Center for Disease Control and Prevention. Physical inactivity. https://www.cdc.gov/chronicdisease/resources/publications/factsheets/physical-activity.htm. Accessed 20 May 2022.
11. Chaput J-P, Willumsen J, Bull F, Chou R, Ekelund U, Firth J, et al. 2020 WHO guidelines on physical activity and sedentary behaviour for children and adolescents aged 5-17 years: summary of the evidence. Int J Behav Nutr Phys Act. 2020;17(1):141.
12. Schuermann D, Mevissen M. Manmade electromagnetic fields and oxidative stress-biological effects and consequences for health. Int J Mol Sci. 2021;22(7):3772.
13. Wheeler SM, Bryant AS. Racial and ethnic disparities in health and health care. Obstet Gynecol Clin N Am. 2017;44(1):1–11.
14. Center for Disease Control and Prevention. Health disparities. https://www.cdc.gov/healthyyouth/disparities/. Accessed 20 May 2022.
15. Thornton RLJ, Glover CM, Cené CW, Glik DC, Henderson JA, Williams DR. Evaluating strategies for reducing health disparities by addressing the social determinants of health. Health Aff. 2016;35(8):1416–23.
16. Schillinger D. Social determinants, health literacy, and disparities: intersections and controversies. Health Lit Res Pract. 2021;5(3):e234–43.
17. Timoneda J, Rodríguez-Fernández L, Zaragozá R, Marín MP, Cabezuelo MT, Torres L, et al. Vitamin A deficiency and the lung. Nutrients. 2018;10(9):1132.
18. NIH O. Vitamin A. A fact sheet for health professionals. https://ods.od.nih.gov/factsheets/VitaminA-HealthProfessional/.
19. Holick MF. The vitamin D deficiency pandemic: approaches for diagnosis, treatment and prevention. Rev Endocr Metab Disord. 2017;18(2):153–65.
20. Mora JR, Iwata M, von Andrian UH. Vitamin effects on the immune system: vitamins A and D take centre stage. Nat Rev Immunol. 2008;8(9):685–98.
21. Lewis ED, Meydani SN, Wu D. Regulatory role of vitamin E in the immune system and inflammation. IUBMB Life. 2019;71(4):487–94.
22. Supplements NI of H-O of D. Vitamin C: a fact sheet for consumers. https://ods.od.nih.gov/factsheets/Vitaminc-Healthprofessional/.
23. Carr AC, Maggini S. Vitamin C and Immune Function. Nutrients. 2017;9(11):1211.

24. Rayman MP. Selenium intake, status, and health: a complex relationship. Hormones. 2020;19(1):9–14.
25. Center for Disease Control and Prevention. Get the facts about sugars. https://www.cdc.gov/nutrition/data-statistics/added-sugars.html.
26. Petruk G, Puthia M, Petrlova J, Samsudin F, Strömdahl A-C, Cerps S, et al. SARS-CoV-2 spike protein binds to bacterial lipopolysaccharide and boosts proinflammatory activity. J Mol Cell Biol. 2020;12(12):916–32.
27. Guevara-Cruz M, Flores-López AG, Aguilar-López M, Sánchez-Tapia M, Medina-Vera I, Díaz D, et al. Improvement of lipoprotein profile and metabolic endotoxemia by a lifestyle intervention that modifies the gut microbiota in subjects with metabolic syndrome. J Am Heart Assoc. 2019;8(17):e012401.
28. Roy R, Tiwari M, Donelli G, Tiwari V. Strategies for combating bacterial biofilms: a focus on anti-biofilm agents and their mechanisms of action. Virulence. 2018;9(1):522–54.
29. Herringa RJ. Trauma, PTSD, and the developing brain. Curr Psychiatry Rep. 2017;19(10):69.
30. Corrigan FM, Fisher JJ, Nutt DJ. Autonomic dysregulation and the Window of Tolerance model of the effects of complex emotional trauma. J Psychopharmacol. 2011;25(1):17–25.
31. Dai S, Mo Y, Wang Y, Xiang B, Liao Q, Zhou M, et al. Chronic stress promotes cancer development. Front Oncol. 2020;10:1492.
32. Yao B-C, Meng L-B, Hao M-L, Zhang Y-M, Gong T, Guo Z-G. Chronic stress: a critical risk factor for atherosclerosis. J Int Med Res. 2019;47(4):1429–40.
33. Richardson JR, Fitsanakis V, Westerink RHS, Kanthasamy AG. Neurotoxicity of pesticides. Acta Neuropathol. 2019;138(3):343–62.
34. Leung MCK, Meyer JN. Mitochondria as a target of organophosphate and carbamate pesticides: revisiting common mechanisms of action with new approach methodologies. Reprod Toxicol. 2019;89:83–92.
35. Peillex C, Pelletier M. The impact and toxicity of glyphosate and glyphosate-based herbicides on health and immunity. J Immunotoxicol. 2020;17(1):163–74.
36. Omotayo OP, Omotayo AO, Mwanza M, Babalola OO. Prevalence of mycotoxins and their consequences on human health. Toxicol Res. 2019;35(1):1–7.
37. Liew W-P-P, Mohd-Redzwan S. Mycotoxin: its impact on gut health and microbiota. Front Cell Infect Microbiol. 2018;8:60.
38. Lawrence GD. Perspective: the saturated fat-unsaturated oil dilemma: relations of dietary fatty acids and serum cholesterol, atherosclerosis, inflammation, cancer, and all-cause mortality. Adv Nutr. 2021;12(3):647–56.
39. Wang W, Yang H, Johnson D, Gensler C, Decker E, Zhang G. Chemistry and biology of ω-3 PUFA peroxidation-derived compounds. Prostaglandins Other Lipid Mediat. 2017;132:84–91.
40. Nurchi VM, Djordjevic AB, Crisponi G, Alexander J, Bjørklund G, Aaseth J. Arsenic toxicity: molecular targets and therapeutic agents. Biomolecules. 2020;10(2):235.
41. Arsenic and Drinking Water. https://www.usgs.gov/mission-areas/water-resources/science/arsenic-and-drinking-water.
42. Yang L, Zhang Y, Wang F, Luo Z, Guo S, Strähle U. Toxicity of mercury: molecular evidence. Chemosphere. 2020;245:125586.
43. Austin DW, Spolding B, Gondalia S, Shandley K, Palombo EA, Knowles S, et al. Genetic variation associated with hypersensitivity to mercury. Toxicol Int. 2014;21(3):236–41.
44. Roy C, Tremblay P-Y, Ayotte P. Is mercury exposure causing diabetes, metabolic syndrome and insulin resistance? A systematic review of the literature. Environ Res. 2017;156:747–60.
45. Dufault R, Berg Z, Crider R, Schnoll R, Wetsit L, Bulls WT, et al. Blood inorganic mercury is directly associated with glucose levels in the human population and may be linked to processed food intake. Integr Mol Med. 2015;2(3)
46. Gidlow DA. Lead toxicity. Occup Med (Lond). 2015;65(5):348–56.
47. O'Connor D, Hou D, Ye J, Zhang Y, Ok YS, Song Y, et al. Lead-based paint remains a major public health concern: a critical review of global production, trade, use, exposure, health risk, and implications. Environ Int. 2018;121(Pt 1):85–101.

48. Hanna-Attisha M, LaChance J, Sadler RC, Champney Schnepp A. Elevated blood lead levels in children associated with the flint drinking water crisis: a spatial analysis of risk and public health response. Am J Public Health. 2016;106(2):283–90.
49. Poleksic A, Xie L. Database of adverse events associated with drugs and drug combinations. Sci Rep. 2019;9(1):20025.
50. Coleman JJ, Pontefract SK. Adverse drug reactions. Clin Med. 2016;16(5):481–5. https://pubmed.ncbi.nlm.nih.gov/27697815.
51. FDA. Preventable adverse drug reactions: a focus on drug interactions. 2018. https://www.fda.gov/drugs/drug-interactions-labeling/preventable-adverse-drug-reactions-focus-drug-interactions#ADRs:%20Prevalence%20and%20Incidence.
52. Stastista. Total number of retail prescriptions filled annually in the United States from 2013 to 2025 (in billions)*. https://www.statista.com/statistics/261303/total-number-of-retail-prescriptions-filled-annually-in-the-us/.
53. U.S. Food and Drug Administration. Current Good Manufacturing Practices (CGMPs) for food and dietary supplements. https://www.fda.gov/food/guidance-regulation-food-and-dietary-supplements/current-good-manufacturing-practices-cgmps-food-and-dietary-supplements. Accessed 21 May 2022.
54. Ronis MJJ, Pedersen KB, Watt J. Adverse effects of nutraceuticals and dietary supplements. Annu Rev Pharmacol Toxicol. 2018;58:583–601.
55. An K-J, Liu Y-L, Liu H-L. Relationship between total polar components and polycyclic aromatic hydrocarbons in fried edible oil. Food Addit Contam Part A: Chem Anal Control Expo Risk Assess. 2017;34(9):1596–605.
56. Miglani K, Kumar S, Yadav A, Aggarwal N, Ahmad I, Gupta R. A multibiomarker approach to evaluate the effect of polyaromatic hydrocarbon exposure on oxidative and genotoxic damage in tandoor workers. Toxicol Ind Health. 2019;35(7):486–96.
57. Rocha PRS, Oliveira VD, Vasques CI, Dos Reis PED, Amato AA. Exposure to endocrine disruptors and risk of breast cancer: a systematic review. Crit Rev Oncol Hematol. 2021;161:103330.
58. Hampl R, Stárka L. Endocrine disruptors and gut microbiome interactions. Physiol Res. 2020;69(Suppl 2):S211–23.
59. Bruner-Tran KL, Osteen KG. Dioxin-like PCBs and endometriosis. Syst Biol Reprod Med. 2010;56(2):132–46.
60. Heindel JJ, Blumberg B. Environmental obesogens: mechanisms and controversies. Annu Rev Pharmacol Toxicol. 2019;59:89–106.
61. Darbre PD. Endocrine disruptors and obesity. Curr Obes Rep. 2017;6(1):18–27.
62. Tang Z-R, Xu X-L, Deng S-L, Lian Z-X, Yu K. Oestrogenic endocrine disruptors in the placenta and the fetus. Int J Mol Sci. 2020;21(4):1519.
63. Rattan S, Zhou C, Chiang C, Mahalingam S, Brehm E, Flaws JA. Exposure to endocrine disruptors during adulthood: consequences for female fertility. J Endocrinol. 2017;233(3):R109–29.
64. Rattan S, Flaws JA. The epigenetic impacts of endocrine disruptors on female reproduction across generations†. Biol Reprod. 2019;101(3):635–44.
65. Center for Disease Control and Prevention. Deaths from excessive alcohol use in the United States. https://www.cdc.gov/alcohol/features/excessive-alcohol-deaths.html. Accessed 21 May 2022.
66. Center for Disease Control and Prevention. Alcohol use. https://www.cdc.gov/nchs/fastats/alcohol.htm. Accessed 21 May 2022.
67. Center for Disease Control and Prevention. Overdose death rates. https://nida.nih.gov/drug-topics/trends-statistics/overdose-death-rates. Accessed 21 May 2022.
68. A A. World Services. Alcoholics anonymous. https://www.aa.org/. Accessed 21 May 2022.
69. National Institute on Drug Abuse. Methamphetamine research report. https://nida.nih.gov/publications/research-reports/methamphetamine/overview.
70. Ciesielski AL, Wagner JR, Alexander-Scott M, Smith J, Snawder J. Surface contamination generated by "one-pot" methamphetamine production. J Chem Health Saf. 2020;28(1):49–54.

71. Center RR. Crystal meth long term health effects. https://reflectionsrehab.com/blog/crystal-meth-long-term-health-effects-dangerous-chemicals-found-in-methamphetamine/.
72. Center for Disease Control and Prevention. Fentanyl facts. https://www.cdc.gov/stopoverdose/fentanyl/index.html.
73. Merino R, Bowden N, Katamneni S, Coustasse A. The opioid epidemic in West Virginia. Health Care Manag. 2019;38(2):187–95.
74. Center for Disease Control and Prevention. Smoking and tobacco use. https://www.cdc.gov/tobacco/index.htm.
75. Medicine NL of. The 1964 report on smoking and health. https://profiles.nlm.nih.gov/spotlight/nn/feature/smoking.
76. Smith ML, Gotway MB, Crotty Alexander LE, Hariri LP. Vaping-related lung injury. Virchows Arch. 2021;478(1):81–8.
77. Bern C, Messenger LA, Whitman JD, Maguire JH. Chagas disease in the United States: a public health approach. Clin Microbiol Rev. 2019;33(1):e00023.
78. Lantos PM. Chronic Lyme disease. Infect Dis Clin N Am. 2015;29(2):325–40.
79. Manini I, Montomoli E. Epidemiology and prevention of human papillomavirus. Ann Ig. 2018;30(4 Supple 1):28–32.
80. Crosbie EJ, Einstein MH, Franceschi S, Kitchener HC. Human papillomavirus and cervical cancer. Lancet. 2013;382(9895):889–99.
81. Schenkein HA, Papapanou PN, Genco R, Sanz M. Mechanisms underlying the association between periodontitis and atherosclerotic disease. Periodontol. 2020;83(1):90–106.
82. Carrizales-Sepúlveda EF, Ordaz-Farías A, Vera-Pineda R, Flores-Ramírez R. Periodontal disease, systemic inflammation and the risk of cardiovascular disease. Heart Lung Circ. 2018;27(11):1327–34.
83. Zeisel SH, Warrier M. Trimethylamine N-oxide, the microbiome, and heart and kidney disease. Annu Rev Nutr. 2017;37:157–81.
84. Gershon AA, Breuer J, Cohen JI, Cohrs RJ, Gershon MD, Gilden D, et al. Varicella zoster virus infection. Nat Rev Dis Prim. 2015;1:15016.
85. Center for Disease Control and Prevention. Sexually transmitted disease/syphilis. https://www.cdc.gov/std/syphilis/default.htm. Accessed 21 May 2022.
86. He C, Liu Z, Wu J, Pan X, Fang Z, Li J, et al. Future global urban water scarcity and potential solutions. Nat Commun. 2021;12(1):4667.

Chapter 5
Assessment of the Patient

Diagnosis in naturopathic medicine follows the same principles that physicians of all orientations use. It is a process of observation and ratiocination that goes back to Greek physicians 2400 years ago. Disease states, pathological lesions, and biochemical imbalances are states of affairs that can be observed and measured. They have implicit hazards and sometimes require immediate action.

In naturopathic medicine, diagnosis is one component of an overall understanding of the patient. The pathogenesis of many diseases is quite well mapped out in the biomedical literature. But how and why that pathogenesis occurred in a specific patient is a matter of importance in naturopathic medicine. What is the overall state of that patient's health? What anomalies and imbalances are present in their immune system, gut microbiome, extracellular matrix, nutritional status, toxin load, and more?

This is critical information. Sometimes, addressing these generative factors can help extinguish the pathology. Many disease states have progressed too far to self-extinguish when their root causes are addressed. But even in those cases, the intensity, and the persistence of a disease in spite of the best medical and naturopathic therapy, can be reduced by addressing this ground state.

Whole-person systems of traditional and complementary medicine, such as (but not limited to) Ayurveda and acupuncture, look at complete patterns. What is the relationship of organs to each other? What pernicious influences on health and what deficits in health and nutrition led to an imbalance?

Naturopathic medicine is somewhat unique, in that the practitioner simultaneously apprehends the pathological disease diagnosis facts about the case and investigates whole system imbalances, including their generative factors where knowable.

This is not only a broader interpretation of symptoms. This assessment of the patient sets the stage for the therapeutic approach described in this book. That approach entails optimizing function, rehabilitating degenerative tissues, and attempting to create the conditions for health.

F. Smith, *Naturopathic Medicine*, https://doi.org/10.1007/978-3-031-13388-6_5

Negating the precise dysfunction, extinguishing maladaptive responses in a disease situation is of course incredibly helpful. But this is only helpful in the long run if the system in question—cardiac, hepatic, pulmonary, etc.—is capable of establishing a homeostatic environment. Often it can, but very often the restoration of function, even with the most precise disease-oriented therapy, is partial. Naturopathic medicine does not enshrine the pathological lesion with absolute importance in the overall therapy. It does gain total priority in emergency and end-stage situations of course. But in the more common, chronic, and challenging situations of ill health, targeting the end result, the consequence of a state of affairs in the body, without addressing the terrain, yields only partial results.

The physical examination has lost some of its importance as laboratory and imaging diagnosis have become more accessible, affordable, and reliable (Table 5.3). This does not mean that there is no value in the data acquired by examining a patient. In an attempt to be "evidence based," some research reviews on the physical examination compare disease recognition statistics with or without a physical examination and have concluded that there is no better outcome from doing a physical examination. This is particularly true of a complete screening examination. That may be true, in that a head to toe physical examination without guidance based on a patient interview and patient health history might not be the best investment of time. The Cochrane Database Systematic Review on the Annual Physical Examination does conclude that:

> Health checks have little or no effect on total mortality and probably have little or no effect on cardiovascular mortality, and probably no little effect on fatal and non-fatal ischaemic heart disease on fatal and non-fatal stroke. General health checks are unlikely to be beneficial [1].

An annual health check, in the time spent and reimbursement model of contemporary practice, is a cursory affair. A brief auscultation, an abdominal palpation, a few neurological tests, etc., and the examination is over. The in-depth, head to toe examination of internists during the era of Sapira or Osler or Cabot is long gone. However, these results suggest that screening that is disconnected from a history or a patient complaint might not really have a high level of detection. Unfortunately, with the downgrading of the annual health screen, as perfunctory as it has become, many physicians do not examine their patient throughout the rest of the year. Again, this may have, outside of an urgent care situation, little impact in a system that uses medications to manage disease. In a system of medicine that seeks to build up resilience and perform very early detection of imbalances and disruptions to homeostasis and function, the data from actually observing the patient takes on new relevance.

On the other hand, not examining a patient would seem to be a drain on time and resources in that errors in the way of missed diagnoses, and the ordering of unnecessary tests might go up in the case of not performing simple office examinations [2]. The hypothesis-driven physical exam [3] is one contemporary way to express the relevance of this skill, which is really what it has been for its history (Fig. 5.1).

In a disease-based model, where the focus is on detecting treatable pathologies, the value of surmising the patient's level of health seems to decrease. In a model of

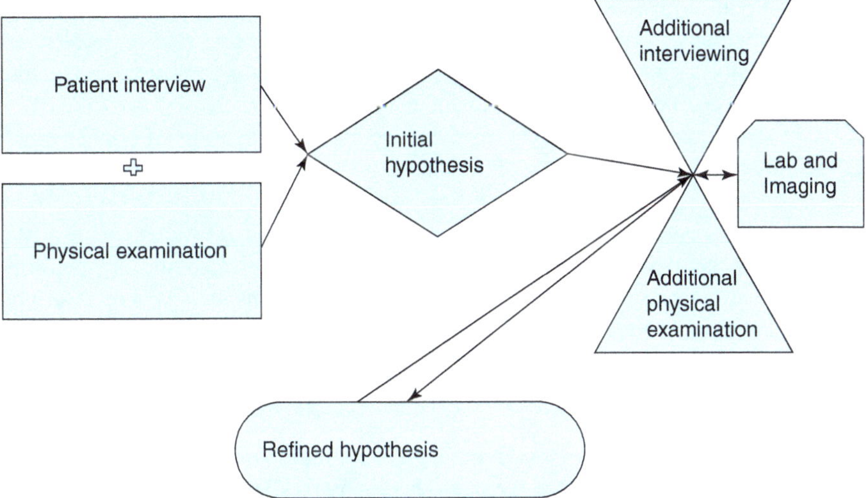

Fig. 5.1 Hypothesis-driven physical examination: The patient interview and physical examination are needed to create an initial hypothesis. Additional question, examination, and lab/imaging can be used to test that hypothesis

care that places importance on understanding the state of each individual patient's health, taking a few moments to meaningfully examine them becomes more relevant.

There are emotional and relationship reasons for conducting a physical examination. The work of Abraham Verghese has helped bring this to the forefront [4]. Touch is reassuring. A doctor who takes time to examine their patient conveys interest and competence. Some visits and some specialities lend themselves more to examination of the patient than others, but the principle is the same. The act of respectfully and thoughtfully examining the patient has been at the heart of medicine for thousands of years. As advanced as medicine is becoming in the dawning age of informatics and genomics/proteomics medicine, it remains a human-centered endeavor.

The techniques of performing the physical examination are described in detail in many other textbooks. In this section, we will examine some of the pertinent infor mation that can be derived by a close examination of each region and system.

Ocular Examination

A general physician can do a fair amount of ocular exam, both the anterior and posterior aspects (with ophthalmoscope). Ongoing care, at the least an annual examination by an eye care specialist (an ophthalmologist or optometrist), is an important aspect of keeping eyes as healthy as possible. Any sudden loss of vision, or abrupt change to visual acuity, or peculiar aspects to the field of vision (sudden appearance of many floaters, changes to hue, sparks, etc.) demand immediate evaluation by an eye care specialist. One reason for annual examinations is that slowly developing, but eventually sight-destroying issues such as macular degeneration and ocular hypertension can be found early and managed.

A general exam of the eye can reveal quite a bit. Depositions of copper in the cornea, due to congenital copper imbalances (Wilson's disease) or dietary/hydrological copper exposure, can create a ring around the cornea. Very dry eyes can be due to a lack of essential fatty acids and vitamin A. The lack of an adequate tear film and a more sensitive cornea can be a vitamin A issue but can also raise the possibility of autoimmune issues. Eyes that appear sunken can be due to loss of retro-orbital fat pads. When someone has calorie or protein-calorie malnutrition, this area loses fat. This may happen due to a metabolic or neoplastic disease, a malabsorption issue, or simply lack of food intake.

In an outpatient setting, corneal and conjunctival problems can present for any number of reasons. The simplest to manage is conjunctivitis. The conjunctiva will be injected (red) but in a diffuse manner. There may be slightly more redness in one area, especially if the patient scratches there. The pain level is low, more of a soreness, but the pruritus can be high, with patients reporting a feeling of warmth or itchiness. A bland and sticky discharge will be found if the conjunctivitis is bacterial. A viral conjunctivitis—pink eye—lacks the discharge and tends to have less pruritus. It is easily transmitted, and for either type of conjunctivitis, wearing gloves and handwashing before and after the exam are important.

If the cornea is irritated, the pain level will be high. A classic example is a corneal abrasion from something as simple as a tree branch scratching the eye while cycling, or a baby reaching out to touch a caregiver and scratching the cornea with their nail. These will heal in about a day, but deeper scratches can become infected. Any injury to the cornea will be painful, with photophobia and lacrimation. The more irritated the cornea becomes, the more that any injection (redness) will be more intense in a ring around the cornea (perilimbal). Bacteria and fungi can unfortunately gain a foothold in the cornea. This requires rapid treatment. Although some herbal poultices and homeopathic drops can be excellent for conjunctivitis, corneal infection must be resolved quickly. Infection will destroy the precisely arrayed collagen stroma of the cornea and heal with fibrosis, causing opacities that can decrease visual acuity. Some contact lens wearers can get amoebic infections, which will be difficult to treat but can cause chronic pain and visual loss.

Extreme pain and perilimbal injection can also be due to iritis or uveitis. This can occur spontaneously but is more likely to be found in those with autoimmune diseases such as ulcerative colitis. This is a medical emergency and prompt treatment with steroids is needed to preserve sight.

The lens of the eye may have lost luster and may have an area of opacity. This is the formation of a cataract, which is a sign of photo-oxidation of the lens. This happens with aging and is accelerated by sun exposure, smoking, diabetes, and lack of sources of vitamin C and carotenoids in the diet.

The vitreous humor, formed embryologically, can oxidize and harden with age. It might contain blood cells from a leak in a retinal blood vessel. The vitreous can

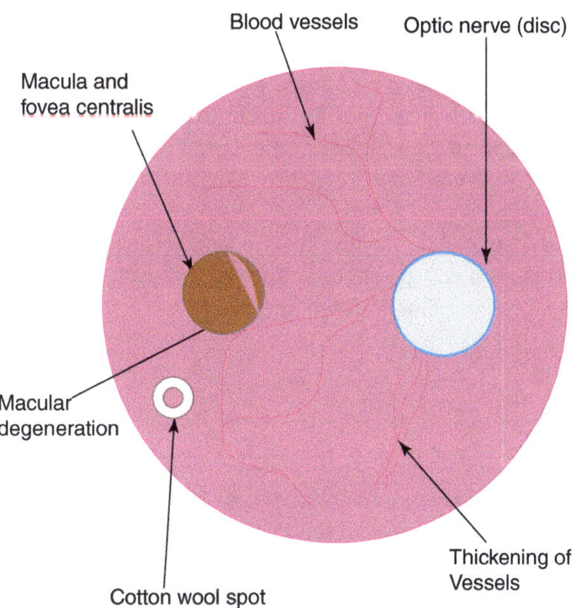

Fig. 5.2 The retinal examination. Local and systemic (such as cardiovascular or metabolic) issues can lead to specific findings in the retina

also coagulate and form a lump-like mass in sections. This can obscure vision. If a vitreous lump is near the retina, the pressure it causes can induce macular edema, rendering vision blurring. It can lead to retinal damage or detachment.

The retina itself contains information relating to local and systemic (such as vascular) health (Fig. 5.2). In retinas that are losing their attachment, the vitreous can traction the retina and accelerate detachment. In an outpatient setting, with the use of cycloplegic drops, it is possible to get a sense of the hue of the retina and to inspect for blood vessel integrity. If the retinal vessels are thickened (copper wire), it may be a proliferative effect of vascular hypertension. If there are signs of fibrosis (cotton wool spots), previous hemorrhages might have healed and left behind a collagen scar, but not normal retinal tissue. Bright red hemorrhages (wet retinopathy), as found in diabetes, are another reason for immediate referral.

Retinal detachment is more common in myopes, due to the egg shape of the eyeball, and the fraying that can occur around the edges of the retina. The matrix that holds the retina in place does weaken with age. Vascular disease and diabetes (which has the combination of vascular deterioration, protein glycation, and sorbitol accumulation in the retina and optic nerve and lens). A patient that complains of sudden visual loss, or a perception of a curtain or shade being pulled over their visual field, needs immediate referral to an ophthalmologist for immediate examination or a hospital. The eyes are a window to the soul, as it has been said, and they are also a window into the vascular system. A patient with signs of vascular disturbance in the eye should not only see an eye specialist, but should be evaluated for cardiovascular disease and diabetes mellitus, if this has not been done. A urinary microalbuminuria test might also reveal accelerated aging of the vascular system.

Glaucoma, a chronic condition due to elevated intraocular pressure, can cause pressure on the optic nerve. Some medications can cause this, and for some patients it is idiopathic. Acute-angle glaucoma is due to a shallow anterior chamber—the patient uses medicines that cause the pupil to dilate (mydriasis) and this blocks the drainage of that anterior chamber. Anticholinergic agents, such as the botanical *Atropa belladonna*, can provoke this problem in those with shallow anterior chambers.

A swollen optic disc, papilledema, is a sign that intracranial pressure is elevated. This would suggest some kind of drainage issues in the cerebral aqueducts, or a space-occupying lesion in the cranium.

Nose

Nasal examination includes both external and internal. External findings might include hemorrhaged blood vessels (telangiectasia) or even rhinophyma as evidence of excessive alcohol intake over a long period of time. Alterations to skin appearance such as moles, erosions, or papules will require referral to a dermatologist to screen for skin cancer (such as basal cell carcinoma).

Intranasal examination shows the state of the nasal turbinates. There might be edema, puss, or growths. Sinus palpation and transillumination might show tenderness and increased density. Often a sinus CT scan is done subsequently to confirm fluid and exudate accumulation. It is also common in a patient with inhalant allergies, poor home allergen control, rhinitis, and sinus tenderness and opacity to transillumination to be treated for presumptive sinus infection.

Mouth and Tongue

Examination of the oral cavity is performed by physicians and dentists. It is a site for cancers, including tonsillar cancer that can be driven by human papillomavirus infection. A number of nutritional deficiencies can manifest in the oral cavity. Scurvy, due to vitamin C deficiency, will lead to loose teeth and spongy, easily bleeding gums. Cracks on the tongue can be due to deficiency of riboflavin or iron. Sometimes an issue such as improper oral hygiene can lead to gum disease. Some patients cannot afford regular dental care. Others consume too much sucrose and do not brush and floss enough. A thick coating on the tongue can be a manifestation of overgrowth of the yeast *Candida albicans*. This yeast is a commensal, but is opportunistic. A *Candida* overgrowth can be a sign of immune deficiency.

Ears

An irritated external ear canal is found in those who swim and those susceptible to skin infections including those from yeast and fungi. Diabetics can be more prone to this. The tympanic membrane usually reflects the light of an otoscope back at the observer, but a dull tympanic membrane can indicate fluid buildup in the middle ear (Fig. 5.3). In small children, the persistence of inflammation due to otitis media leads to fluid buildup and hearing impairment. Pediatricians will sometimes insert myringotomy tubes to drain the middle ear fluid.

In general practice, it is possible to screen for hearing loss, but audiological testing is necessary to provide precise data. A vibrating tuning fork that is placed at the vertex of the head (or high on forehead) is known as the Weber test. This action will transmit sound waves via bone conduction. If this vibratory sound lateralizes to one ear, it suggests that there is sensorineural loss in the ear that did not pick up the vibration. Placing a vibrating tuning fork in front of the ear can screen for issues with hearing—in the case of an intact nervous apparatus on an impaired ear, it should not result in lateralization in the bone conduction Weber test. Ultimately, these are screening tests, but can be important ways to catch on to a deficit that can be better analyzed with auditory tests involving various frequencies and decibel volumes.

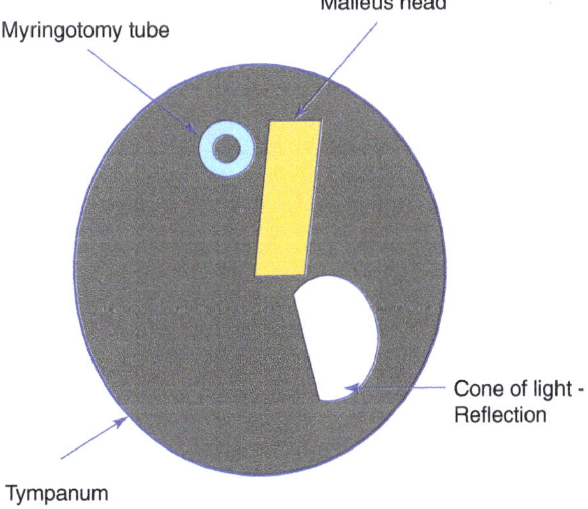

Fig. 5.3 The location of a myringotomy tube: Drainage of built up fluid in the middle ear is done to relieve the pressure and reduce risk of chronic infection

Neck

The neck in the physical exam can be divided into the anterior and posterior triangles and the anterior aspect of the trachea. When lymph nodes in these areas are palpated, it is a good idea to also palpate the submandibular area. Lymph node enlargement is going to occur due to infections in the mouth and gums and even due to pharyngitis caused by self-limiting infections. However, some cancers, such as breast cancer, tonsillar, pharyngeal, laryngeal, and lymphomas, are going to present with lymph node enlargement in the neck. Some serious lung infections, such as tuberculosis, will also cause lymphadenopathy. Tracheal deviation is a noticeable impact of soft tissue swelling. Any investigation of this region should involve gentle examination of the thyroid gland for size, symmetry, tenderness (provided the technique is very gentle), texture, and presence of nodules (Fig. 5.4).

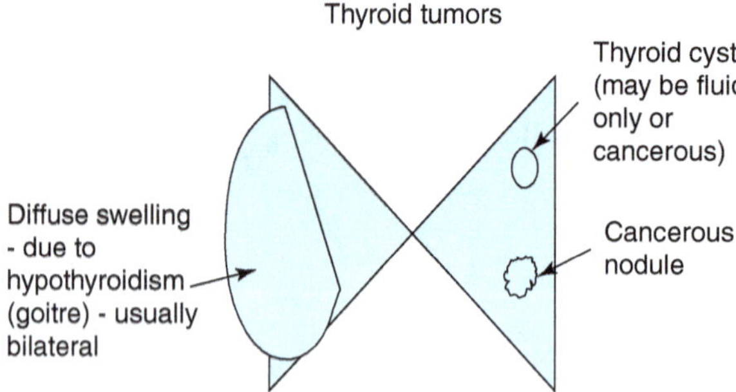

Fig. 5.4 Lesions on the thyroid: Obvious swellings and distortions of the thyroid gland can be visible, and some lesions such as cysts or tumors are detected on a gentle palpation of the gland. Although imaging and biopsy will lead to a precise diagnosis, patients may not be aware of these lesions which are uncovered in a physical examination

Heart and Lungs

The examination of the thoracic region begins with inspection. Increased anterior to posterior diameter is found in chronic obstructive pulmonary disease. The use of accessory muscles of breathing, such as the scalenes, is found in this condition. The apical impulse of the heart can be found in very thin persons.

Auscultation is done across a wide range. Posteriorly, it is done from upper lung fields (on the trapezius muscle) down to the lower lung fields (above the diaphragm) (at thoracic vertebrae 10 in the central/spinal plane but down to T12 more laterally). Auscultation should be done with the patient breathing through a relaxed open mouth, deeply but in a relaxed manner. Breath sounds are adventitious as a soft rumble. Coarser sounds, whistles, wheezes, and gurgling suggest some form of restriction or obstruction due to airway narrowing, swelling, mucus, or fluid accumulation. Percussion of the posterior lung can reveal areas of increased density where the sound is normal tympanic (so not above bone or organ). This can be due to fibrosis or tumor, but more commonly due to accumulation of fluid and exudate. The clinical term is consolidation.

Palpation and percussion can also compare the extent of diaphragmatic excursion on both sides of the back.

Auscultation on the anterior thorax also includes a series of vertical points to listen to breath sounds (Fig. 5.5). The heart auscultation points are found below the second rib, one either side of the sternum, and below the third, fourth, and fifth ribs with the fifth intercostal space point being at the midclavicular line. Percussion of the chest might reveal dullness more laterally than normal, which would be the case in left ventricular enlargement.

Even though the vital signs are done on their own and often in the absence of a heart and lung exam, the information gathered there does pertain to these organs. Pulse rate, blood pressure, and respiration rate in particular provide baseline data about heart function and oxygenation of the blood and about lung function at least indirectly.

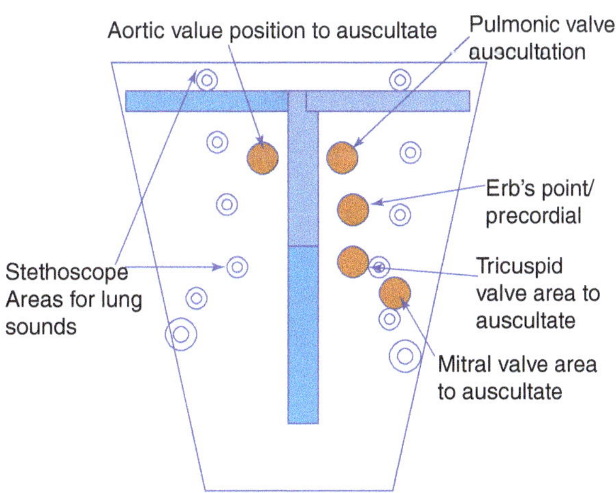

Fig. 5.5 Auscultation of the anterior chest: A pattern that covers breath sounds from various aspects of the lungs and the sounds created by the valves of the heart

The Abdomen

Abdominal exam includes signs and elicited symptoms (such as tenderness) from organs such as the liver, spleen, kidney, and uterus and from the bowel.

The examination begins with inspection. This should be done with the patient lying supine. The examiner should look at the abdomen from different angles. In thinner persons the pulsations of the aorta might be seen. A scaphoid abdomen has a C shape to it. In contrast, some patients have excessive extra-abdominal fat, which is in the tissue layer between the fascia and dermis. For others, much of the adiposity is around the organs, which might not be palpable. This is highly correlated with metabolic syndrome and diabetes. Shining the examination light in a tangential manner can bring out contracts. Blood vessel patterns, such as enlarged veins, which might accompany a protruding fluid-filled abdomen, can be a sign of liver failure. Noting the patient's facial expression is valuable as well, as peritoneal pain, or colicky pain (such as an acute episode of cholecystitis), can cause an expressionless appearance, due to the extreme discomfort.

Abdominal auscultation is done in a wide pattern that can pick up sound from some very different underlying structures (Fig. 5.6). Auscultation of the abdomen will normally pick up various bowel sounds often referred to as borborygmi. This can be rushes, pings, gurgles, etc. as fluids, semifluid chyme, and gas make their way through the intestines. Auscultation should be done in all quadrants of the abdomen and, to be thorough, should be in 12 areas. Excessive borborygmi might be heard during colonic spasm, diarrhea, or soon after a meal. A silent abdomen for a least a minute (but listening for 2 min is advised) can indicate ileus or paralysis of the bowel. This can occur due to infection, infarction, or intussusception. Bruit, a coarse vascular noise, might be detected over the aorta, renal or iliac arteries bilaterally, hepatic artery, or splenic artery.

Percussion is performed by a rapid tap. One common method is to place the distal interphalangeal joint of one middle finger on a spot and then briskly strike it in a "swinging hammer"-type movement with the tip of the other middle finger. This should be repeated across the abdomen. Different areas normally have a distinct sound. The liver should be flat, but this should end before or by the right lower costal margin. The ascending colon should be tympanic, but the terminal descending colon might be dull due to the presence of stool. If the abdomen is swollen due to fluid accumulation, as such ascites in liver failure, percussion will result in small ripples across the area. Percussion might elicit tenderness, the location of which should be noted. Percussion can show that fluid is accumulating the abdomen, or that a solid mass is encroaching on normally present structures.

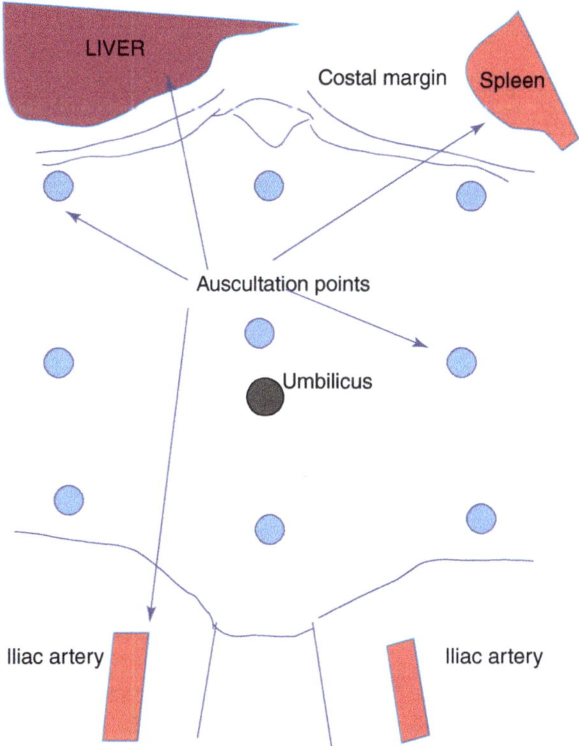

Fig. 5.6 Abdominal auscultation: Preceding percussion and palpation, the abdominal auscultation can detect bowel, vascular, and even the rub (friction produced by inflamed serosal membrane) sounds of inflamed organs

The span of the liver in various superior to inferior lines (such as the midclavicular) and the span of the spleen are suggested by this test.

Light palpation is performed after the preceding steps, and tenderness is noted (Fig. 5.7). Peritoneal irritation might lead to tenderness even in some quadrant that is not directly affected by something like an infection. One method is to put the finger pads on the abdomen and gently depress about 2 cm.

Deeper palpation, which the patient should be informed about first, can elicit information about some deeper structures. This too can elicit tenderness. The inferior surface of the liver can often be palpated. Most people will find palpation of the gallbladder region uncomfortable but not frankly painful. In patients with gallbladder disease, this can elicit sharp pain. A thorough coverage of the abdomen is worth doing. If the previous steps indicated a widening or tortuous route of the aorta, this area should not be palpated deeply because of the possibility of an aortic aneurysm.

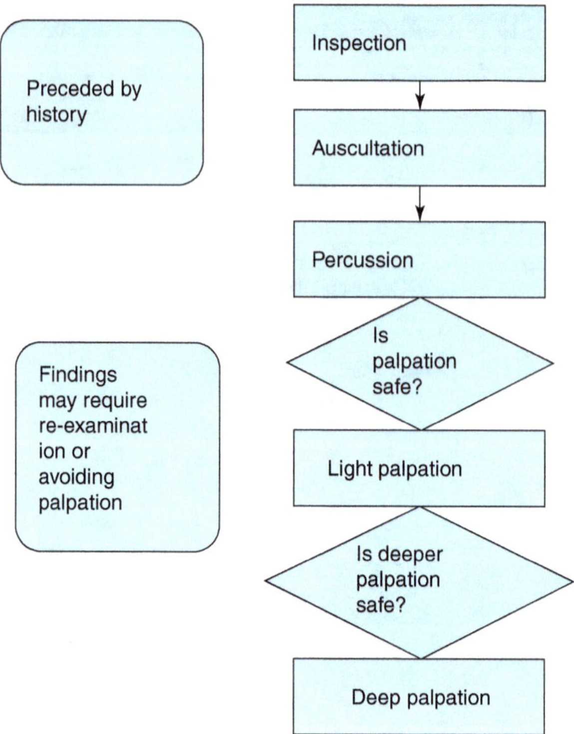

Fig. 5.7 The abdominal examination is done in a purposeful order. Auscultation can detect widening of the aorta, and the pressure of the stethoscope or very light percussion will elicit pain when the peritoneum is inflamed. This is a situation where deep palpation could cause injury. Palpating can activate bowel activity can alter the findings of auscultation, which is performed prior. This does not preclude the examiner from repeating certain maneuvers, but the introduction of each step should follow the sequence

Pulses

Peripheral pulses are an important extension of the cardiovascular examination; some of the common palpated ones are as follows:

Brachial artery—medial arm, below the biceps muscle belly.
Radial and ulnar arteries—anterior wrist (lateral and medial/radial and ulnar sides, respectively).
Popliteal artery—posterior knee.
Tibialis anterior—posterior to the ankle, anterior to the Achilles tendon.
Dorsalis pedis—dorsum of the foot.

Pulses may be detected as normal–relatively full and easy to detect pulse rate; weak and easily compressed; faint and difficult to detect; warm, tender, and edematous area (possible deep vein thrombosis); and full and bounding.

Muscles

Muscle strength can be graded by the examiner (Table 5.1). Muscle strength can be tested at various joints and joint integrity can be assessed by the following:

Asking the patient to perform full range of motion of that joint—observe for complete range of motion and smooth movement and ask the patient if there is pain.
By holding the patient's limb, move it through the full range of motion of that joint, and note restriction, pain, and a spring or resistance toward the end of the range of motion.
Stabilize the joint and then have the patient resist your pressure in one vector—note pain and relative strength.
The physician should compare the functions on all of these sides.

Muscles to test are as follows:

- Trapezius (shoulder elevators).
- Deltoid middle (shoulder abductors).
- Biceps brachii (elbow flexors).
- Wrist extensors (pronation).
- Wrist flexors (supination).
- Iliopsoas (hip flexors).
- Quadriceps femoris (knee extensors).
- Ankle dorsiflexors.
- Neck flexors.

Table 5.1 Manual muscle testing procedures

Key to muscle grading				
	Function of the muscle	Grade		
No movement	No contractions felt in the muscle	0	0	Zero
	Tendon becomes prominent or feeble contraction felt in the muscle, but no visible movement of the part	T	1	Trace
Test movement	*Movement in horizontal plane*			
	Moves through partial range of motion	1	2–	Poor –
	Moves through complete range of motion	2	2	Poor
	Antigravity position	3	2+	
	Moves through partial range of motion			
Test position	*Gradual* release from test position	4	3–	Fair –
	Holds test position (no added pressure)	5	3	Fair
	Holds test position against slight pressure	6	3+	Fair +
	Holds test position against slight to moderate pressure	7	4–	Good –
	Holds test position against moderate pressure	8	4	Good
	Holds test position against moderate to strong pressure	9	4+	Good +
	Holds test position against strong pressure	10	5	Normal

Modified from 1993 Florence P. Kendall. Author grants permission to reproduce this chart

- Gluteus medius (hip abductors).
- Neck extensors.
- Gluteus maximus (hip extensors).
- Hamstrings (knee flexors).
- Ankle plantar flexors.

https://www.niehs.nih.gov/research/resources/assets/docs/muscle_grading_and_testing_procedures_508.pdf [5].

Neurological Exam

Although imaging and special tests are often used to isolate a neurological lesion and form a specific diagnosis, the neurological exam is an important first step (Fig. 5.8). Various body regions correspond to certain levels of the spinal cord. Certain functions relate to a specific brain region or spinal cord tract.

In dermatome testing, light touch across different limb and trunk segments can confirm that dermatome innervation and CNS reception of that information is intact.

Muscle testing can not only reveal joint information but show that the myotome is intact.

Dull versus sharp (being careful to use a sterilized or single-use object) discrimination on fingers or toes and on limbs, relate to the spinal-thalamic tract.

Vibration can be tested on metacarpal-phalanges and metatarsal-phalangeal joints with a tuning fork.

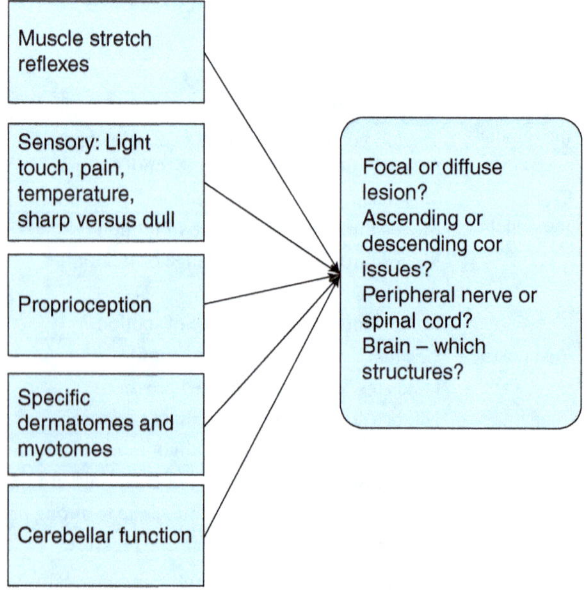

Fig. 5.8 Information derived from neurological examination: The various components of the exam, such as sensory information or cerebellar function tests, can provide evidence about the possible location of lesions in the nervous system

Proprioception can be tested by deviating the patient's great toe from flexion to extension with the patient's eyes closed and asking them to locate it.

Stereognosis can be tested by having the patient identify a common object in hand with their eyes closed.

The Rhomberg test is done with feet shoulder width apart and eyes closed. Swaying or instability (barring joint issues in the legs) suggests proprioceptive or vestibular issues.

Deep tendon reflexes are elicited by a rapid strike of certain tendons such as the patella, Achilles, triceps, biceps, and brachioradialis with a queen's hammer or less reliably with a rubber triangle. A rapidly appearing countermovement/muscle contraction is normal. Excessive movement, such as a kicking out of the leg during patellar reflex testing is noted as sluggish movement. Absence of reflexes suggests a lower motor neuron issue. Spasmodic reflexes suggest an upper motor neuron issue.

Cerebellar tests include having a patient put their finger on their nose and then touching the examiner's finger, which is held about 18 in. from their face. This target can be moved. Overshoot could suggest visual acuity issues but also implicates the cerebellum.

Some blanket tests such as tandem walking, toe walking, or squats involve multiple sensory and motor pathways.

The cranial nerves are a special group of tests and are valuable in many situations, from post-concussion examination to screen for multiple sclerosis.

Cranial nerve I: The olfactory nerve is tested when a patient sniffs a commonly recognizable odor with eyes closed (i.e., coffee grounds).

Cranial nerve II: The optic nerve can be tested with vision; in a screening sense, a basic reading chart, and a confrontation/visual field examination can suggest normal or abnormal function. Ophthalmoscopy can pick up papilledema (swelling of the optic disc) and retinal degeneration, hemorrhage, or detachment. But these screening tests ought to be followed immediately by examination by an eye specialist.

Cranial nerves III, IV, and VI are the oculomotor, trochlear, and abducens nerves. Eye movements in an even way, without excessive saccades, are the expected result. Pupillary reaction to light involves both CN II and III.

Cranial nerve V: The trigeminal nerve controls facial sensory function at the temple/forehead, malar, and mandible areas as part of screening. A cotton ball is often used. The corneal reflex depends on the CN V input.

Cranial nerve VII. The facial nerve controls the muscles of facial expression, so various expressions (smile, grimace) can test this. Although an important motor nerve, the taste receptors in the anterior two-thirds of the tongue are innervated by CN VII.

Cranial nerve VIII: The vestibulocochlear nerve receives auditory information from receptors in the auditory canals including the cochlear and positional information from the trochlea.

Cranial nerve IX: The glossopharyngeal nerve helps to control swallowing, innervating cranial muscles in the mouth and throat.

Cranial nerve X: The vagus nerve travels into the thorax and then the abdomen and has important parasympathetic (automatic) signals for the heart, intestine, and other tissues. It also has swallowing/pharyngeal functions.

Cranial nerve XI: The accessory nerve supplies the sternocleidomastoid and trapezius muscles.

Cranial nerve XII: The hypoglossal nerve supplies the tongue and some hyoid area muscle fibers.

History Taking

There are many excellent resources about how to create patient chart notes. This text will not replicate them, but some important points deserve mentioning.

The chief complaint (or complaints) should be filled out with specific attributes as possible. This should not be at the expense of allowing a patient to fully express the nature of their issue without frequent interruptions. If the interviewing style is too interrogative and brusque, the patient presenting complaints may come to reflect what the doctor led the patient to say. For example, a patient is attempting to describe a symptom presentation that is erratic, but their rather assertive clinician asks "So it's really a nighttime problem, right?" Some patients will continue, or will negate this kind of attempt (premature) at clarification, but others will let it pass.

As much as time permits, scanning for associated symptoms or other issues will help to create a well-rounded differential diagnosis.

A review of general symptoms, such as body temperature, energy levels, digestion, etc., is important for ascertaining health status, further inquiries about the determinants of health (Table 5.2), and selecting some remedies.

A medical history, past, recent, and present, is needed to put problems in context and to get to know what the patient is dealing with. Medical histories also help describe how the patient arrived in their current situation.

Current medication: This should include both prescribed and self-purchased over-the-counter medications.

Current supplements: Some patients use a very extensive array of nutrients, botanicals, homeopathics, etc.

Psychosocial history: Current or past, such as depression, anxiety, social isolation, abuse, addiction, etc.

Goals of patient care: Immediate and long term.

Concerns of patient: Past negligence of physician, financial issues, family support, or opposition to seeking naturopathic assistance.

Other health-care providers: Role, visit frequency, treatments.

Table 5.2 Overall inventory of determinants of health

Determinant	Considerations	Impact
Mother's prenatal health	Nutritional status, stress level, existing health conditions, toxin exposure, and pregnancy history	Development, birth weight, and future health risks can be influenced by prenatal health
Birth history (trauma, hypoxia, premature)	Pregnancy history, maternal health, placental position, health-care access	Developmental delays, injuries
Childhood illnesses and environment including possible toxin exposures	Infections, adverse reactions to immunization, home and water lead exposure, smoking at home	Impacts on growth, immune and allergy, CNS development
Sleep	Average hours per night, interruptions/waking, snoring and apnea, nocturia, nighttime routines, BMI	Deficient sleep increases inflammation and cardiovascular disease risk and reduces growth hormone secretion and CNS repair
Diet	Adequate nutrients, digestion and eating patterns, presence of harmful foods and take out foods	This can lead to nutritional deficiencies, burdens on the body from sugar, trans fats, chemical additives, proinflammatory foods
Hydration	Volume of water consumed per day, heat exposure, activity, diuretics, non-water beverages	Dehydration impacts brain, mucus membranes, kidneys, and muscles and increases pain
Movement, exercise	Hours moving per day, level of exertion, type of exercise (general activity, aerobic, strength, flexibility, endurance, etc.)	Movement is required to maintain circulation and keep myofascial system tuned, and health outcomes are worse with lack of movement
Breathing, allergy	Air quality in neighborhood, at work, in school, or at home, pets in home, exposure to mold	Oxygenation, stress on lungs, and exacerbation of allergy impacted by these factors
Stress levels	Mental outlook, perceptions of circumstances	High cortisol levels and chronic stress can impact immunity and health
Life satisfaction	Contentment with current circumstances	Dissatisfaction is not inherently wrong, but a chronic sense of dissatisfaction with life can lead to pessimism, perhaps poor choices about health
Socioeconomic factors	Food budget and access, economic stress, health insurance and access	Lack of food and health-care access can impact health at many levels; economic struggle, marginalization, and discrimination can take their own toll on health
Nighttime light and noise exposure	Disruption to sleep quality and regulation of circadian rhythms due to noise pollution and bedroom light exposure	Circadian dysregulation can impact various body systems

(continued)

Table 5.2 (continued)

Determinant	Considerations	Impact
Sun exposure and reaction to seasons	Sunlight activates the retinal thalamic tract and helps set circadian rhythms, creates vitamin D, and improves mode	Synchronicity with seasons in one's locality brings harmony with earth
Exposure to nature	Spending time in environments that are not human engineered	Linked to happiness and lower stress
Toxin exposure	Multiple industrial, agricultural, household, pharmaceutical, lifestyle-dietary, and natural toxins	Toxins that overwhelm the body's detoxification mechanisms can damage genes, cells, and extracellular matrix
EMF exposure	Power lines, appliances, phones	May be damaging to the central nervous system at high exposures
Viral exposure	A natural event but some viruses leave the person permanently changed	Long-term sequelae (such as post-COVID syndrome), latent infections (such as varicella zoster, measles morbillivirus)
Iatrogenic exposures	Exposure to radiation, pharmaceuticals, vaccines	Not intrinsically harmful to all, but some will have long-term damage, immune dysfunction, and mutations
History of illness and legacy	Illness and clinical course	Deficits, chronic inflammation, and compensations to illness have to be taken into consideration

Patient Experience, Goals, and Concerns

Every patient has a story to tell. It may be a short story about an acute trauma and their desire to completely recover from it. Or it may be a much longer one. If patients are given the right signals from their physician, such as an open manner, good listening, encouraging gestures, a lack of overt disapproval (which can be conveyed unconsciously by physicians), etc., they may share many things about themselves. This can include their fears and concerns about their health, or other things about their life. They may have goals such as a higher level of health. If they have not worked with a naturopathic doctor before, they may not be familiar with a model of care that not only addresses acute illness of the moment, but also seeks to work with the patient for ongoing improvement.

Informed Consent

While not strictly an assessment activity, it is part of a treatment plan, and obtaining informed consent is aided by knowledge of the patient's concerns and history. They may have had adverse outcomes from other treatments and other practitioners. They might have particular health issues, risk factors, medical conditions, etc. that factor into informed consent. For example, if they have had a history of allergic reactions to plants, gardens, fields, etc., when we prescribe an herbal medicine, we should mention that depending on the taxonomic family the herb is from, the patient may be sensitive to it.

Assessing Hypofunction

Determining that an organ or physiological process is hypofunctioning can be as straightforward as taking a careful history, performing relevant physical examination, and ordering a simple laboratory test (Table 5.3). But in some cases, the hypofunctioning of a system is below the detection of some types of tests that are calibrated to detect more advanced pathology (Table 5.4).

Table 5.3 Laboratory testing

Test or panel	Components	Purposes
Comprehensive metabolic panel	Albumin, a liver protein Alkaline phosphatase (ALP) Alanine aminotransferase (ALT) Aspartate aminotransferase (AST) Blood urea nitrogen (BUN) Calcium Carbon dioxide, an electrolyte Chloride, an electrolyte Creatinine Glucose Potassium, an electrolyte Sodium, an electrolyte Total bilirubin Total protein	Screen for hepatic dysfunction Screen for electrolyte imbalances Check albumin protein levels (low liver disease or negative nitrogen balance due to malabsorption, renal losses, poor intake) Screen for kidney function, muscle damage Detect extremes in glucose levels Screen for overhydration or dehydration
Complete blood count	White blood cells Red blood cells Hemoglobin Hematocrit Mean corpuscular volume Mean corpuscular hemoglobin Mean corpuscular hemoglobin concentration Platelets	Number of white blood cells (depressed or increased due to infection or neoplasia) Screen for anemia due to lack of red blood cells but ultimately lack of hemoglobin Red blood cell average volume and variety of sizes as clues about the etiology of anemia (i.e., microcytosis/small-volume RBC could be due to iron deficiency) Platelets to detect hyper- or hypocoagulability states Polycythemia states (too many RBCs) * There are male and female differences with RBC and hemoglobin
White blood cell differential	Neutrophils Lymphocytes Monocytes Eosinophils Basophils	Can show immune activation or lack of function Particular type might suggest bacterial, allergic, parasitic/helminthic infection
Prothrombin time (PT)	Extrinsic pathway (factor VII) and common pathway	Prolonged in vitamin K deficiency, vitamin K antagonist therapy (warfarin), and factor VII deficiency
Diabetic diagnosis	Fasting blood glucose Random blood glucose Glycosylated hemoglobin 2-h 75-g oral glucose tolerance test (OGTT)	All can be diagnostic although fasting blood glucose and HA1c are the most reliable and practical

(continued)

Table 5.3 (continued)

Test or panel	Components	Purposes
Extended hepatic screen	PT/INR Serum albumin Serum bilirubin (total) Serum bilirubin (direct) Alanine aminotransferase (ALT) Aspartate aminotransferase (AST) Alkaline phosphatase (ALP) Gamma-glutamyl transferase (GGT)	Clotting problems due to liver disease Destruction of liver cells (transaminases) Protein synthesis
Lipid panel	Total cholesterol LDL cholesterol HDL cholesterol Triglycerides	Shows overall lipid levels, potentially atherogenic low-density lipoprotein and triglycerides and protective high-density lipoproteins. The HDL ratio (total cholesterol divided by HDL) or the non-HDL cholesterol level (everything except HDL) are often used as risk predictors
Thyroid panel	Thyroid-stimulating hormone (TSH) T4 (thyroxine) T3 (triiodothyronine)	Used as a group to determine if thyroid hormone levels are too high or low, if the problem is primary (gland) or secondary (pituitary), and if sufficient convection to T3 is happening
Thyroid immune markers	Thyroid peroxidase antibody, thyroglobulin antibody, and TSH receptor antibody	Screens for autoimmune thyroid conditions including processes that destroy thyroid gland tissue and those that cause agonism or antagonism to the TSH receptor
Cortisol test	Blood Urine Saliva	Can help in the diagnosis of hyper or hypo adrenal states, as well as prolonged general adaptation syndrome and decompensation states associated with chronic stress
C-reactive protein	CRP hsCRP	Different assay methods have different reference ranges. C-reactive protein is elevated in inflammation, which can be due to infection or autoimmune activity. It is a good predictor of cardiovascular morbidity and mortality, especially in conjunction with other risk factors
Hormone panel female	Estradiol, total estrogens, DHEA, total testosterone, free testosterone, progesterone (may also include luteinizing hormone and follicle stimulating hormone)	The day of the menstrual cycle (if applicable) is relevant to the choice of reference ranges. This panel can reveal deficiencies, excess, and imbalances
Hormone panel male	Total testosterone, free testosterone, androstenedione, estradiol, DHEA, progesterone (may also include luteinizing hormone and follicle stimulating hormone)	This panel can reveal deficiencies, excess, and imbalances

Table 5.3 (continued)

Test or panel	Components	Purposes
Heavy metal screens	Arsenic Lead Mercury	In addition to serum screens for these heavy metals, complete blood counts, with examination of red blood cell morphology (and in the case of lead, basophils)
Lyme disease panel	Serology testing for *Borrelia burgdorferi*: Sensitive enzyme immunoassay (EIA) or immunofluorescence assay, followed by a Western immunoblot assay for specimens yielding positive or equivocal results. Follow-up may be a second EIA DNA testing for the presence of *Borrelia burgdorferi*	Simple screen tests lack sensitivity, and results should be clinically correlated
Babeosis	*Babesia microti* IgG Ab *Babesia* DNA *Babesia* FISH assay	Microscopic examination of blood samples is diagnostic
Rheumatoid arthritis panel	Anti-cyclic citrullinated peptide Carbamylated protein (CarP) antibody, IgG Rheumatoid factor	Needs to be clinically correlated with physical exam and radiological findings
Nutritional panel bariatric surgery	Vitamin D Folate B12 Ferritin Albumin Zinc	Malabsorption issues may lead to other nutritional deficiencies
Celiac antibodies	Antibodies: antigliadin; deamidated gliadin peptide; anti-transglutaminase 2; transglutaminase 2; anti-reticulin; R1-type reticulin; endomysial	There is a wide variety in serology and clinical presentations, a trial of a completely gluten free diet is necessary

*Females have an average hemoglobin 12% lower than the male average. The average male has 5 million RBCs and the average female has 4.5 million RBCs

Table 5.4 Examples of hypofunction across organ systems

Tissue or organ system	Signs of hypofunction
Cardiovascular	F2 isoprostane test—reveals increased oxidative stress in the arterial environment
Pulmonary	Mild aberrations on spirometry; pulse oximetry
Small intestine	Dyspepsia or mild malabsorption
Large intestine	Constipation
Liver	Fatigue or headache on exposure to environmental toxins (household cleaning chemicals, diesel fumes, volatile organic compounds)
Central nervous system	Slight decreases in working memory, slight losses in learning efficiency
Renal system	Small decreases in glomerular filtration rate, barely detectable microalbuminuria
Musculoskeletal system	Myofascial tightness, physical deconditioning on physical examination

Assessing Lack of Circulation and Communication

Circulation and communication issues can emerge subtly, but at this stage, the right tests can detect changes in flow, secretion, perfusion, etc. (Table 5.5). This level of dysfunction can exist alongside other types of dysfunction, but it may manifest earlier in the long disease process.

Table 5.5 Examples of lack of communication and circulation across organ systems

Tissue or organ system	Signs of lack of circulation and communication
Cardiovascular	Decreased peripheral circulation on Doppler test, decreased performance on treadmill test
Pulmonary	Ratios on spirometry indicate obstructive, restrictive, and capacity issues
Small intestine	Stool elastase test; secretin stimulation test; lactulose-mannitol test for excess permeability
Large intestine	Sitz marker colonic transit time study; scintigraphic emptying and transit
Liver	Ultrasound to detect hepatic steatosis
Central nervous system	Ultrasound testing of carotid blood flow; intracranial pressure monitoring; EEG (seizure disorders)
Renal system	GFR calculation; ultrasound of kidney, ureter, and bladder (volume)
Musculoskeletal system	Nerve conduction velocity

Assessing Inflammation

Inflammation is a natural response to injury. It facilitates remodeling of damaged or dysfunctional tissue. When inflammation is becoming a clinical issue, there are observable and measurable changes in tissues and organs (Table 5.6). Sometimes the intensity of the inflammation is higher than normal, and it may persist longer than a normal inflammatory process which is self-limiting and resolves itself once the tissue has healed.

Table 5.6 Examples of inflammation across organ systems

Tissue or organ system	Signs of inflammation and immune involvement
Cardiovascular	High-sensitivity C-reactive protein Asymmetric dimethylarginine Oxidized LDL
Pulmonary	Sputum culture; chest radiograph
Small intestine	Breath test for methane, CO_2, hydrogen
Large intestine	Stool analysis; urinary organic acid tests
Liver	Transaminase levels: AST, ALT
Central nervous system	CSF analysis
Renal system	Microalbuminuria; urinalysis; cystoscopy
Musculoskeletal system	Nerve biopsy

Deeper Inflammation and Immune Involvement

What sets deeper inflammation apart is the more aggressive actions by the immune system (Table 5.7). More destructive processes can begin, which unfortunately can attract yet more attention from the immune system. This stage of dysfunction will be very noticeable on imaging or laboratory testing, and with a few exceptions (atheromas in the cardiac arteries can proceed silently to a point), the patient will report signs and symptoms that suggest a deeper inflammation.

Table 5.7 Examples of deeper inflammation and immune involvement across organ systems

Tissue or organ system	Signs of deeper inflammation and immune involvement
Cardiovascular	Myeloperoxidase; lipoprotein-associated phospholipase A2
Pulmonary	Bronchoscopy/bronchial lavage; lung CT scan; fractional exhaled nitric oxide (FeNO) tests
Small intestine	Tissue transglutaminase; upper endoscopy/capsule endoscopy
Large intestine	Colonoscopy, large intestine CT scan, stool analysis; fecal blood
Liver	Gamma glutamyl transferase; lactate dehydrogenase, conjugated and unconjugated bilirubin
Central nervous system	Lumbar puncture with cell count, cell types, glucose, protein, and culture; head CT; head MRI; blood tests for pathogens depending on patient history
Renal system	Microalbuminuria to creatinine ratio
Musculoskeletal system	Muscle biopsy; creatine kinase or creatine phosphokinase, aldolase, lactate dehydrogenase, myoglobin

Assessing Fibrosis, Tissue Damage, and Extracellular Matrix Degeneration

A reaction to injury that physically and often permanently alters the structure of the organ or tissue is the hallmark of stage (Table 5.8). Sometimes the reaction is exaggerated, but often, the damaging factor (such as alcohol intake that precedes cirrhosis) has been chronic. When this stage of dysfunction is reached, the extracellular matrix has degenerated and changed in function. This ensures that a chronic, degenerative process has begun. This can be mitigated and resolved to some extent.

Table 5.8 Examples of fibrosis and extracellular matrix degeneration across organ systems

Tissue or organ system	Signs of fibrosis, tissue damage, matrix degeneration
Cardiovascular	Heart CT, heart biopsy, angiogram
Pulmonary	Lung biopsy, lung CT
Small intestine	Small intestine biopsy, barium X-ray
Large intestine	Barium X-ray, colonoscopy and biopsy, colon CT; fecal blood
Liver	Hepatic ultrasound, hepatic CT, liver biopsy
Central nervous system	MRI of head and spinal cord
Renal system	Kidney biopsy
Musculoskeletal system	Muscle biopsy, bone DEXA scan

Decline of Function

This level of dysfunction results in clinical syndromes that require medical attention (Table 5.9). They are threatening to life and can decompensate rapidly. They often lead to situations where some extrinsic support is needed to maintain homeostasis.

Table 5.9 Examples of decline of function across organ systems

Tissue or organ system	Signs of decline of function
Cardiovascular	Left ventricular ejection fraction; nuclear heart scan
Pulmonary	Lung diffusion capacity test; lung volume test, lung volume test
Small intestine	Serum levels of protein and nutrients; xylose absorption test
Large intestine	Colonoscopy, fecal analysis for proteins, fats, parasites, and yeast
Liver	Serum ammonia; serum albumin; clotting time tests (i.e., PT)
Central nervous system	Mental status tests; cognitive performance tests; positron emission tomography (PET)
Renal system	Urine albumin, glomerular filtration rate
Musculoskeletal system	Electromyography; muscle and nerve biopsy

Neoplasm and Screening or Diagnostic Tests

Neoplasm, or cancer, is not always the direct outcome of degenerative changes. A mutation that creates a lineage of cells that eventually transform into neoplastic cells can occur within an otherwise healthy organ (Table 5.10). The degenerative organ however is one with disturbed extracellular matrix, poor circulation and immune access, and often a fair amount of cellular damage.

Table 5.10 Examples of tests to detect neoplasm across organ systems

Tissue or organ system	Tests that are used for investigating cancer (note: these are sometimes done in a screening setting in general practice; others are performed by an oncologist to arrive at a definitive diagnosis, with typing and staging of cancer)
Cardiovascular [6]	MRI, CT, biopsy
Pulmonary [7]	CT, chest X-ray, PET/CT scan, thoracocentesis, sputum cytology, fine-needle aspiration biopsy (transtracheal/bronchial/thoracic); molecular tests EGFR, ALK, KRAS
Small intestine [8]	CT, MRI, barium X-ray, endoscopy, capsule endoscopy, biopsy
Large intestine [9]	Fecal immunochemical test (FIT), guaiac-based fecal occult blood test (gFOBT), stool DNA test, colonoscopy, CT colonography (virtual colonoscopy)
Liver [10]	Angiography, biopsy: Laparoscopic, needle, surgical; ultrasound, CT, MRI; alpha-fetoprotein blood (AFP)
Central nervous system [11, 12]	MRI; magnetic resonance angiography (MRA) and magnetic resonance venography (MRV); magnetic resonance spectroscopy (MRS); magnetic resonance perfusion; functional MRI; CT angiography; PET scan; stereotactic (needle) biopsy; surgical or open biopsy (craniotomy); lumbar puncture Children, above plus: Gliomas: IDH1 or IDH2 gene mutations Oligodendrogliomas: 1p19q co-deletion In high grade gliomas: MGMT promoter methylation
Renal system [13]	Urine cytology, MRI, CT, angiography, ultrasound, biopsy/Fuhrman grade
Musculoskeletal system [14, 15]	Muscle biopsy; radiograph, CT, MRI, PET scan Biopsy: Core-needle, fine-needle aspiration, open surgical
Hematologic [16]	

References

1. Krogsbøll LT, Jørgensen KJ, Gøtzsche PC. General health checks in adults for reducing morbidity and mortality from disease. Cochrane Database Syst Rev. 2019;1(1):CD009009.
2. Artandi MK, Stewart RW. The outpatient physical examination. Med Clin North Am. 2018;102(3):465–73.
3. Garibaldi BT, Olson APJ. The hypothesis-driven physical examination. Med Clin North Am. 2018;102(3):433–42.
4. Russell SW, Garibaldi BT, Elder A, Verghese A. The power of touch. Lancet. 2020;395(10230):e63.
5. Sciences NI of EH. Manual muscle testing procedures [Internet]. https://www.niehs.nih.gov/research/resources/assets/docs/muscle_grading_and_testing_procedures_508.pdf.
6. Hudzik B, Miszalski-Jamka K, Glowacki J, Lekston A, Gierlotka M, Zembala M, et al. Malignant tumors of the heart. Cancer Epidemiol. 2015;39(5):665–72.
7. American Cancer Society. Lung cancer diagnosis [Internet]. https://www.cancer.org/cancer/lung-cancer/detection-diagnosis-staging/how-diagnosed.html.
8. American Cancer Society. Tests for small intestine cancer [Internet]. https://www.cancer.org/cancer/small-intestine-cancer/detection-diagnosis-staging/how-diagnosed.html.
9. American Cancer Society. Colorectal cancer: early detection, diagnosis, and staging. https://www.cancer.org/cancer/colon-rectal-cancer/detection-diagnosis-staging.html.
10. American Cancer Society. Tests for liver cancer [Internet]. https://www.cancer.org/cancer/liver-cancer/detection-diagnosis-staging/how-diagnosed.html.
11. American Cancer Society. Tests for brain and spinal cord tumors in adults [Internet]. https://www.cancer.org/cancer/brain-spinal-cord-tumors-adults/detection-diagnosis-staging/how-diagnosed.html.
12. American Cancer Society. Tests for brain and spinal cord cancer in children [Internet]. https://www.cancer.org/cancer/brain-spinal-cord-tumors-children/detection-diagnosis-staging/how-diagnosed.html.
13. Capitanio U, Montorsi F. Renal cancer. Lancet. 2016;387(10021):894–906.
14. American Cancer Society. Bone cancer diagnosis [Internet]. https://www.cancer.org/cancer/bone-cancer/detection-diagnosis-staging/how-diagnosed.html.
15. American Cancer Society. What is rhabdomyosarcoma [Internet]. https://www.cancer.org/cancer/rhabdomyosarcoma/about/what-is-rhabdomyosarcoma.html. Accessed 21 May 2022.
16. Huntington S. Blood cancers [Internet]. https://www.yalemedicine.org/conditions/blood-cancers. Accessed 21 May 2022.

Further Reading

Davis JL, Murray JF. History and physical examination. In: Murray and Nadel's textbook of respiratory medicine; 2016. p. 263–77. https://doi.org/10.1016/B978-1-4557-3383-5.00016-6.

Khattak ZE, El Sharu H, Bhutta BS. Overview on ordering and evaluation of laboratory tests [Internet]. https://www.ncbi.nlm.nih.gov/books/NBK570615/.

Papadakis MA, McPhee SJ, Rabow MW. Current medical diagnosis and treatment 2020. New York: McGraw Hill; 2020. https://accessmedicine.mhmedical.com/content.aspx?bookid=2683§ionid=222924373. Accessed 21 May 2022.

Smith F. Introduction to principles and practices of naturopathic medicine. Kingston: CCNM Press; 2008.

Chapter 6
Therapeutics within a Naturopathic Approach

Botanical Medicine

Relation to Determinants of Health

Botanical medicines can act much like a food, and some of them are commonly eaten foods, such as artichoke, dandelion, and garlic. As a by-product of other effects—essential functions such as sleep, digestion, and breathing can be improved with botanical medicine.

The line between plants as medicines and foods is often difficult to see. Historically, in Hippocratic medicine, and in many other systems, such as Traditional Chinese Medicine, Ayurveda, and Unani, food was considered therapy. Biochemically, the body does not differentiate between an active molecule that was eaten as food or taken in a capsule. But there are differences in dose and delivery. Biologically active molecules in a food are embedded in a matrix of cellulose, tannins, lipids, etc. In medicines that are prepared for use in botanical therapy, these substances are usually extracted in some way, with water (as in an infusion) or with ethanol and water, as in an herbal tincture. Some preparations go even further and concentrate certain molecules in the medicine.

Some foods that are both edible and easy to obtain that have powerful phytochemical effects include the following:

- *Cynara scolymus* (artichoke): hepatoprotective, hypolipidemic [1].
- *Taraxacum officinale* (dandelion): hepatoprotective, diuretic, chemopreventive [2].
- *Vaccinium* species: *V. macrocarpon* (cranberry), bladder antiseptic [3]; *V. myrtillus* (bilberry), vascular tonic, astringent [4].
- *Glycine max* (soy): phytoestrogen [5].

F. Smith, *Naturopathic Medicine*, https://doi.org/10.1007/978-3-031-13388-6_6

Botanical Medicine: Relation to Hormetic Applications to Support Adaptive Responses

Botanical medicines contain numerous compounds that are active in the body. Many of these actions are of a hormetic nature. Hormetins work in the very-low-dose zone and exert an effect that is about 120%–150% above control value [6]. This action is on a J- or U-shaped curve, with a different possible action than what is typically considered to be the effect (at larger doses) of the substances (Fig. 6.1). Note that these are not ultradilutions, just small doses between 0 and the amount at which observable adverse effects are possible. Hormetic effects are not present in all substances, but approximately 40% of herbal extracts and drugs exhibit some hormetic effects in bioassay.

Some botanical extracts exert an antioxidant effect that goes beyond the common (and indeed very useful) action as a free-floating antioxidant. For example, in *Brassica oleracea* (broccoli), an antioxidant is an inducer of an antioxidant response element via NRF2 [7]. Small amounts of *Cruciferae* can activate (via dissociation from the protein KEAP) NRF2 to migrate the nucleus and bind to the antioxidant response element. This leads to greater expression and transcription of genes that lead to the production of an antioxidant, or "phase 2" enzymes, such as glutathione synthase.

Neuroprotective hormetins introduce a mild stressor to the neurologic tissues [8] (Fig. 6.2). The adaptive response that this creates is defined by the expression of pro-survival proteins. An example is the expression of genes that lead to

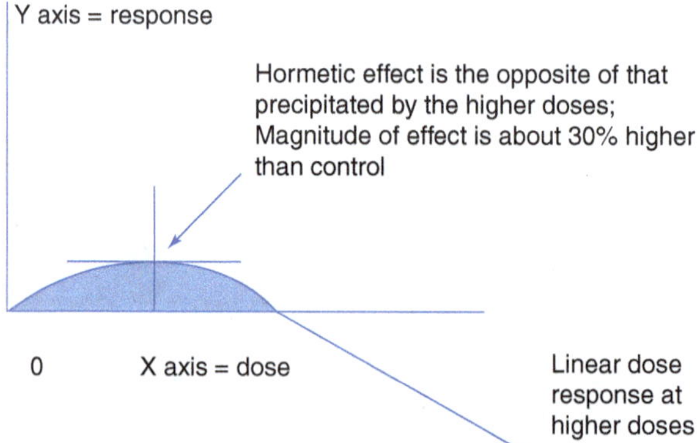

Fig. 6.1 Hormetic dose–response curve: As described by Calabrese [6], the hormetic dose–response is found in a significant number of substances. It is characterized by a modest stimulatory effect in the low-dose range, often peaking at a midpoint between a dose of zero and the dose at which observable adverse effects could theoretically be seen. The J- or U-shaped dose–response curve is biphasic, with the hormetic effects (which can be adaptive, preconditioning, etc.) seen in the lower-dose range and a linear effect at higher doses. These linear effects can proceed for some range of doses that are still at a generally tolerable level and comprise what is typically thought of as the effect of a substance (at least based on bioassays and therapeutics that do not measure for or consider the hormetic zone)

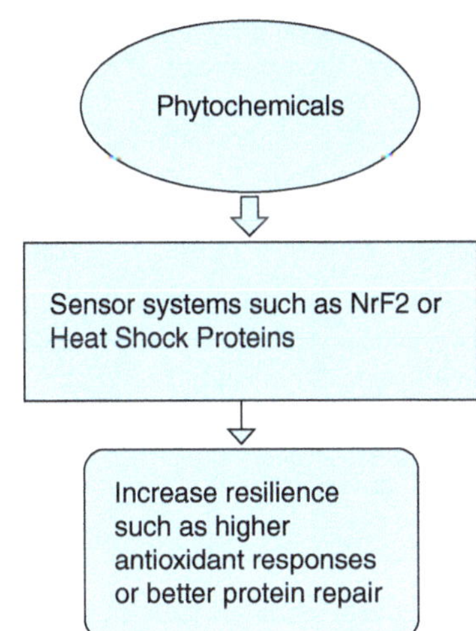

Fig. 6.2 As Calabrese, Mattson, and others have outlined [7–9], the cellular response to essentially benign phytochemicals can elicit gene expression that is protective and adaptive, with benefits for many systems including the nervous system

neurotrophic factors in the brain, as a response to exercise, or botanical hormetins [9]. Another is the activation of repair processes to deal with misfolded proteins [10]. Some herbal extracts can precondition the body to better withstand future stressors. *Ginkgo biloba* has the ability to precondition neural tissue in the central nervous system to ischemia [11].

In this way, botanical hormesis is a way of switching on *pro-survival responses that* strengthen the body.

Botanical Medicine: Relation to Specific Biochemical Support of Adaptive Responses

Botanical extracts can elicit a variety of adaptive resources at the cellular and extracellular matrix level. Below are examples of major organs and tissues.

Digestion

Botanical medicines that support digestion can be meant to enhance normal functions such as secretions and muscle contraction and peristalsis. They can also be used to relieve muscle spasm or colic and reduce nausea. These two uses can be mutually reinforcing.

Digestive stimulation often comes in the form of compounds that bind to bitter taste receptors (Fig. 6.3). These include the TAS receptors [12]. These are located on the tongue, but also throughout the gastrointestinal tract. Bitter taste receptors are also found in other tissues such as the lung. Binding leads to increased secretions and peristalsis. This is facilitated by the release of the hormone

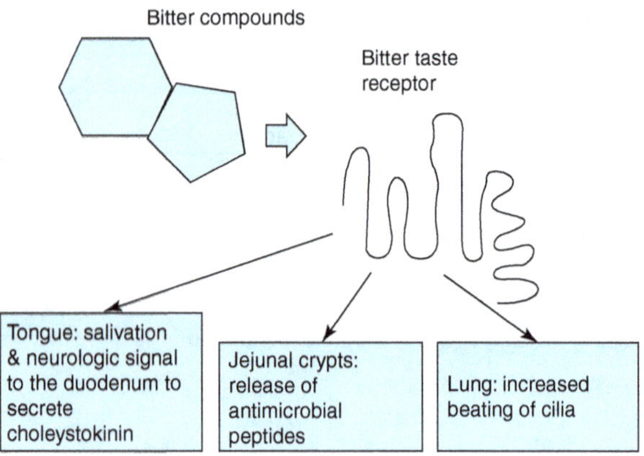

Fig. 6.3 Bitter taste receptors: The activity and actions of bitter compounds go far beyond the tongue. Digestive activation, as well as protective responses, such as increased pulmonary cilia beating, or the release of antimicrobial compounds in the jejunal crypts, results from the binding of specialized receptors to bitter compounds

cholecystokinin, which activates the stomach, small intestine, gallbladder, and pancreas. For this reason, the same bitter compounds that increase salivation and stomach acid secretion will also encourage the gallbladder to contract and release bile.

Carminative herbs have compounds that often relax smooth muscle and have an antispasmodic effect on the gastrointestinal tract [13]. They also have aromatic compounds that stimulate secretions in the mouth (saliva and digestive enzymes) and gastric acid and pepsin.

The support of digestion goes very far beyond the utility of relieving symptoms for those who suffer from dyspepsia. Some botanical substances have a sensitizing effect on the insulin receptor. This can lead to a reduction in insulin resistance.

Liver: Biliary Functions

Biliary flow is necessary for both disposal of waste products that have been processed by the liver and for the digestion of fat. Although the gallbladder will store bile and release larger quantities of it when stimulated by bitter taste receptor binding or the presence of fat in the mouth and stomach, the bile is produced by hepatocytes. A drainage effect of thousands of small channels, the bile canaliculi, creates a *flow* of bile through the liver. If this is obstructed, it can lead to hepatitis and become a medical emergency.

Liver Detoxification–Biotransformation

The actual chemistry of what the hepatocyte accomplishes is remarkable. The mixed-function oxidase—cytochrome P450—will act on substrates that are taken up in the cell. This immediately creates an intermediary that is reactive due to an unpaired electron. The intent of this reaction is to then pair that radical molecule with a side chain and, in so conjugating the two, create a water-soluble and nontoxic compound that can be disposed of in the bile, or the urine.

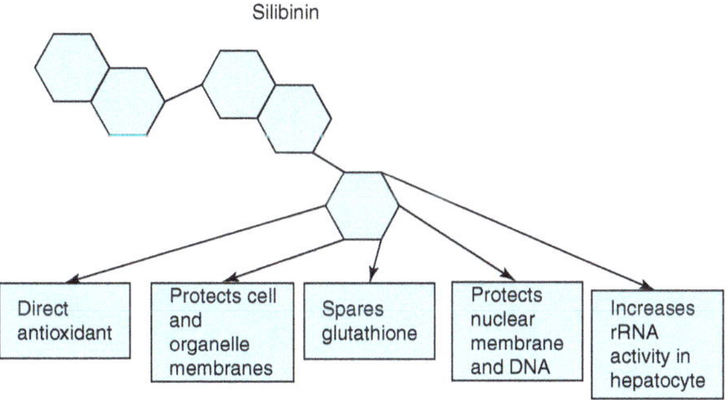

Fig. 6.4 Silibinin, a flavonolignan from *Silybum marianum*: Silymarin, a group of flavonolignans that include silibinin, protect hepatic cells at a number of levels—direct free radical scavenging and the sparing of glutathione, protection of organelle membranes including nuclear membranes, cell membrane stabilization, and increased of transfer RNA

To do this successfully requires conjugation of side chains, such as acetyl and methyl groups, amino acids, sulfur, glucuronic acid, and glutathione. It also requires bystanding antioxidants. Not all electrophilic species produced by P450 reactions instantly find their way to a conjugate molecule. Damage to the hepatocyte can occur if this is not squelched. There are many herbal compounds, including the polyphenolic herbs, that are excellent at protecting the liver cell from free radical damage. Other substances have an additional effect of stabilizing and protecting organelle, nuclear, and cellular membranes. An example is the well-known botanical *Silybum marianum* or milk thistle (Fig. 6.4). This plant contains flavonolignans that stabilize membranes and protect them from the kind of dissolution that leads to cell death. The crude extracts of the plant contain far less of the active constituents than the commonly used, and thoroughly studied, standardized extract (which contains 80% silymarin—the flavonolignans considered the active compounds).

There are many other herbs that have *hepatoprotective* properties. *Cynara scolymus* (artichoke), *Schisandra chinensis* (magnolia berry), and *Taraxacum officinale* (dandelion) [14].

Arteries

Arterial impact of herbal medicines range from decreasing autonomic–sympathetic tone to protecting the endothelium from oxidation. The actions on the inside of the vascular system is critical. The oxidation of low-density lipoprotein creates more opportunities for oxLDL to damage the intima of the arteries. This is followed up by white blood cell migration into the artery to attempt to mop up the oxidized LDL particles. These scavenging macrophages often die, full of cholesterol, and begin creating what becomes an atheromatous plaque. This "foreign body" in the intima of the artery does not go unnoticed by the immune system. Neutrophils attack, and their inflammation actually creates more plaque growth including more oxidized

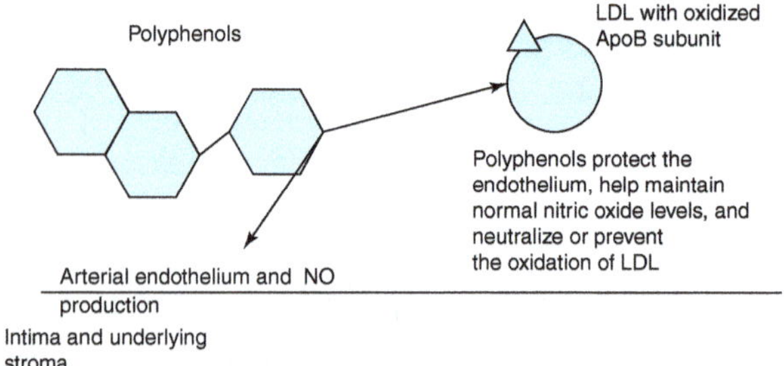

Fig. 6.5 Polyphenols and vascular protection: Polyphenolic molecules directly protect the vascular endothelium and neutralize oxidized LDL that can damage the endothelium

LDL. A positive feedback loop ensues. Plant-derived antioxidants, polyphenols, flavonoids, and terpenes can all work to lower oxidized LDL, quell inflammation, and support healing and restoration of function (Fig. 6.5) [15]. This effect is not an absolute one, and there is no plant-derived substance that simply "switches off" atherosclerosis. However, as evidenced by the many benefits seen in a Mediterranean diet, these plant-derived compounds (in addition to other benefits of that dietary pattern, including consumption of healthy fats) can decrease inflammation and promote cardiovascular health.

Myocardium

The myocardium is an energy powerhouse, depleting its ATP every few seconds. This requires superactive mitochondria that burn up fatty acids as well as glucose. This also requires a blood supply that can deliver the nutrients and oxygen necessary for this level of aerobic metabolism. Botanicals such as *Crataegus oxyacantha* can both vasodilate the coronary arteries and support the aerobic metabolism of heart muscle cells [16]. *Panax ginseng* [15] can support cardiac output, and *Astragalus membranaceus* can reduce cardiac enlargement (a reaction to declining function), inflammation, and cell death [17].

Pulmonary Epithelium

The lining of the lung is a specialized tissue. It must be in contact with the outside world, and therefore, it is capable of rapid inflammatory responses. Cilia help move mucus out of the bronchi and bronchioles. Mast cells release histamine as a frontline defense. Herbs that help expel mucus include *Prunus serotina* (cherry bark), *Pulmonaria officinalis* (lungwort), and *Eriodictyon californicum (*yerba santa). These botanicals usually contain a resin or a sapoin that irritates the esophagus and promotes the cough reflex. Other expectorant herbs can work by loosening secretions and relaxing bronchial smooth muscle. Herbs that contain terpenes such as

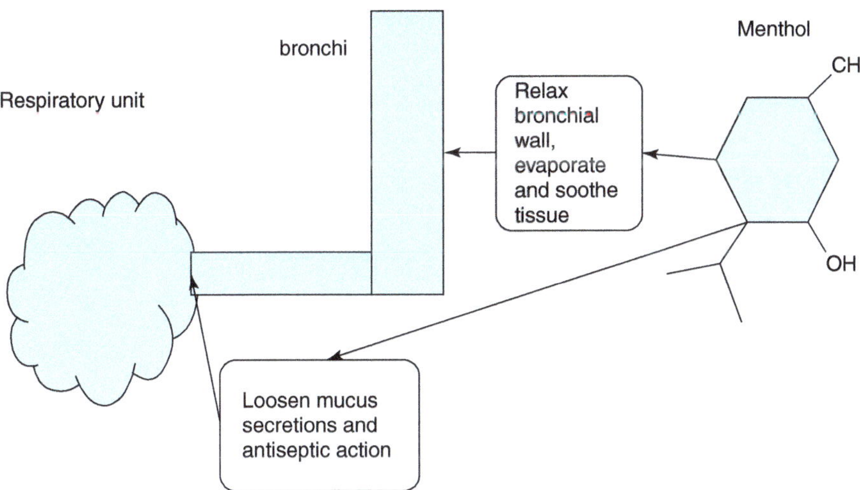

Fig. 6.6 Terpenes and the lung: Monoterpenes such as menthol and eucalyptol have multiple actions on the bronchi and smaller airways. They are cooling, antispasmodic–bronchodilating, and antiseptic and can loosen tenacious mucus

Eucalyptus globulus and *Mentha piperita* (peppermint) can do this by the relaxing effect of monoterpenes and diterpenes on the bronchial smooth muscle. These "essential oils' 'can also have a cooling and soothing effect on the bronchi (Fig. 6.6). Many plant extracts have an antioxidant effect that is directly beneficial to the lung [18].

Central Nervous System

Many herbs act on the central nervous system. Very often, these plants contain alkaloids. These are compounds that contain nitrogen and are synthesized from amino acids (Fig. 6.7). Alkaloids have an affinity for receptors of the nervous system. Another example would be the harman alkaloids from *Passiflora incarnata* (passion flower) which have a relaxing effect [19]. Alkaloids such as codeine from *Papaver somniferum (*poppy) [20] are well known for their central nervous system action. Other compounds, such as valerianic acid from *Valeriana officinalis* (valerian) can bind to GABA (gamma-aminobutyric acid) receptors, inducing a state of relaxation [21].

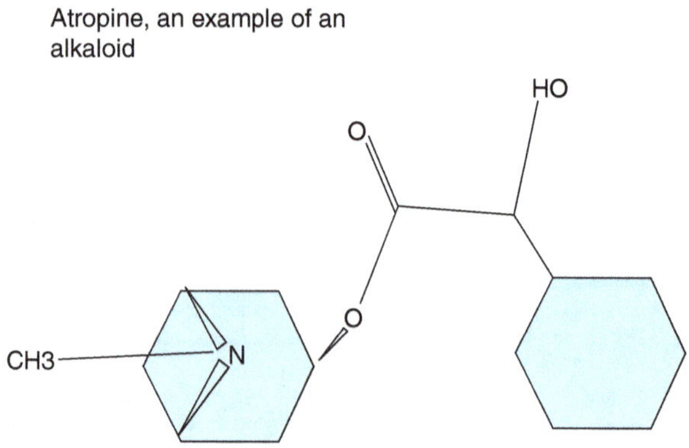

Fig. 6.7 Atropine: This alkaloid contains nitrogen, is basic, and when precipitated is a white powder. Alkaloids generally have these traits with a few exceptions

Atropine, an example of an alkaloid

Hippocampus

Some plant extracts have been shown to have a protective effect on the hippocampus and midbrain structure essential to learning and memory. *Ginkgo biloba, Panax ginseng, Hypericum perforatum,* and *Bacopa monnieri* are examples [22]. These herbs sometimes have compounds that actively boost certain aspects of brain processing—such as increasing catecholamine or acetylcholine concentrations in the brain. But in a protective sense, preventing oxidative stress, programmed cell death, and the accumulation of amyloid protein in the hippocampus is important for long-term brain health (Fig. 6.8).

Another example is Melissa officinalis, or lemon balm [23]. This herb is calming to the mind and helps relax the enteric nervous system, which makes it useful in irritable bowel syndrome in patients who have anxiety. It has also been found to be neuroprotective, even improving cognitive skills in patients with early dementia. The plant has a strong antioxidant effect (which makes it helpful for hypertension, relaxing blood vessels and providing antioxidant support).

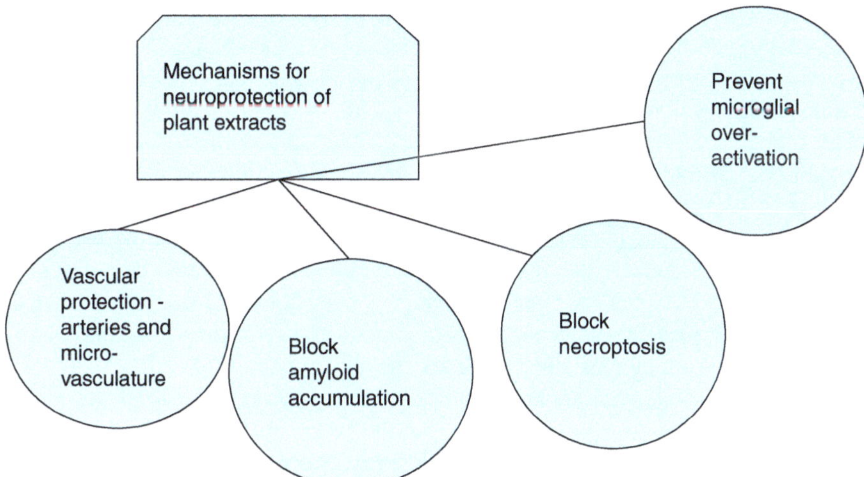

Fig. 6.8 Neuroprotection from plant extracts: Some of the compounds from plants appear to have antioxidant but also inflammation attenuating effects that could benefit the brain

Botanical Medicine: Generalized Support

Adaptogens

The term adaptogen was first proposed in 1940 by a scientist from the USSR, namely, N. Lazarev, when he described *Schisandra chinensis* (Turcz.) Bail. and other herbs with the following definition: plant-originated adaptogens that can non-specifically enhance the human body. These substances must meet three criteria: first, adaptogens must be nonspecific and must assist the human body in resisting a wide range of adverse conditions, such as physical, chemical, or biological stress. These may include environmental pollution, climate change, radiation, infectious diseases, and interpersonal disharmony. These substances must meet three criteria: first, adaptogens must be non-specific and must assist the human body in resisting a wide range of adverse conditions, such as physical, chemical or biological stress. Second, adaptogens must support homeostasis, the ability of the body to stay in a state of balance. Third, adaptogens must not harm the normal functions of the human body. Brekhman and Dardymov, 1969, added to this that plant-originated adaptogens must reduce the harm caused by stressed states, such as fatigue, infection, and depression; plant-originated adaptogens must have positive excitatory effects on the human body; in contrast to traditional stimulants, the excitatory effects produced by plant-originated adaptogens must not cause side effects such as insomnia, low protein synthesis, or excessive energy consumption; and fourth, plant-originated adaptogens must not harm the human body [24].

As the physiology of stress and adaptation became better understood, newer and more precise mechanistic explanations for the observable effects of adaptogens were proposed. In the 1990s, Hildebert Wagner, George Wikman, and Alexander Panossian stated that adaptogens are natural bioregulators that increase the ability to adapt to environmental factors and avoid the damage caused by those factors. Wagner and colleagues also said that the advantage of adaptogens is they minimized the bodily response to stress, reducing the negative reactions during the alarm phase and eliminating, or at least decreasing, the onset of the exhaustion phase that is part of the so-called general adaptation syndrome [24]. This clearly builds upon the work of Nobel laureate Dr. Hans Selye, who pioneered the stress concept and research, including the model of the general adaptation syndrome [25]. In 1998, the American Food and Drug Administration (FDA) defined an adaptogen as a new kind of metabolic regulator that has been proved to help in environmental adaptation and to prevent external harms. Adaptogen has been generally used as a functional term.

Yance and others added to this understanding an ability of adaptogens to tune the hypothalamic–pituitary–adrenal axis [26]. He stated that adaptogen functions mainly by affecting the hypothalamic–pituitary–adrenal (HPA) axis in response to stimulation by external stress. Primary adaptogens can not only maintain or recover homeostasis and allostasis but can also promote anabolic recovery. Primary adaptogens can produce positive stress response and the associated hormone expression.

Immunomodulators

Immunomodulating herbs typically work by providing an input to some aspects of the immune system, which causes a signaling effect, which in turn influences the actions of an immune response. Botanical extracts do not program the immune system the way that natural encounters with antigens and with nature do, or in a narrower sense, the way that vaccinations do. They do not give someone immunological memory. But they can stimulate the response.

One example that is widely used is *Echinacea* species. This plant is native to North America. The Lakota nation used it, and later, the Eclectic physicians adopted it. Three species are commonly used: *E. purpurea*, *E. angustifolia*, and *E. pallida*. It was used for fevers, relapsing infections, and indigenous medicine for snakebite. The herb was in the National Formulary well into the twentieth century. Interest in it declined as allopathic medicine made its leap from using natural products and semisynthetics to using mostly synthetic substances (which were deemed de facto superior as medicines for both acute and chronic issues). *Echinacea* sp. contains polysaccharides and a type of compound called alkylamides [27]. The polysaccharides bind to the surfaces of T cells and various scavenger cells—and can cause upregulation of the immune response but, in some cases, a dampening of excess inflammation. The alkylamides are interesting in that they are taken up by macrophages and then can reduce inflammatory responses, including the production of NfκB, which can drive up inflammation. Perhaps this explains *Echinacea*'s symptom reduction effect in viral and bacterial infections. One of the polysaccharides, Echinacoside, has anti-hyaluronidase effects. This can reduce the extent of inflammatory damage to connective tissue. Speculatively, this might have helped in cases of snakebite, where powerful enzymes in the venom that include hyaluronidase can melt away skin to allow a neurotoxin to penetrate through to the bloodstream.

Mushrooms and fungi contain polysaccharides, which can be broken down to beta-glucan molecules. These are usually 1,3- and 1,6-beta-glucans. There are receptors for these molecules on many types of immune cells (Fig. 6.9). The glucans are taken up by antigen-presenting cells, including dendritic cells and then presented to white blood cells. They can in some cases act via the complement receptor as well [28].

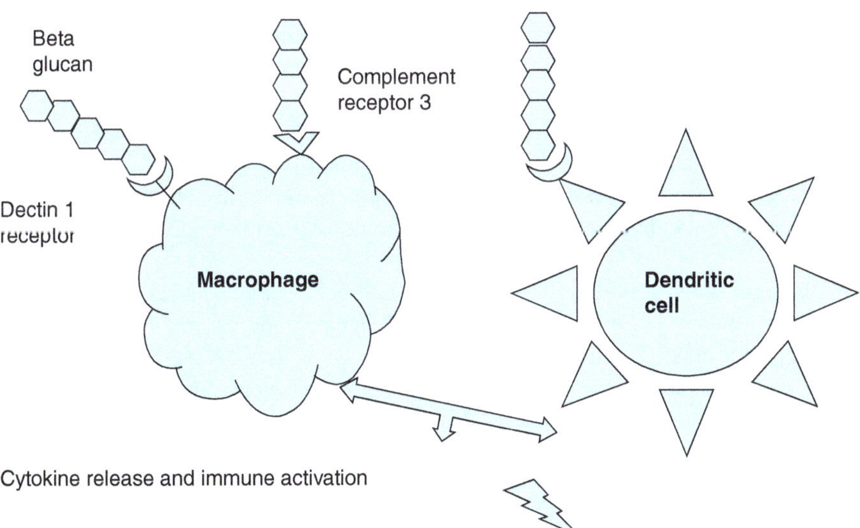

Fig. 6.9 Beta-glucans and antigen-presenting cells (APCs): Beta-glucans can bind to APC at dectin-1 or complement receptor 3 sites. This can upregulate an immune response

Mushrooms can also contain terpenes and proteins. An example of a terpene-containing mushroom is *Grifola frondosa*, or reishi mushroom, which has benefits for metabolic syndrome and has hepatoprotective actions [29]. Mannose-binding lectins and other proteins found in many mushrooms, including the edible mushroom, *Agaricus bisporus*, can block viral binding in the human body [30]. Interestingly, the plant *Ginkgo biloba* also contains similar lectins.

Mushrooms have a complex action on the immune system, generally upregulating function. However, some doses of mushrooms can elicit cytokines that are associated with the downregulation of inflammation. This may be due to either a complex entourage effect of mushroom compounds or a type of U-shaped curve to doses—a biphasic effect [31].

Botanical Medicine: Relation to Dampening Maladaptive Responses

Botanical medicines can be important tools to support patients who are suffering with a pathological state and to limit damage. An example would be the substance resveratrol, a stilbene molecule found in many plant foods and in high amounts in grapes. Resveratrol acts as an antioxidant but it can do more. It can recondition the vascular endothelium. It will work to restore eNOS in the endothelium, leading to more nitric oxide availability, which increases blood flow to the heart and makes blood vessels less stiff. It can reduce inflammation and tone down white blood cell attacks in the vicinity of atherosclerotic lesions (a process which leads to more inflammation, more damage to the artery, and more white blood cell response).

Anti-inflammatory effects abound in herbal medicine. Some of these are due to mild hormetic inputs or general antioxidant functions, as mentioned above. But botanical extracts can be more pointedly anti-inflammatory. *Curcuma longa* can directly inhibit NfκB and reduce inflammation [31]. Certain fractions of *Astragalus membranaceus* and *Ganoderma lucidum* (a fungus) [32] can exert an antifibrotic effect. So can *Silybum marianum,* more specifically the highly concentrated flavonolignan in a standardized extract of this plant (milk thistle) known as silymarin [31].

Curcuma longa act through a remarkable number of targets and cell signal transduction pathways and work to alleviate renal, hepatic, and cardiac fibrosis. This is of great importance, as in many disease processes; as the oxidative stress in a diseased tissue increases and the extracellular matrix that nourishes and protects this tissue becomes inflamed, the matrix metalloproteinases will become activated. The extracellular matrix, which is contiguous with the cells of that tissue type, becomes rigid and less adept at bringing nutrients in and removing wastes and toxins. This is a major event not only in aging and slowly degenerating diseases such as osteoarthritis, but also reactive and often lethal diseases of the organs.

Autonomic Nervous System

Some of the nervine herbs mentioned above are excellent tonics for the autonomic nervous system. These induce relaxation. Some botanicals directly impact the ANS. For instance, *Rauwolfia serpentina* (*Rauwolfia/Rauvolfia*) contains an alkaloid—reserpine—that can reduce the formation of norepinephrine-containing vesicles in the diencephalon [33] (Fig. 6.10). This leads to less adrenergic activity, and this is why *Rauwolfia* is used to lower blood pressure. This action is at a higher center of control. The pure alkaloid reserpine is a blood pressure medication for third-line use. The drug can deplete norepinephrine in the brain too efficiently, leading to severe depression. This is why an herb like *Rauwolfia*, while safe at typical herbal doses, is considered more along the lines as an agent to dampen maladaptive resources versus true biochemical support.

Some herbal substances have the opposite effect and are adrenergic in nature. They bind to adrenergic receptors in the sympathetic nervous system. An example, which is off the market due to abuse in weight loss products, is *Ephedra sinica,* which was used to suppress appetite and induce thermogenesis. *Ephedra* species contain two important alkaloids: ephedrine and pseudoephedrine [34]. These alkaloids in pure form are used as drugs for asthma and nasal congestion. They are also the original template for amphetamine. In the United States, pseudoephedrine tablets must be purchased across the counter from a pharmacist, versus off of the store shelf. This is because it is relatively simple to convert ephedrine and pseudoephedrine into methamphetamine, a potent drug of abuse.

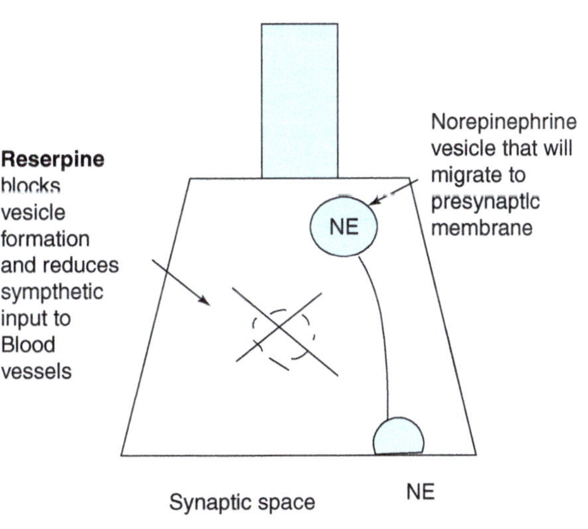

Fig. 6.10 Reserpine: The alkaloid reserpine can lower the available norepinephrine for sympathetic nervous system activation at the level of the diencephalon. This reduces blood vessel tone. High amounts of reserpine, as that used in pharmacological preparations, can impact mood, especially in those already suffering from a depressive disorder

Ephedrine will bind to the sympathetic nervous system receptor at an allosteric site and make that receptor more activated by its natural ligands: norepinephrine and epinephrine. Hence, taking ephedrine in a case of bronchospasm has a sympathomimetic effect and causes bronchodilation.

Botanical Medicine: Creation of Physiological Constants in Situations Where the Body System Cannot Do So Independently

Some botanical medicines can act as true natural pharmacology, more or less rivaling pharmaceutical preparations in their ability to create a predictable effect due to binding at a specific receptor site. Pharmaceutical preparations have a much wider range of selections and a very deep evidence base for this action. Sometimes the physiology, structure, and biochemistry of the body are so damaged that an external agent is needed to create a homeostatic balance. The use of herbs at a nutritive and supportive level aims at creating a homeostatic state. In the use of higher-dose herbs that have specific site binding and pharmacological actions (and this is true for most pharmaceuticals), the aim is to fix certain physiological constants in place. A pharmaceutical example would be a sodium-depleting diuretic for a patient with hypertension who is a natural high renin secretor. This diuretic will reduce sodium levels in the body, with the secondary action of lowering blood pressure.

The compounds from herbs that can in a sense override certain processes and enforce a given state have a strong receptor agonism or antagonism. In the case of agonism, they bind to a receptor, and much like the natural ligand, they elicit the second messenger effects that are naturally an extension of that receptor. Antagonists bind to the receptor, but do not elicit the normal effects. But they do prevent the natural ligand from binding at that site.

The assertive biological effects are often due to the presence of alkaloids, but there are other important compounds as well. Alkaloids are a group of plant compounds that contain nitrogen, are basic, and precipitate into a white powder (there are exceptions). Much of modern synthetic pharmacology is derived from alkaloids. For example, *morphine* is an alkaloid from the plant *Papaver somniferum* (opium poppy) [35]. The "*-ine*" suffix is the typical ending for the name of an alkaloid: morphine, colchicine, and epinephrine are all alkaloids. These compounds have a high affinity for receptors in the nervous system, both central and peripheral, which have a lot to do with their efficacy.

Anticholinergic Alkaloids

This are often called "belladonna alkaloids" because they are naturally present in the plant *Atropa belladonna* [35]. They are found in other plants such as *Datura stramonium*. The botanical *Atropa belladonna* (belladonna, deadly nightshade) contains tropane alkaloids such as hyoscyamine and its derivative scopolamine and, notably, atropine. These alkaloids, atropine being a prime example, are anticholinergic medicines. Atropine binds to muscarinic receptors in the parasympathetic nervous system. This makes atropine selective for terminal or effector-level parasympathetic synapses—where the nerve meets the organ or tissue. It is used to raise the heart rate in some emergency settings. It is also carried by military personnel in theaters of war where nerve agents might be used, as atropine is an antidote for some of these poisons. Scopolamine is used for motion sickness and to prevent postanesthesia nausea and vomiting.

Atropine does not bind to nicotinic receptors in the ganglia. This is advantageous, as ganglionic blockers are too diffuse in their actions and too dysregulating to be practical in day-to-day medicine. When atropine binds to a muscarinic receptor in the bronchi, or gut, or sphincter of Oddi, it blocks out (competitively antagonizes) the neurotransmitter acetylcholine. This leads to less parasympathetic activity and more sympathetic effects.

These alkaloids are the original anticholinergic agents. They are selective for the postsynaptic neurons of the parasympathetic nervous system, specifically the muscarinic receptors at target tissues. It is used to raise the heart rate in some emergency settings. It is also carried by military personnel in theaters of war where nerve agents might be used, as atropine is an antidote for some of these poisons. Scopolamine is used for motion sickness and to prevent post anesthesia nausea and vomiting.

This specificity for muscarinic receptors versus receptors at the ganglionic level is what makes them practically useful, atropine being a prime example of a useful and muscarinic-binding anticholinergic medicine (Fig. 6.11). Ganglionic blockers, on the other hand, are too wide ranging and disruptive. An anticholinergic drug has a specific downregulating effect on parasympathetic activity. The herb *Atropa belladonna* is used to relieve gastrointestinal spasm. If the slow-wave actions of the colonic muscle are disorganized, and a high level of tonicity is creating smooth muscle spasms and pain, then anticholinergics will constrain this action. Of course, this is not a curative measure; it is a palliative one that alters physiology. Another use of *Atropa belladonna* would be to relieve spasm of the sphincter of Oddi (gallbladder). This herb has more affinity for the enteric system, versus the neuromuscular junction. But synthetic anticholinergics such as benztropine do work more in this area, hence its use for tremor and spasm in patients with Parkinson's disease.

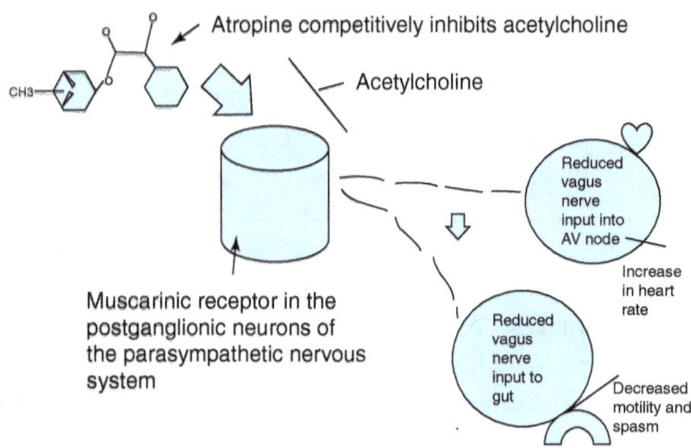

Fig. 6.11 Atropine and parasympathetic nervous system: Atropine binds to the muscarinic receptors in the parasympathetic nervous system and competitively inhibits atropine at those sites. This can reduce parasympathetic input into the particular organ or tissue, such as reducing vagus nerve input at the AV node, which causes heart rate to rise

The atropine from *Atropa belladonna* was well known to cause mydriasis, or dilation of the pupil, which was in fact a cosmetic use of the herb in the past. Modern cycloplegic drugs used in a dilated fundus exam use isomers of this same substance. Anticholinergics were used, in very small and probably hormetic-level doses, to treat mania and agitation in mental health facilities in the early twentieth century.

The toxicity of belladonna alkaloids includes tachycardia, which results from the inhibition of the vagal nerve input to the AV node (which normally acts to slow the heart rate), dry mouth, dilated pupils, and the progression to agitation, delirium, and fatal arrhythmias.

In the nineteenth and early twentieth century, small doses of *Atropa belladonna* was used to combat opium poisoning as well as withdrawal symptoms from opium and alcohol [36].

Monoamine-Enhancing Compounds

Monoamine oxidase alkaloids are a class of compounds that block the enzyme that breaks down monoamines such as serotonin, dopamine, and norepinephrine. Drugs that block monoamine oxidase are an earlier form of treatment for depression. *Hypericum perforatum* (St. John's wort) has this action, but the mood effects of *Hypericum perforatum* come from a variety of compounds that act synergistically. The traditional Iranian herbal medicine *Peganum harmala* (African rue, Syrian rue) has very strong monoamine oxidase inhibition attributed to its harmine alkaloids. This plant can be hallucinogenic [37].

MOA inhibition from herbs can have an additive effect with that of drugs, and MOA inhibition itself can interact with certain drugs. Patients consuming a large amount of vasoactive amines, such as tyramine from aged cheddar cheese, might experience toxicity due to their inability to break the monoamines from the food source down at the synaptic level.

Blood Pressure-Lowering Alkaloids

Essential hypertension can be such a persistent problem that some chemical intervention becomes necessary, even after sodium restriction, magnesium and calcium supplementation, and stress management have been employed. While there are certainly effective pharmaceuticals for this situation, including older classes of drugs such as diuretics, beta-adrenergic blockers, and calcium channel blockers and angiotensin-converting enzyme inhibitors and angiotensin receptor blockers, there are herbal medicines that can control blood pressure. Because these herbal compounds tend to work through the nervous system, they have limits in the case of patients who have high renin and aldosterone levels, which are not amenable to adjustments to the sympathetic nervous system.

Rauwolfia serpentina

As mentioned above, the autonomic nervous system effects of *Rauwolfia* have been observed for a long time. *Rauwolfia serpentina* or snakeroot has been used in traditional Ayurvedic medicine for centuries. It was used as a sedative, in accordance with the principles of Ayurveda. In the twentieth century, one of the most bioactive compounds in the plant, the indole class alkaloid reserpine, was studied as a blood pressure drug [33]. The herb already had been used by eclectic physicians for high blood pressure and as a mental calming agent in mental health hospitals. Published research in the 1940s and 1950s and further chemical analysis showed promise, with substantial scientific work done in the native country of the plant—India. Reserpine is a powerful alkaloid, but it acts more gradually in lower concentrations in an herbal extract, than in the purified alkaloid used as a pharmaceutical agent. This furthered its use as an antihypertensive. The most recent systematic review of reserpine shows that it is an effective medicine for hypertension. Reserpine blocks adrenergic activity in the presynaptic neurons that control blood vessel tone. This is accomplished by blocking vesicular monoamine transporters, so that norepinephrine in the presynaptic neurons cannot be packaged into vesicles which would normally migrate to the presynaptic cell membrane when a depolarizing wave arrives, fuse with the membrane, and release norepinephrine into the synapse. This heralds the main problem with reserpine, in which it can worsen or in some cases induce (at higher doses) depression. The action of reserpine is not so selective that it only targets the presynaptic neurons in the autonomic nervous system. This decrease in an important catecholamine can impact mood, an effect that is in opposition to the effects of a drug such as atomoxetine. While *Rauwolfia* tincture (whole plant extract) is much safer, it is not an herb for those with depression or at risk for depression.

Viscum album

This herb is commonly known as mistletoe. It has been used as an adjunctive cancer treatment in Germany for over 100 years, and it has shown some efficacy in blocking kinase enzymes towards an antiproliferative effect on tumor cells. Current research on this plant is focused on its role in adjunctive care in conditions such as breast cancer, used in addition to standard medical treatments. Much modern use and research are ongoing, and at the very least, it has a well-established use in countries, where it can be given intravenously, to support immune function and improve quality of life for those undergoing chemotherapy [38].

The tinctures of the whole plant can have a positive effect on blood pressure. *Viscum album* can increase nitric oxide synthase, which dilates blood vessels [39]. Nitric oxide can desensitize muscle contractile fibers towards calcium and decrease intracellular calcium. This is an effect that is opposite to what we see with the steroidal glycosides of *Digitalis purpurea* and *D. lanata*. *Viscum album* compounds, including oleanic acid, directly block calcium channels as well, resulting in a dual action in combination with increased nitric oxide synthase activity. This herb can therefore vasodilate in a powerful way. The increase in nitric oxide production suggests that this herb is protective to the vascular endothelium as well. Because of its antiproliferative properties, *Viscum album* is absolutely contraindicated in pregnancy—a blocking of mitosis could be catastrophic for a developing human.

Assertive Pain-Blocking Compounds

Piscidia erythrina, also known as Jamaican dogwood, is a potent pain relief (anodyne in herbal medicine nomenclature) and sedative. While not as efficacious as drugs from the opioid class, it does have strong pain relief. This herb might be used for a patient with migraine, or with craniofacial or peripheral nerve pain, or insomnia due to pain [40].

BacterioStatic Compounds in High Doses

Berberine-containing herbs such as *Hydrastis canadensis, Mahonia aquifolium, Mahonia vulgaris,* and *Coptis chinensis* contain a type of isoquinoline alkaloid that can be inhibitory to the growth of bacteria [41]. The alkaloid include berberine and hydrastine. Very high doses for too long a period of time can elevate transaminase levels, perhaps due to the stress of detoxifying the quinone aspect of these alkaloids. These bacteriostatic botanical extracts are not actual antibiotics but, at higher doses, have some ability to reduce microbial activity. The purified alkaloid, berberine sulfate, is used as a supplement (Fig. 6.12). Interestingly, a study that fractionated the herb *Hydrastis canadensis* into components and then tested pairs of compounds to look for synergy in the inhibition of *Staphylococcus aureus* determined that a flavonoid in the herb works synergistically with the alkaloid. *S. aureus* has an antiporter

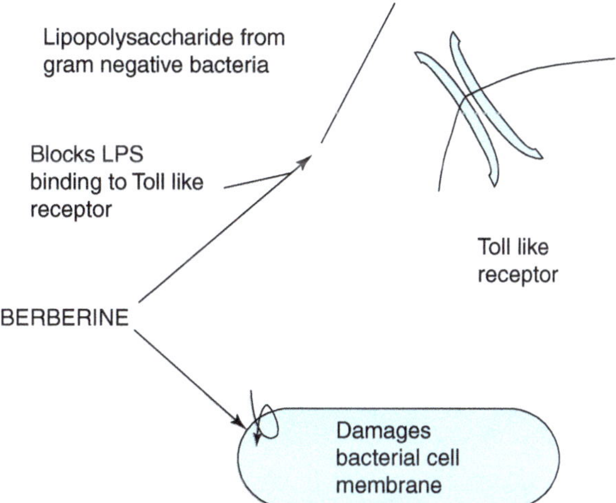

Fig. 6.12 Berberine: An isoquinoline alkaloid found in plants such as *Hydrastis canadensis*, *Mahonia aquifolium*, *M. vulgaris*, and *Coptis chinensis*, berberine can inhibit the growth of some bacteria. It can also block binding of lipopolysaccharides (a toxic compound from gram-negative bacteria) to toll-like receptors, preventing the inflammation that this activates

mechanism, an efflux pump that would normally remove some of the berberine and hydrastine from the bacterial cell. This flavonoid inhibits the efflux pump, rendering the *S. aureus* more vulnerable to the action of the alkaloids. Thus, the complexity of plant medicines in this case, and in many other instances, enhances the efficacy of whole extracts of the herb versus isolated compounds.

Laxative Effects of Anthraquinone-Containing Herbs

Botanical laxatives are commonly used, and the most reliable mode of action is the presence of anthraquinone glycosides. These molecules contain anthrones, a quinone-containing molecule. When ingested, they pass to the large intestine where they have their sugar molecule removed by gut bacteria. This is the point at which they become activated. Examples of sources include *Rhamnus purshiana* and *Cassia acutifolia* (*Cascara sagrada* and *Senna*—which are both readily available as over-the-counter preparations) [42]. These activated anthrones will stimulate nerve endings in the colon (enteric plexus) but will not damage them. A more important action is chloride secretion into the gut lumen. This causes water to follow. The rush of more water into the colon leads to distention and peristalsis, which result in more bowel movements (Fig. 6.13). Although some concern about increased risk of colon cancer exists, a systematic review indicates this is not supported. Long-term use is not advised, as this can deplete electrolytes from the body, including potassium. It can also impart a dark pigment to the colonic epithelium, which might make a colonoscopy exam more difficult to do. These compounds, since they have a quinone molecule, do put some burden on the hepatic detoxification systems, which is another reason to avoid long-term use. For those with neurologic damage which might necessitate some laxative effect for life, these herbs should be used at lower doses and rotated with other types of laxatives, such as magnesium salts.

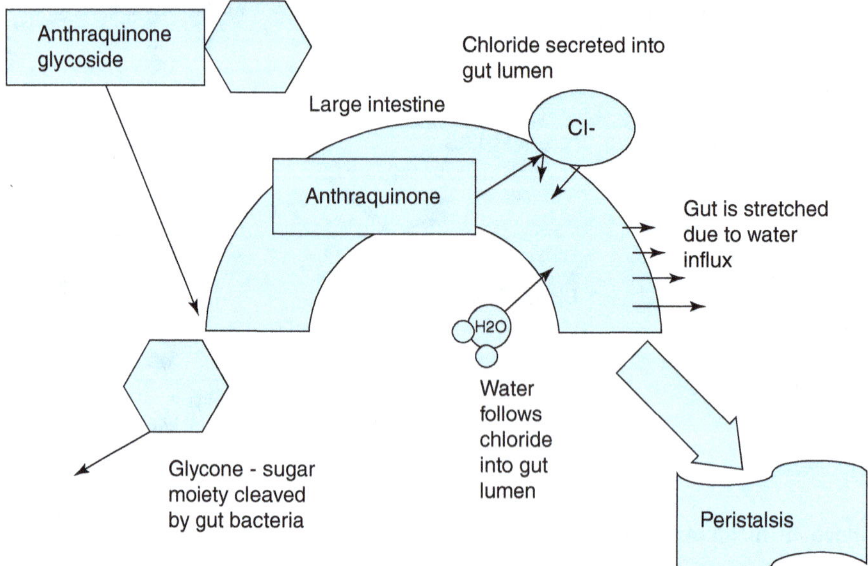

Fig. 6.13 Anthraquinone laxatives: Plants such as *Cascara sagrada* contain glycoside molecules that become active when gut bacteria cleave them, releasing an anthracene molecule. This compound can cause chloride secretion into the gut, which water follows, leading to expansion of the colon and peristalsis

Cardiac Stimulation: The Cardiac Glycosides

Digitalis lanata and *Digitalis purpurea* are plants that are native to the Mediterranean region and Western Europe [43]. They are found worldwide now and have a long history of use for cardiac illness, particularly heart failure. These plants contain steroidal glycosides. *Digitalis lanata* contains other steroidal saponins, one called digoxin, and *Digitalis purpurea* contains digitoxin. Both are available as prescription medications with the more tolerable digoxin being prescribed far more commonly. Digoxin is used for heart failure and certain arrhythmias. These steroidal saponins have the ability to increase the concentration of calcium in the cardiac myocyte (Fig. 6.14). This leads to more calcium binding to the actin–myosin binding site of troponin in these cells—which leads to more forceful contractions. The manner in which this increase in calcium is achieved within the muscle cells of the heart is key to understanding the potential (and easily induced) toxicity of digoxin (or in the case of *Digitalis purpurea,* digitoxin). Digoxin inhibits the sodium/potassium ATPase in the cell membrane of these heart muscle cells. This alters the balance of cations—with the concentration of potassium intracellularly decreasing. This does not eliminate the gradient (of more sodium outside the cell, more potassium inside), but it does make the concentration gradient less steep. The cell membrane has an exchanger protein that will allow a sodium ion to enter the cell and ejects a calcium ion at the same time. With the concentration gradient disturbed, the

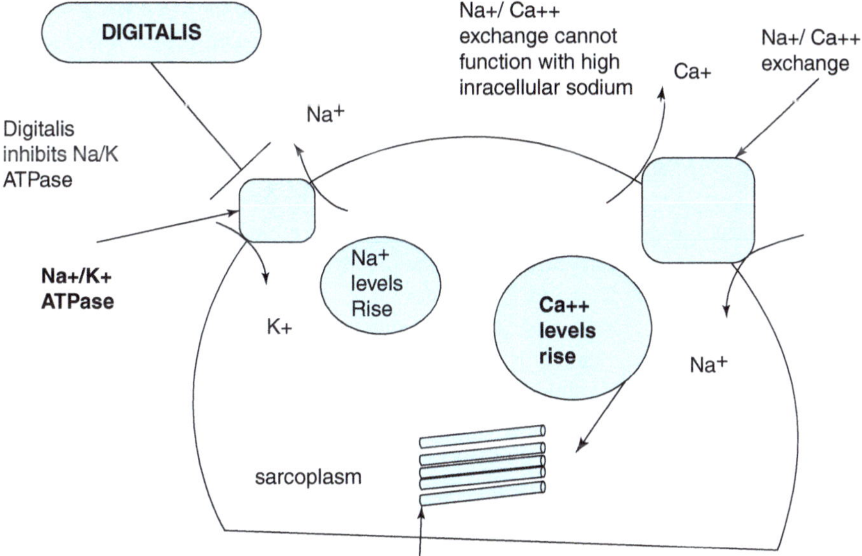

Fig. 6.14 Mechanism of digoxin: Digoxin, one of the compounds found in *Digitalis lanata* and *D. purpurea*, increases the force of cardiac contraction. Calcium is sequestered in the myocytes, due to blockade of the Na + K+ ATPase. The increase in calcium can lead to greater actin–myosin binding and more cardiac work. *Digitalis* species must be used with great care. One mode of toxicity comes from the disabling of Na + K+ ATPase, which all cells, especially those with excitable membranes, depend upon to maintain the normal gradients of intracellular and extracellular sodium and potassium

motive force for sodium is decreased, and so with sodium entering the cell less readily, there is less ejection of calcium ions. This is where the calcium concentration in the heart muscle cells can increase.

While the idea of forcing the heart muscle cell to contract more forcefully for patients with left ventricular dysfunction seems like an ideal solution, it has its drawbacks. One of them has to do with the very mechanism of inhibition of the sodium/potassium ATPase. This protein is ubiquitous in the body and is a major aspect of the maintenance of homeostasis. Any excitable membrane, nerves, and muscles are very sensitive to fluctuations in these concentrations. The fact that digoxin can deaden transmission of depolarizing signals is one important way in which it can help with certain types of arrhythmias. By reducing excessive or chaotic depolarization in the heart, it can reduce risks in some types of arrhythmias. If this inhibition of the sodium/potassium ATPase goes further, it can start to cause electrically dysfunction, including cardiac arrhythmias (which lower doses might have helped) and lead to hospitalization and death. Another is the very long half-life of these molecules. These molecules tend to bioaccumulate. Anyone taking cardiac glycosides such as digoxin needs to have their blood levels monitored regularly, as they can gradually build up to toxic levels. If this happens, the patient will at first experience nausea, the strange visual disturbances, and it can progress to cardiac arrest. Low serum levels of potassium prior to starting the drug, which is found in some patients taking diuretics for the treatment of hypertension, can make the digoxin more toxic.

Another drawback is that there are diminishing returns to stimulating cardiac output. This is why the pharmacological treatment of heart failure shifted in the 1970s to reducing peripheral resistance, with the eventual arrival of drugs such as angiotensin-converting enzyme blockers. Some morphological issues such as a calcified aortic valve can make digoxin dangerous.

Still, digitalis has in the past and continues to be used in situations where an uptick in cardiac output can be therapeutically advantageous. The left ventricle has the responsibility for pumping oxygenated blood to the organs, limbs, and head. If the pump action of the left ventricle is not strong enough, a series of adaptations such as increased renin release by the kidneys will ensue. Gains in performance by digitizing a patient can pay off in cardiac output and increase quality of life.

The herbal medicine, the diluted (traditionally a 1 in 10 dilution) tincture of *Digitalis lanata,* can be used effectively, in conjunction with an overall plan of treatment. The lower amounts of cardiac glycosides in a judiciously used tincture (provided that caution is taken) might allow for more latency between the beginning of symptoms such as nausea and dangerous cardiac electrical disturbance. This allows for adaptation to dose or even cessation of the medicine. *Digitalis* steroid glycosides are an excellent example of herbally derived products that can lock biological processes into place, to maintain homeostasis. It illustrates that these higher-force treatments must be done carefully and can lead to unwanted or toxic effects by virtue of their mechanism.

Nutritional Medicine

Relation to Determinants of Health

Nutritional medicine is a significant component of naturopathic treatment. This therapeutic category has both the required nutrients for proper physiological function and the use of certain nutrients beyond what is considered the minimum sufficient quantity to address specific disease conditions. This superuse of nutrients is not always indicated. But it can be effective because:

(a) Individuals vary in their biological requirements for nutrients.
(b) Individual needs change during disease states and when under stress.
(c) The sheer number of toxins and disturbances to natural living in our society create nutritional demands.
(d) Upregulating certain biochemical pathways can be supportive of healing.

In naturopathic treatment, with the sometimes exception of acute illness treatment, we examine the food intakes, biochemical nutritional status, digestive function, and, of course, the intake of water and other beverages that can enhance or deplete hydration status. Because nutrients and water are such fundamental requirements for life that to consider health, disease, and healing as a process entails nutritional analysis and often corrections.

Energy

One of the important functions of food is simply providing energy. The potential energy within the bonds of food molecules can be turned into ATP in the mitochondria. This is preceded by an amazing array of enzymes and transport proteins that ingest, digest, absorb, transport, and transform foods.

Human energy goes into three major uses. The largest is resting energy expenditure (Fig. 6.15). This is the sum total of all energy used to power cells, the nervous system, homeostatic mechanisms, etc. It occurs 24 h a day, including when our bodies appear to be at rest. This is a stable consumption rate, but it can be modulated by the basal metabolic rate. For example, patients with low thyroid activity will see their resting energy expenditure decline. Children and adolescents have a higher metabolic rate than older adults. The second category is that of exercise and voluntary activity. This can add to our total energy requirements. People who engage in

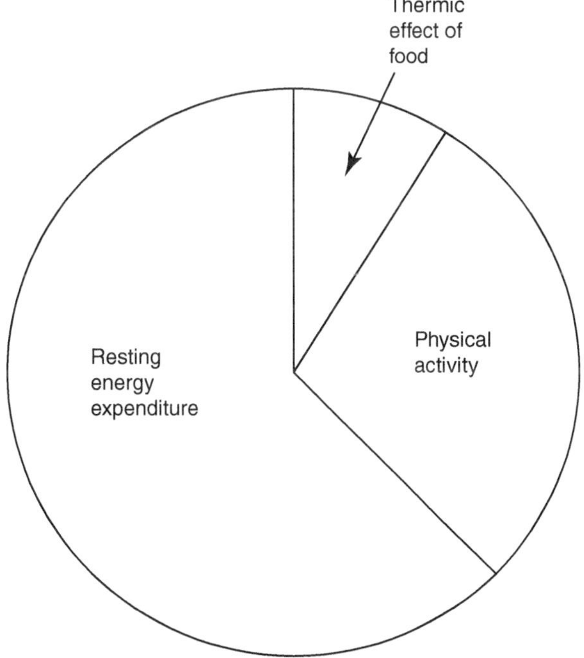

Fig. 6.15 Resting energy expenditure: Resting energy expenditure, which is the energy needed to maintain body systems and homeostasis, is a constant, 24 h a day demand, accounting for the majority of energy utilization in the body, even in those who are extremely physically active

heavy work and exercise will need to consume more energy sources than those who do light exercise or are sedentary. The third use is the thermic effect of food. It takes energy to harvest energy and nutrients from food [44].

Energy is measured in calories, but to keep numbers simple without using exponents, the common unit for human nutrition is actually the kilocalorie. kCal is the amount of energy needed to raise 1 g of water to 1 °C.

Carbohydrates are built from sugars, five or six carbon molecules, such as glucose. Longer-chain carbohydrates are known as complex carbohydrates. Many of these molecules serve as highly available energy sources. Others are indigestible to humans, but serve an important role as dietary fiber. Simple carbohydrates include monosaccharides (glucose, fructose, galactose). Disaccharides including sucrose, lactose, and maltose are made from two monosaccharides. Sucrose is made from glucose and fructose. Lactose is composed of glucose and galactose, and maltose is simply two glucoses. Oligosaccharides have from three to ten sugar molecules. Longer-chain carbohydrates are found in many foods, including whole grains.

In terms of pure energy, carbohydrates yield 4 kcal/g. That is lower than fats, but carbohydrates are often easier to digest and can be more abundant. The brain, heart, and skeletal muscles require a lot of glucose. Carbohydrates provide glucose that does not have to be synthesized in the liver (gluconeogenesis). Excessive carbohydrate intake is a problem in many societies. In North America, the extensive availability of corn, wheat, rice, and other grain products, in addition to massively consumed sweeteners such as sucrose, fructose, and high-fructose corn syrup, creates a major stress on the metabolisms of many people. In some countries, for the poor in any country, and definitely in human history, starches and sugars were easy to store and help feed people through times of scarcity. But in industrialized societies, or places where the food system has started to mimic such societies, an overabundance of refined and mostly low-cost carbohydrates can create dietary imbalances. A prime example is nonalcoholic fatty liver disease (NAFLD). Excessive carbohydrates in the diet lead to insulin resistance, building up of glucose in the bloodstream, and eventual buildup of triglycerides (stored fatty acids) in the liver. In the past, ethanol (which has an energy value of 7 kcal/g) was the major cause of fatty liver disease. This has been surpassed by NAFLD.

Dietary intake of carbohydrates is valuable, but across a wide range of dietary plans and specific therapeutic interventions, naturopathic physicians will guide patients about what quantity and quality of carbohydrates they should select. In some dietary plans, a restriction of not only sugars, but also oligosaccharides, is made to reduce proliferation of bacteria in the small intestine (FODMAPS diet). Carbohydrates might appear in the diet in highly manipulated forms such as high-fructose corn syrup. But they also appear bundled with proteins, fats, and many nutrients.

During the golden age of vitamin discovery, the nutrient thiamine (B1) was isolated by Casimir Funk. It was noted by Christiaan Eijkman and Takaki Kanehiro that people eating highly refined diets developed the condition known as "beriberi," which was later found to be curable with B1. As other B complex vitamins were discovered, food authorities began to require the enrichment of many foods that were made from grains. For example, rice that is steam polished and depleted of nutrients will introduce glucose molecules into human metabolism without contributing the cofactors needed to process them. Enrichment adds some of these required nutrients, such as B1, B2, B2, and iron, back into foods such as pasta, bread, and rice.

Proteins

Proteins in the diet are composed of amino acids, which are nitrogen (amine)-containing molecules with various characteristics (sulfur containing, aromatic, branched chain, etc.). Amino acids are the building blocks of proteins and needed for the production of neurotransmitters. Some amino acids cannot be synthesized by humans and are essential in the diet (also known as indispensable amino acids). These are:

- Phenylalanine.
- Valine.
- Tryptophan.
- Threonine.
- Isoleucine.
- Methionine.
- Histidine.
- Leucine.
- Lysine.

There are amino acids able to be synthesized from other amino acids and are nonessential or "dispensable." These are:

- Alanine.
- Arginine.
- Asparagine.
- Aspartic acid.
- Cysteine.
- Glutamic acid.
- Glutamine.
- Glycine.
- Histidine.
- Proline.
- Serine.
- Tyrosine.

Of the dispensable or conditional amino acids, there are some which the human body can synthesize, but under certain conditions of stress, disease, and increased metabolic demand, these will need to be supplemented by dietary sources (Fig. 6.16):

- Arginine.
- Cysteine.

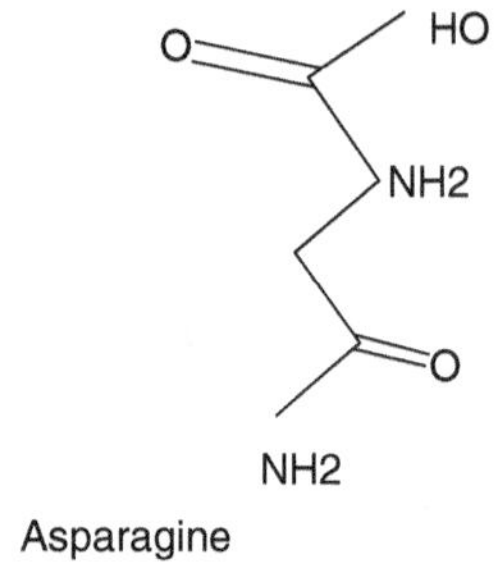

Fig. 6.16 Asparagine: A nonessential amino acid that can be produced by conversion of oxaloacetate

- Glutamine.
- Glycine.
- Proline.
- Serine.
- Tyrosine.

Protein is lost daily due to exfoliation of skin, shedding of intestinal epithelial cells, excretion in the urine (often in a further broken down form called urea), and disposal of compounds from the liver into the bile. If the intake of amino acids is adequate to replace the loss of amino acids, that person is said to be in a positive nitrogen balance. If they are taking in less than they need, it is a state of negative nitrogen balance. Protein malnutrition will at first lead to depletion of skeletal muscle mass, as well as decreased immune function. Over time, it will lead to loss of internal organ integrity [45].

Amino acids can be used to supply energy to the body, yielding 4 kcal/gram. Many diets in North America have more than adequate amounts of amino acids. In therapy, higher protein diets come into play when a person is healing from surgery, or during times of rapid growth, such as childhood. Some therapeutic diets elevate protein as a way to glycemically balance the diet. This can be helpful to those who are very insulin resistant and who react to too many carbohydrates in the diet with a surge of insulin secretion.

In certain diseases, the amount of protein in the diet must be monitored more closely. In some renal diseases, excessive protein can be harmful because of the burden of nitrogen it imposes on the body. The nitrogen aspect of amino acids can become ammonia, which might not be properly detoxified into urea. In other renal diseases, such as nephrotic syndrome, massive losses of protein in the urine might necessitate a higher protein diet to stay in positive nitrogen balance. Patients with liver failure will need a certain amount of protein in order to prevent muscle wasting. But that intake must not be excessive, or the levels of toxic ammonia in their blood will rise, leading to hepatic encephalopathy.

Dietary sources of amino acids are found in both plant and animal foods. Meat, fish, dairy, and eggs are considered high biologic value proteins, because they contain all of the indispensable (essential) amino acids in adequate quantities to allow for protein synthesis in the body to proceed. However, combinations of foods that contribute some of the essential amino acids can provide the same needs. For example, corn combined with legumes, wheat combined with legumes, and rice combined with legumes were the basis of many traditional diets and are today (notwithstanding the fact that the hybridized and genetically modified versions of corn, wheat, and soy found in stores and in animal feed today are quite different than what was grown traditionally). The body does maintain an amino acid pool and foods with various amino acid contributions can be eaten asynchronously.

Fats

Fats are an integral part of the structure of the body. Cell, organelle, and nuclear membranes all have lipids as their core (but not sole) component. Important signaling mechanisms, prostaglandins and thromboxanes, are derived from fats. Fat provides cushioning for the body. And very significantly, fat is an important energy source. Fatty reserves in the body, including the fat stored around organs, are important for survival. In times of scarcity, fat storage has helped the human race survive, including the ability of mothers to feed their children. In not so scarce circumstances, particularly with the overconsumption of carbohydrates, the fat content of the body, including intra-abdominal fat, can build up to levels that disturb health. Overconsumption of fat can lead to energy excesses, but the judicious use of fats provides an energy source that does not trigger immediate oversecretion of insulin the way that large boluses of carbohydrates can. Fats have an energy value of 9 kcal/g, making them the most energy-dense macronutrient (still beating out ethanol, which has 7 kcal/g).

Fatty acids are stored in the body as triglyceride, composed of three fatty acids attached to a glycerol backbone. Free fatty acids are found in the bloodstream, and lipoprotein particles are a way of moving fatty acids and cholesterol around the body. The liver packages these fats along with lipoproteins. The dietary fatty acids, many of them released from triglyceride form during digestion, are absorbed into lymphatic channels, forming large particles called chylomicrons. This is a different route of absorption than other nutrients, which are collected into the portal venous system.

There are several ways of classifying fatty acids. One classification is by the chain length of that fatty acid, a single carbon unit, with a carboxyl group. Butyric acid has two carbons. Palmitic acid has 16. Arachidonic acid has 20. Fatty acids can be saturated or unsaturated. The saturated fatty acids have all available bonding sites, aside from the carbon to carbon bonds that form (aside from the carboxyl group) saturated with hydrogen. That means that the carbon to carbon bonds are single bonds. An unsaturated fatty acid has at least one double bond between carbons. This introduces a kink of sorts into the structure of the fatty acid. The 16-carbon fatty acid linoleic acid is one example.

One nomenclature system for fatty acids is to label the carbon atom that is in the chain immediately after the carboxyl group at alpha and the terminal carbon as omega. That terminal carbon is part of a methyl group that is at the very end of the chain. In terms of unsaturated fatty acids, an omega-3 unsaturated fatty acid has the first double bond, counting from the terminal methyl carbon back towards the alpha carbon and carboxyl group, at the third carbon down the chain. An omega-6 fatty acid has the first double bond at the sixth carbon in the chain, counting from omega back towards alpha. Eicosapentaenoic acid is a 22-carbon polyunsaturated (five double bonds), omega-3 fatty acid [46].

Fatty acids have an important role to play in therapy. Some diets are designed to be very low in fat, such as a diet for those with acute gallbladder disease. For many years, low-fat diets were a strategy to reduce serum cholesterol. The evidence around the use of the Mediterranean diet supports the concept that while limiting saturated fats has utility, a diet with unsaturated, particularly omega-9, and omega-3 fats in addition to omega-6 fats has excellent cardiovascular and metabolic benefits.

The diet in North America, and many other regions with industrialized agriculture and food processing systems, has a high preponderance of omega-6 fatty acids. This is a direct result of the emergence of processed seed oils in both cooking and food processing. There are two major issues with this. One is the imbalance that results from a diet with a ratio of omega-6 to omega-3 fatty acids. The other is the pro-oxidant effect of the oil products themselves, due to their chemical processing and loss of natural antioxidants as found in a food context.

Specific nutrients, examples:

Fat-Soluble Vitamins

Vitamin A

Vitamin A is an isoprenoid molecule. Vitamin A is the name of a group of fat-soluble retinoids, including retinol, retinal, and retinyl esters [47]. It plays a vital role in vision, immune system, reproduction, and cellular communication. Vitamin A is critical for vision as an essential component of rhodopsin, a protein that absorbs light in the retinal receptors, and because it supports the normal differentiation and functioning of the conjunctival membranes and cornea [2–4]. Vitamin A also supports cell growth and differentiation, playing a critical role in the normal formation and maintenance of the heart, lungs, kidneys, and other organs. Vitamin A derivatives are used in various dermatologic treatments (Fig. 6.17).

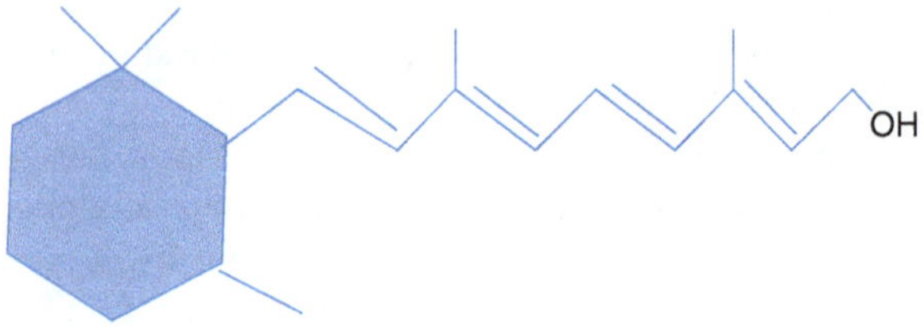

Fig. 6.17 All-trans-retinol: A derivative of vitamin A that is used for dermatologic applications

Vitamin D

It starts off as 25-cholecalciferol in the skin from ultraviolet light and calcifediol. It is hydroxylated in the liver and then kidneys to form calcitriol (1,25-(OH)2D3) or "25-hydroxycholecalciferol." This is the active form. Vitamin D is necessary for absorbing calcium in the gut and reducing its excretion in the kidney. It has nuclear binding sites in the cell and is an immunomodulating hormone. It is found in fish liver oils and is added to some foods such as dairy products and, more recently, some orange juices. Lack of vitamin D can worsen inflammatory conditions and will certainly lead to demineralization of bones.

Vitamin E

Alpha-tocopherol is found with other tocopherols in nature. It protects polyunsaturated fats. All cell membranes need vitamin E, which also serves in the reduction (recycling) of glutathione. Lack of vitamin E will lead to damage to the nervous system, including the appearance of ataxia, extreme incoordination in walking and moving. Sources include raw nuts, pure cold pressed vegetable oils, wheat germ, and eggs.

Vitamin K

This vitamin is a group of similar compounds that are necessary for normal blood clotting. They are 2-methyl-1,4-naphthoquinone (3-) derivatives. Vitamin K includes two subtypes: vitamin K1 (phylloquinone) and vitamin K2 (menaquinone), which itself has a number of subtypes. It is found in leafy greens, asparagus, blueberries, chicken, clams, and broccoli. Gut microbiomes also produce it. People at risk of deficiency and therefore easy bleeding are those who have dietary lack of greens and those who have used antibiotics recently. Newborns do not have good vitamin K levels and can develop a hemorrhagic disease. This is why many newborns are given a vitamin K injection.

Folic Acid

Folic acid is found in the diet and is converted in the body to tetrahydrofolic acid. This very important methylation agent is used in amino acid, purine, and thymidine synthesis. It is needed for the conversion of homocysteine to methionine in the synthesis of S-adenosyl-methionine which is integral for DNA synthesis and detoxification reactions. A deficiency is noticeable in the blood, as a megaloblastic anemia. Folic acid deficiency has a major consequence in pregnancy, most notably neural tube defects. This includes spina bifida and anencephaly. This is primarily why folate is added to some foods and has been since the 1990s. Population studies indicated enough marginal folate status to warrant this. Folic acid is found in leafy green vegetables, meats, grains, seafood, some fruits, and eggs. Some individuals have a defect in the genes encoding for methylenetetrahydrofolate reductase. They will have homocysteinemia due to difficulty breaking it down. Their need for folate, particularly methylfolate, will be greatly increased. Those who smoke, use oral contraceptives, and take the anticancer/antirheumatic drug methotrexate will have increased folate needs [48].

Cobalamin: Vitamin B12

B12 is needed to synthesize the amino acid methionine. It also is required for the isomerization of methylmalonyl-CoA, a by-product of amino acid and fatty acid degradation. While the anemia that results from B12 deficiency, a megaloblastic anemia, is well known, an insidious and serious effect of B12 deficiency is degeneration of the nervous system. When methylmalonyl-CoA cannot be broken down to succinyl-CoA, fatty acids that do not belong in the cell membrane will accumulate, particularly in neurons, leading to pathology.

This vitamin appears in supplements often with a cyanide group in the form cyanocobalamin. In the body, to become an active coenzyme, the cyanide is replaced with 5′-deoxyadenosine, or a methyl group (rendering 5′-deoxyadenosyl-cobalamin and methylcobalamin, respectively).

Only microorganisms produce B12. Animals obtain it from their microflora. Humans and their commensal flora, and plants, do not produce it. Deficiency can arise in those who eat no animal source foods and who do not supplement. Those who have had a disease of the ileum or stomach may not absorb B12. The vitamin is actually absorbed in the ileum, but it must be paired with a special protein known as "intrinsic factor," which is made in the stomach. Some people develop an autoimmune disorder that targets the stomach and they cannot make an intrinsic factor. This will lead to anemia and then nervous system symptoms of increasing severity. This condition is called pernicious anemia. Meats, dairy, clams, fish, and liver are good sources [48].

Vitamin B1

Thiamine was one of the first vitamins to be discovered and its ability to reverse the state known as "beriberi" was demonstrated in the early twentieth century. The active form of B1 is thiamine pyrophosphate. It is a vital part of energy-producing reactions in the cell. Thiamine serves as a cofactor for enzymes that perform some of the key conversions in the energy cycle. This includes alpha-ketoglutarate to succinyl-CoA and pyruvate to acetyl-CoA. When these enzymes cannot function, there is a lack of energy. Tissues that are extremely energy-hungry such as the heart, and other muscles, will suffer. The condition beriberi presents with cardiomyopathy and extreme weakness. Tachycardia (with poor ejection fraction) and convulsion can lead to death [48].

A tragic outcome of prolonged alcoholism is the Wernicke–Korsakoff syndrome. The brain suffers a global deterioration with memory, especially for new events (anterograde amnesia), and difficulty with orientation to place and time, confabulation, and aberrant eye movements are all seen. Alcohol is a source of energy that lacks any nutritional cofactors for its own metabolism, it can displace nutritious foods in the diet, and it irritates the gastrointestinal tract when consumed at abuse levels. This all works to create thiamine deficiency [49].

Thiamine does not seem to be toxic. It is usually supplemented with other B1 vitamins as part of a strategy to support metabolism especially when the body and mind are under stress. Given the extreme amount of refined carbohydrates and sugars that are in the American diet, which do not really provide the cofactors that support their own metabolism (such as thiamine, riboflavin, niacin, etc.), it seems that assuming that all patients other than alcoholics or those with starvation situations are in optimal B1 status is a mistake. The original field experiment for the discovery of the cause of beriberi was to feed one group of chickens a whole-grain rice diet and then the other the steam polished rice (that many local people with beriberi were using as a dietary staple). The refined rice chickens all became immobilized and died. This is a reminder that the feeding of large amounts of sugars that are divorced from any nutrients is a recipe for metabolic catastrophe.

Vitamin B2 Riboflavin

Riboflavin has two biologically active forms: flavin mononucleotide and (FMN) and flavin adenine dinucleotide (FAD).

These molecules are important for electron transport. Deficiency is not common because B2 is so widely distributed in foods, and in a starvation situation it will be one of the many B vitamins that are deficient. Deficiency signs include dermatitis and angular stomatitis, a cracking in the corners of the mouth [48].

Vitamin B3 Niacin

This vitamin has two forms in the diet: nicotinic acid and nicotinamide. The latter is deaminated in the body to form nicotinic acid. The active forms of this vitamin in the body are nicotinamide adenine dinucleotide (NAD+) and nicotinamide adenine dinucleotide phosphate (NADP+). It is also involved in electron transfer. It is also involved in hundreds of other reactions in the body. It is found in whole grains, meats, legumes, nuts, and seeds. Deficiency leads to pellagra, which is famous for the "3Ds" of dermatitis, dementia, and diarrhea [48].

Niacin, but not niacinamide, has a direct pharmacologic effect of lowering lipids when taken in large amounts, such as 3 g per day. It will cause a flushing reaction. Psychiatrists and other physicians who use the approach of orthomolecular medicine have used niacin to treat patients with schizophrenia and bipolar disorder, in large doses [50]. This form of treatment appears to pertain to a subset of schizophrenics who have unusually high needs for niacin. This approach has been very well documented. Recently, a large study of over 1000 patients with schizophrenia in India that included genetic analysis found that NAPRT1, a gene that is important for niacin metabolism, was associated with schizophrenia. There are probably other such genes in other populations as well.

Vitamin B6

B6 is found as pyridoxine, pyridoxamine, and pyridoxal. It is needed for amino acid metabolism, including the transaminase, deamination, decarboxylation, and condensation reactions that allow the body to convert one amino acid to another. It is found in the same kinds of foods that other B vitamins are found in such as whole grains, meats, legumes, etc. Deficiency is not common but it can present with neuropathy. There is treatment for infection with *Mycobacterium tuberculosis* that has been in use since the mid-twentieth century—isoniazid. This drug binds to B6 and inactivates it, so it must be supplemented during such treatment. Another sign is glossitis, a smooth and shiny red tongue [48].

Biotin

This nutrient is considered part of the “B” group. It is a carrier of carbon dioxide in carboxylation reactions. It is widely found in many foods and it is produced by gut bacteria. There is a protein in raw egg white called avidin that can bind biotin. This would take a couple of dozen of eggs per day to cause a deficiency, which remains extremely rare [48].

Pantothenic Acid

This is part of the thiol-containing coenzyme A, which carries acyl groups. A key citric acid cycle molecule such as succinyl-CoA contains this complex. Liver, yeast, and egg have higher amounts, but pantothenic acid is found across many foods [48].

Vitamin C

Vitamin C, ascorbic acid, is not synthesized by humans. It is a needed cofactor for the hydroxylation reaction. In the formation of collagen, the hydroxylation reactions of proline creates hydroxyproline and, for lysine, creates hydroxylysine. This makes the connective tissue that collagen is involved in much looser and lacking integrity. The cross-linkages created by hydroxylation will bind collagen fibrils together. The vitamin is found in citrus and other fruits and vegetables including peppers, herbs, and potatoes. Those who do not eat many plant foods, or are in a starvation situation, can become deficient. Gingivitis and retraction of the gums, difficulty healing, immune depression, and bleeding from minor bruising are all hallmarks of deficiency [48].

Vitamin C has many uses in therapeutics. It is often given for overall detoxification support, because it is both a free-floating antioxidant in water-soluble compartments such as the cytosol, and it helps to recharge glutathione. Vitamin C is needed more by people who smoke, who are exposed to a lot of environmental toxins, and those with chronic inflammatory and immune issues, including cancer. The ultra-high doses of vitamin C can be administered intravenously. Oral vitamin C is very tolerable, with loose stools or mild gastric irritation being the main issue. There is a slight increase in the chance of oxalate kidney stones with long-term high-dose [51] (over 1000 mg per day) use of C, and that is easily offset with magnesium supplementation.

Magnesium

Magnesium is a cofactor in over 300 enzymes, including those involved in energy metabolism, hepatic detoxification, and muscle conduction. It also has a role in protein synthesis, bone development, and DNA synthesis. It aids potassium and calcium transport across excitable cell membranes, which is critical in nerve conduction, muscle activation, and regulation of cardiac activity [52].

Zinc

Zinc is a catalyst of hundreds of enzymes. It is critical for growth, immunity, wound repair, and cellular metabolism. It is found in meat, eggs, shellfish, nuts, legumes, whole grains, dark chocolate, shiitake mushroom, green peas, and spinach. Zinc deficiency will impair immune function and, in children, delay growth [53].

Iron

Iron is a critical part of hemoglobin, which binds oxygen in red blood cells. It is also found in myoglobin, which binds a single oxygen in muscle cells. Normal growth, brain development, and immune function are also reliant on iron. Dietary sources include both heme and non-heme. The heme form of iron is from animal sources and finds the iron element in a matrix of protein, such as muscle tissue with myoglobin in it. Non-heme iron is from vegetable sources, such as leafy green vegetables, beans, and chocolate. The non-heme iron is less absorbable but it is still a good source. Gastric acid and a low gastric pH help with absorption because it reduces the iron from the Fe++ to Fe+++ state which is easier to transport into epithelial cells. Ascorbic acid also helps with absorption. People with iron deficiency will have disturbances in growth, brain function, and immune function and will eventually develop iron deficiency anemia when their iron stores run out [54].

Nutritional Medicine: Relation to Hormetic Applicants to Support Adaptive Responses

Hormesis is the mechanism whereby small amounts of a substance cause a lower magnitude but significant effect, which is opposite of what higher doses result in. In the case of hormesis, the higher doses are not the generally toxic ones, but often are the dose considered to actually be effective. Hormesis, for example, where a small dose stimulates and a larger dose inhibits, will produce a J- or U-shaped dose–response curve. The explanation can be due to a modest overcompensation response to a mild stimulation, or to a preconditioning response [6].

In general, many nutrients are understandable on a U-shaped dose–response curve. Suboptimal amounts lead to deficiency. Supernormal amounts can lead to toxicity. Lower-dose amounts can produce beneficial cellular effects. However, this is sometimes easily attributable to the fact that the vitamin or mineral is a necessary cofactor in some metabolic pathways [55].

Vitamin C, ascorbic acid, has some hormetic properties with regards to cancer cells. At lower doses, it might actually encourage tumor cell growth. At very high levels achievable by intravenous administration, some tumor cells that express sodium-dependent vitamin C transporter family-2 will accept a large amount of ascorbic acid. This will lead to increased cell death of the cancer cells.

More generally, many nutrients provide a small amount of stimulation to cells and activate the NRF-2–KEAP pathway, leading to more expression of genes that code for antioxidant enzymes (Fig. 6.18) [7].

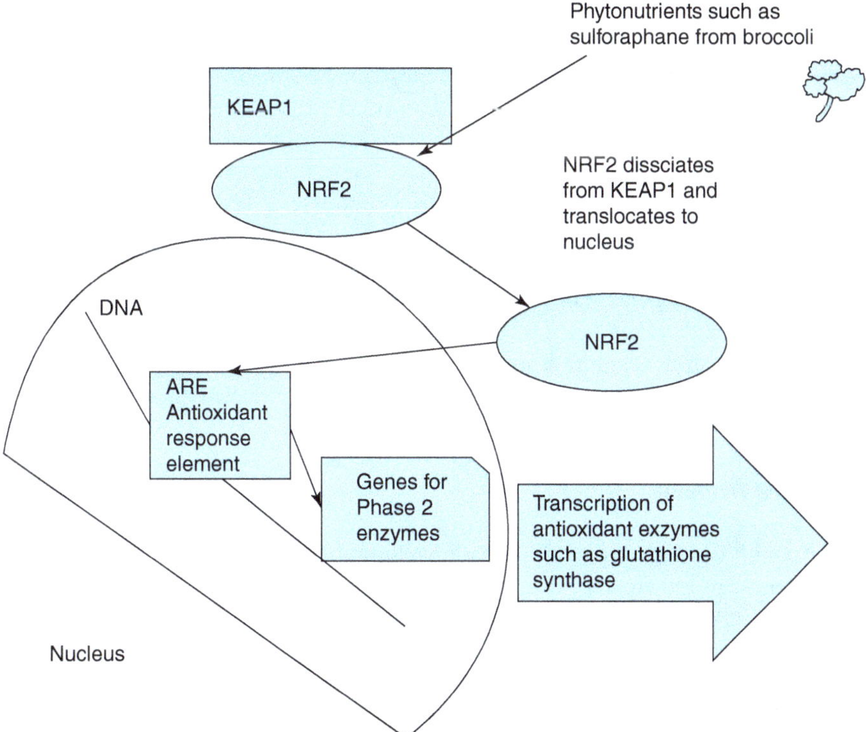

Fig. 6.18 Nuclear factor erythroid 2-related factor 2 (NRF2): This protein acts as a sensor for oxidative stress. When cellular oxidative stress increases, it translocates to the cell nucleus and binds to the antioxidant response element of the DNA. This leads to increased transcription of genes that code for proteins central to protection from oxidative stress and detoxification, such as glutathione synthase. Some plant compounds can activate NRF2, without any real cost to the cell

Nutritional Medicine: Relation to Specific Biochemical Support of Adaptive Responses

The use of food, vitamins, minerals, and special compounds (enzymes, coenzymes, antioxidants) to support a weakened system is often a very good idea. The ways that these nutrients can be helpful are in the following ways:

The Nutrient Can Make Up for a Deficiency

This is closer to the idea of creating the basis for health. But some marginal deficiencies of nutrients are tolerable until the person is under the stress of illness. In some cases, the marginal deficiency might have contributed to developing the illness. Some deficiencies are more pronounced. Severe nutrient deficiencies are not found only in impoverished or famine-stricken areas, or history books. They are quite common in the United States. The fact that people can carry on for a time with these issues is a testament to human adaptation and resilience. Some disease conditions create deficiencies. For example, most patients with ulcerative colitis (UC) will not be iron deficient when they first present with the illness, but they will be at very high risk of developing iron deficiency if they have a severe bout or chronic recurrence of UC due to the bleeding. Some deficiencies are relative to the individual.

Increased Demand

Some conditions and stages of life require additional nutrients. When someone is in a rapid phase of growth, they need plenty of zinc, protein, and essential fatty acids—virtually everything. Pregnant patients have additional needs. Patients who have suffered burns to their body will need a lot of protein to offset loss. Patients with diabetes need additional support for glucose metabolism and insulin receptor—GLUT4—function. Patients in midlife and beyond will typically need more vitamin D and calcium to protect bone density.

Optimal Amounts

Providing a person with amounts of nutrients that go over and above the amounts they need for body growth or maintenance can be beneficial in some cases. The drawback of this approach is that sometimes, this additional amount may not really confer much benefit. Occasionally it can cause harm. A solid scientific question to ask about this is: if nutrients have a well-defined biochemical role, and a certain range allows a person's metabolism to function, why would amounts that exceed the dietary reference intake (RDI) really make a difference?

One reason is that a certain magnitude of benefit can be obtained by giving beyond the RDI, sometimes. Vitamin C, ascorbic acid, is an example. The DRI for adults (over 19 years of age) is as follows: males, 90 mg; females, 75 mg; pregnancy, 85 mg; and lactation, 120 mg. According to the Office of Dietary Supplements, National Institutes of Health, approximately 70%–90% of vitamin C is absorbed at moderate intakes of 30–180 mg/day [56]. This drops to 50% at doses over 1 g a day and the urine will show ascorbic acid in higher amounts. It appears that doses of

1.25 g/day ascorbic acid produce mean peak plasma vitamin C concentrations of 135 μmol/L, which are about two times higher than those produced by consuming 200–300 mg/day ascorbic acid from vitamin C-rich foods [57].

What happens with higher vitamin C levels? Some enzymes will become saturated, and the higher intake will have no impact on their function. In another sense, the higher amount of vitamin C can function as a free-floating antioxidant in plasma and in cell cytoplasms. Ascorbic acid will act to recharge glutathione along with vitamin E. The oxidation of the LDL (low-density lipoprotein) particle makes LDL more atherogenic. Vitamin C reduces this oxidation. People who eat a higher plant food diet consume more dietary vitamin C than most who do not and also obtain many polyphenolic molecules and other food-derived antioxidants. Vitamin C has many other reported effects. In a 2019 study, patients with type 2 diabetes experienced improved postprandial and 24-h glycaemia and decreased BP after 4 months of ascorbic acid supplementation as compared to placebo [58].

Intravenous ascorbic acid can create plasma concentrations of vitamin C that rise faster and higher than the oral route. There are reports of improved recovery from sepsis with intravenous vitamin C, and yet larger trials have not confirmed that.

The basic model for nutritional science, which grew as a discipline in the early twentieth century, has been the prevention of deficiency. This is a useful standard, as demonstrating that a disease state can be prevented or reversed by a known nutrient is rather straightforward. However, this model is incomplete. The aggregate of human metabolism and biochemistry is extensive. Biochemical pathways, and nutrients, interact with each other. What might prevent a deficiency at one dose can confer additional benefits at a higher dose.

Individual Variability

The RDI is meant to account for the majority of people. For example, the daily recommended allowance (one of the RDI indices) is meant to pertain to 96%–98% of the population [59]. This is a good safety margin, but the 4% whose diets do not provide their body with enough of a vital nutritional substance may suffer from this fact. In recent years, the role of genetic variability and single-nucleotide deletions has gained prominence. For instance, defects in methylenetetrahydrofolate reductase (MTHFR) can reduce someone's ability to break down homocysteine [60]. But it has wide-ranging effects on the nervous system. Some people have minor alterations in this function and for others it is profound. For them, the amount of dietary folic acid that works well for the large majority of people is insufficient to maintain health [60]. The amount of vitamin D that they need is well above that of the average requirement, because they simply do not respond to lower plasma levels of D.

Nutritional Medicine: Generalized Support

There are some agreed-upon principles of a healthy diet, and they have a qualitative and quantitative side. Quantitatively, a diet that supports overall health must provide adequate levels of nutrients. Adequate is a term that can be questioned, in the sense that it is adequate to prevent deficiency (the classical test of something being a required nutrient, such as thiamine). And it is adequate in the sense of preventing disease. The latter is much harder to prove, and even in large population groups followed for long periods of time, it is sometimes only likely that a dose of a nutrient higher than that known to prevent deficiency can prevent a disease.

There are some practical reasons why encouraging patients to consume more than the bare minimum amount of nutrients in their diet is important. One is that nutrients can be studied in isolation, but diets are complex wholes that interact. For example, a patient who consumes a lot of unsaturated fatty acids ought to consume more vitamin E, which protects them from oxidation. A patient who derives all of their iron as non-heme (vegetable) sources will need more ascorbic acid unless their menu is replete with many iron sources.

Another reason is that individual circumstances vary. A person who works in painting and wood floor finishing and who inhales and absorbs a lot of volatile organic compounds needs more cofactors for detoxification. Some people have partial enzyme deficiencies, and they need more than the average requirement.

Just as the connection of a dietary pattern and a disease prevention outcome can be tenuous, so is the assumption that the amount of a nutrient needed to prevent a deficiency disease in a short-term observational study is automatically adequate to support optimal functioning of the body over years, or decades. This has not been proven, although in an indirect sense, narrow or no gaps in health outcomes between those with average intakes and high intakes provide a form of evidence that base amounts are adequate. Still, dietary reference intakes provide a useful goalpost, for both advising individuals and considering the needs of populations.

Qualitative measures of eating for health are another type of puzzle to solve. Large and long-term observational studies also provide data here. The Mediterranean diet is one example of a diet that has distinct qualitative features. For instance, lipids—fats and oils—tend to be found directly from foods, such as fish and walnuts. There is also extra virgin olive oil, a cold pressure oil with an array of types of fatty acids and rich in antioxidants. There is less wheat and less saturated fat-laden protein sources. Polyphenolic molecules, including flavonoids, are plentiful. Mediterranean diets (variations on them with many common denominators) seem to deliver good results.

Quality can also relate to the growing, storage, processing, and cleanliness of food. Some foods are labeled organic due to the nature of their cultivation, and this is favored by consumers who want to avoid foods sprayed with pesticides or herbicides. They may also approve of the way that the soil is tended to in the organic model. Foods that are minimally processed are more likely (but not always) lower on the glycemic index and contain fewer processing agents (such as sodium inosinate for flavor). Handling of food, such as butchering of animals and processing of meat, is an overdue topic of interest. In the United States, meat processing facilities (which are also called slaughterhouses) run animals through at a much faster rate than in Europe. This is dangerous for workers, can make for an even more traumatic end for the animals, and can lead to fecal contamination of meat. At the time of this writing, using beef as an example, four corporations/companies who collectively own about 60 facilities are responsible for 80% of all cattle slaughtered and processed in the United States [61]. This is again in contrast to other countries where meat is derived from smaller-scale and often local sources. There are arguments for cost and consumer access, especially in a country as large as the United States.

Midway between quantity and quantity are issues of proportionality (Table 6.1). For instance, should a diet derive 30% of the calories from fat, or should it be 20% to lower the risk of heart disease? If the energy is not from fat, will it be from carbohydrates, and will that increase the risk of metabolic syndrome and type II diabetes? Or if it is from protein, does that not put strain on the liver and kidneys, and what about the impact on the microbiota of all that protein?

Not surprisingly, the USDA published *ranges* that are thought to promote good health. For example, the current advice is as follows [62].

These are wide ranges, but the fact is that people can adapt to different proportions. And as is well known in the world of food sciences, requirements change based on energy expenditure, stage of life, and physical activity. A patient recovering from surgery needs more than the bare minimum of protein. A woman breastfeeding her child should not take in the bare minimum of fat. On the other hand, someone with familial hypercholesterolemia and a strong family history of heart disease should probably not do the upper limit of percentage energy from fat. A person with certain types of renal failure should not take in 35% of their energy from protein. And of course, an athlete that engages in prolonged aerobic activity can burn through more energy from carbohydrates than someone who is sedentary—they have the use for the ATP that their mitochondria could produce from this readily available energy from carbohydrates. A patient with nonalcoholic fatty liver disease ought not get 65% of their energy from carbohydrates. Not when their liver is also filled up with triglyceride that is formed from acetate units that carbohydrates provide.

There are other general frameworks for eating than the much studied (and useful) Mediterranean diet of course. In terms of quality and quantity of research, the DASH (Dietary Approaches to Stop Hypertension) [63] stands out. It has many shared traits with the Mediterranean diet [64], with controls on sodium and good

Table 6.1 Ranges of calorie sources

Macronutrient (adults)	Recommended percentage range of energy
Carbohydrates	45–65%
Fats	20–35%
Proteins	10–35%

sources of other cations such as potassium. The flexitarian diet [65] allows for some animal-derived foods, with no strict prohibitions on such things, but encourages and emphasizes (for personal and planetary health) plant-derived foods that require less energy and water to create. The Nordic diet [66] has an emphasis on fish, berries, whole grains such as rye, canola oil, and traditional Scandinavian foods.

These diets tend to provide a lot of nutritionally dense foods, good fiber, a healthy omega-3 to omega-6 balance, and lots of phytonutrients such as polyphenols. There is a lack of burnt food, saturated fat, sugar, processing (with exceptions, such as the aforementioned canola oil), and added chemicals.

There are hundreds of dietary plans, and each year, new apps, books, and websites appear that provide a plan for eating. This can be motivational for many, and they provide structure in a world of too many choices and many antinutrient temptations. Many people and families never abandoned cooking and traditional dishes. But many people are now reclaiming their cooking and, after two or three generations of mass-marketed processed foods (and a mind-boggling level of restaurant/takeout food), are seeing the value of preparing their own dishes. Ready-to-cook boxes with the prep and portions already taken care of are a growing industry. Cookbooks, websites with recipes, and cooking shows are all a reflection of the growth in interest in skill in preparing one's own food. This bodes well for the future, in spite of the fact that according to the CDC, in the 2013–2016 period, 37% of adults consumed fast food every day [67]. This has probably not changed much, and with the advent of mobile apps that allow for restaurant to door delivery, it might have gone up.

The downside, as many have remarked (including the very articulate Michael Pollan), of all of the information, options, and "diets" is a certain degree of complexity that does not necessarily have to be there. That is not to say that all diet plans are complicated. But the constant rotation of multiple programs of eating, and the surge in popularity of some (coincident with the derogation of out-of-fashion diets and foods), brings an unreality to it. Someone who is out of touch with their body's own needs might feel overwhelmed. And it is worth noting that in many societies, nutrition in the home is not a complicated matter. There is traditional cooking, there is balance, there are treats and festive occasions, and it works pretty well. The nutrition *industry* in advanced economies/nations, complete with gurus and guides, creates a hypercomplexity that need not be there. Conservative nutritional scientists and dieticians, while sometimes overlooking the need for innovation, have a solid point when they decry "fad" diets and the consumers' wish for a magical solution to health problems.

A grounding in simpler, natural ways of eating never really goes out of style. The Weston Price Foundation is an organization and network that provides resources and advocates for a very local, unprocessed, and nutrient dense way of eating. This organization traces its roots to dentist and researcher Dr. Weston Price who traveled the early twentieth-century globe meticulously studying traditional diets and the health of those who ate them, compared to groups that had recently adopted Western/processed modes of eating [68]. An avoidance of processed oils and refined carbohydrates and inclusion of fermented foods and some animal products are hallmarks.

A popular educator about nutrition is Dr. Catherine Shanahan, a physician who has written books such as *Deep Nutrition* [69]. Dr. Shanahan has her own metabolic center and has in the past been a nutritional consultant to the LA Lakers. She refers to the "four pillars" of traditional diets:

Fruits and vegetables—plant food.
Organ meats.
Fermented foods.
Meat on the bone (which include nutrients derived from the breakdown of marrow and cartilage).

Dr. Shanahan cites Dr. Price and add much modern information and her own considerable experience to her educational resources. Her more recent focus has been on the quality of fats in the modern diet, including the adverse effects of mass ingestion of processed vegetable/seed/grain oils.

It is interesting to look at societies where the traditions of eating nutrient-dense, cultured, local, and varied food still holds sway. In many communities in France, both rural and urban, there is a heavy emphasis on small-scale and local food production. Fish markets, cheeses that are from traditional cultures, and small portions are very common. Of course, with some of the world's best pastries, it is possible in France to do some of the wrong things. The French diet varies by region and definitely has aspects of what is more broadly referred to as the Mediterranean diet (even in non-Mediterranean regions of that country).

It is not surprising that France was the center of a major study on the value of whole foods. In the NutriNet-Santé cohort (2009–2017), 104,980 participants aged at least 18 years (median age 42.8 years) from the French dietary intakes were collected using repeated 24-h dietary records, designed to register participants' usual consumption for 3300 different food items. These foods were sorted by the NOVA classification (developed by researchers from the University of São Paulo) which differentiates unprocessed, processed, and ultraprocessed foods (Table 6.2). In the study, a 10% increase in ultraprocessed foods led to an 10% increase in cancer,

Table 6.2 NOVA classification system [72]

Group	Description	Example
1	Unprocessed or minimally processed foods	Grains, vegetables, meat, fruits, juices (no sugar added), herbs, mushrooms
2	Processed culinary ingredients: Oils, sugars, fats, salt	Vegetable oil, butter, salt, sugar, honey
3	Processed foods	Canned vegetables, canned meat, fresh cheese, fresh bakery bread, smoked meats
4	Ultraprocessed foods	Pastries, snack foods, salted snack meats, breakfast cereals, fast foods, packaged bread, sweetened and colored sports drinks, sweetened yogurts, infant formulas, protein shakes, breakfast bars

including breast cancer [70]. Additionally, higher consumption of ultraprocessed foods was associated with higher risks of cardiovascular, coronary heart, and cerebrovascular diseases [71].

Ultraprocessed foods have become so pervasive, in the diets of developed and high-income countries, including the United States, that the health effects of their overconsumption will be felt for decades. These foods are becoming dominant in middle-income countries and, astoundingly, are catching on in low-income countries. Of course, some modes of this eating incur costs, but many ultraprocessed foods are unfortunately in a price range that they can displace traditional, natural, nutrient-dense foods. The global burden of disordered and unnatural eating is felt now and will increasingly be seen in the mid-twenty-first century.

Vegetarian Diets

Meatless diets are one form of vegetarian eating. The lacto-ovo vegetarian does not consume flesh foods of any kind, but does incorporate cheese, mild, yogurt, etc. [73]. This allows for a wider variety of foods including some B12 from these animal source foods.

Vegan diets eliminate any animal-sourced products as well. These diets can have a wide number of health benefits derived from many servings of vegetables, fruits, grains, and legumes each day. This diet will have to supplement B12 as far as the current literature would indicate.

Risks of cancer and cardiovascular disease decrease in this diet.

Flexitarian Diet

This umbrella term includes those who eat various quantities of animal foods including meat. This might be several times per week instead of daily. This diet is looking to maximize the benefits of plants as food and minimize any of the downsides of animal-derived food [65].

Both flexitarian and vegetarian diets are generally more sustainable in the sense that meat, particularly beef, requires large amounts of water, and grains, to produce. There are exceptions such as the free-ranging, pastured, and local poultry. Cattle do require a lot of resources to produce, ultimately, slaughtered and butchered meats. Their waste (hogs as well) places a burden on their locality. There are ethical situations that arise from animals as food. Some people outright reject the concept. Others look at the conditions in which the animals are raised and slaughtered. Crated pigs that cannot move, chickens that are literally wing to wing, and cattle that are overfed grain in a pen are all examples of animals raised in unnatural and often inhumane conditions. The slaughterhouses and processing plants for these meats have undergone consolidation in the past several decades. At present, four companies control 70% of the beef packing plants of the United States. It is no wonder that many consumers want to purchase smaller or less frequent quantities of meat from more local vendors that have more direct relationships with farmers. This smaller-scale, less complex model was the traditional one. The fact that mega pro cessors are needed to sustain the demand for restaurants, food processors, grocery stores, etc. raises the question, "do we need that many sources of meat?" This dovetails with an increasing consciousness that not only are ways of eating based on highly processed foods, which were developed in the twentieth century, not very sustainable for the resources to share on planet earth, but they have generally negative effects on people's health.

Nutritional Medicine: Relation to Dampening Maladaptive Resources

Ketogenic Diet

This diet obtains 10% or less of calories from carbohydrates in the diet. This means that the liver will be converting fatty acids to acetoacetic acid and beta-hydroxybutyrate. Numerous studies in children and adults find that the ketogenic diet reduces seizure activity in patients with epilepsy [74]. Up to a third of patients do not respond adequately to antiseizure medicine. They may get some control but need more, or they may obtain very little control. Ketogenic diets are used in children after two antiseizure drugs have failed and in some cases earlier. This type of fasting from carbohydrate intake, and metabolizing ketone bodies, seems to contribute to the opening of potassium ion channels. This leads to some reduction in depolarization (due to a hyperpolarization) and this leads to less neuron activity. The modified Atkins diet (MAD) and low glycemic index therapy (LGIT) diet are also used in the treatment of epilepsy [75]. The evidence is less convincing over the traditional ketogenic diet; however, some children tolerate the variants of ketogenic diets such as MAD or LGIT better.

Not everyone can undergo a ketogenic diet. There are a number of metabolic subtypes who should avoid it. One example is carnitine palmitoyltransferase (CPT) I or II deficiency. These people will be unable to send fatty acids for beta-oxidation in the mitochondria. Their symptoms, including muscle weakness, will be much worse if they attempt a ketogenic diet.

In addition to the treatment of epilepsy, ketogenic diets have been found beneficial for weight loss and diabetic control.

Low-Purine Diet

This is recommended for sufferers of gout. This painful condition results from the accumulation of uric acid in the body. This is usually due to enzyme defects in the body including the renal urate transporter system. A diet very high in alcohol, meat, seafood, liver, fruit juice, and high-fructose corn syrup will exacerbate this. Purines are broken down to uric acid, but if it cannot be eliminated, it will build up in parts of the body with a lower circulation. The distal foot, particularly the great toe, is a known common site for gout attacks. The uric acid crystalizes and triggers immune activation and neutrophil responses. A massive inflammatory response creates swelling and intense pain. Limiting these foods is part of treatment for gout [76].

Phenylalanine

Phenylketonuria is an "inborn error of metabolism," a genetic condition where the patient cannot process the amino acid phenylalanine. It is an autosomal recessive condition where a lack of the enzyme phenylalanine hydroxylase leaves a person unable to convert phenylalanine to tyrosine. It can cause extensive nervous system damage. The patient must adhere in their lifetime to a very-low-phenylalanine diet. This includes avoiding the artificial sweetener aspartame [77].

Methylmalonic and Propionic Acidemia

These are both rare, autosomal recessive, multisystemic inborn errors of metabolism. These patients have difficulty metabolizing branched-chain amino acids. It can be lethal in infancy and childhood and cause organ damage to older patients. Mitochondria have difficulty in creating coenzyme A-activated carboxylic acids, due to impairment in using branched-chain amino acids [78].

Gluten-Free Diet

Gluten is a protein found in wheat, containing two subunits: gliadin and glutenin. Some people develop a hypersensitivity reaction to these proteins. It will lead to cytotoxic reactions at the gut epithelium. Celiac disease is a severe form of this hypersensitivity, and it can present in children or adults. Malabsorption occurs because of the wearing down of the small bowel epithelium. The "brush border," which contains villi and microvilli, will appear smooth, due to loss of architecture and loss of active cells. Reduced absorbed surface area and enzyme activity cause loss of digestive and absorptive capacity. The patient has loose stools, abdominal bloating, and fatigue with various nutritional deficiencies. Although once thought of as a pure type, celiac disease has gradations of severity. There are certainly classical presentations of this malady, including children with failure to thrive. But

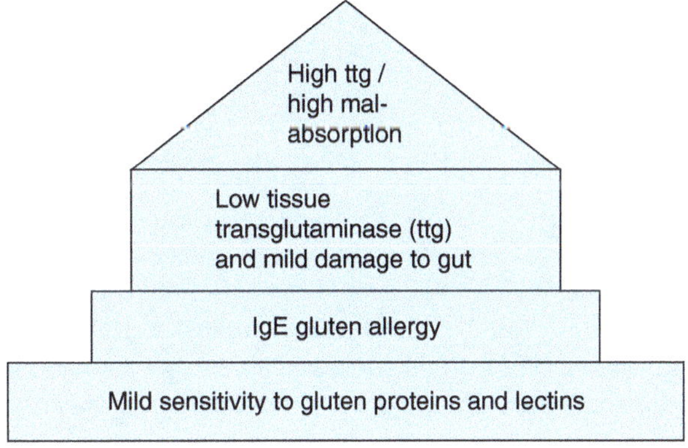

Fig. 6.19 Gluten allergy: Reactivity to gluten is a spectrum, with classically presenting celiac disease being just one, albeit clinically significant, presentation

adult-onset and some subacute presentations comprise a spectrum of severity (Fig. 6.19). A great number of people probably find that gluten is somewhat proinflammatory to their gut and that it causes spikes in blood sugar and insulin, but they are not celiac. Wheat that is consumed in the United States is mostly from a hybridized dwarf wheat plant that was developed in the mid-twentieth century. It is more tolerant of various weather patterns and it produces plenty of protein. Unfortunately, most of this protein is gluten.

In a gluten-free diet, patients avoid wheat (bread, noodles, pastries) products [79, 80]. They must avoid foods that are cooked with wheat, such as gravy with flour as a thickening agent. Grains that are milled or cut with tools that also worked on wheat can cross-contaminate the grain. Oats can have this problem. Rye and barley do not contain gluten but have similar enough proteins that they should be avoided by those with celiac disease. In the past, patients with celiac could simply stick to foods such as rice, meat, beans, fruits and vegetables, fish, etc. Or if they wanted products that were similar to more popular foods, they could get pasta or bread made from rice starch. This was a fairly limited selection. These days, there are many gluten-free options in most food stores. Gluten-free certification is also on products that are safe. The Gluten-Free Certification Organization is one such group (https://gfco.org/).

The celiac disease foundations list the following grains as gluten-free:

- Amaranth.
- Arrowroot.
- Beans.
- Buckwheat groats (also known as kasha).
- Cassava.
- Chia.
- Corn.
- Flax.
- Gluten-free oats.
- Millet.
- Nut flours.

- Potato.
- Quinoa.
- Rice.
- Sorghum.
- Soy.
- Tapioca.
- Teff.
- Yucca.

Like any trend in the nutritional industry, gluten sensitivity and gluten-free products are promoted and some consumers do not have specific issues. But many do, and some have a more generalized allergy to wheat, just as allergy can develop to any food that has proteins in it. The nature of hybridized wheat, and its high gluten content, is that it causes insulin spikes for some people. This might be due to lectins from wheat (wheat germ agglutinin). Various herbicides and pesticides tend to be used on wheat, with some strains being resistant to glyphosate, so that they can receive a substantial amount of it. Mycotoxins can also develop on stored wheat.

Farmers are a small percentage of the US population, and they feed this populous country and many people around the world. This is done with amazing efficiency. In the science-informed practice of naturopathic medicine, we want to avoid overgeneralizations and simplistic solutions. But we must look at the way that the techniques and financing structures of modern agriculture promote monoculture and the use of chemical additives. This is important in advising people to eat a variety of foods, to eat sustainable and low-toxin foods, and to identify those in any population who are the most sensitive and vulnerable to certain foods to which they suffer an adverse reaction.

Alkalizing Diet/PRAL Diet

Patients with tendency to form calcium citrate stones benefit from eating more alkalizing foods. Most foods are categorized in terms of how much they contribute to acidosis in the blood, or are alkalizing, or are neutral. Because the body has buffering systems, eating these foods do not immediately shift the pH of blood or tissues. But the stress on buffering systems, and on the kidneys, is something to consider. The potential renal acid load or PRAL is a measure of how acidifying a food is [81]. For example, beef has a higher PRAL value, and buckwheat has a lower PRAL. Eating whole grains, vegetables, and fruits tends to have an alkalizing effect. There are reports of joint pain, fatigue, and gastrointestinal problems being improved by lowering the PRAL value of foods in the diet.

Nutritional Interventions That Create Temporary Homeostatic Balance

Total Parenteral Nutrition

Circumstances arise where an individual cannot adequately digest and absorb enough nutrients to stay alive or function with a minimum of health. TPN is used for patients after extensive surgeries for cancer, such as the Whipple procedure which removes pancreas and proximal duodenum. The patient might transfer to an elemental diet in time. People with extremely active inflammatory bowel disease, or hepatic failure, are put on total bowel rest. Someone who is comatose will be fed this way [82].

Niacin

Vitamin B3 or niacin is an essential cofactor in metabolism. It is also known that doses that are many orders higher than the recommended daily intake, such as 3 g of niacin a day, can lower total cholesterol and triglyceride. In this sense, the niacin is not used just to support normal pathways; it has a pharmacologic effect that is used to the patient's benefit [83].

In a related way, orthomolecular psychiatrists have used high-dose niacin in some patients with schizophrenia and bipolar disorder [50]. These individuals presumably have extraordinary requirements for the vitamin.

Physical Medicine

This modality is a traditional approach in naturopathic medicine. Early twentieth-century naturopaths used "nature's agents," a practice rooted in hydrotherapy, and the "nature cure" movements of the late nineteenth century. These agents of nature include touch, electricity, water, hot and cold, sunshine, air, and sound energy.

In modern naturopathic medicine, this continues in therapies such as hydrotherapy, bodywork, joint adjustive technique, rehabilitative therapies, and exposure to nature. These approaches all have different effects.

Hydrotherapy

Hydrotherapy is the use of water therapeutically. This is a form of treatment that has roots so deep across so many cultures that its origination cannot be determined. People have used bathing and the pouring of water on painful parts intuitively. Water has soothing and invigorating effects that people can directly experience. Many traditions in medicine reference hydrotherapy. Unani (traditional Islamic medicine) makes use of water therapy. In ancient times, people in Egypt bathed in the Nile river to purify their body, as did people in India using the Ganges River. Hippocrates, who is a direct forerunner of the naturopathic approach, wrote about the use of water, including bathing in mineral springs. The Hippocratic school saw disease as a process with a crescendo, a "healing crisis," where toxins were "cooked" off (coction) [18].

Hydrotherapy was a major thread of the development of naturopathy. A long history of the use of hydrotherapy in Europe culminated in several nineteenth-century practitioners of the water cure. Father Sebastian Kneipp was a Bavaria-based (part of modern Germany) healer, who eventually was allowed by his church to devote his work to healing. He had an incredibly busy retreat where people came from far away for treatment. He worked with the wealthy and powerful and provided treatment for the poor. Kneipp had used hydrotherapy to recover from tuberculosis as a young priest. He had read the works of Johann Hahn, a prominent hydrotherapist of an earlier generation.

There were different styles of practice. Some historical practitioners such as Vincenz Priessnitz, a farmer by trade, used cold water mainly. Inspired by the way that animals seek out cool streams to wade in when in pain, Priessnitz developed a system with cold immersion and cold pours. This was obviously easier to do on some of the robust constitutions that showed up in a rural setting in central Europe in the nineteenth century. Not everyone could endure this treatment. A bland diet with whole grains and vegetables accompanied the treatment [84, 85, 87].

A contemporary of Priessnitz, Johan Scroth used warmth, steam, etc. in more of a Hippocratic approach. This would have been appealing to those who are cold sensitive, or with decreased circulation due to atherosclerosis or diabetes. Scroth also used a bland diet, and he did a peculiar thing. On some days patients had a total fast, with just a few sips of weak wine. Water restriction is a physiologically harmful practice, so it is probably that Scroth was judicious about this kind of restriction [87].

Father Kneipp combined these two approaches. Over the years, he found that alternating hot and cold—contrast—could stimulate blood circulation. He found that shortening the cold phase of treatment usually provided equal or better effects. Although the science of autonomic nervous system control of circulation was in its infancy and likely not known to Father Kneipp, he was tapping into an important fact. When the skin, or a body region, is exposed to a short burst of cold, it leads to vasoconstriction. This is a physical effect of the cold. This leads to reflex activation via the spinal cord for the body to attempt to shunt more blood to the area. If the

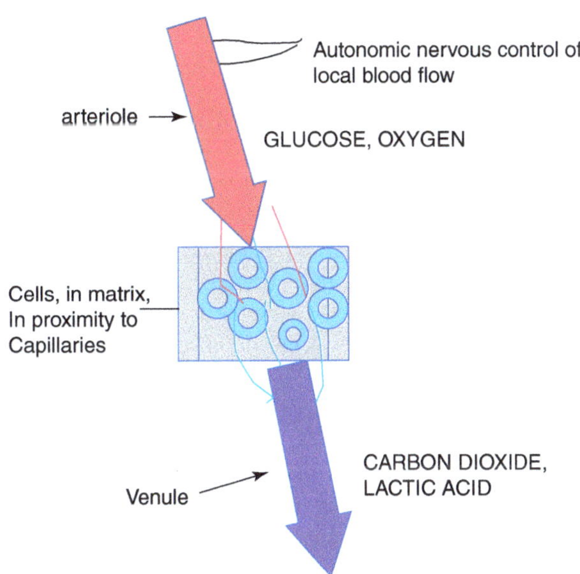

Fig. 6.20 Effect of circulation on cellular metabolism: Under autonomic control, arterial blood with oxygen and nutrients enters the area of a cellular cluster, and venous blood with carbon dioxide and waste materials flow away. Hydrotherapy, with the use of various warm or cold applications, can alter local circulation

cold is removed, this response by the body can assert itself. The tissue in question will receive an influx of circulation [86, 87].

If the cold exposure to a tissue is maintained for a long time, it can suppress circulation. For instance, putting ice on an injured tendon or ligament for 10 min can reduce acute inflammation. But keep replacing the ice and freeze the area for hours, it can start to do damage. By contrast, if heat is put on a part of the body for a short time, it opens up local circulation through its physical effect. If heat is applied for a long time, then spinal reflexes lead to a decrease in local circulation. This creates stagnation.

The promotion of circulation leads to healing. The flooding in of oxygen, glucose, and other nutrients helps tissues to heal and the immune system to act there. The exit of carbon dioxide, lactate, and other waste products is important for the tissue to function properly (especially to avoid acidic conditions) (Fig. 6.20).

As Kneipp developed his work, he found that shorter and even smaller surface area treatments were just as or more effective in many cases. He had found that leveraging the autonomic nervous system and adjusting circulation was key. Kneipp had three students who had a major impact on the development of naturopathic medicine. The students and successors of these doctors adapted hydrotherapy in ways that were well suited to a twentieth-century practice. It is important to realize, however, that nature cure and hydrotherapy spas exist today. In Europe, many people take a week or more to attend such a facility and build up their health or recover from illness. In North America there are the famous Hot Springs, Arkansas, and Warm Springs, Georgia. The latter was owned by US President Franklin Delano Roosevelt. He had used the facility as a part of his efforts to recover from polio [88]. He went from being basically supine to being able to sit with ease and stand, and even perambulate, with leg braces. He built up his health with exercise and hydrotherapy to the point that he could be elected four times to the office of president and led the country through the Great Depression and World War II. In Canada, there are facilities such as Manitou Waters, at Lake Manitou, Saskatchewan, founded by Dr. Sussanna Czeranko, who is one of the foremost scholars of the history and philosophy of naturopathic medicine.

David Ruggles was an African-American businessman, first a grocer and then bookseller. He was born in Connecticut in 1810 [89]. He was very involved in the abolitionist movement, helping many escaped slaves. He was secretary of the New York Vigilance Committee, which was composed of both black and white Americans. He helped organize the legal defense for those slaves who had fled to northern states. In September 1838, Ruggles assisted Frederick Washington Bailey, who later changed his name to Frederick Douglas.

Ruggles suffered from several health issues, including visual deterioration. He learned of hydrotherapy and, after 18 months of treatment, regained his health and much of his eyesight. He set out to practice it and quickly developed a large clientele. In 1846, Ruggles purchased land and built a hydrotherapy (hydropathic as it was then called) facility. This is the first full-service hydrotherapy inpatient facility in the United States.

Kneipp to Lust, Lindlahr, and Howard

Father Kneipp was struggling with "consumption," about the time that David Ruggles was developing his skills in hydrotherapy. Kneipp went on to have an incredible body of work, with many books written for the public. He was known in many countries, and due to the preponderance of German immigrants to the US Atlantic coast, such as Philadelphia and New York City, as well as the Upper Midwest, home Kneipp methods were quite common.

In the 1890s, a young German named Benedict Lust traveled home to Germany from New York City. He had been working in a high-end hotel restaurant, but contracted tuberculosis. As a last resort, he took a steamer home. His father sent him to the Kneipp facility in Bad Wörishofen, in Bavaria where Kneipp treated thousands of patients a year. Lust regained his health and became a very vital, energetic person. He stayed on and learned the methods of detoxification, gentle use of herbal medicines, hydrotherapy, the use of sun and air, and other aspects of Kneipp's methods. Lust desired to return to the United States. Father Kneipp commissioned him to bring his way of doing "spa cure" to America [87, 90].

This put Lust in the midst of an already large community of Kneipp cure enthusiasts. He found himself busy, but wanted more. He took up the study of osteopathic manipulation and massage. Lust had a vision of a type of doctor who combined the best of the emerging natural therapies, a knowledge of the science of the human body and its biochemistry, and traditional nature cure. The United States at this time was a ferment of natural approaches. Osteopathic medicine, as developed by Andrew

Taylor Still, was growing with its emphasis on circulation and visceral–nervous connections. D.D. Palmer was launching chiropractic as a healing profession. Homeopathic medicine had been well established for two generations and many medical doctors considered themselves primarily homeopathic in orientation to treatment. A small number of medical doctors, particularly in the Midwest, were members of the eclectic school of herbal medicine. They studied the chemistry of herbs, made incredibly potent extracts, and documented their effects in great detail. Indigenous healers, including Native Americans, had an incredibly rich materia medica of plants, which was made use of by the eclectics in addition to other sources. African-American medicine had developed a deep treasury of herbal medicines and other treatments, in part due to lack of access to medical doctors and due to insights and experimentation with the herbs of North America. Curanderismo, from Mexico, fused Galenic, Arabic, and Indigenous medicines with many spiritual beliefs.

Lust decided to embark on creating a fusion of some of these threads and purchased rights to the term "naturopathy." It was a portmanteau word from a Latin root (naturo, for nature) and a Greek one (pathos, for suffering or disease). The idea was to remove the roots of disease and cure using nature's methods and according to precepts that were in agreement with natural laws and natural tendencies of healing.

Kneipp had some other impressive students. Henry Lindlahr was a German immigrant to the United States [87, 90, 91]. He was a baker and brewing chemist, with a knowledge of using yeasts and bacteria to create ferments and flavors. He was successful in this and an astute businessman. He made a great deal of money in real estate speculation, buying land that he guessed the ever-expanding railroads would want in order to build tracks. By his mid-30s, he was mayor and owner of many enterprises in Kalispell, Montana. He was also dying of type II diabetes. He was very overweight and indulged in a hard driving life with excess food, liquor, and tobacco. Having amassed quite a bit of money, he was able to make the rounds and consult with some of the leading physicians of the time. Nobody was able to help him. He found himself, in his late 30s, "a wreck, with neither faith in God nor myself." He decided to travel to Germany and seek the assistance of the famous Father Kneipp. Once there, Kneipp took charge of his case, and within the year, Lindlahr had lost a large amount of weight, and the sugar had disappeared from his urine.

Lindlahr stayed to learn from Kneipp and then returned to the United States. He entered medical school, the National Medical University, in Illinois, a respectable MD granting school of the time. He opened a large clinic in Chicago, on Ashland Avenue, in 1902. Lindlahr's facility had diagnostic facilities, including X-ray machines and some in-house laboratory instruments. He had a food preparation staff that made diets per physician orders, as it was an inpatient facility. Dentists checked for tooth abscess and periodontal infection, very common problems of the time. There were hydrotherapy treatments, but also many other modalities. Later, Lindlahr opened a summertime live-in facility in Elmhurst, Illinois, that in a sense replicated the return to nature and more rural (at that time) experience he had had in Bavaria.

Lindlahr has a local associate and former Kneipp patient, Dr. John Howard, who was the founding president of the National College of Chiropractic in Iowa and then shortly thereafter in Chicago, Illinois [92]. Howard had sought out Father Kneipp for health issues, recovered his strength, and then studied chiropractic at the first such school in Des Moines, Iowa. Wanting to expand the practice to include the "physiological adjustment," he started his own school in Chicago. This facility grew to prominence and was located on Ashland Street, not far from the Lindlahr facility. Howard and his successors, including the legendary Dr. Joseph Janse, wanted to train chiropractors to be diagnosticians and to use the broader array of nature's agents to treat disease.

When Lindlahr died in 1925, he had developed a school that granted degrees in "nature cure"—probably under an osteopathic degree. He bequeathed this operation to NCC, and the curriculum at that school received an influx of hydrotherapy, botanical medicine, and more. NCC, or National, granted an ND (Doctor of Naturopathy) degree, as well as "Drugless Therapy" degrees for its chiropractors, until 1952. At that time, pressure from the office of education (later becoming the US Department of Education) on all chiropractic programs to drop "spurious degrees" led to the National ending its naturopathic program in 1952.

In 2006, under the leadership of President James Winterstein, the National, now known as the National University of Health Sciences, launched a naturopathic medicine degree. By this time, the naturopathic profession and education system had made a resurgence, with accredited (at federal and regional levels) programs across North America [93].

There are many, many aspects to the development of naturopathy, the history of hydrotherapy, and many healers who built this movement. But hydrotherapy deserves some special mention because it is integral to naturopathic medicine. This is true historically and philosophically.

Addressing Determinants of Health

Movement is a fundamental requirement for health. In general, physical therapies help to restore function and structural abilities to permit movement without pain and undue restriction. This has knock-on effects of improved circulation, lymph flow, myofascial conditioning, and the sensory effects of movement that go to the brain.

Movement also occurs between joints in ways that allow for fluid circulation. Cramer et al. have shown that spinal manipulation leads to zygapophyseal joint (facet joint) gapping and becoming mobilized [94]. This was shown with Magnetic Resonance (MR) technology. Cramer et al. are currently completing a human trial building on previous work that shows that accelerometry can show that movement has occurred in the Z joint [95]. This is important in that they have demonstrated that crepitus prevalence decreased pre–post spinal manipulation therapy. This is important work that is showing in detail how mobilization at this small synovial joint level can occur. Demobilized joints with high crepitus and poor motion are more likely to degenerate.

Many physical medicine treatments involve touch. This touch is delivered with the patient's consent and safely. The human need for touch is known at an experiential and intuitive level. Neurodevelopment is touch dependent. Current literature confirms that compassion expressed through touch makes patients feel safe. It strengthens the doctor and patient bond.

Biochemical Support

Laser Therapies

Lasers vary in frequency and intensities. They are typically used in naturopathic medicine and physical rehabilitation to stimulate circulation, mitochondrial function, and mitosis. Or they are used for analgesic effects [96, 97]. Other types of lasers used for ablative or coagulation treatments are not discussed here as they are more germane to ophthalmology as a specialty or dermatology. Low-power laser light has been shown to reduce joint inflammation and enhance the circulation needed for healing [98]. Higher-intensity laser energy penetrates more deeply into tissue, but must be used with its own precise settings and precautions.

Centripetal Massage

Bodywork as a whole comprises many techniques and, globally, many traditions. The use of hands to heal is ancient. The kneading and stretching of tissues during bodywork can help with myofascial function and decrease hypertonicity. Whole body massage that rolls and pushes the tissues in a centripetal direction (towards the center of the body) helps lymph flow back to the vena cava. In terms of draining tissues, improving circulation, and stimulating the sensory system, bodywork is a very direct approach that can add to the healing process [99].

Hormetic Effect

Sauna is a great example of how inputs of a physical agent, heat in this case, can promote pro-survival responses. Sauna is used in many societies and can be a rock sauna, as is popular in Nordic countries, or an infrared sauna, which is a self-contained unit that creates sustained heat. A series of sauna treatments has a preconditioning response that is hormetic in nature. A low-dose stimulation (or low intensity in this case) leads to a modest overcompensation response that elicits pro-survival mechanisms [100]. This has bodily repair and antiaging aspects. Although exercise is a common example, sauna has interesting advantages in its focus on the heat-shock protein, as well as being a more passive treatment, which is helpful for those with advanced arthritis and pain.

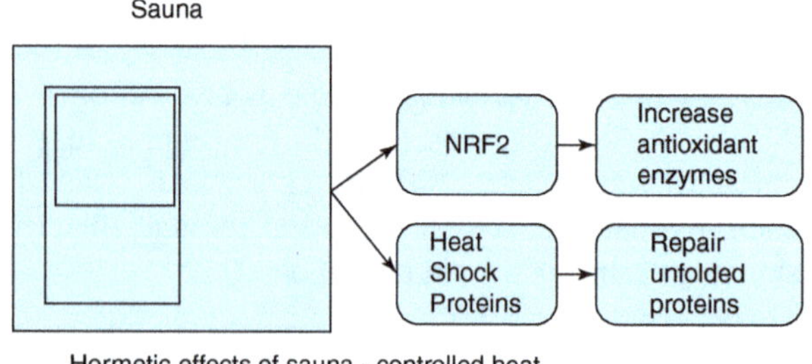

Fig. 6.21 Effects of sauna therapy: The sustained heat of a sauna can activate heat-shock proteins and NRF2 pathways. If the sauna treatment is within tolerance limits for an individual, it could be said to have a hormetic effect

Genomically, the expression of heat-shock proteins and antioxidant proteins arise from heat treatment. These are hormetic effects that are designed to limit damage to the organism. All cells have heat-shock proteins. They are linked to a variety of tasks such as cell signaling, cell cycle regulation, and proteome homeostasis. Heat-shock proteins prevent protein aggregation and disruption of the proteasome. They repair damaged proteins and may preserve muscle mass. Stress such as oxidative stress, nutritional deficiency, and environmental shocks such as extreme heat or cold, toxins, etc. can damage proteins causing them to unfold and lose their tertiary structures. Heat-shock proteins (HSP) can ameliorate this.

Under stressful environmental conditions, cellular proteins can unfold or become damaged, impairing their normal functions and further increasing their vulnerability to change. During exposure to environmental stressors such as temperature extremes, caloric restriction, certain plant compounds, or even hypoxia, cells increase expression of HSPs to stabilize unfolded proteins and repair or resynthesize damaged proteins. In therapy, we avoid the extremes that the HSP system was designed for, but give a subthreshold (of harm) exposure to elicit the adaptive responses.

The heat of a sauna, or for that matter other hydrotherapy treatments, in measured exposures, can activate heat-shock proteins (Fig. 6.21). This begins in the first 30 min of heat treatment. Another effect of this exposure is activation of Nuclear factor erythroid 2–related factor 2 (Nrf2). As is often the case with hormetins, heat can cause Nrf2 to translocate to the nucleus, switch on the antioxidant response element, and lead to transcription of antioxidant/detoxification enzymes such as glutathione synthase. Sauna and whole-body hyperthermia can both elicit Nrf2 activation. Balneotherapy, such as immersion in a hot tub, has many of the same benefits [101].

Therapeutic Ultrasound

This therapy uses low-intensity ultrasound waves. This is produced by a piezoelectric crystal inside the head of an applicator. This produces sound waves that are far beyond human hearing. Therapeutic ultrasound is a form of acoustic energy. There are high-intensity forms that can be used to ablate tissue or shatter nephrolithiasis (kidney stones).

Low-intensity ultrasound can generate heat and cause a thermal effect. The ultrasound waves pass through tissues, but do not push or pull molecules along. Instead, they cause them to vibrate in place. This has a beneficial effect on stimulation. But the nature of the response to this jarring motion of the ultrasound appears to be hormetic in nature. A low-dose stimulation leads to a second effect. High doses will melt away tissue and cause injury. Bone, ligament, tendons, and any higher protein tissue will respond most to ultrasound. Adipose tissue responds less. Pulsed ultrasound has become more commonly used as it allows for more space in between acoustic bursts, not necessarily a lower wavelength but pauses. This permits heat to evaporate, reducing the change of thermal injury in tendons, ligaments, periosteum of bone, etc. [102].

Some of the effects of therapeutic ultrasound include a stimulation of cell regeneration. Production of extracellular matrix proteins in connective tissue as well as bone and cartilage (chondrocyte activation) can occur with low-intensity ultrasound. Mesenchymal stromal cells that become the basis of tissue parenchyma, including bone and intervertebral discs, increase after ultrasound treatment [103]. This energy also reduces the enzymes that degrade the matrix, and while these are important for remodeling, they appear to frustrate long-term repair. These include MMP-3 (matrix metalloproteinase-3) expression. Type II collagen is produced in higher amounts. Ultrasound also creates stimulation of cells via the integrin proteins and MAPK activation (a normal mechanotransduction mechanism whereby an extracellular matrix can interact with integrins in the cell membrane and stimulate growth) [103, 104].

Ultrasound encourages collagen-producing cells such as osteoblasts and epithelial cells to migrate to treatment areas. In an acute treatment of ultrasound, inflammation may increase, including mast cell degranulation and immune cell activation. This may not be the best therapy for many acute inflammations. But for a stalled healing process, the acoustic stimulation of ultrasound provides a small stimulation that leads to extracellular matrix formulation, increased cellular activity, and migration of needed tissue progenitor cells to an area needing reconstruction.

Short-Term Warm and Cold Application

Short-term warmth is used as a circulatory stimulation. For example, a 5-min foot bath is used to relax muscles in the foot, or to draw circulation to the lower extremity away from the head (called "derivation" in the past and used for sinus congestion or headache) [106]. Foot baths can also help relax someone and improve sleep [105]. These must be done with care especially for those with diminished sensation in their feet (as in diabetes) as they might not realize they are getting burned if the temperature is too high.

Short-term cold is of course used for its analgesic and anti-inflammatory effect. It is used to numb pain and after acute tendon or ligament sprain. Although the value in the immediate suppression of inflammation with cold is debated, a brief burst of cold, used according to traditional hydrotherapy principles, would bring down swelling.

A cold application that is left on for a long time, such that the body warms it up, will bring circulation to the area. This assumes that the source of cold is left to be warmed up by the arrival of circulation and the compresses or towels are not replaced with new cold ones. A continual cold treatment created by replacing compresses frequently or with ice immersion will slow down cellular metabolism and at some point might thwart healing by overly suppressing the normal inflammatory response and even injuring cells due to lack of circulation and depressed cellular metabolism.

Whole-Person Therapy

Constitutional Treatment

An in-office adaptation of hydrotherapy was developed by naturopathic physician O.G. Caroll. This was done alone with food sensitivity testing, use of herbs to support detoxification, and other natural therapies as needed [106].

The constitutional method is done on a treatment table, with available hot and cold water at hand. The concurrent use of gentle sine wave electrical stimulation to the abdomen and the thoracic spinal junction provides additional input to the digestive and detoxification organs (Fig. 6.22). The basic steps are as follows:

Complete a history and examination of the patient—identify any special needs:

- Take body temperature and urinary specific gravity.
- Patient supine.
- Apply hot towels over the chest and abdomen (double hot towels, four layers) for 5 min.
- Apply a new hotel towel, and then cover with a cold towel, warn patient, and flip—with cold towel still on top of patient's chest and abdomen.
- Cover with a blanket and allow patient's own circulation to warm up the cold towel for at least 20 min. Apply sine wave to solar plexus and thoracolumbar function for the final 10 min (midpoint).
- Have patient turn to lie prone.
- Apply two hot towels at the back for 5 min.

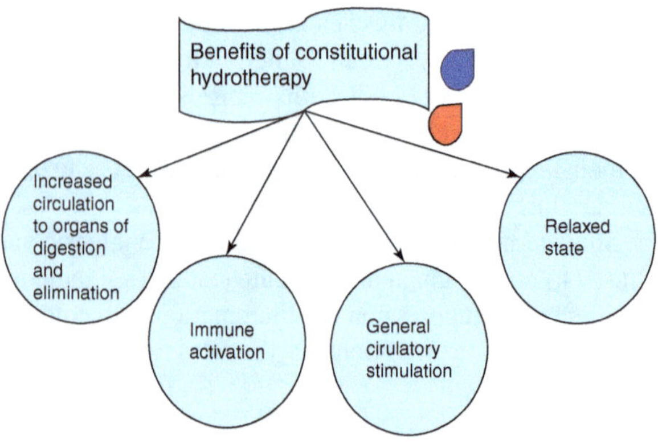

Fig. 6.22 Constitutional hydrotherapy: This treatment delivers circulation enhancing alternation of warmth and cold to the core of the body and has generalized effects such as improved circulation to organs of digestion and elimination

- Prepare a new hot towel and cold towel, apply in sequence, and then with a warning, flip towels to leave the cold towel on patient's back.
- Cover up with blanket and allow patient's circulation to warm up with a cold towel for at least 10 min.
- The patient's temperature is taken again, along with a second urine sample.

There are numerous modifications based on the patient's starting temperature. Patients with low body temperature receive extra warmth and less intense cold. Those with elevated temperatures receive less intense heat and prolonged cold (and the perspiration that occurs along with it).

There are many other modifications to this treatment that would be included in appropriate training in this modality that includes supervised practice actually performing the treatments.

Wet Sheet Pack

This is a very traditional hydrotherapy approach where the patient is wrapped in cold sheets and then in wool blankets [106]. In the first 5–20 min, the patient slowly vasodilates and begins to feel less cold, as their circulation is activated. In the time frame from 20 min into the treatment to 1 h, the person moves from not feeling chilly to actually feeling warm. If the treatment is continued to a third hour, the patients sweats profusely into the sheets.

This treatment follows a progression from stimulating a first to relaxing to the nervous system as the temperature of the sheets because neutral with body temperature. It then begins to stimulate metabolism and elimination.

So a short wet sheet application might be helpful for those who need a boost for energy and circulation. A moderate-length treatment (about 30–40 min) is mentally calming and stress reducing. A longer treatment where the patient begins to sweat is helpful for chronic gastrointestinal and hepatic disturbances. Even longer treatments are helpful in metabolic syndrome, obesity, and toxin deposition (including those who are going through smoking cessation).

Immersion: Balneotherapy

Bath therapy is sometimes partial immersion, such as a sitz bath for hemorrhoids, pelvic pain, or episiotomy pain. Full immersion can be used for strengthening the body and relieving stress [101]. Neutral baths have been known for a long time to have a calming effect. In a small clinical trial in 2018, participants who receive immersion bathing fill out a Profile of Mood States (POMS), in short form before and after 2 weeks of treatment. Scores were significantly lower for tension–anxiety, depression–dejection, and anger–hostility during bathing intervention than a non-bathing group that did a showering intervention [101].

Bone metabolism (growth and mineralization), muscle pain, and arthritis pain have all been shown to improve with balneotherapy. This continues to be a powerful treatment in naturopathic medicine and many other systems of medicine.

Spinal Manipulation

Spinal manipulation is a powerful tool that has both whole-person effects and local pain relief. Mobilizing the neuromuscular segment of a joint allows muscle spasms to abate, creates mobility at joint surfaces, and allows better biochemical function. This therapy can be done safely with proper training. It has strong evidence for relief from low back pain and evidence that varies in quality for other issues and sources of pain [107–109]. When incorporated into a whole-person approach, it can help with resetting biochemical and myofascial patterns.

Rehabilitative Therapies: Exercise and Reconditioning

Naturopathic physicians recommend rehabilitative exercises, recognizing that complex cases due to certain injuries such as trauma, post cerebral vascular accident, pediatric developmental, and many other situations require more precise intervention from physicians and doctors of physical therapy who specialize in this area (which some naturopathic physicians certainly do).

Rehabilitative exercises such as gradual strengthening, stretching, and proprioceptive training (regaining joint to brain communication and control) are sometimes recommended to patients.

Exercise in general is often recommended to patients, including aerobic, strength, endurance, flexibility, and more. Specific schools of exercise that also incorporate breath, mindfulness, and myofascial mobility, such as Pilates, yoga, and tai chi, are also important recommendations [110].

Dampen Symptoms

Interferential Current Therapy

This is an electrical therapy that consists of two sinusoidal alternating currents of slightly different frequencies. One is set at 4000 Hz and the other at 4001–4250 Hz. These currents are generated in a crossing pattern, with a zone of overlap which

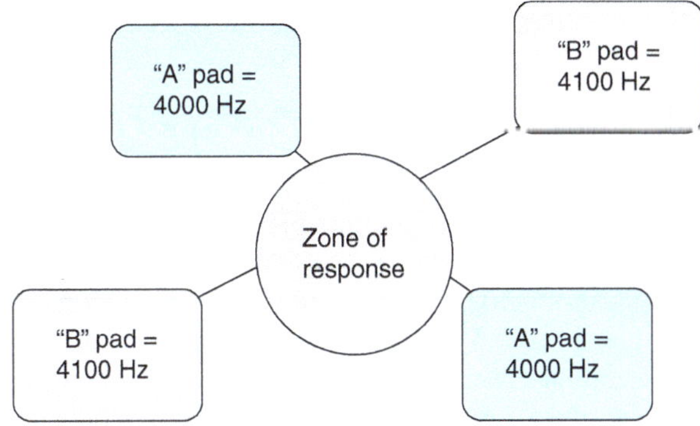

Fig. 6.23 Interferential current therapy: The pads of the IFC treatment are placed in a crisscross pattern, with pads of the same level of Hz opposite each other. The zone in the center of the pads exhibits the physiological effects. These can vary depending on the setting, but improved circulation, reduced edema, and reduction in pain are common indications for this treatment

creates the therapeutic effect (Fig. 6.23). IFC therapy has been used for neuropathies and to stimulate bone healing. One of its uses is to reduce pain. It is unclear precisely why it has analgesic effects. It may activate large-diameter nerve fibers and suppress the processing of afferent pain signals from other nerves (gate control theory of pain). It might also cause release of spinal cord endogenous opioids (endorphins). It might also block transmission of some pain fibers, which would be a very transient benefit, unless that blockage during therapy led to a quiescent period of those afferent nociceptive fibers post treatment [111–113].

Steam Inhalation with Essential Oils

Steam itself is a thermal therapy, but it can also be used to ventilate and soothe the bronchial surfaces. This can have a mucus loosening effect which is beneficial to those with lower respiratory infections, chronic obstructive lung disease, and asthma. Essential oils can be added to the water mixture that will become vaporized. Thymol from *Thymus vulgaris*, rosmarinic acid from Rosmarinus officinalis, eucalyptol from *Eucalyptus globulus*, and menthol from *Mentha piperita* are just some of the options. These plants are sources of terpene molecules which are cooling to the surface of the bronchi, due to their lower latent heat evaporation (compared to water). They relax smooth muscle, dissolve and loosen mucus, and are antiseptic [114, 115].

Trigger Point Therapy

Trigger points are small, hypertonic knot-like areas of myofascial tissue. When pressed, they cause a referred pain. They can be found across the myofascial–muscular system, but are often paraspinal. Although they are similar to tender points, such as one might find in patients with fibromyalgia, they are found in many people with chronic stiffness and pain and have a radiating effect. Manual manipulation of trigger points can make them less tender, and this is an effect that seems to keep increasing with ongoing manual manipulation and release [116].

Injection of trigger points can also yield results. In more conventional approaches to treatment, local anesthetic agents such as lidocaine and novocaine, plus a corticosteroid, are used. Naturopathic physicians might also use a sterile, diluted homeopathic medicine (such as *Hypericum* or *Arnica*), or solution–/injection-grade vitamin B12 [117].

Induce Homeostasis

Transcutaneous electrical stimulation, or TENS, is the application of a mild electrical current across the skin. It involves a small current generator and pads attached to the skin. It is often used for long periods of time and hours at a time. Patients are given a TENS unit to block pain signals and raise endorphin levels (Fig. 6.24). It has been shown to reduce pain and increase quality of life. It may also reduce inflammatory cytokines. While not a causal treatment, it is a relief-giving and harmless

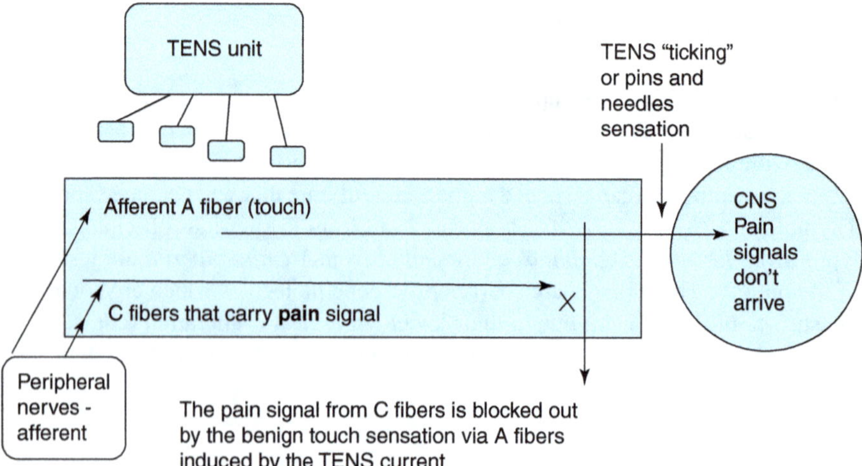

Fig. 6.24 Transcutaneous electrical nerve stimulation (TENS) therapy: The mild current from the applicator sends a signal down afferent A fibers that suppresses the impact of the pain signals that travel to the spinal cord from C fibers

therapy. There are contraindications. Patients with implants such as pacemakers, pregnant patients, those with cancer, or those with deep vein thrombosis should not apply this current. Also, those with bleeding near the site should avoid it. Patients with epilepsy should not put the unit in the shoulders, neck, face, or head. Cardiac patients who have arrhythmias, even if they do not have a pacemaker, should avoid TENS [113].

Special Section on Whole-Person Therapies

Some therapies used by naturopathic physicians are based on a whole-person response. That does not mean that they cannot be used for specific symptoms or locally. But their framework is based on treating the whole person. As the science of whole systems as applied to biology and medicine continues to evolve, so will guidance as to how to use these therapies. This is not to say that other therapeutics do not have whole-person effects. Botanical medicines, as much as we might seem to categorize them, can have broad effects. Diet is a foundational building block of metabolism and it influences the microbiome. Physical medicine, and even touch itself, has a global beneficial effect, even if it is via the lessening of anxiety and the reassurance that comes from attention and respectful and healing touch by a physician.

Deep Meditation, Prayer, Faith

While these acts differ in their nature, they involve an inward focusing on the sacred, divine, and universal that a person can sense. Meditation can take many, many forms. Some people repeat certain word sequences; others visualize something. For example, a person who slows their breathing and focuses on how they are one cell among all human cells and tries to recall all the times in their life they felt loved could be said to be meditating. There are also structured forms of mediation that can be presented in an educational manner.

Prayer, again, has a multiplicity of forms. It usually involves speaking to, communing with, and raising feelings and thoughts to what one considers a higher power. That concept differs between people. Some prayers are intersessional, such as asking for help for one's self or others. Prayers can be directional, asking for guidance and discernment. Prayer can also be gratitude and thanksgiving.

Faith is a broad concept. The term can be used to refer to a specific belief system (i.e., "I am of the _______ faith"). But in a health-related sense, faith is some belief in the goodness of the universe and the positive intentions and acts of the human family as they operate in harmony with that goodness.

The medical literature refers to religiosity/spirituality as one way to categorize research on this area. They are separated somewhat with religiosity being defined as belonging to a group that has shared beliefs and practices. Spirituality is a more commonly appearing term and relates to personal beliefs, values, and meaning.

It is worth nothing that in many traditional medicine systems, spirituality is front and center. That does not mean that behavior factors and remedies are disregarded. But resolving spiritual and inner tensions or suffering is a vital part of healing. This often involves restitution or reconciliation with others in the family or community. Many traditional systems do not fully differentiate between mind and body.

In the Western Medical tradition, there is a separation of mind and spirit from body and neurochemistry in Western medicine. This arose out of a drive to explain disease and its cures on a rational basis and using the scientific process to slowly accrue knowledge. This is not a bad thing in itself. The problem was that clinical medicine involves working with human beings and their self, their personhood, their beliefs, and inner experience are simply a huge part of the experience. These might shrink in relevance in emergency situations where events proceed in seconds and a reliable and fast treatment is required to save a life. But in the long haul of illness, chronic illness, and even terminal illness, these verities of our existence rise back to the surface.

In the twentieth century, movements such as holistic nursing have worked to spring spirituality back into view. The cancer surgeon Bernie Siegal, with his books such as "Love, Medicine, and Miracles" and "Peace, Love, and Healing," brought this issue further into the public consciousness [118]. He was a cancer surgeon, using the most modern methods, giving case history after case history of how people's lives were dramatically altered by finding a connection with an inner consciousness of the sacred. Sometimes that meant inexplicable healing or resolve to endure a painful series of treatments and defy a prognosis, or a quiet and serene acceptance (stages of grief notwithstanding) of the dying process.

Published first in 1986, there is Reed's Spiritual Perspective Scale. The National Institute of Aging published research on the Multidimensional Measure of Religiousness/Spirituality (MMRS). There are well over 20 such instruments. Some focus on overall spiritual well-being. Others look at how beliefs and practices can be relied upon when a health crisis intervenes in a person's life. Some are tailored to those recovering from alcoholism, addiction, etc. [119].

One practical interviewing tool that is in common use originated at Brown University. The HOPE model is something that is simple to integrate into the flow of a patient intake where:

H = sources of hope, meaning, comfort, strength, peace, love, and connection [120].
O = organized religion.
P = personal spirituality and practices.
E = effects on medical care and end-of-life issues.

Homeopathy

Homeopath is a widely used therapy by naturopathic physicians. It was initially a very minor part of naturopathy. In the mid-twentieth century, the influence of Dr. John Bastyr, who had trained at a homeopathic hospital as a young man, helped integrate this therapy into naturopathic training and practice. Currently, it is becoming less used. One reason is that the thought process and reasoning methods differ from other therapies. Another is that outside of acute−/first aid-type prescribing, homeopathic medicine can require longer visits. A third reason is that the preparation of many homeopathic remedies is controversial. It involves for many remedies an extreme dilution (alongside the input of kinetic energy) to the point that very few or no molecules of the substance are being diluted out to remain.

Homeopathy was developed by Dr. Samuel Hahnemann, a German physician who was born in 1755. He was trained at the University of Leipzig and was a medical doctor trained in the therapies of his time. A series of events left him rather disillusioned with practice of the time, which was based on prevailing theories and employed, among other agents, mercury. He worked as a medical textbook translator for some years, being fluent in several languages and knowing Latin. He ran across reports by the Scottish physician John Cullen of cinchona bark (*Cinchona officinalis*) being curative of malaria. We know that this bark contains quinine, which is toxic to the parasite *Plasmodium falciparum* (although resistance to this class of drugs is quite common now). Cullen attributed its action to the herb's bitter taste. This was unsatisfactory, so in an effort to test the herb, Hahnemann took it himself. He developed alternating fever and chills, which is recognized as having a periodicity very similar to actual malaria. This intrigued him and he spent several years investigating the possibility that a substance could cure diseases that had a similar symptom presentation to the effects of the would-be remedy [121, 122].

The physician, philosopher, and alchemist Paracelsus had written about using similar (to the symptom picture in question) medicines to treat disease. Hippocrates wrote a little about similars, such as this quote from his aphorisms:

> The pains (complaints) will be removed by means of their opposite, each according to its own characteristics. Thus, heat corresponds to a hot constitution that has been made ill by the cold, and so on for the others. Another way of removing pain is the following: a disease develops by means of its like and is cured by means of the use of its like. Thus, what causes urinary tenesmus in health cures it in disease. Cough is caused and cured by means of the same agent, as in the case of urinary tenesmus. Another method: the fever causing the development of inflammation will be caused and cured by the same agent.... [Littre's Oeuvres Completes d'Hippocrates, VI, 334, Paris, 1839, cited in (2), p. 9] [123].

Hahnemann set out to test various substances on himself or colleagues, to get a sense of what their effect was (based on signs and symptoms) on the healthy. He then attempted to see if these substances were therapeutic when given to a sick person who displayed a similar set of signs and symptoms. He found this was the case, and over the years, he developed, and practiced, the system he called homeopathy.

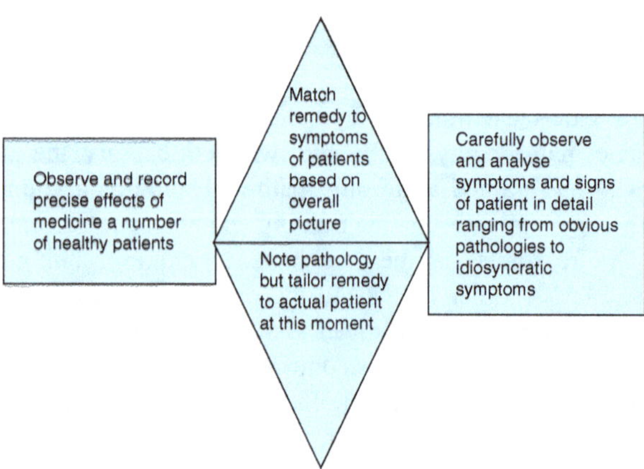

Fig. 6.25 Concept of homeopathic similar principle: Remedies are studied closely for their fullest range of effects, by observing their actions on the healthy. Patient symptoms and signs in their broadest sense are recorded by the physician. The prescription takes pathology into account, but the goal is to find a remedy based on some substance in nature which would cause a similar symptom picture in the healthy and deliver that substance (almost always in some dilution) to the patient

This was based on what Hahnemann called the law of similars or "like cures like." The term "homeopathy'" literally means similar suffering. He contrasted this with antipathy, treating with opposites. He also made a point of describing the mercury and bloodletting doctors of the time as "allopathy"—treating to create a different disease state in the patient that displaced the original disease (or to put it another way, to trade in your current unpleasant situation for a different but unknown situation). Finally, he identified "isopathy" as treated with not similar, but the same agents.

He also proposed using the minimum dose. Any plant, mineral, or animal substance could be used in this framework, so some of these, such as arsenic, had to be diluted to be tolerable. Hahnemann found over time that a very dilute medicine could provide the necessary "similar effect" input. This was in contrast to the prevailing philosophy of meeting aggressive diseases with even more aggressive treatments.

Hahnemann also developed very detailed descriptions of remedies. The point was to have the healthy, those who were not in a drastic state of imbalance, take the remedies and then meticulously record the observed effects (Fig. 6.25). This created a profile of effects, signs and symptoms, of various agents that could be compared to clinical presentations by individual patients, in order to find a match between similar disease presentation in a specific patient and a remedy. This he called "provings" based on the German word "prober" or to experiment.

Hahnemann continued to develop these medicines and started to share this way of treating patients with certain colleagues. In time, this homeopathic method began to attract many users in the European medical profession. This spread to the Americas and across the world. Homeopathy had a lot of success in the United States. By 1900, one in five medical doctors identified as a homeopath. This was in spite of fierce opposition from local medical societies and a national association known as the American Medical Association that was initially formed to combat the surge of homeopathic practice in the 1840s.

Homeopathy developed into a large system with many hundreds of remedies. Some have received good provings (tests to outline their range of effects) and some have had rather incomplete provings. Indexes where symptoms can be correspondent with possible remedies used to be in rather large books. Now they are in computerized databases.

In the later nineteenth century, American homeopaths were a house divided. Some homeopaths wanted to belong to those county medical societies, they are, after all, MD, and it was good for business to have referrals from colleagues. This meant using more patent drugs and fewer homeopathic remedies. The way of prescribing became more routine, with a top five approach to common conditions. They also used homeopathic medicines that had only been slightly diluted. That was not far off from many of the emerging drugs of the time, which were purified extracts from herbs, such as atropine, morphine, scopolamine, etc., which are all alkaloids from plants.

A smaller but very influential group stuck to a very Hahnemann-based approach, taking a complete inventory of symptoms of each patients and trying to really apply the principle of similars in earnest. They tended to use very, very dilute medicines. Some of these were diluted 1 in 100 so many times that they no longer likely contained any of the starting substance. This taking of serial dilution to the point that the solution of the solvent and the concentration of the herb, mineral, etc. in it passed Avogadro's number actually started with Hahnemann. Later in his long career (he practiced into his 90s), he had taken dilutions to this point.

Homeopathy presents something of a conundrum for naturopathic medicine today. It has a vast clinical experience, around the world. Millions of treatments back up the observations of homeopaths that it is a therapy that can help people "reboot" the system and heal. Hahnemann stated that an "untunement" in the "Dynamis," the inherent principle of adaptation and repair, led to true chronic disease. The point of a homeopathic medicine was to lift a person out of this counterproductive loop they were stuck in.

Homeopathy has been studied scientifically. It has many positive studies. It also has negative ones. Systematic reviews of homeopathy tend to find too high a risk of bias and small sample size. The idea of using something that dilute is outside of the current paradigm of chemistry and physics. The fact that a truly testable hypothesis about these dilutions, a falsifiable hypothesis, is not yet at hand has not helped homeopathy.

In many countries, physicians incorporate it into practice. In France, about 10% of oncologists recommend homeopathy as adjunctive care for their patients. In Switzerland, about 30% of outpatient (ambulatory) physicians recommend some homeopathy. In India, there are over 225 colleges that offer homeopathy.

For naturopathic physicians, homeopathy is a conundrum because they are attempting to show through research that naturopathic therapies work. Homeopathic research tends to be weak or hard to replicate. Pure science research into ultrahigh dilutions is always interesting, but not conclusive and sometimes not replicable. And yet homeopathy continues to have positive studies. A 2020 study that was three-armed found that in patients with non-small cell lung cancer, quality of life and survival improved (435 days of survival for the homeopathic treated group versus 225 for placebo). This was add-on care, not the main form of care for this type of cancer [124].

Systematic reviews on homeopathy typically show unclear results and a conclusion of not sufficient evidence or "cannot be recommended." This is partly due to issues such as study size or risks of bias. On the other hand, homeopathic medicine is a highly individualized form of therapy, with remedy selection based on idiosyncratic attributes of a patient at one moment in time. This does not excuse homeopathy from the need to be a subject of research. But it underscores the inherent shortcomings of the randomized controlled trial/systematic review (RCT/SR) approach for dynamic types of therapy such as homeopathy. The massive replication of effects from thousands of cases, which homeopaths have documented over the years, is also a kind of evidence. The trend in medicine at this time is to not see or acknowledge evidence that does not fit an RCT/SR pure model, even if rigorous replication shows an effect. In spite of the fact that bias and generally the post hoc *ergo propter hoc* fallacy of the human mind can indeed distort experience, the general agnosticism about the value of clinical experience says more about the current state of medical research than homeopathy.

Homeopathic medicine can be used for specific ailments or even first aid (Table 6.3). It is best applied based on an individual symptom picture based on a carefully taken patient history. Some homeopathic prescriptions are meant to match the overall symptoms of the person. In this way, it is a whole-person therapy. This is true because it is based on treating the whole person. Hahnemann taught that in order to establish an accurate portrait of a specific patient at a precise moment in time, it was necessary to consider the "totality of symptoms." It is also premised on the idea that a similar chosen remedy will act to stimulate the self-healing mechanism. Given that the human body has a complex and self-regulating network of systems, and stimuli to these systems can reset them, the central idea of homeopathy as a way to tune this complex organism is ahead of its time.

The above remedies are examples only. There are hundreds more. Homeopathic treatment is often done for chronic conditions, and the prescription includes consideration of local or pathological symptoms but also general symptoms such as body temperature, sleep, food aversions, etc. and what are called mental symptoms, such as emotional states.

It is interesting to note that Hahnemann started out simply diluting substances to a subtoxic dose. He was in all likelihood giving a material dose at first, but it was micrograms of some of these toxic substances. The late nineteenth-century and early twentieth-century homeopaths were using low doses of botanicals and minerals, in drop dose form. They were giving these medicines, but in an attenuated, but still measurable form.

Table 6.3 Examples of homeopathic remedies used in acute or first aid care [125, 126]

Remedy	Homeopathic indication	Natural effects in high dose versus low dose
Arnica montana a flower used in herbal medicine	Bruises, injuries to soft tissues, or overall trauma (like a fall on ice)	Can bc in high doscs, causc gastrointestinal upset, skin irritation, hypersensitivity reactions, cardiac arrhythmias
Apis mellifica—Venom of the honey bee	Pain, swelling/edema, pruritus (inflammatory events in joints, swelling in an area that is traumatized, and insect bites)	Pain, edema, white blood cell migration to an area, histamine release
Aconitum napellus—The mountain-growing herb wolfsbane, also known as monkshood	Fever, pain, sleepless with pain and excitation during fever, especially those fevers that come on suddenly and forcefully; panic attacks	Poisoning due to paralysis (lack of depolarization) of all nerves and excitable membranes. Aconitine (an alkaloid) causes sodium channels to stay open. The patient may remain conscious as they find their nervous system not responding. Cardiac arrhythmias
Arsenicum album—Arsenic trioxide	Burning pains, fever with chills, anxiety	Blocks oxidative phosphorylation and causes hypoxia, abdominal pain, and cardiac arrhythmia (chronically: Damage to multiple organs, glycemic issues, skin lesions, and increased cancer risk). Provokes dysglycemia at sublethal but chronic levels
Atropa belladonna—From the deadly nightshade plant	Fever, migraines, sunstroke or heat exhaustion with mental confusion	Anticholinergic toxidrome with dry mouth, hot skin, tachycardia, and then cardiac arrhythmias. Delirium due to anticholinergic (antagonist at acetylcholine receptors)
Calendula officinalis—Marigold	Skin abrasions, or aphthous ulcers in the mouth	Photosensitizing thiophene derivatives that lead to irritation of the skin on sun exposure; smaller amounts of the marigold extract are conditioning to the skin
Hepar sulphuricum (calcium sulfide)	Sores in mouth, wounds, tonsillitis, pharyngitis, feeling as if a foreign body is embedded in tissue	Appears rather inert. Related but not identical calcium sulfate will irritate all mucus membranes and as will sulfur
Nux vomica (from *Strychnos nux-vomica*)	Spasms of the gut, headache, neuralgias, withdrawal from stimulants or alcohol	Botanical source of strychnine, which blocks inhibitory neural pathways, leads to hyperexcitement of muscles, spasticity, convulsions, and death by respiratory paralysis

(continued)

Table 6.3 (continued)

Remedy	Homeopathic indication	Natural effects in high dose versus low dose
Phosphorus	Cough, bronchitis	Actual phosphorus exposure as a gas causes extreme burning in the skin, eyes, mucus membranes and internally extensive organ damage
Rhus toxicodendron—Poison ivy plant	Painful joints which improve with continued motion, warm pains that do not improve or get worse with warm applications	The plant contains urushiol, a compound that can cause delayed hypersensitivity reactions and very extensive erythema, skin wheals, and serous exudate

Acupuncture

Acupuncture is a treatment modality that is a part of a larger system of medicine. Actually, several medical systems use it. Traditional Chinese Medicine, which spans about 3000 years and in canonical form, about 1500 years, developed this therapy. There are Korean and Japanese systems of acupuncture. It involves inserting a needle into a specific, and mapped out, series of precise points on the surface of the body. These points are arrayed in linear patterns, or "channels" that travel from the hand and foot to the trunk or head. The theory behind acupuncture is complex and ancient. It is based on a Taoist concept of balancing Yin and Yang energies in the body. Acupuncture points are one way to influence this balance and the flow of the body energy, "qi," through these channels and the organs they are associated with [127].

In the twentieth century, physicians of different types began to incorporate some limited acupuncture, in order to treat conditions such as shoulder pain, headache, nicotine addiction, etc. This is known as medical acupuncture. It is an abridged form of delivering acupuncture. Likewise, ear acupuncture is sometimes used for anxiety or posttraumatic stress disorder [128, 129].

Some naturopathic physicians use acupuncture, either in a more limited form (but still informed by the traditional theory they are trained in) or by pursuing a professional degree in acupuncture in addition to their naturopathic medical degree. Although it can be used for painful or tender points, almost as a form of physical medicine, it is much more. Acupuncture and other therapies and practices such as Tai Chi, Qi Qong, Tui Na, and Chinese herbal medicine are used extensively in China and around the world. The research on these practices is growing daily. It is truly a whole-person system, because it considers the interconnectedness of organs and the effect of modes of living and the environment on a person's health. Although mind and body can be distinguished in Traditional Chinese Medicine, they are not separate entities in the way that they are thought of in Western medicine. It truly is a medicine that is hardwired to be holistic.

References

1. Ben Salem M, Affes H, Athmouni K, Ksouda K, Dhouibi R, Sahnoun Z, et al. Chemicals compositions, antioxidant and anti-inflammatory activity of Cynara scolymus leaves extracts, and analysis of major bioactive polyphenols by HPLC. Evid Based Complement Alternat Med. 2017;2017:4951937.
2. Lis B, Jedrejek D, Rywaniak J, Soluch A, Stochmal A, Olas B. Flavonoid preparations from Taraxacum officinale L. fruits—a phytochemical, antioxidant and hemostasis studies. Molecules. 2020;25(22):5402.
3. Bruyère F, Azzouzi AR, Lavigne J-P, Droupy S, Coloby P, Game X, et al. A multicenter, randomized, placebo-controlled study evaluating the efficacy of a combination of Propolis and cranberry (Vaccinium macrocarpon) (DUAB®) in preventing low urinary tract infection recurrence in women complaining of recurrent cystitis. Urol Int. 2019;103(1):41–8.
4. Pires TCSP, Caleja C, Santos-Buelga C, Barros L, Ferreira ICFR. Vaccinium myrtillus L. fruits as a novel source of phenolic compounds with health benefits and industrial applications—a review. Curr Pharm Des. 2020;26(16):1917–28.
5. Chen L-R, Chen K-H. Utilization of Isoflavones in soybeans for women with menopausal syndrome: an overview. Int J Mol Sci. 2021;22(6):3212.
6. Calabrese EJ, Dhawan G, Kapoor R, Iavicoli I, Calabrese V. HORMESIS: a fundamental concept with widespread biological and biomedical applications. Gerontology. 2016;62(5):530–5.
7. Calabrese EJ, Kozumbo WJ. The hormetic dose-response mechanism: Nrf2 activation. Pharmacol Res. 2021;167:105526.
8. Calabrese EJ, Dhawan G, Kapoor R, Mattson MP, Rattan SI. Curcumin and hormesis with particular emphasis on neural cells. Food Chem Toxicol. 2019;129:399–404.
9. Calabrese EJ, Kozumbo WJ. The phytoprotective agent sulforaphane prevents inflammatory degenerative diseases and age-related pathologies via Nrf2-mediated hormesis. Pharmacol Res. 2021;163:105283.
10. Moore MN. Lysosomes, autophagy, and Hormesis in cell physiology, pathology, and age-related disease. Dose Response. 2020;18(3):1559325820934227.
11. Calabrese EJ, Calabrese V, Tsatsakis A, Giordano JJ. Hormesis and Ginkgo biloba (GB): numerous biological effects of GB are mediated via hormesis. Ageing Res Rev. 2020;64:101019.
12. Jeruzal-Świątecka J, Fendler W, Pietruszewska W. Clinical role of extraoral bitter taste receptors. Int J Mol Sci. 2020;21(14):5156.
13. Kelber O, Bauer R, Kubelka W. Phytotherapy in functional gastrointestinal disorders. Dig Dis. 2017;35(Suppl 1):36–42.
14. Madrigal-Santillán E, Madrigal-Bujaidar E, Álvarez-González I, Sumaya-Martínez MT, Gutiérrez-Salinas J, Bautista M, et al. Review of natural products with hepatoprotective effects. World J Gastroenterol. 2014;20(40):14787–804.
15. Shaito A, Thuan DTB, Phu HT, Nguyen THD, Hasan H, Halabi S, et al. Herbal medicine for cardiovascular diseases: efficacy, mechanisms, and safety. Front Pharmacol. 2020;11:1–32.
16. Wang J, Xiong X, Feng B. Effect of crataegus usage in cardiovascular disease prevention: an evidence-based approach. Evid Based Complement Alternat Med. 2013;2013:149363.
17. Zang Y, Wan J, Zhang Z, Huang S, Liu X, Zhang W. An updated role of astragaloside IV in heart failure. Biomed Pharmacother. 2020;126:110012.
18. de Llano DG, Moreno-Arribas MV, Bartolomé B. Cranberry polyphenols and prevention against urinary tract infections: relevant considerations. Molecules. 2020;25(15):3523.
19. Janda K, Wojtkowska K, Jakubczyk K, Antoniewicz J, Skonieczna-Żydecka K. Passiflora incarnata in neuropsychiatric disorders—a systematic review. Nutrients. 2020;12(12):3894.
20. Dhaliwal A, Gupta M. Physiology, opioid receptor. Treasure Island, FL: StatPearls; 2022.
21. Shinjyo N, Waddell G, Green J. Valerian root in treating sleep problems and associated disorders—a systematic review and meta-analysis. J Evid Based Integr Med. 2020;25:2515690X20967323.

22. Meeusen R, Decroix L. Nutritional supplements and the brain. Int J Sport Nutr Exerc Metab. 2018;28(2):200–11.
23. Noguchi-Shinohara M, Ono K, Hamaguchi T, Nagai T, Kobayashi S, Komatsu J, et al. Safety and efficacy of Melissa officinalis extract containing rosmarinic acid in the prevention of Alzheimer's disease progression. Sci Rep. 2020;10(1):18627.
24. Todorova V, Ivanov K, Delattre C, Nalbantova V, Karcheva-Bahchevanska D, Ivanova S. Plant adaptogens—history and future perspectives. Nutrients. 2021;13(8):2861.
25. Szabo S, Yoshida M, Filakovszky J, Juhasz G. "Stress" is 80 years old: from Hans Selye original paper in 1936 to recent advances in GI ulceration. Curr Pharm Des. 2017;23(27):4029–41.
26. Yance DR, Tabachnik B. Breakthrough solutions in herbal medicine adaptogenic formulas: the way to vitality. In: Townsend Letter: The Examiner of Alternative Medicine, vol. 282; 2007. p. 86–90. https://link.gale.com/apps/doc/A157081507/AONE?u=anon~9b440f6e.
27. Saunders PR, Smith F, Schusky RW. Echinacea purpurea L. in children: safety, tolerability, compliance, and clinical effectiveness in upper respiratory tract infections. Can J Physiol Pharmacol. 2007;85(11):1195–9.
28. Xu X, Yan H, Chen J, Zhang X. Bioactive proteins from mushrooms. Biotechnol Adv. 2011;29(6):667–74.
29. Iu Z, Zhong D, Yang B. Preventive and therapeutic effect of Ganoderma (Lingzhi) on liver injury. Adv Exp Med Biol. 2019;1182:217–42.
30. Ismaya WT, Tjandrawinata RR, Rachmawati H. Lectins from the edible mushroom Agaricus bisporus and their therapeutic potentials. Molecules. 2020;25(10):2368.
31. Trovato Salinaro A, Pennisi M, Di Paola R, Scuto M, Crupi R, Cambria MT, et al. Neuroinflammation and neurohormesis in the pathogenesis of Alzheimer's disease and Alzheimer-linked pathologies: modulation by nutritional mushrooms. Immun Ageing. 2018;15:8. https://pubmed.ncbi.nlm.nih.gov/29456585.
32. Stanković V, Mihailović V, Mitrović S, Jurišić V. Protective and therapeutic possibility of medical herbs for liver cirrhosis. Rom J Morphol Embryol. 2017;58(3):723–9.
33. Lobay D. Rauwolfia in the treatment of hypertension. Integr Med (Encinitas). 2015;14(3):40–6.
34. Odaguchi H, Hyuga S, Sekine M, Nakamori S, Takemoto H, Huang X, et al. The adverse effects of ephedra herb and the safety of ephedrine alkaloids-free ephedra herb extract (EFE). Yakugaku Zasshi. 2019;139(11):1417–25.
35. Rauf A, Akram M, Semwal P, Mujawah AAH, Muhammad N, Riaz Z, et al. Antispasmodic potential of medicinal plants: a comprehensive review. Oxid Med Cell Longev. 2021;2021:4889719.
36. Ganguli MN. Cases illustrating the benefit of belladonna in opium-poisoning. Ind Med Gaz. 1880;15(5):134–5.
37. Herraiz T, Guillén H. Monoamine oxidase-a inhibition and associated antioxidant activity in plant extracts with potential antidepressant actions. Biomed Res Int. 2018;2018:4810394.
38. Oei SL, Thronicke A, Kröz M, von Trott P, Schad F, Matthes H. Impact of oncological therapy and Viscum album L treatment on cancer-related fatigue and internal coherence in non-metastasized breast cancer patients. Integr Cancer Ther. 2020;19:1534735420917211.
39. Khan T, Ali S, Qayyum R, Hussain I, Wahid F, Shah AJ. Intestinal and vascular smooth muscle relaxant effect of Viscum album explains its medicinal use in hyperactive gut disorders and hypertension. BMC Complement Altern Med. 2016;16:251.
40. Meolie AL, Rosen C, Kristo D, Kohrman M, Gooneratne N, Aguillard RN, et al. Oral nonprescription treatment for insomnia: an evaluation of products with limited evidence. J Clin Sleep Med. 2005;1(2):173–87.
41. Wang A-Q, Yuan Q-J, Guo N, Yang B, Sun Y. Research progress on medicinal resources of Coptis and its isoquinoline alkaloids. Zhongguo Zhong Yao Za Zhi. 2021;46(14):3504–13.
42. Cirillo C, Capasso R. Constipation and botanical medicines: an overview. Phytother Res. 2015;29(10):1488–93.
43. Kreis W. The foxgloves (digitalis) revisited. Planta Med. 2017;83(12–13):962–76.

44. Agriculture USD of Dietary Guidelines [Internet]. https://nal.usda.gov/legacy/fnic/dietary-guidelines. Accessed 24 May 2022.
45. Hoffer LJ. Human protein and amino acid requirements. J Parenter Enteral Nutr. 2016;40(4):460–74.
46. Russo GL. Dietary n-6 and n-3 polyunsaturated fatty acids: from biochemistry to clinical implications in cardiovascular prevention. Biochem Pharmacol. 2009;77(6):937–46.
47. Stevens SL. Fat-soluble vitamins. Nurs Clin North Am. 2021;56(1):33–45.
48. Lykstad J, Sharma S. Biochemistry, water soluble vitamins. In: StatPearls [Internet]. Treasure Island, FL: StatPearls; 2022.
49. Chandrakumar A, Bhardwaj A, 't Jong GW. Review of thiamine deficiency disorders: Wernicke encephalopathy and Korsakoff psychosis. J Basic Clin Physiol Pharmacol 2018;30(2):153–162.
50. Xu XJ, Jiang GS. Niacin-respondent subset of schizophrenia—a therapeutic review. Eur Rev Med Pharmacol Sci. 2015;19(6):988–97.
51. Jiang K, Tang K, Liu H, Xu H, Ye Z, Chen Z. Ascorbic acid supplements and kidney stones incidence among men and women: a systematic review and meta-analysis. Urol J. 2019;16(2):115–20.
52. NIH. Magnesium Fact Sheet for Health Professionals [Internet]. https://ods.od.nih.gov/factsheets/Magnesium-healthProfessional/.
53. Ogawa Y, Kinoshita M, Shimada S, Kawamura T. Zinc and skin disorders. Nutrients. 2018;10(2):199.
54. Pasricha S-R, Tye-Din J, Muckenthaler MU, Swinkels DW. Iron deficiency. Lancet. 2021;397(10270):233–48.
55. Cho S, Chae JS, Shin H, Shin Y, Song H, Kim Y, et al. Hormetic dose response to (L)-ascorbic acid as an anti-cancer drug in colorectal cancer cell lines according to SVCT-2 expression. Sci Rep. 2018;8(1):11372.
56. Office of Dietary Supplements. Vitamin C [Internet]. https://ods.od.nih.gov/factsheets/Vitaminc-Healthprofessional/. Accessed 25 May 2022.
57. Lykkesfeldt J, Tveden-Nyborg P. The pharmacokinetics of vitamin C. Nutrients. 2019;11(10):2412.
58. Mason SA, Rasmussen B, van Loon LJC, Salmon J, Wadley GD. Ascorbic acid supplementation improves postprandial glycaemic control and blood pressure in individuals with type 2 diabetes: findings of a randomized cross-over trial. Diabetes Obes Metab. 2019;21(3):674–82.
59. Supplements NI of H-O of D. Nutrient recommendations: dietary reference intakes [Internet]. https://ods.od.nih.gov/HealthInformation/Dietary_Reference_Intakes.aspx. Accessed 25 May 2022.
60. Zaric BL, Obradovic M, Bajic V, Haidara MA, Jovanovic M, Isenovic ER. Homocysteine and hyperhomocysteinaemia. Curr Med Chem. 2019;26(16):2948–61.
61. Successful Farming. How four big companies control the U.S. beef industry [Internet]. https://www.agriculture.com/markets/newswire/explainer-how-four-big-companies-control-the-us-beef-industry. Accessed 25 May 2022.
62. USDA, HHS. Dietary Guidelines for Americans [Internet]. https://www.dietaryguidelines.gov/resources/2020-2025-dietary-guidelines-online-materials. Accessed 25 May 2022.
63. Filippou CD, Tsioufis CP, Thomopoulos CG, Mihas CC, Dimitriadis KS, Sotiropoulou LI, et al. Dietary approaches to stop hypertension (DASH) diet and blood pressure reduction in adults with and without hypertension: a systematic review and meta-analysis of randomized controlled trials. Adv Nutr. 2020;11(5):1150–60.
64. Davis C, Bryan J, Hodgson J, Murphy K. Definition of the Mediterranean diet; a literature review. Nutrients. 2015;7(11):9139–53.
65. Derbyshire EJ. Flexitarian diets and health: a review of the evidence-based literature. Front Nutr. 2016;3:55.

66. Berild A, Holven KB, Ulven SM. Recommended Nordic diet and risk markers for cardiovascular disease. Tidsskr den Nor laegeforening Tidsskr Prakt Med ny raekke. 2017;137(10):721–6.
67. Center for Disease Control and Prevention. Fast food consumption among adults in the United States, 2013–2016 [Internet]. https://www.cdc.gov/nchs/products/databriefs/db322.htm. Accessed 22 Apr 2022.
68. Weston Price Foundation. The Weston Price Foundation for wise traditions in food, farming, and the healing arts [Internet]. https://www.westonaprice.org/. Accessed 25 May 2022.
69. Shanahan C. Deep nutrition: why your genes need traditional food. New York: Flatiron Books; 2017.
70. Fiolet T, Srour B, Sellem L, Kesse-Guyot E, Allès B, Méjean C, et al. Consumption of ultra-processed foods and cancer risk: results from NutriNet-Santé prospective cohort. BMJ. 2018;360:k322.
71. Srour B, Fezeu LK, Kesse-Guyot E, Allès B, Méjean C, Andrianasolo RM, et al. Ultra-processed food intake and risk of cardiovascular disease: prospective cohort study (NutriNet-Santé). BMJ. 2019;365:l1451.
72. Monteiro CA, Cannon G, Moubarac J-C, Levy RB, Louzada MLC, Jaime PC. The UN decade of nutrition, the NOVA food classification and the trouble with ultra-processing. Public Health Nutr. 2018;21(1):5–17.
73. Parker HW, Vadiveloo MK. Diet quality of vegetarian diets compared with nonvegetarian diets: a systematic review. Nutr Rev. 2019;77(3):144–60.
74. Ułamek-Kozioł M, Czuczwar SJ, Januszewski S, Pluta R. Ketogenic diet and epilepsy. Nutrients. 2019;11(10):2510.
75. Sondhi V, Agarwala A, Pandey RM, Chakrabarty B, Jauhari P, Lodha R, et al. Efficacy of ketogenic diet, modified Atkins diet, and low glycemic index therapy diet among children with drug-resistant epilepsy: a randomized clinical trial. JAMA Pediatr. 2020;174(10):944–51.
76. Zhang C, Tan Y, Feng J, Huang C, Liu B, Fan Z, et al. Exploration of the effects of substrate stiffness on biological responses of neural cells and their mechanisms. ACS Omega. 2020;5(48):31115–25.
77. Wiedemann A, Oussalah A, Jeannesson É, Guéant J-L, Feillet F. Phenylketonuria, from diet to gene therapy. Med Sci (Paris). 2020;36(8–9):725–34.
78. Baumgartner MR, Hörster F, Dionisi-Vici C, Haliloglu G, Karall D, Chapman KA, et al. Proposed guidelines for the diagnosis and management of methylmalonic and propionic acidemia. Orphanet J Rare Dis. 2014;9:130.
79. Caio G, Lungaro L, Segata N, Guarino M, Zoli G, Volta U, et al. Effect of gluten-free diet on gut microbiota composition in patients with celiac disease and non-celiac gluten/wheat sensitivity. Nutrients. 2020;12(6):1832.
80. Rostami K, Bold J, Parr A, Johnson MW. Gluten-free diet indications, safety, quality, labels, and challenges. Nutrients. 2017;9(8):846.
81. Trinchieri A, Maletta A, Lizzano R, Marchesotti F. Potential renal acid load and the risk of renal stone formation in a case-control study. Eur J Clin Nutr. 2013;67(10):1077–80.
82. Ayers P, Adams S, Boullata J, Gervasio J, Holcombe B, Kraft MD, et al. A.S.P.E.N. parenteral nutrition safety consensus recommendations. JPEN J Parenter Enteral Nutr. 2014;38(3):296–333.
83. Schandelmaier S, Briel M, Saccilotto R, Olu KK, Arpagaus A, Hemkens LG, et al. Niacin for primary and secondary prevention of cardiovascular events. Cochrane Database Syst Rev. 2017;6(6):CD009744.
84. Czeranko S. Vincent Priessnitz (1799-1851). Integr Med (Encinitas). 2019;18(4):25.
85. Hydropathy; or the cold water cure, as Practised by Vincent Priessnitz, at Gräeffenberg, in Silesia. Med Chir Rev. 1842;36(72):362–8. https://pubmed.ncbi.nlm.nih.gov/29918622.
86. Czeranko S. Father Sebastian Kneipp (1821-1897). Integr Med (Encinitas). 2019;18(4):24.
87. Boyle W, Kirchfeld F. Nature doctors: pioneers in naturopathic medicine. Portland, OR: NCNM Press; 1994.

88. Rogers N. Polio chronicles: warm springs and disability politics in the 1930s. Asclepio. 2009;61(1):143–74.
89. David Ruggles Center for History and Education. David Ruggles [Internet]. https://davidrugglescenter.org/david-ruggles/. Accessed 25 May 2022.
90. Cody GW. The origins of integrative medicine-the first true integrators: the philosophy of early practitioners. Integr Med (Encinitas). 2018;17(2):16–8.
91. Czeranko S. Henry Lindlahr (1862-1924). Integr Med (Encinitas). 2019;18(3):49.
92. Beideman RP. The role of the encyclopedic Howard system in the professionalization of chiropractic National College, 1906-1981. Chiropr Hist Arch J Assoc Hist Chiropr. 1996;16(2):29–41.
93. Dynamic Chiropractic. First Graduates of Naturopathic Degree Program at National [Internet]. https://www.dynamicchiropractic.com/mpacms//dc/article.php?id=54413. Accessed 25 May 2022.
94. Cramer GD, Cambron J, Cantu JA, Dexheimer JM, Pocius JD, Gregerson D, et al. Magnetic resonance imaging zygapophyseal joint space changes (gapping) in low back pain patients following spinal manipulation and side-posture positioning: a randomized controlled mechanisms trial with blinding. J Manipulative Physiol Ther. 2013;36(4):203–17.
95. Cramer GD, Budavich M, Bora P, Ross K. A feasibility study to assess vibration and sound from zygapophyseal joints during motion before and after spinal manipulation. J Manipulative Physiol Ther. 2017;40(3):187–200.
96. Choi H-W, Lee J, Lee S, Choi J, Lee K, Kim B-K, et al. Effects of high intensity laser therapy on pain and function of patients with chronic back pain. J Phys Ther Sci. 2017;29(6):1079–81. https://pubmed.ncbi.nlm.nih.gov/28626329.
97. Avci P, Gupta A, Sadasivam M, Vecchio D, Pam Z, Pam N, et al. Low-level laser (light) therapy (LLLT) in skin: stimulating, healing, restoring. Semin Cutan Med Surg. 2013;32(1):41–52. https://pubmed.ncbi.nlm.nih.gov/24049929.
98. Cotler HB, Chow RT, Hamblin MR, Carroll J. The use of low level laser therapy (LLLT) for musculoskeletal pain. MOJ Orthop Rheumatol. 2015;2(5):68. https://pubmed.ncbi.nlm.nih.gov/26858986.
99. Barreto DM, Batista MVA. Swedish massage: a systematic review of its physical and psychological benefits. Adv Mind Body Med. 2017;31(2):16–20.
100. Patrick RP, Johnson TL. Sauna use as a lifestyle practice to extend healthspan. Exp Gerontol. 2021;154:111509.
101. Gálvez I, Torres-Piles S, Ortega-Rincón E. Balneotherapy, immune system, and stress response: a hormetic strategy? Int J Mol Sci. 2018;19(6):1689.
102. ter Haar G. Therapeutic applications of ultrasound. Prog Biophys Mol Biol. 2007;93(1–3):111–29.
103. Tsai W-C, Chen JY-S, Pang J-HS, Hsu C-C, Lin M-S, Chieh L-W. Therapeutic ultrasound stimulation of tendon cell migration. Connect Tissue Res. 2008;49(5):367–73.
104. Ennis WJ, Lee C, Gellada K, Corbiere TF, Koh TJ. Advanced technologies to improve wound healing: electrical stimulation, vibration therapy, and ultrasound-what is the evidence? Plast Reconstr Surg. 2016;138(3 Suppl):94S–104S.
105. Rahmani A, Naseri M, Salaree MM, Nehrir B. Comparing the effect of foot reflexology massage, foot Bath and their combination on quality of sleep in patients with acute coronary syndrome. J Caring Sci. 2016;5(4):299–306.
106. Boyle W, Saine A. Lectures in naturopathic hydrotherapy. Sandy, OR: Eclectic Medical; 1988.
107. Rubinstein SM, de Zoete A, van Middelkoop M, Assendelft WJJ, de Boer MR, van Tulder MW. Benefits and harms of spinal manipulative therapy for the treatment of chronic low back pain: systematic review and meta-analysis of randomised controlled trials. BMJ. 2019;364:l689.
108. Masaracchio M, Kirker K, States R, Hanney WJ, Liu X, Kolber M. Thoracic spine manipulation for the management of mechanical neck pain: a systematic review and meta-analysis. PLoS One. 2019;14(2):e0211877.

109. Driehuis F, Hoogeboom TJ, Nijhuis-van der Sanden MWG, de Bie RA, Staal JB. Spinal manual therapy in infants, children and adolescents: a systematic review and meta-analysis on treatment indication, technique and outcomes. PLoS One. 2019;14(6):e0218940.
110. Geneen LJ, Moore RA, Clarke C, Martin D, Colvin LA, Smith BH. Physical activity and exercise for chronic pain in adults: an overview of Cochrane reviews. Cochrane Database Syst Rev. 2017;4(4):CD011279.
111. Fuentes JP, Armijo Olivo S, Magee DJ, Gross DP. Effectiveness of interferential current therapy in the management of musculoskeletal pain: a systematic review and meta-analysis. Phys Ther. 2010;90(9):1219–38.
112. Rampazo ÉP, Liebano RE. Analgesic effects of interferential current therapy: a narrative review. Medicina (Kaunas). 2022;58(1):141.
113. De ACC, Da SVZM, Júnior GC, Liebano RE, Durigan JLQ. Transcutaneous electrical nerve stimulation and interferential current demonstrate similar effects in relieving acute and chronic pain: a systematic review with meta-analysis. Braz J Phys Ther. 2018;22(5):347–54.
114. Asif M, Saleem M, Saadullah M, Yaseen HS, Al ZR. COVID-19 and therapy with essential oils having antiviral, anti-inflammatory, and immunomodulatory properties. Inflammopharmacology. 2020;28(5):1153–61.
115. Ichiba T, Kakiuchi K, Suzuki M, Uchiyama M. Warm steam inhalation before bedtime improved sleep quality in adult men. Evid Based Complement Alternat Med. 2019;2019:2453483.
116. Dayanır IO, Birinci T, Kaya Mutlu E, Akcetin MA, Akdemir AO. Comparison of three manual therapy techniques as trigger point therapy for chronic nonspecific low Back pain: a randomized controlled pilot trial. J Altern Complement Med. 2020;26(4):291–9.
117. Hammi C, Schroeder JD, Yeung B. Trigger point injection. In: StatPearls. Treasure Island, FL: StatPearls; 2021.
118. Siegel B. http://berniesiegelmd.com/. Accessed 25 Oct 2021.
119. Monod S, Brennan M, Rochat E, Martin E, Rochat S, Büla CJ. Instruments measuring spirituality in clinical research: a systematic review. J Gen Intern Med. 2011;26(11):1345–57. Epub 2011 Jul 2. PMID: 21725695; PMCID: PMC3208480. https://doi.org/10.1007/s11606-011-1769-7.
120. Brown University. TIME—toolkit of instruments to measure end of life care: spirituality [Internet]. http://www.chcr.brown.edu/pcoc/Spirit.htm. Accessed 21 Oct 2021.
121. AIH. American Institute of Homeopathy [Internet]. https://homeopathyusa.org/. Accessed 26 May 2022.
122. Weir J. Samuel Hahnemann and his influence on medical thought. Proc R Soc Med. 1933;26(6):668–76. Available from: https://pubmed.ncbi.nlm.nih.gov/19989242
123. Boyd LJ. A study of the simile in medicine. Philadelphia: Boericke and Tafel; 1936.
124. Frass M, Lechleitner P, Gründling C, Pirker C, Grasmuk-Siegl E, Domayer J, et al. Homeopathic treatment as an add-on therapy may improve quality of life and prolong survival in patients with non-small cell lung cancer: a prospective, randomized, placebo-controlled, double-blind, three-arm, multicenter study. Oncologist. 2020;25(12):e1930–55.
125. Boericke W, Boericke O. Materia Medica. Santa Rose, CA: Boericke and Tafel; 1927.
126. Hershoff A. Homeopathic remedies. New York: Avery; 2000.
127. Maciocia G. The foundations of Chinese medicine. New York: Churchill Livingstone; 1989.
128. Vickers AJ, Vertosick EA, Lewith G, MacPherson H, Foster NE, Sherman KJ, et al. Acupuncture for chronic pain: update of an individual patient data meta-analysis. J Pain. 2018;19(5):455–74.
129. Yuan Q-L, Wang P, Liu L, Sun F, Cai Y-S, Wu W-T, et al. Acupuncture for musculoskeletal pain: a meta-analysis and meta-regression of sham-controlled randomized clinical trials. Sci Rep. 2016;6:30675.

Chapter 7
States of Ill Health: The Ground of Clinical Presentations

Inflammation, Microbiome

Positive Feedback-Driven: Uncontrolled Inflammation

Inflammation is a process that is normal and necessary for life. It has upregulators and downregulators. For a number of reasons, inflammation can become out of control. Most of the bioregulatory systems of the human body are subject to negative feedback. In a cybernetic system, there are switches to start a process, and the control of the process is governed by some factor that downregulates it. It might be the actual product of the process, a hormone, for example, that acts as the inhibitor. Thyroid hormone is like this. It inhibits the thyroid gland, until it cannot because its levels are dropping. When inflammation is poorly kept in check, it can start to permanently alter tissues—reducing the number of viable cells and degrading the extracellular matrix. Some forms of inflammation become so aggressive, that they become positive feedback systems that simply fire up their own activity [1] (Fig. 7.1).

Imbalances in cell death pathways are one way that the inflammation can become overly exuberant. The common form of cellular turnover, apoptosis, programmed cell death, results in an involution of the cell. Its demise is relatively quiet, and its proteins and other cell structures are consumed by phagocytes, which are attracted by very specific protein markers. This is a generally noninflammatory event, and immunological tolerance is normal. If the clearance of apoptotic cells is not efficient, the presence of the particles of these dead cells can induce membrane permeability in surrounding cells and lead to a secondary necrosis. Bystanding cells that were earlier in their life cycle perish because of the debris of apoptosis.

This secondary necrosis can start to activate immune responses. Damaged associated molecular patterns (DAMP) are released by necrotic cells. Instead of a controlled phagocytosis of cellular debris, this process is known as necroptosis

F. Smith, *Naturopathic Medicine*, https://doi.org/10.1007/978-3-031-13388-6_7

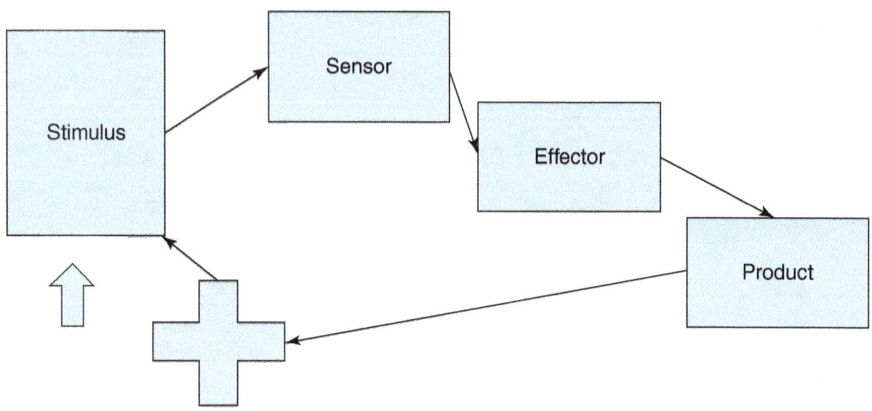

Fig. 7.1 Positive feedback loop: Some processes break away from inhibitory constraints, and the product of the processes spurs on more activity of the process. This is found in a very few normal physiological situations, such as oxytocin release in childbirth. But generally, positive feedback loops are a sign of imbalance and can have damaging effects

(Fig. 7.2). It is mediated by a number of agents including RNA-editing factor interacting protein 1 (RIP1). This will cause more aggressive white blood cell migration and activity [2].

Other forms of cell death can be even more pro-inflammatory. Pyroptosis is reaction to cellular death by bacterial infection. Not only are DAMP factors present but also pathogen-associated molecular patterns (PAMP) such as terminally mannosylated and polymannosylated compounds (which bind the mannose receptor) and various microbial components, such as bacterial lipopolysaccharide, hypomethylated DNA, flagellin, and double-stranded RNA (all of which bind to Toll-like receptors). Pyroptosis is mediated by caspase-1.

When an inciting source of damage in the body continues to generate necrosis, it can lead to more cellular damage, more activation of necrosis via cell permeability and signaling cascades via caspase or RIP proteins, and more DAMP and Toll-like receptor binding [3]. A simple example is periodontal disease or low-grade dental abscess. A persistent source of infection can create ongoing inflammation. Excessive oxidative stress, due to exogenous free radical generating chemicals and/or a lack of intrinsic or nutritional antioxidant systems, can also trigger inflammation.

Aberrations in the gut microbiome, and defects in cell junctions in the gut, can be an ingress for antigens and even entire microorganisms, which can be inflammation upregulators [4]. Regulatory T cells in the lymphatics of the gut perform the role of dampening inflammation, a completely necessary action given the massive antigen traffic in the gut epithelium, lamina propria, and lymphatics. But these

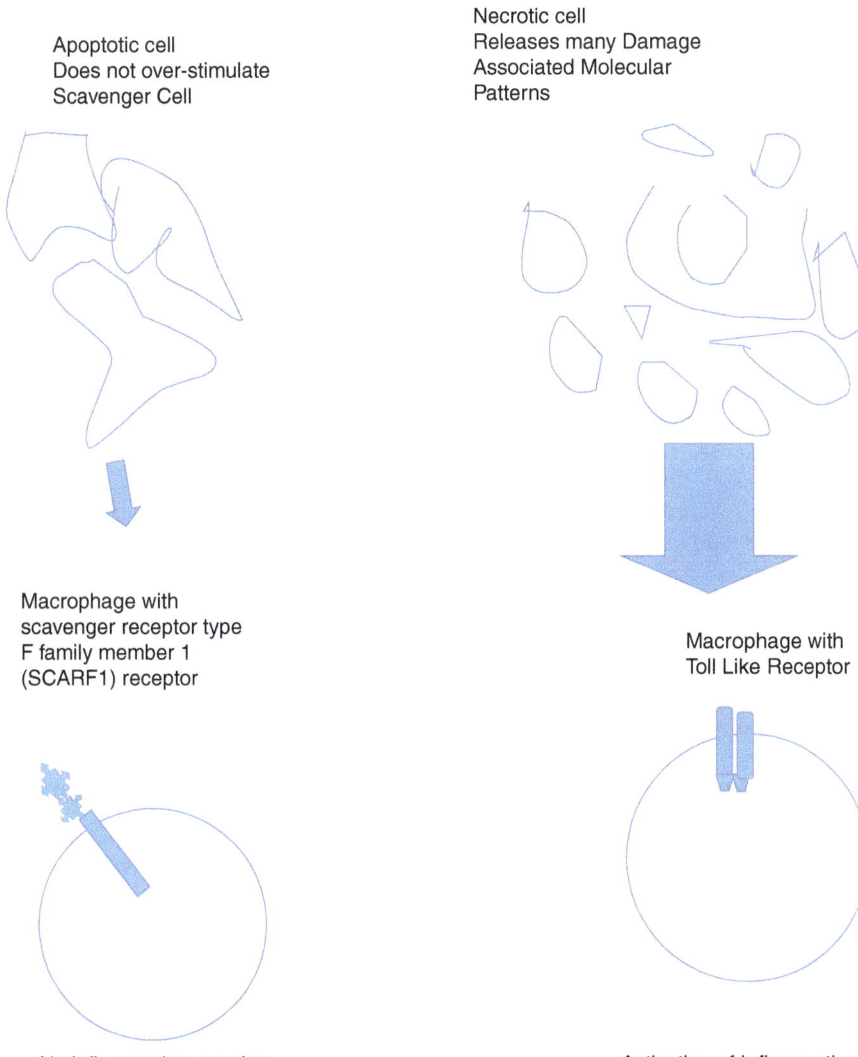

Fig. 7.2 Apoptosis versus necroptosis: Damage-associated molecular patterns can activate inflammation in a way that normal apoptotic end products will not

regulatory or suppressive functions can be overwhelmed. Glycation of cells in diabetes can again create new structures in molecules that unfortunately set up inflammatory reactions. Nutritional imbalances such as a low ratio of omega 3 fatty acids to omega 6 fatty acids, or vitamin D deficiency, can make inflammatory processes more prolonged and forceful, and not in a defensive way, but a destructive one.

Neuroinflammation

There are genetically and virally influenced pathways that cause some of the common presentations of neurodegeneration. In Alzheimer's disease, there is the initial insult to the tissue from amyloid protein. Once this protein has entered the brain, it causes damage to microtubule structures in the neuron. These fragments of Tau protein can then oligomerize and then form longer neurofibrillary tangles. This leads to more localized immune activity in the brain, more inflammation, more damage, and so on.

The gut can play a role in triggering this process. Lipopolysaccharide is a powerful proinflammatory molecule from the cell walls of Gram-negative bacteria [5]. The substance, independent of the bacteria that produce it, can find its way into the blood stream and cause inflammatory reactions in the border of the brain and sometimes within the brain.

Bacteria can translocate from the gut to the bloodstream and trigger inflammation. *Escherichia coli*, *Salmonella enterica*, *Bacillus subtilis*, *Mycobacterium tuberculosis*, and *Staphylococcus aureus* are species of bacteria that can produce amyloid protein that can then find its way into the bloodstream and at times the brain [6].

What are the consequences of neuroinflammation beyond the very serious degenerative process associated with dementia? This problem seems to impact mood and may be implicated in depressive and anxiety disorders [7, 8].

Microbiota Disturbance: Composition, Byproducts, and Conditioning Impact on Immune System.

The human microbiome begins to establish itself at birth. Vaginal births and Cesarean section births follow different trends. The skin, mouth, eyes, ears, respiratory tract, and of course the gastrointestinal tract all allow in commensal organisms. The microbiome interacts with the immune system and in fact makes products that communicate with the human body as a whole, with gut-derived serotonin being an example. Aberrants in the microbiome can take many forms such as the following: [9, 10].

(a) Overabundance of pathogenic and immunoprovocation species.
(b) A lack of microbiome diversity (not enough types of families/genera/species).
(c) A lack of symbiotic organisms.
(d) A change of the cross talk of immune system and microbe to become less tolerant and more reactive.

This microbiome, not only in the gut, but across the body, changes with time, due to diet, physiology, medications, and stress levels. The composition is becoming clearer due to DNA analysis, but the range of normal and the implications of what various species do to the human body and to each other is very complex. Certainly, when very out of balance, depleted, or supplanted with more pathogenic organisms, the microbiome can drastically impact health [11].

Mitochondrial, Genetic, and Cellular Protein Degradation

Mitochondrial Dysfunction

Mitochondria are the basis of aerobic metabolism. They are the site of oxidative phosphorylation and are a site of consumption of NADP and fatty acid oxidation. Mitochondria are evolutionary vestiges of prokaryotes, and they have a subset of their own DNA which is maternally derived.

Mitochondrial dysfunction is seen across a spectrum of diseases. It is not always clear if this problem is a consequence of deterioration of the organ or if the decay of mitochondrial function was an inciting factor in the decline of the health of a tissue or organ. It is probably that even when mitochondrial dysfunction was not a primary cause of a pathological state, once the dysfunction sets it, an acceleration of pathology sets in. Mitochondrial dysfunction occurs across a number of aspects of this organelle.

Mitophagy is a natural process of apoptosis of mitochondrial cells. This is a normal regulatory function that removes damaged mitochondria [12]. If mitophagy is overactive, deleting still-functioning mitochondria too early, it can attrit the mitochondrial population, leading to a lack of energy production.

Mitochondrial and the endoplasmic reticulum (ER) distance is in close proximity to each other. The proteins created in the ER are needed by the mitochondria. The human mitochondrial proteome is composed of nearly 1500 different proteins, only 13 of which are encoded by the maternally inherited mitochondrial genome (mtDNA) [13]. Although the mitochondria can transcribe and translate many of the mitochondrial genes, using "mtRNA" and "mt-tRNA," many proteins must be imported into the mitochondria. Just as the cell has a dependency on the mitochondria for ATP, the organelle must import certain proteins in order to function. The proximity of the ER is an important factor in the availability of some needed proteins and communication. The mitochondria and the ER can drift apart, which stresses the organelle.

Control of oxidative stress is important for maintaining stability of the mitochondria. Oxidative stress is a byproduct of the chemistry that occurs in the organelle. Electron transport and the presence of oxygen can lead to unpaired electrons. These are hopefully intercepted by some form of antioxidant enzyme or nutrient. If this fails, then the mitochondrial genetic material, proteins, or membranes are damaged. The inner and then outer mitochondrial membrane can be damaged. This can have serious consequences. There is a gradient of protons across the inner mitochondrial membrane, and if this is disturbed by defects in the membrane, the efficiency of ATP production will decline.

ATP demand-production balance is important to avoid a backlog and buildup of transferred electrons. The demand for ATP needs to match the production, because production involves electron transfer and the potential for increased oxidative stress. Overfed individuals who do not exercise are at risk for underutilization of electron transport chain products. Those who limit or restrict calories and remain active will use up the mitochondrial products.

Reverse flow in the electron transport chain can occur in response to bacterial infection. This is where electrons flow backward down the enzyme assembly line in the mitochondria. Electrons from ubiquinol are transferred back to respiratory complex I, reducing NAD+ back to NADH. This event will create a lot of free radical stress (Fig. 7.3).

Fusion/fission ratio is another aspect of mitochondrial dysfunction [14]. Mitochondria have a protein signaling pathway for fissioning. This pinches the mitochondrial membrane and creates smaller units. This appears naturally on the more peripheral aspects of muscle fibrils. In more energy intense areas, the mitochondria can undergo a protein-driven fusion of membranes. When membranes are knitted together, the resulting larger organelle can become more efficient at energy generation. When imbalances occur, extreme fission of the mitochondria can lead to loss of efficiency. This is noted in many disease states, and whether it is a more fundamental cause or later effect, it is a serious sign of degeneration.

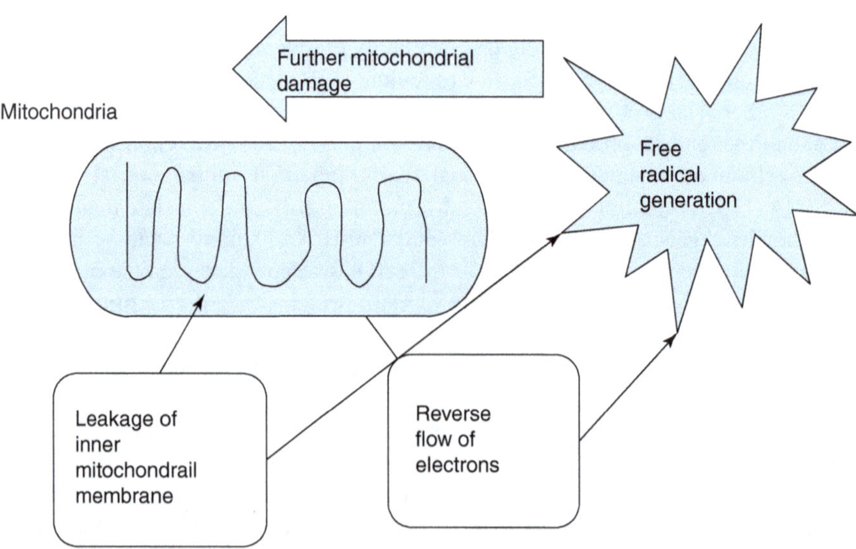

Fig. 7.3 Mitochondria can begin to malfunction, and when electrons flow in the wrong direction, or protons begin to leak within the organelle, increased oxidative stress can create damage

Autophagy Defects

Although the human body is built to last, all proteins are only meant to function for a limited period of time. Then they must be replaced. The damaged, oxidized, or chemically substituted protein must be broken down by the cell. This is done via the proteasome. Selected proteins are "ubiquitinated," and this tagging with special marker proteins sends them for degradation in lysosomes or proteasomes. There are different pathways to this, and some people have deficits in what is known as "autophagy." Autophagy is the breakdown of self-proteins. Part of the packaging—the taking out of the trash—is the formation of a small vesicular sac called a phagophore. The phagophore pinches off a tiny amount of cytoplasm to form a double-membrane structure called an autophagosome. Various genetic anomalies can limit a person's ability to do this molecular clean up. If there is a severe limitation, it will express as early-onset neurodegeneration. But there are various degrees of impairment in autophagy, and some defects mildly advance the aggregation of molecular junk in the body, including neurons. Defective autophagy has been linked to heart disease risk, as well as cancer, and neurodegenerative disease risk [12, 15, 16]. Exercise, fasting, and ketogenic diets are under investigation for being able to switch on autophagic mechanisms, as these are known to upregulate phagophore production.

Genetic Damage

Genetic damage is inevitable in our cells due to oxidative stress, solar radiation, chemical carcinogens from the environment and diet, and even other spectrum energies such as cosmic rays and radioactive particles from the earth (uranium, radon gas, etc.). Damage can be repaired to some extent by excision and dimerizing enzymes. Some polymerase enzymes, in the nucleus and the mitochondria, have proofreading capabilities. Unfortunately, mutations can persist and become integrated into the cell's DNA [17]. Some of these are immediately fatal to the cell. Others create ongoing mistakes, and this might activate genes that cause the cell to shut down, a process known as apoptosis. Sometimes, a mutated cell will continue to replicate, and subsequent generations are increasingly dedifferentiated. These cells might progress to being neoplastic cells, which can become clinical cancer. This process has a genetic core of events, but the context in which it occurs is important. The extracellular matrix provides growth regulation to cells, partly through the connections between matrix proteins, the integrin proteins in cell membranes, and the microtubule assembly within the cell itself. The immune system can, and usually does, detect and eliminate nascent cancer cells. But those that persist will actually try to reorder the extracellular matrix in order to stimulate their own uncontrolled growth and to facilitate the traveling of cancer cells to new sites [18].

The health defining issues described in this textbook, and being researched across the world, and applied to clinical practice by naturopathic physicians and others, are extremely important example of what genetic damage can become. Toxin exposure, our ability to manage those chemical compounds, our biochemical equipment that depends on our nutrient intake to run, the supply of antioxidant enzymes and compounds in the body, our overall determinants of health and their adequacy, the normal structure and function of our extracellular matrix, and the strength of the immune system all impact the fate of our cells and bodies due to genetic damage. There are numerous factors that make cancer development more likely, and many ways to reduce this risk. The fact that inborn and random events can give rise to cancer should not promote a nihilist or blind attitude about the many circumstances that surround this phenomenon. Early cancer researchers in the nineteenth century, long before so much was known about the molecular cell biology of this disease, referred to "seed and soil" as two aspects of this disease. The twenty-first century naturopathic physician can take this simple concept into the present and consider both the seed (mutations) and soil (context of cell, matrix, immunity, and other sites) and work to better equip patients to be as highly functioning as they can be.

Bioregulatory Disturbance and Metabolic Disturbance

Control Systems

What happens when bioregulatory systems, such as various endocrine feedback loops, autonomic nervous system controls, or central pathways of metabolism, cease to function normally? When these systems function weakly, or too forcefully, or erratically, they create circumstances that disease symptoms can arise from. Most control systems have the ability to absorb disturbances [19, 20]. For example, if a person is exposed to heat, they perspire. If heat is prolonged and their hypothalamus is sending a signal to exhale forcefully and perspire abundantly, the person is now in a high state of activation. Once they go into some air conditioning, hydrate, and relax, their temperature set point is easily achieved and the regulatory system stops sending those signals that it was out in the heat (Fig. 7.4). Systems can tolerate changes to oscillatory activity.

Cortisol levels peak in the morning and decline at night (Fig. 7.5). If a person is under prolonged stress, those cortisol levels persist late in the day [21]. Over time, this can suppress the immune system. If the stressors are removed and the overall state of adaptation decreases, cortisol secretion returns [22].

What if the person stays in that adaptive state? Other systems have to compensate, even if by simply operating in the presence of an abnormal condition [23]. This adaptation is sometimes called an allostatic state. Allostasis is something we see in chronic disease. When a person doesn't have enough ventricular output from their heart because of some sort of damage (perhaps a myocardial infarction in the recent

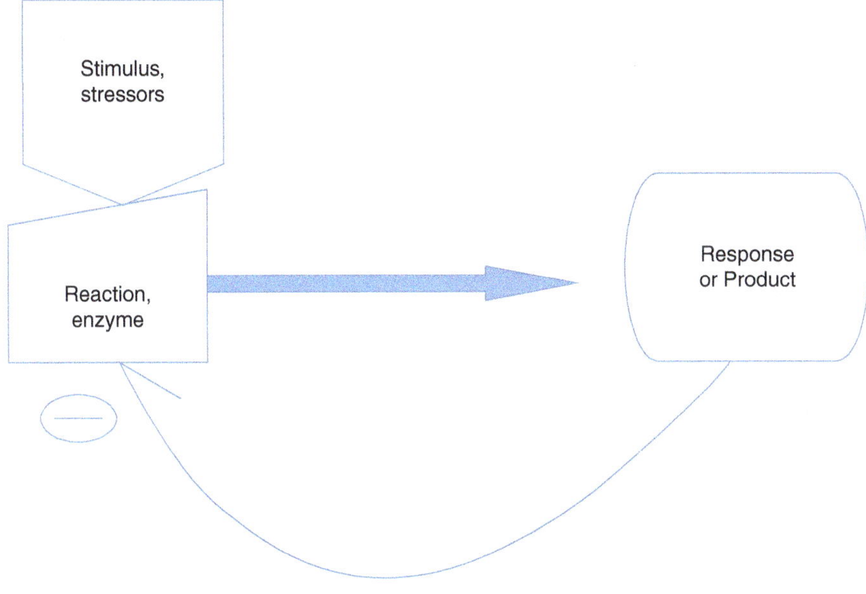

Fig. 7.4 Bioregulatory system: In normal homeostasis, once a system has acted to return to a level of activity that is near its set point, the activity decreases

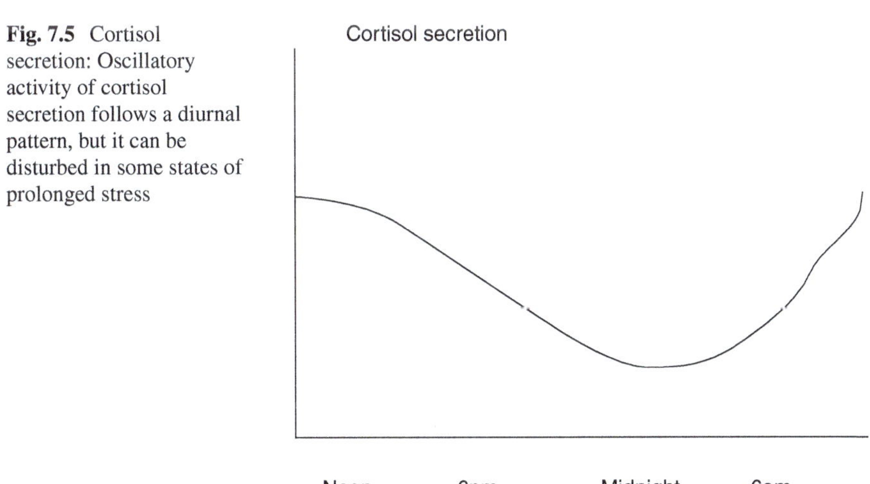

Fig. 7.5 Cortisol secretion: Oscillatory activity of cortisol secretion follows a diurnal pattern, but it can be disturbed in some states of prolonged stress

past or viral myocarditis), their organs and brain could shut down. The body will create hormones that increase adrenergic activity (sympathetic nervous system), which temporarily helps the heart to do more. Over time, this allostatic adaptation becomes a problem too. The adrenergic effects can increase the chances of sudden cardiac death [24].

Some systems have a buffering capacity. Humans do not have many buffers against cold exposure, notwithstanding the clothes they fabricate and wear, but many animals have a fur coating. Drops in blood volume lead to a number of long-term changes, but thirst may occur almost immediately. Buffering is only a protection against stressors, but we cannot avoid them. The use of adequate nutritional support, attention paid to requirements of health, and the use of hormetic stimulation to capitalize adaptive responses are some of the recording treatment tactics of naturopathic physicians.

Autonomic Neuropathy

With enough damage due to trauma, toxicity, or diabetes, the autonomic nervous system can become dysfunctional. In the case of autonomic neuropathy, there are losses to the postganglionic neurons that efface the organs and tissues under their control [25]. These nerves have long axons and are susceptible to damage. An example is in poorly controlled diabetes. Damage to the supporting Schwann cells from sorbitol accumulation and glycation of neuron proteins, as well as underlying microvascular disease, will cause loss of nervous input. This can impact the sensory or even motor neurons. In the case of autonomic losses, key functions such as the emptying of the stomach into the duodenum (controlled by the pyloric valve), the coordinated actions of the colon, or the coordination of blood flow into the penis to maintain an erection will also become erratic or impaired. Damage to the autonomics can happen at a higher level. When someone suffers from a spinal cord trauma, it is not just the motor neurons that are transected. The branches of the sympathetic and parasympathetic nervous system can also lose some of their preganglionic neurons.

Neurotransmitter Deficiency or Dysfunction

Poor nutritional status can result in a lack of amino acids for proper structure and for normal neurotransmitter function. Most people eating a mixed diet who have adequate digestion tend to get the amino acids they need. This is especially true in the protein-heavy diets of today that many people consume. However, individuals vary in their needs at the moment and in their genetic structure and expression. Some people simply need more of an amino acid to get something done in their basic chemistry including neurochemistry.

In other situations, the problem is that the person lacks the enzymes to transform an amino acid into a needed product, such as a neurotransmitter. That may be due to an inherent deficiency of enzymes or a lack of the cofactors that help power that enzyme as catalysts.

The contribution of the gut microbiome to our neurotransmitter pool is something that has gained attention in twenty-first century physiology [26]. For example, gut bacteria create a significant amount of serotonin that finds its way into circulation [27]. The bloodstream serotonin from the gut might impact the autonomic nervous system, but does not seem to cross the blood brain barrier. However, gut bacteria can modulate the amounts of tryptophan (precursor enzyme for serotonin) in the bloodstream [27]. Tryptophan crosses the blood-brain barrier, and it is from this amino acid that the brain synthesized serotonin. Increased inflammation in the body, such as the generation of lipopolysaccharide from microflora, can change the way that tryptophan is taken up into the brain. A high amount of inflammation may in fact disrupt the blood-brain barrier and allow some bloodstream products to enter the brain. Thus, the gut microbiome is not without agency when it comes to impact brain chemistry.

Metabolic Derangements

Dysglycemia and Insulin Resistance

Insulin resistance is a symptom of sorts, but it is part of a chronic state that is the precursor to many pathophysiological consequences. Insulin resistance arises as the insulin receptor on muscles becomes less efficient. The decreased insulin-stimulated glucose uptake is due to impaired insulin signaling and multiple postreceptor intracellular defects including impaired glucose transport and glucose phosphorylation and reduced glucose oxidation and glycogen synthesis (Fig. 7.6). Genetic predispositions are one cause [28]. Elevated levels of insulin which impact the receptor are

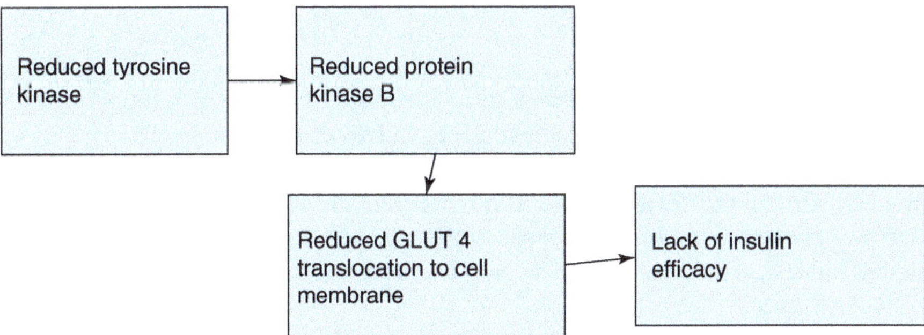

Fig. 7.6 Insulin resistance: The breakdown in responsiveness of GLUT 4 production and migration to the muscle cell membrane will allow serum glucose levels to stay elevated, leading to more insulin secretion

another. Very high free fatty acid concentrations in the bloodstream can damage the receptor. The amount of fat in the muscle is another factor that can damage the receptor.

Malabsorption and Cachexia

The human gastrointestinal tract has many functions that ensure that the body is properly nourished. It secretes acid, enzymes, bile, and special chemicals such as bicarbonate, in order to break down food. It can absorb nutrients (especially after digestion of foods to transform them into small components). Absorption can be passive diffusion across cell membranes of the epithelium of the gut, diffusion through specialized channels through the membrane, active transport using a protein as carrier and expending energy to pull something into the epithelium, and even pinocytosis where a cell engulfs its target.

The gut also has an important motility function. Food and the consecutive broken down and liquified food mass, chyme, must be propelled forward through the various stages of digestion. From the coordinated swallowing in the esophagus and lower esophageal sphincter to the pylorus and from the small intestine to large intestine, a movement through the process occurs. That movement also dissects food into smaller portions. The stomach can pinch and squish food, and the small intestine can pinch but also roll food forward in a twisting motion. This maximizes the amount of food material that can be exposed to enzymes. The large intestine reclaims water but also moves that residue from digestion forward and out of the body. This waste excreting function is also a function of the gut. The residue is disposed of, but along the way, it provides a substrate for the trillions of bacteria that have a critical metabolic, physiologic, and immunological role.

Malabsorption can occur due to a breakdown in any aspect of digestion and absorption [29]. Because the human body is efficient at digesting many things and there is a certain redundancy built into the system, people can sustain losing some of it and still function. For example, people have had 1 or 2 ft of their small bowel removed due to cancer, or trauma, and still regain health. A malabsorptive issue might be due to the specific part of the gastrointestinal tract that was damaged. If a portion of the duodenum is removed, this can reduce fat or iron absorption.

The stomach can decrease in its efficiency due to aging, with gradual atrophy of the mucus membranes and reduced secretion of hydrochloric acid and pepsin/pepsinogen. The stomach can also lose its motor activity to some degree. Damage to the nerves that control the stomach, as one might see in autonomic neuropathy (secondary to diabetes, spinal cord damage, etc.) can lead to delayed gastric emptying and a sluggish, atonic stomach.

The small bowel can be injured by inflammatory bowel disease. Crohn's disease can create lesions that dig into the bowel and are replaced by fibrotic tissue. Any such area will be unable to absorb nutrients at that particular spot of scar tissue. The epithelium of the small intestine has specific enterocytes that are able to absorb many nutrients. These are arrayed in a way that maximizes surface area. The cells are aligned around capillaries and lymph vessels on very tiny microvilli (small fingerlike projections). Numerous microvilli populate a larger fingerlike projection known as a villus. In celiac disease, immune reactions to the presence of gluten cause attrition of the microvilli and villi. An endoscopy will reveal villous atrophy. In this case, in a similar manner to Crohn's disease, there is poor absorption through this area. Water and glucose might pass, but many other nutrients cannot. Moreover, the epithelial cells create certain enzymes that break down small amino acid sequences and carbohydrate sequences to their terminal forms. The loss of some of these enzymes further decreases digestion and therefore absorption.

Excessive motility can cause chyme to travel through the gut too quickly. Likewise, a pyloric valve that allows all stomach contents to rush into the duodenum all at once (dumping syndrome) will overwhelm the digestive machinery with sugars and fats typically ending up in the colon and causing loose stools and bloating.

Some malabsorption is intentionally created. The Roux-en-Y procedure, a form of bariatric surgery, bypasses the duodenum, in addition to other structural changes, such as partitioning the stomach. The bypass of the duodenum drastically reduces the amount of fat absorption. It also means that digestive enzymes and bile join the chyme a bit later than normally would occur.

Pancreatic exocrine deficiency will lead to malabsorption. The pancreas enzymes are necessary for breaking down all macronutrients: fats, carbohydrates, and proteins. Bile that was stored in the gallbladder can emulsify fat. It is possible to live without a gallbladder and to absorb fat fairly well. Sometimes the quality of bile is poor and not very helpful for fat digestion.

Not all patients who appear to be losing weight in spite of eating are malabsorbing. Cachexia is really a form of wasting [30, 31]. It is seen in cancer, palliative situations, heart disease, and other situations. Cachexia is from the Greek word "kakos" meaning "bad things" and "hexus," meaning "state of being." The causes seem to be a combination of factors. Increased inflammation, driven by tumor necrosis factor, is part of the problem. A heightened metabolic rate in cancer seems to be due to increases in aerobic metabolism (which might be due to oncogene expression) and anaerobic metabolism of the cancer cells themselves. These cells obtain about 80% of the massive amount of energy they consume via fermentation of glucose, the Warburg effect. It is also easy to see that cancer cells are thieves, taking as much energy as they can from the host.

This can be so extreme that even providing cancer patients with supplemental and parenteral nutrition does not for long prevent cachexia. In 2008, Evans et al., at a gathering in Washington, DC, proposed a new definition for cancer cachexia. This was weight loss with or without the loss of fat with the presence of an additional three of the following criteria: decreased muscle strength, reduced muscle mass, anorexia, symptoms of fatigue, or biochemical abnormalities including anemia, evidence of inflammation, or low albumin level.

There are many ways that someone can starve—malabsorption, cachexia, and of course protein-calorie malnutrition itself due to lack of intake. But when these conditions exist, the adaptive resources that we count on to promote healing will begin to fail. Maladaptive responses remain, and simple failure of function develops rapidly and directly. This state is an ideal example of a ground or fundamental state. Innumerable disease conditions can arise from it. Immune deficiency, infections, hypersensitivity reactions, poor wound healing, anemia, breakdown of hepatic protein synthesis, cardiac arrhythmias, and possible hemorrhages are just some examples. In situations like this, in addition to attempt to address causes, naturopathic physicians have to do all that they can to improve nutritional status.

Toxin Deposition and Extracellular Matrix Degeneration

Hypersensitivity, Environmental Toxin Sensitivities

Any processing system in the body can become saturated. For example, if someone consumes far too many carbohydrates and cannot burn them in aerobic metabolism, they convert to acetate, which ends up becoming fatty acids. These are stored in the liver, and throughout the body, as triglyceride. This can lead to fatty liver disease.

The human body processes toxins in a number of nodes, with the liver being the key player in the system [32]. Any chemical compound will start with an enzyme that starts the processing of it. The cytochrome P450 group of enzymes is a family of isozymes that are mixed function oxidases. There are other hepatic enzymes that are the first to encounter a chemical compound. Quinone reductase and alcohol dehydrogenase are examples of these.

Any of these enzymes can become saturated, if the substrate, that is, the chemical compound they are supposed to process, is superabundant. There may be over 100 cytochrome P450 isozymes, but there are thousands of chemicals that need to be broken down. Therefore, several chemical compounds may be found all being processed by the same isozyme.

Even when this frontline system can keep up, the process has just begun. The product of P450 processing is a reactive molecule that has an unstable electron. This is meant to rapidly be conjugated with a secondary molecule to make a nonreactive and water-soluble product. That product can then be eliminated through emunctory systems: urine, bile, sweat, breath, tears, and gastrointestinal secretions. The conjugation system attaches side groups such as sulfur, acetyl and methyl groups, amino acids such as cysteine, and glutathione.

Bystander antioxidants must be present during this chemical process, because even under optimal conditions, some of the products of P450 will naturally react with whatever is in proximity, such as an organelle membrane or proteins within the cell. Glutathione is an important antioxidant, as is the versatile superoxide dismutase. Food-derived antioxidants, including vitamins such as ascorbic acid or plant polyphenols, provide a strong layer of protection.

The kinetics of a person's ability to manage toxin exposure versus some kind of spillover or collateral damage is clearly nutritionally related. The enzymes, catalysts, conjugate groups, and antioxidants impose nutritional needs. These kinetics are altered by toxins themselves. For instance, corn syrup, an overused and extremely abundant sweetener in the American diet, is produced using mercury alkali (as are some food colors and chlorinated flour). This is a source of inorganic mercury. Those who eat a diet high in ultra-processed food consumed a harmful level of mer cury. This will suppress methylation systems in the body, which inhibited DNA synthesis and the ability to transcribe proteins. The metabolic poisoning of mercury decreases the net resources that the liver might have to process multiple toxins [33].

In terms of spillover effects, when biochemical pathways are saturated and toxin exposure continues, these compounds can persist in the body. Their effect varies—it can be hormonal dysregulation, increased inflammation, oxidative stress, brain neurotransmitter depletion, or carcinogenicity.

There are also individual ways that people respond to toxin spillover. Two people with the same basic toxin exposure can present with some overlapping issues but also idiosyncratic symptoms. Again, this can depend on what *other* toxins are at work. It also depends on their nutritional status, genetic predisposition, medical history, and current levels of dysfunction.

The intestinal epithelium has an "antiporter" system that can expel some toxins back into the gut. This has its limits, and when a person is in a higher state of inflammation and their redox potential declines due to antioxidant depletion, the gut itself can become inflamed. The immune system as well as some nonspecific, innate, differences can lead to more damage in the gut. This will lead to tight junctions among the epithelial cells, desmosomes, and hemidesmosomes, becoming less numerous. An intestinal epithelium with poor integrity will allow more antigens and toxins, to enter the blood circulation.

Amount of exposure, length of exposure, sudden exposure without any opportunity for preconditioning, and the lack of defensive nutrients can all overwhelm the body [34]. An abundance of toxins can damage target organs. Fortunately, some of it can be eliminated. Most toxins will transit through, and sometimes damage or become stuck (in the case of heavy metals), in the extracellular matrix.

Extracellular Matrix (ECM) Degeneration

The extracellular matrix governs the behavior and survival of cells. The concept of a human cell is a useful construction, since the structure and function of cells is visible and very clearly explained down to the molecular level. However, human cells cannot exist outside of their contextual matrix. The matrix provides a conduit for oxygen from nearby capillaries to diffuse into proximity to cells and for carbon dioxide to diffuse out. The matrix is a transit zone for nutrients in proximity to cells where passive and active transport mechanisms can acquire the nutrients. It is also an area where waste products and toxins can transit out and back into the circulation. The cell, the capillaries, the extracellular matrix, and fibroblast cells create the environment in which life and metabolism can occur [35–37].

An incredible number of proteins and sugars form this structure. Proteoglycans and glycosaminoglycans are key molecules. Some proteins articulate with the integrin molecules of the human cell. This forms a primary communication network, as the protein scaffolding of the matrix is conjoining with the integrins of cells. Those integrins are themselves connected to the microtubule assemblies within cells. Thus, a transcellular, intracellular, and cohesive structure system augments the very locally acting and functional structure.

About 300 proteins constitute the core matrisome, with a great variety of collagen and glucosaminoglycan subtypes. Collagen provides structural strength. Proteoglycans act like a sponge and hold water in this space. Glucosaminoglycans, such as heparin sulfates, also bind to many growth factors. This turns the ECM into a repository of growth factors and may help to create a regular and stable pattern to growth. Glycoproteins (laminins, elastin, fibronectins, thrombospondins, tenascins, and nidogen) are important for binding to the integrin proteins. Other glycoproteins have a less structural role and are there to bind hormones, neurotransmitters, etc. Other visitors to the ECM include cytokines and white blood cells. Younger people have a lot of elastin synthesis in their extracellular matrix, but this declines as we age.

The extracellular matrix also allows stimuli to be transferred from one area to another [38]. There is the abovementioned structural integration. There is also a certain electrical charge that is the product of proteoglycans. When a perturbation to one area occurs, the change in potential is transmitted widely. It is quite possible that the communication across extracellular matrix is a more primitive form of communication in animal cells preceding the nervous system as we know it. Bacteria have similar sugars on their exterior cell way to the type that multicellular organisms have in the ECM, and bacteria can communicate via quorum sensing. Human cells have second messenger systems that can be activated by matrix activity.

One of the functions of this connectivity is the control over growth. The proliferation of cells and their growth in a purposeful direction is guided by the matrix. When a tissue recovers from injury, the matrix allows the new cellular growth to proceed but controls and limits it. Tissue remodeling is very much brokered by the matrix.

Damage to the matrix occurs due to excessive oxidative stress. This can occur due to a lack of intrinsic antioxidant capacity. It can also occur due to extensive exposure to chemicals that generate free radicals, often but not always in the diet. It can also occur during diabetes mellitus, where advanced glycation end products directly damage the proteins that make up the matrix.

One unfortunate result of this damage is the overactivation of an enzyme called matrix metalloproteinase (MMP) [39]. This enzyme can dissolve some of the proteins of the matrix including collagen and is important for turnover and remodeling. All tissues have a turnover, a steady-state of creation and destruction—anabolic and catabolic functions. MMP will overactivate under these conditions of runaway oxidative stress, depletion of endogenous antioxidant defenses, and constant damage by glycation and inflammation as seen in diabetes. This very dangerous destabilization of the extracellular matrix will loosen the connections between cells and the matrix, and indirectly to each other. The coordination of cell proliferation or even

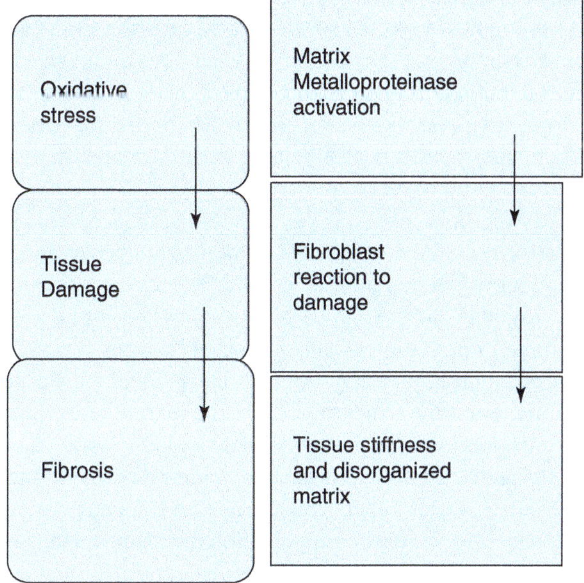

Fig. 7.7 Extracellular matrix stiffness: a prolonged and overly exuberant response to injury can create fibrosis and disorganization of the extracellular matrix

migration is coordinated through the matrix—the loss of cohesion is analogous to a number of traffic lights in a city malfunctioning at the same time. Confusion reigns.

Another pernicious outcome of this matrix dissolution is the counterreaction by the matrix leading to increased density and stiffness [40]. Fibroblastic cells are found in this area, and they will start to overactivate. This leads to a stiffening and clogging of the matrix with fibrotic tissue—much like a scar that has exceeded its needed function and now causes restriction (Fig. 7.7). It must be kept in mind that the ECM is contiguous with cells, so that the state of health and function of a tissue is bound up with activities in the matrix as well as intracellularly. Although the matrix may appear to be random in the array of collagen, there is a variable but recurring structure that seems ideal for the ECM functions. It seems to have at its core hyperbolic shapes that have a twist, which appears to be very energetically stable. As this becomes too loose, due to enzymatic degradation, or too dense due to fibroblastic overactivity, the matrix becomes less effective to support our cells. A balance between macrophages and fibroblasts is thus important for homeostasis. Imbalances and loss of homeostasis can be seen in the local matrix of various tissues and organs: liver, kidney, lung, heart, brain, etc., as disease and degeneration set in.

An example is matrix activation in the heart in patients with diabetes. This can lead to fibrosis of the heart tissue, leading to a stiff heart that cannot properly fill with blood and contract to eject that blood.

Toxin exposure can generate free radicals, and some toxins themselves can simply block enzymatic activity (lead, mercury, arsenic, etc.) can cause direct damage to the body and in particular to the ECM. A person in reasonably good health, particularly a younger person under the age of 40, can tolerate quite a bit of this attrition and deformation to the ECM without appearing to suffer any ill effects. They might smoke, eat burnt food, be exposed to all sorts of off-gassing compounds from human-made environments, etc. As they age, however, the matrix loses its basic architecture and becomes rigid as more collagen and less elastin accumulate. Some toxins are stored in the ECM, but to the extent that they pass through or chemically alter it before being removed to the lymph or blood circulation, they can lead a trail of damage.

By the time many people present for naturopathic treatment and are using conventional medical treatment, in their fifth decade and beyond, the ECM is already showing dysfunction (Table 7.1). The communication from cell to cell via the microtubule-integrin-ECM protein network is impaired. Drainage to and from the capillary circulation is not optimal. Elastin is replaced with collagen, and a more acidic environment may occur. It has been demonstrated that cancer cells have the ability to rearrange nearby ECM. The matrix adjacent to a cancer cell can turn from being hyperbolic shapes with some randomly arrayed proteins (a bit like a haystack, but somewhat like tree branches) to being oddly aligned with parallel proteins that are close to each other. This creates an even stiffer matrix. Cancer cells are stimulated by this, via the communication mechanisms intrinsic to cell-ECM interactions, and it can enhance even more proliferation of the cancer cells. There is also evidence that cancer cells can begin to manipulate the ECM in areas to which they will send metastatic tumor cells [39].

It is not surprising that the early naturopathic doctors found that constitutional hydrotherapy, or wet sheet pack therapy, combined with fasting, herbs that open the pathways of elimination, very simple diet, and avoidance of toxins led to clinical improvement. To a degree they did not realize that they were given the patient's ECM a chance to heal. It was able to discharge toxins, reduce inflammation, and start to circulate more like a younger, healthy ECM. That has a direct effect on the ability of cells to function. Human cells do not exist outside of an optimized environment any more than single-celled organisms in the ocean do. We create our own ocean, our own *milieu interior* as what Claude Bernard called it [41].

Levels of Dysfunction and Relation to Ground States

These generalized states that are disease precursors can exist at all levels of dysfunction (Table 7.1). For illustrative purposes, some examples of how these states relate to levels of dysfunction are given below, keeping in mind that an entire range of manifestations of these morbid states are possible.

Table 7.1 Levels of Dysfunction

Level of dysfunction	Example of a damaged state that can induce this dysfunction[a]	Comments
Hypofunction	Early stages of insulin resistance due to high glycemic diet and mercury	Ultra-processed foods can accelerate this process
Impaired coordination and circulation	Defective autophagy	Tau protein begins to accumulate in CNS
Inflammation	Pyroptosis	DAMPs and PAMPs begin to recruit immune cells
Deeper inflammation and immune involvement	Activation of AGE receptors by advanced glycation end products	Accelerates diabetic complications
Fibrosis and extracellular matrix degeneration	Excessively dense and oxidized matrix	End result of numerous toxin exposure and in particular sustained oxidative stress
Decline of function	Mitochondrial dysfunction	Advanced cardiac and other diseases can exhibit extensive mitochondrial fusion and decrease in numbers of functioning mitochondria
Neoplasm	Mutations induced by carcinogens	Potential cancer blocking defenses were overwhelmed by too many xenobiotics

[a]Note: States of ill health can lead to consequences at all levels of dysfunction. Examples above are selected for illustrative purposes

References

1. Wu H, Wang Y, Zhang Y, Xu F, Chen J, Duan L, et al. Breaking the vicious loop between inflammation, oxidative stress and coagulation, a novel anti-thrombus insight of nattokinase by inhibiting LPS-induced inflammation and oxidative stress. Redox Biol. 2020;32:101500.
2. Mihm S. Danger-associated molecular patterns (DAMPs): molecular triggers for sterile inflammation in the liver. Int J Mol Sci. 2018;19:E3104.
3. Yuan J, Amin P, Ofengeim D. Necroptosis and RIPK1-mediated neuroinflammation in CNS diseases. Nat Rev Neurosci. 2019;20(1):19–33.
4. Doney E, Cadoret A, Dion-Albert L, Lebel M, Menard C. Inflammation-driven brain and gut barrier dysfunction in stress and mood disorders. Eur J Neurosci. 2022;55:2851–94.
5. Catorce MN, Gevorkian G. LPS-induced murine neuroinflammation model: main features and suitability for pre-clinical assessment of nutraceuticals. Curr Neuropharmacol. 2016;14(2):155–64.
6. Trovato Salinaro A, Pennisi M, Di Paola R, Scuto M, Crupi R, Cambria MT, et al. Neuroinflammation and neurohormesis in the pathogenesis of Alzheimer's disease and Alzheimer-linked pathologies: modulation by nutritional mushrooms. Immun Ageing. 2018;14(15):8. https://pubmed.ncbi.nlm.nih.gov/29456585
7. Troubat R, Barone P, Leman S, Desmidt T, Cressant A, Atanasova B, et al. Neuroinflammation and depression: a review. Eur J Neurosci. 2021;53(1):151–71.
8. Zheng Z-H, Tu J-L, Li X-H, Hua Q, Liu W-Z, Liu Y, et al. Neuroinflammation induces anxiety- and depressive-like behavior by modulating neuronal plasticity in the basolateral amygdala. Brain Behav Immun. 2021;91:505–18.

9. Lloyd-Price J, Abu-Ali G, Huttenhower C. The healthy human microbiome. Genome Med. 2016;8(1):51.
10. Dominguez-Bello MG, Godoy-Vitorino F, Knight R, Blaser MJ. Role of the microbiome in human development. Gut. 2019;68(6):1108–14.
11. Weiss GA, Hennet T. Mechanisms and consequences of intestinal dysbiosis. Cell Mol Life Sci. 2017;74(16):2959–77.
12. Oka T, Hikoso S, Yamaguchi O, Taneike M, Takeda T, Tamai T, et al. Mitochondrial DNA that escapes from autophagy causes inflammation and heart failure. Nature. 2012;485(7397):251–5.
13. Ruan L, Zhou C, Jin E, Kucharavy A, Zhang Y, Wen Z, et al. Cytosolic proteostasis through importing of misfolded proteins into mitochondria. Nature. 2017;543(7645):443–6.
14. Meyer JN, Leuthner TC, Luz AL. Mitochondrial fusion, fission, and mitochondrial toxicity. Toxicology. 2017;391:42–53.
15. Huang T, Song X, Yang Y, Wan X, Alvarez AA, Sastry N, et al. Autophagy and hallmarks of cancer. Crit Rev Oncog. 2018;23(5–6):247–67.
16. Cerri S, Blandini F. Role of autophagy in Parkinson's disease. Curr Med Chem. 2019;26(20):3702–18.
17. Chang MT, Asthana S, Gao SP, Lee BH, Chapman JS, Kandoth C, et al. Identifying recurrent mutations in cancer reveals widespread lineage diversity and mutational specificity. Nat Biotechnol. 2016;34(2):155–63.
18. Pickup MW, Mouw JK, Weaver VM. The extracellular matrix modulates the hallmarks of cancer. EMBO Rep. 2014;15(12):1243–53.
19. Gonze D, Ruoff P. The Goodwin oscillator and its legacy. Acta Biotheor. 2021;69:857–74.
20. Franco E, Galloway KE. Feedback loops in biological networks. Methods Mol Biol. 2015;1244:193–214.
21. Spiga F, Walker JJ, Gupta R, Terry JR, Lightman SL. 60 Years of neuroendocrinology: glucocorticoid dynamics: insights from mathematical, experimental and clinical studies. J Endocrinol. 2015;226(2):T55–66.
22. Gjerstad JK, Lightman SL, Spiga F. Role of glucocorticoid negative feedback in the regulation of HPA axis pulsatility. Stress. 2018;21(5):403–16.
23. Goldstein DS. Concepts of scientific integrative medicine applied to the physiology and pathophysiology of catecholamine systems. Compr Physiol. 2013;3(4):1569–610.
24. Parmley WW. Pathophysiology of congestive heart failure. Clin Cardiol. 1992;15(Suppl 1):I5–12.
25. Kaur D, Tiwana H, Stino A, Sandroni P. Autonomic neuropathies. Muscle Nerve. 2021;63(1):10–21.
26. Dinan TG, Cryan JF. The microbiome-gut-brain axis in health and disease. Gastroenterol Clin North Am. 2017;46(1):77–89.
27. O'Mahony SM, Clarke G, Borre YE, Dinan TG, Cryan JF. Serotonin, tryptophan metabolism and the brain-gut-microbiome axis. Behav Brain Res. 2015;277:32–48.
28. Brown AE, Walker M. Genetics of insulin resistance and the metabolic syndrome. Curr Cardiol Rep. 2016;18(8):75. https://pubmed.ncbi.nlm.nih.gov/27312935.
29. Montoro-Huguet MA, Belloc B, Domínguez-Cajal M. Small and large intestine (I): malabsorption of nutrients. Nutrients. 2021;13(4):1254.
30. Dev R. Measuring cachexia-diagnostic criteria. Ann Palliat Med. 2019;8(1):24–32.
31. Evans WJ, Morley JE, Argilés J, Bales C, Baracos V, Guttridge D, et al. Cachexia: a new definition. Clin Nutr. 2008;27(6):793–9.
32. Liska DJ. The detoxification enzyme systems. Altern Med Rev. 1998;3(3):187–98.
33. Dufault R, Berg Z, Crider R, Schnoll R, Wetsit L, Bulls WT, et al. Blood inorganic mercury is directly associated with glucose levels in the human population and may be linked to processed food intake. Integr Mol Med. 2015;2(3).
34. Rea WJ. History of chemical sensitivity and diagnosis. Rev Environ Health. 2016;31(3):353–61.
35. Karamanos NK, Theocharis AD, Piperigkou Z, Manou D, Passi A, Skandalis SS, et al. A guide to the composition and functions of the extracellular matrix. FEBS J. 2021;288:6850–912.

36. Theocharis AD, Manou D, Karamanos NK. The extracellular matrix as a multitasking player in disease. FEBS J. 2019;286(15):2830–69.
37. Hynes RO. The extracellular matrix: not just pretty fibrils. Science. 2009;326(5957):1216–9.
38. Pischinger A. In: Heine H, editor. The extracellular matrix and ground regulation. Berkely: North Atlantic Books; 2007.
39. Wight TN, Kang I, Evanko SP, Harten IA, Chang MY, Pearce OMT, et al. Versican—a critical extracellular matrix regulator of immunity and inflammation. Front Immunol. 2020;11:512.
40. Bonnans C, Chou J, Werb Z. Remodelling the extracellular matrix in development and disease. Nat Rev Mol Cell Biol. 2014;15(12):786–801.
41. Bernard C. An introduction to the study of experimental medicine. Chelmsford: Courier Corporation; 1957.

Chapter 8
Organ Systems

Cardiovascular System

The cardiovascular system is the conduit for living giving oxygen and nutrients to the body's tissues. The blood that is moved in this system delivers glucose, hormones, and various proteins and carries many active components of the immune system. It removes CO2 and waste products [1]. The vascular aspect of this system has a treelike, branching structure, with ramifications that perfuse the entire body. The more oxygen demanding the tissue, the more intense the perfusion. These terminal points of gas exchange, the capillaries, allow oxygen to be released from hemoglobin into areas of relatively lower oxygen pressure. Carbon dioxide and lactic acid can enter the system at this point and be carried along in the venous circulation. This venous system returns the blood to the heart. At that point, the right side of the heart pushes blood into the pulmonary vasculature, where CO_2 can be released and O_2 collected. This blood then moves to the left side of the heart, where the left ventricle ejects it into the aorta. The aorta has major branches, very large arteries, which distribute blood into the branching structure.

The large- and medium-sized arteries have a muscular layer that is influenced by the autonomic nervous system. This allows them to dilate and accommodate the flow of pressurized blood coming through the system. It also allows them to stiffen up and increase blood pressure and resistance against the flow of blood coming from the heart. Although the kinetic energy released by the left ventricle, in a way of fluid motion as blood is ejected, carries much of its own momentum, it is augmented by the arteries. The muscular arteries have elastic properties—absorbing kinetic energy and returning it. This elasticity helps the arteries accommodate a high-pressure fluid without tearing. Their ability to constrict lets them maintain pressure at a constant, in between ventricular ejections.

The inner lining of the arteries, the "intima," has a specialized tissue called the "endothelium." This is a very responsive tissue that can heal from minor traumas

F. Smith, *Naturopathic Medicine*, https://doi.org/10.1007/978-3-031-13388-6_8

due to turbulent blood flow. Transient influences, such as prostaglandins, leukotrienes, and oxidative stress, can change endothelial function.

Hypofunction

An early occurring state of hypofunction in the cardiovascular system is in the endothelium itself. This tissue has been extensively studied because it is the site of lipid and collagen deposits that can lead to gradual obstruction. This is the process known as atherosclerosis, and it not only chokes off blood flow but can lead to acute events.

Oxidative stress can damage the endothelium, leading to changes in endothelial interaction with lipoproteins. It also damages the ability to produce nitric oxide from the amino acid L-arginine. Nitric oxide can lower inflammation, strengthen the junctions between endothelial cells, and relax blood vessels [2–4].

The contractile function of the heart might hypofunction when certain cofactors for muscular and electrical function, or ATP production, are lacking. This can include magnesium [5], potassium, more rarely sodium, and protein. B complex vitamins such as B1 (thiamine) are necessary for the mitochondria in cardiac muscles to function. The heart burns through its own ATP every few seconds, so the powering of central metabolism pathways such as the Kreb's cycle will sharply decrease if those cofactors are missing.

Impaired Communication and Circulation

Constricted vessels can be of various diameters. Larger blood vessels such as major coronary arteries will deliver less blood to major sections of the heart when they are constricted. But the dispersion of blood into the heart tissue, via smaller ramifying vessels and capillaries, is vital for oxygen and nutrients to reach the heart. If these microcirculatory vessels become inflamed and constricted, the heart muscle will not be evenly and adequately supplied with blood [6, 7]. This limits the work that the heart can do and, if severe enough, can cause ischemia in stressful situations.

As endothelial degradation proceeds, the way in which it interacts with lipoprotein particles begins to change. There is more intrusion of cholesterol and free fatty acids from lipoprotein particles, particularly LDL, through the endothelial and into the underlying arterial intima (Table 8.1). This is more likely with oxidized LDL and in particular oxidized polyunsaturated fatty acids within the LDL particular, such as linoleic acid [8].

Table 8.1 Clinical monitoring of cardiovascular disease

Turning point	Threshold measurement	Implications	Reversal
Damage to endothelium and plaque establishment	F2 isoprostanes, CT scan, ASDM	Normal regulation is lost at this point, and progression to active, inflammatory atherogenesis can happen easily from this point on	Reduction in oxidative stress, normal nitric oxide levels, appropriate endothelial function
High inflammation and plaque progression	hsCRP, myeloperoxidase, lipoprotein-associated phospholipase A2, angiogram	A self-propagating cycle of inflammation, damage, ineffectual repair, plaque growth, and plaque instability will result from progression to this stage	Reduction in inflammatory biomarkers, cessation of plaque expansion, increased plaque stability
Left ventricular output	Ejection fraction <50%	A series of compensations including high renin release may occur next. This is just one presentation of heart failure	Improvement in ejection fraction, decrease in blood pressure, decrease in pulmonary edema, improved exercise tolerance and quality of life

Inflammation

Once the endothelium is damaged and an atheroma is established, an ongoing inflammatory process is underway. This is evidenced by elevated hsCRP levels and appearance of indicators of poor nitric oxide status, including asymmetric dimethylarginine [9, 10] (Table 8.2). This inflammation is the primary driver of the pathology. Increased LDL levels, high insulin levels, appearance of linoleic acid in the lipoprotein in excessively high amounts, lack of antioxidants, and lack of HDL (or dysfunctional HDL) will certainly promote the disease process. The heart muscle itself is not immune to this degeneration. Macro- and microvascular impairment can damage the heart, both its myocytes and the electrical system that coordinates their actions [7].

Table 8.2 Levels of dysfunction in the cardiovascular system

Levels of dysfunction	Tests to consider
Hypofunction: oxidative stress, early endothelial dysfunction	F2 isoprostane Lipid panel
Impaired circulation and communication: vessel constriction, early plaque formation	Oxidized LDL Asymmetric dimethylarginine
Inflammation: establishment of atheroma and change to intima	High-sensitivity C-reactive protein
Deeper inflammation and intrusion of the immune system: rapid plaque progression, cardiac output decline	Myeloperoxidase Angiogram (for higher risk score patients) Coronary nuclear scan Coronary artery CT scan Carotid artery ultrasound Doppler echocardiogram
Fibrosis and extreme compensations: left ventricular dilatation, plaque thickening, plaque instability	Doppler echocardiogram Lipoprotein-associated phospholipase A2 Angiogram
Deterioration of function: cardiomyopathy, rigid heart muscle	Doppler echocardiogram (including measurement of preload) CT scan of heart PO_2 and oxygen saturation

Deeper Damage and More Aggressive Intrusion by the Immune System

Hemorrhage can occur when a rupture or laceration allows blood to escape from a vessel. This could have minor and local consequences, such as a hematoma from a venipuncture access. It can be catastrophic, as in the case of a cerebral hemorrhage or major blood loss during trauma. Vasculitis presents when blood vessels become inflamed due to infection and the immune response to it or due to autoimmune attack on vascular tissue. This can be found in large blood vessels, such as muscular arteries, or in small ramifying blood vessels such as those that perfuse the heart or the kidney.

Constriction of blood flow can happen because of the narrowing of the arteries due to atherosclerosis. It can also occur due to increased vessel muscular tone, at least in the arteries. This is under the control of the autonomic nervous system.

An injured endothelium is less able to control the intrusion of LDL into the intima. Much of the LDL, under conditions of high oxidative stress and inflammation, became oxidized. This makes it less likely to be returned to the liver (due to dysfunction apo proteins in the LDL particle) and more likely to interact with and enter the intima. This leads to macrophage involvement, and as many macrophages die attempting to remove oxidized fats and cholesterol, they heap up as foam cells and expand the plaque. The liver makes pentameric C-reactive protein in response to TNF and IL-6 (which are elevated as white blood cells detect damage). Monomeric

C-reactive protein activates innate defenses, which leads to accelerated inflammation [11–13].

As atherosclerotic plaques progress, they can become more inflamed and unstable. White blood cells such as neutrophils release myeloperoxidase, "as if" the lesion where a foreign body. But it is not enough to remove it. The plaque grows, and as its core expands, the collagen cap, which no longer has normal endothelium on it, becomes more friable. The day arrives when they rupture, and this activates platelets, leading to a thrombus. While this is a normal reaction to acute injury, it can be disastrous for the body. If the thrombus obstructs blood flow, then any tissue downstream that depends on flow of blood from that area for oxygen will undergo ischemia.

Fibrosis and Breakdown of the Extracellular Matrix

Arteriosclerosis is a more advanced, degenerative, disease that is almost always following on atherosclerotic lesions within the artery (Table 8.2). In arteriosclerosis, the artery is calcified [14–16]. This of course increases the pressure of blood and reduces the flexibility and distension of these vessels—they are stiff instead of elastic. The calcification may also have a beneficial effect of stabilizing intimal atherosclerotic plaques, preventing their rupture. As in many situations of the body, calcium deposition on top of fibrotic tissue has a scarring but stabilizing effect.

The myocardium begins to remodel in later stages of atherosclerosis and cardiomyopathy. The extracellular matrix begins to lose some of its elasticity, with excessive collagen formation. This creates a situation of ventricular and arterial stiffness [17]. This negatively impacts filling of these chambers and can decrease ejection fraction. Sodium retention induced by renal renin secretion will somewhat offset this due to volume overload, as will cardiac dilatation (where possible), but this is only a short-term compensation.

Breakdown of Function

As the compensations in this system fail, the ischemia experienced by remote tissues, such as the extremities, the kidneys, and the brain due to lack of cardiac output, will be found in the heart muscle itself (Table 8.2). Mitochondria begin to display decreased autophagy, and the lack of protein maintenance takes its toll in mitochondrial fission or fusion. The remaining mitochondria begin to uncouple and decrease in numbers [18, 19]. Death of electrical fibers in the heart, or even prominent conduction nodes, will lead to arrhythmias. Destabilization events such as an infarction or even excessive exertion can provoke fibrillation of atria or ventricles. The sodium-retaining aspects of renin will lead to pulmonary edema (Fig. 8.1), and

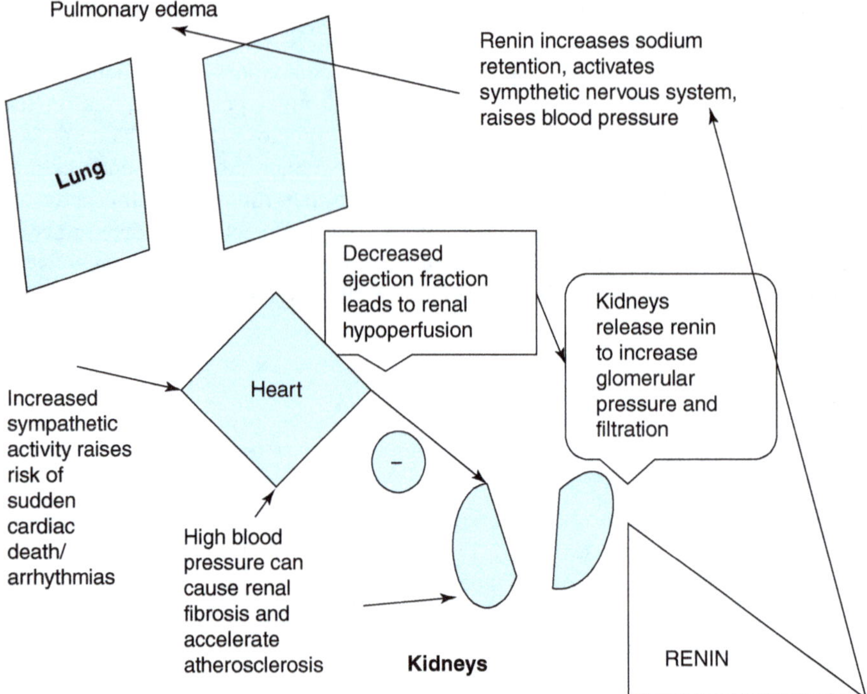

Fig. 8.1 Compensation and decompensation in heart failure: initially helpful compensations such as renin release can in time lead to costly effects, such as pulmonary edema and increased risk of sudden cardiac death

the right ventricle will struggle to move enough blood through the pulmonary vasculature in order to stave off hypoxia.

Neoplasia

Cancer can develop within tissues of the hematological system. A hemangiosarcoma is an example. The blood itself can develop into malignant cells. In a broader sense, the cardiovascular system ends up being a conduit for many cancers. Solid tumors use angiogenesis to sprout a blood supply and very aggressively eat through layers of tissue to find their way to the host's vasculature, for oxygen, glucose, and other nutrients. The circulatory system and lymph are used by metastatic cells to seed new sites for tumors.

Relation to Determinants of Health

The susceptibility to and progression of disease in the cardiovascular system are very connected to disturbances to the determinants of health. Of course, illness can strike due to any number of causes, genetic, environmental, infectious, and traumatic. All cardiovascular disease is not somehow a "lifestyle" issue. However, disturbed determinants make the individual more susceptible. The imbalances that result from disturbed or insufficient determining factors of health can become more serious, and over time, their impact can be magnified. A consequence can be, as seen in the above examples of fibrosis and breakdown, a degenerative tissue structure with cells that can no longer function properly. On the way to that state, loss of balance in bioregulatory systems can also contribute to disease.

Sleep and the Heart

Lack of sleep and poor-quality sleep have been well documented to adversely impact the cardiovascular system. The National Sleep Foundation recommends 7–9 h of sleep per night. The impact of sleep times below and above this amount is a U-shaped curve [20]. Only about half of Americans get this amount, and about a quarter get 6 h or less. There is increased incidence of adverse events *associated with* less than 7 h and typically 10 and up. There are comorbidities associated with both extended sleeping and reduced sleeping, which can also drive some of these adverse cardiovascular events. However, studies that have been large enough to have reliable data sets where these comorbidities can be eliminated still show an association.

In the cardiovascular system, hypertension is linked to both increased and decreased sleep times. Overall vascular health is compromised in these situations. Scans of intimal thickness show progression (which is an indicator of development of atherosclerosis) of thickness in poor sleepers. Vascular compliance decreases—vessel stiffness increases in both under and oversleeping [21, 22]. Cerebrovascular events seem to be more focused on the oversleeping population. It could be that increased norepinephrine secretion is behind some of these effects.

Dysregulation of the circadian rhythms is another important factor in sleep imbalances [23]. The body's physiological processes run on a 24-h cycle. Sleep is an important anchor of that cycle. Circadian disruption brought about by sleep "debt" can start to impact other systems.

Another interesting effect of sleep deprivation over time is increased insulin resistance. Not only does this have implications for diabetes risk, but increased insulin levels, which are often the response to insulin resistance, are known to increase inflammation and damage to the vascular system [24].

Emotions and the Heart

Depression and heart disease are found together—patients with cardiac illness are much more likely to be depressed. While the difficulties and suffering of a cardiac illness can certainly cause or exacerbate depressive feelings, the converse is possible. Depression makes the progression of cardiovascular disease and the possibility of poor outcomes more likely. This is true independently of other risk factors [25–27].

Social Support

In a recent study, individuals with poor social health were 42 % more likely to develop cardiovascular disease, over a 4-year period. A 2010 meta-analysis found across 148 studies (308,849 participants) a 50% increased likelihood of survival for participants with stronger social relationships. This underscores the importance of social support and a sense of belonging [28–30].

Stress

Anxiety and chronic stress are associated with increased risk of cardiovascular disease. Short-term stress does increase heart rate and vessel tone, although this is not in itself harmful. Sustained increased in blood pressure and vessel stiffness are harmful. Poor socioeconomic conditions and discrimination are associated with an increased risk of cardiovascular disease. Experience of these situations does not ensure that a person will develop cardiovascular disease, but it does make it more likely [31–33].

Nutrition

The diet which seems to work against the atherosclerosis process is one that is [34]:

- Reasonably high in omega-3 fats.
- Not disproportionately high in omega-6 fats.
- Comprising mostly low glycemic index meals and foods.
- High in fruits and vegetables and, because of that, high in polyphenols, luteolin, resveratrol, flavonoids, carotenoids, tocopherols, and ascorbic acid.
- High in dietary fiber.

  Low in:

- Saturated fats.
- Refined carbohydrates and added sugars.
- Excessively processed foods.

- Excessive amounts of sodium.

The Mediterranean diet is an important focal point in this discussion, because it has been thoroughly researched. Of course, there are many variants on this diet. Some allow for more whole grains. Others emphasize red wine, and still others put olive oil as a foundational requirement.

Overall, the Mediterranean diet has performed well in a life extension sense. The studies on this diet go back to the 1990s. Most recent meta-analyses indicated reduced mortality and morbidity from cardiovascular disease [35–37].

Benefits for non-insulin-dependent diabetes mellitus and for reducing risk of dementia are also strongly supported. The Mediterranean diet has been extensively studied and held up well to systematic reviews since the 1990s.

More recently, the DASH diet (Dietary Strategies to Stop Hypertension) has good evidence behind it for reducing blood pressure. The diet reduces sodium and increases intake of magnesium, calcium, and potassium [38].

Lack of processed foods is a common denominator in many heart supportive diets. In the 3rd French Individual and National Food Consumption Survey (INCA3) which was conducted in 2014–2015, the associations between health, including risk of cardiovascular disease, and minimally processed, processed, and "ultra-processed" foods were studied. Mortality from cardiovascular disease was decreased by 31% for those eating a minimally processed food diet. Those eating a processed food diet had an 11% increase in cardiovascular mortality, and those eating the ultra-processed food diet had 42% increased risk of dying from cardiovascular disease [39].

This has major implications given the amount of processed food consumed in the American diet and globally. According to the CDC, during 2013–2016, 36.6% of adults consumed fast food on a given day. According to the National Institutes of Health, overall, the proportion of calories in youths' diets that came from ultra-processed foods rose between 1999 and 2018 from about 61% to 67%. The proportion from whole, unprocessed foods dropped from almost 29% to 23.5% during the same time period [40].

Starting in the 1960s, the research into the association of dietary saturated fat, elevated LDL cholesterol (as well as triglycerides), and atherosclerosis and cardiovascular disease has yielded an astounding amount of research [8]. Massive population studies, enormous clinical trials, and incredibly sophisticated statistical analysis of the data have gone into the saturated fat-cholesterol-atherosclerosis hypothesis. Like any good hypothesis, it has served as an excellent vehicle for the scientific process.

In spite of this, cardiovascular disease is the number one cause of mortality. Some of this is attributable to an aging population, which lives longer thanks to many successful diagnostic and therapeutic interventions. Another is the unwillingness or inability of many people in the United States and globally to follow dietary recommendations.

What needs to be asked, however, is *why* higher cholesterol levels are so atherogenic. The role of cholesterol in an atheroma is fairly well understood. Cholesterol enters the arterial intima, and macrophages that might have minded it out themselves die after they become engorged with cholesterol (the well-known foam cells). The assumption is that through the law of mass action, the more cholesterol is floating around, the more the events that drive atheroma formation will occur. While this is generally true, the more pertinent driver of this process is the oxidation of LDL particles. Particularly, when the APO-B subunit is damaged, the LDL particle is unlikely to respond to signals from the endothelium to accept or reject cholesterol from this particle. Under these conditions, the amount of LDL does impact the progression of the disease [13]. But the assumption, one that has been heavily pushed to the public, that saturated fat reduction leads to decreased mortality form atherosclerosis is being reevaluated [41].

A lack of fundamental thinking about why oxidation occurs has arrested therapeutic thinking to mostly relying on statin therapy. Statins are powerful medicines and they have benefits. They do reduce mortality especially in those with developed disease. They seem to lower C-reactive protein, which is a reduction in inflammation that can reduce cardiac risk [6]. The statins are turning out to have plaque stabilization effects, which is of importance is rendering plaques less vulnerable to rupture. But the question is, are there variables that make the LDL particular and its cholesterol more or less of a threat.

It seems that the combination of a lack of dietary and endogenous antioxidants and an oversupply of omega-6 polyunsaturated fatty acids plays a major role. An endothelial environment replete with antioxidants can reduce the levels of oxidized LDL. The higher antioxidant levels might prevent the damage from oxidative stress that led to endothelial dysfunction and great vulnerability of the intima to plaque formation. Linoleic acid is found in many polyunsaturated vegetable oils. These oils have been touted as a health-promoting food that should supplant saturated fat. Americans' consumption of these oils has increased several hundred percent in the past century. This is due to industrial supply of seed oils. Rapeseed, cottonseed, corn, soy, safflower, and other oils are produced in high amounts. Their production often involves a complex process to maximize extraction, stabilize storage, clarify appearance, and improve taste (which can suffer after so much chemical manipulation). These oils lose much of their natural antioxidants along the way and oxidize easily during cooking. In the 1960s to early 1990s, health authorities even encouraged adults to eat margarine which contained vegetable oils and trans fats.

Even when these oils are not overly oxidized during processing or in cooking, they have pro-inflammatory and pro-atheromatous actions in the body. Within the LDL particle, the weak link is in fact linoleic acid. Cholesterol in the LDL particle is initially more stable. Once linoleic acid is oxidized, a propagation reaction that spreads to ApoB and cholesterol, as well as other fats, will occur. The modest reductions in total serum cholesterol derived from eating unnaturally occurring amounts of seed-derived linoleic acid are not worth the increased atherogenicity of the LDL particle [42].

This is one reason that it is no surprise that the Mediterranean diet performs well in studies. The oils in a well-constructed Mediterranean diet are more stable omega-9 oils such as olive oil (particularly extra virgin olive oil which is cold-pressed and contains many polyphenols giving it a greenish appearance and a strong flavor) [43].

Sunlight

Sunlight exposure is inversely correlated with cardiovascular disease risk. Visible light helps set the circadian rhythms, and this may have general health effects that reduce the progression of atherosclerosis [44]. Sunlight, depending on duration of exposure, latitude, time of year, and individual pigmentation and use of sunscreen and clothing, can increase vitamin D production. Many genes (up to 4%) in humans are regulated by vitamin D. Cardiovascular health is increased in the presence of sufficient vitamin D levels in the body [45].

Built spaces, as opposed to natural spaces, may create more risk for cardiovascular disease [46]. Research on nocturnal noise shows elevated inflammation and stress levels, in those exposed to higher levels of night noise that impacts sleep.

Biochemical Support

Collagen Strengthening

The defects in the arterial endothelium that occur in atherosclerosis are driven by inflammation, oxidative stress, and of course, cholesterol deposition. But the integrity of the arterial inner lining is compromised. This can have an accelerating effect on the growth of the atheroma lesion. The loss of structural integrity in the inner lining of the artery allows more cholesterol to enter. It deepens the injury in the local area, intensifying the response to injury that unfortunately leads to atheromas. The magnitude of the increase in the integrity of the vascular endothelium, in the presence of elevated vitamin C levels, is not clear (other benefits of vitamin C notwithstanding). But certain populations who need additional ascorbic acid (smokers, the elderly, those with high oxidative stress) ought to be put on a diet with abundant plant foods or supplemented with vitamin C.

There are other structural issues to consider. Heart valves can become weaker with age and prolapse. Strengthening cerebral vascular pathways are important in stroke prevention. Capillaries and small blood vessels can degenerate, and the bruising and microhemorrhage in the elderly are not always due to blood thinner use; it can be a sign of weakened vascular integrity. On a larger and potentially more catastrophic scale, plaque rupture and delamination of plagued arteries (such as a dissecting event) can be more likely if structural integrity, including collagen, is poor [14].

There does not seem to be one dietary supplement that automatically strengthens these tissues to the point of clinical significance. But diet does seem to be very beneficial. The Mediterranean diet has numerous benefits in this regard, in providing the nutrients to build healthy tissue, reducing vascular inflammation, and avoiding dietary choices that carry atherosclerosis risk [47].

Lipoprotein phospholipase A2 is a long-term inflammatory compound created by macrophages. It shows increased inflammation within an atherosclerotic plaque. This is a predictor of plaque rupture. It also generally shows increased disease activity. The inflammation that this marker represents will in fact further oxidize nearby LDL particles, which increases their ability to bind to and penetrate the artery wall. Thus, a sort of positive feedback loop has established itself when L-PLA2 is high [48].

Myeloperoxidase is created by macrophages that are entering the endothelium. It is a sign of oxidized lipid deposition and plaque progression [48]. Resveratrol has been shown to reduce inflammatory molecules such as myeloperoxidase and to restore nitric oxide function. Antioxidant support in general is important for the prevention of oxidation of LDL and for the reduction in white blood cell-mediated events that lead to atherosclerotic plaques.

In addition to resveratrol, cocoa flavanols have been found effective in blocking the ability of myeloperoxidase to inhibit nitric oxide production in the arterial environment [49].

NO Availability

Nitric oxide is an important signaling molecule that causes vasodilation. The reduction in vessel tone that results from this allows for better local blood perfusion. At the systemic level, more compliant blood vessels reduce blood pressure and reduce peripheral resistance to left ventricular ejection. In states of inflammation in the arteries, particularly those where the inflammatory compound myeloperoxidase (MPO) is released by white blood cells (often due to the attraction of neutrophils to areas of damage due to the deposition of oxidized LDL), there is reduced nitric oxide. Supplementation with the amino acids arginine and L-citrulline can boost NO levels [50]. Nitric oxide-mediated vasodilation is enhanced by the consumption of polyphenols, including those in cherry, blackcurrant, and elderberry. Inflammation in the cardiovascular system is driven down by higher levels of polyphenol anthocyanins from black raspberry, blueberry, cranberry, red raspberry, and strawberry [51]. These compounds, from these foods, can neutralize free radicals and lower oxidative stress. They block the formation of advanced glycation end products.

Vessel Tone: Autonomic Nervous System

Vessel tone can be driven to an imbalance of sympathetic dominant inputs at the expense of parasympathetic inputs. This is driven by hormones such as renin and angiotensin II. The adrenergic increases might help with short-term adaptations to poor cardiac output. But, over time, the increased adrenergic activity can increase mortality [52]. This is one reason why the drug class of beta-adrenergic blockers seems to be helpful for these patients, in spite of the apparent problem with decreasing cardiac output.

There are natural ways to also decrease or level off adrenergic input, which can have beneficial effects on vessel tone. One is the use of nervine herbs, such as *Scutellaria lateriflora* and *Humulus lupulus* to relax the nervous system. The nervine, relaxing herb *Passiflora incarnata* seems to have even more relaxing effects on the blood vessels. Relaxing breathing exercise, positive imagery, and meditation or the modality of biofeedback can also reduce tone.

Mitochondrial Support

Mitochondrial function declines in heart disease—as the tissue with the highest density of mitochondria in the body, this has serious consequences. This can be an indicator of an overall degenerative situation, due to lack of oxygenated blood flow, or residual damage from a previous myocardial infarction, or post-viral infection. Less efficient or reduced numbers of mitochondria will lead to impaired heart function. The heart accounts for only ~0.5% of body weight but is responsible for roughly 8% of ATP consumption. The energy of the heart is exhausted and replaced second to second. Mitochondria can be supported by providing cofactors that are necessary for their performance. Sometimes, providing these cofactors eliminates a deficiency. In other cases it allows for improved performance. Many people with chronic heart conditions do not have all necessary cofactors. For example, magnesium deficiency is very prevalent in adults. Additionally, in some disease situations, requirements of magnesium are increased, because the efficiency of the cells and the mitochondria has declined. In comparing a mature or elderly heart patient with a healthy juvenile, the healthy young person can do more function with less nutritional intake. The other way to support mitochondria is to increase its ability to offset oxidative stress. Because the mitochondria are the center of oxidative phosphorylation, the generation and propagation of oxygen free radicals are inevitable. The body has in-built defenses against this. This includes the enzymes catalase and superoxide dismutase and the antioxidant glutathione. The above measures can also offset the phenomena of uncoupling. This is where electron transport occurs in the mitochondria, but it does not produce ATP. This is always present to some degree, but at a high degree, it impairs the ability to create energy. Brown fat, which infants are known to have, produces heat by a built-in high degree of uncoupling. But this is not a desirable trait in high-performance aerobic tissues such as heart muscle [53, 54].

Coenzyme Q10 or "ubiquinol" is a naturally produced molecule that is found in the inner mitochondrial membrane. It is a component of the electron transport chain. Cells that are more metabolically active and which depend on aerobic metabolism will naturally have higher amounts of coenzyme Q10 in their mitochondria. This is certainly true of myocardial cells. Coenzyme Q10 will help with the process of creating energy. In aging or diseased heart muscle, it is decreased. There are a number of therapeutic benefits to CoQ10. It is important for coupling of electron transport with ATP production. It helps with the left ventricular ejection fraction. Patients who have a myocardial infarction fare better in rehabilitation if supplemented with CoQ10. It has beneficial effects on hypertension. It may help condition the arterial endothelium. It may lower the risk of neuromuscular adverse effects of statin therapy—offsetting the tendency of statin drugs to suppress CoQ10 synthesis in the body [55–57].

D-ribose, a pentose sugar, has been shown to support cardiac function. It can be used in the formation of phosphoribosyl pyrophosphate, which itself is a precursor to ATP. D-ribose can be helpful, especially if combined with CoQ10, for hearts that are struggling to meet their energy needs [58]. It will not help so much if ischemia (due to vasospasm or artery narrowing) is the problem. D-ribose might help improve insulin sensitivity, but it is a sugar. It might have adverse effects in cases of diabetes mellitus if used at very high doses.

Calcium Levels in the Heart Muscle Cell

Taurine is an amino acid that is present in large quantities in the heart. It is mostly obtained from dietary sources, but the heart and brain can manufacture it. Taurine, when absorbed into a cardiac cell, also cotransports sodium. The presence of a sodium-calcium exchanger in the cell means that the elevation in intracellular sodium that results from taurine transport will lead to an intake of calcium when the exchanger transmembrane protein ejects sodium and allows a calcium into the cell. The increase in calcium levels can help with cardiac contractility. Taurine also has antioxidant properties [59].

Magnesium

Magnesium is a critical mineral for heart function. Adequate magnesium can allow vasodilation and relaxation of the ventricles to allow proper diastolic filling. Moreover, magnesium helps to prevent some types of arrhythmias in the heart [5, 28]. Chrysant and Chrysant (2019), in a thorough review of the role of magnesium on heart disease and hypertension, found the great benefits of adequate Mg++ levels [60]. This included vasodilation and arrhythmia risk reduction, as well as atherosclerosis prevention. Less than half of Americans consume the estimated average requirement of magnesium. This can be due to dietary insufficiency, loss through use of diuretics, and the use of proton pump inhibitor drugs. Since atherosclerosis, ventricular function, circulation, inflammation, and electrically stability are all impacted negatively by suboptimal magnesium status, this is a high-priority nutritional factor.

Ginkgo biloba and Blood Flow

Ginkgo biloba is an extract of the maidenhair tree. *Ginkgo biloba* extract (GBE) is concentrated in ginkgo flavone glycans and terpenes. This amazing medicine can increase blood flow in areas where medium-sized, muscular arteries are involved. GBE seems to induce vasodilation and have a local anti-inflammatory effect (Table 8.3). It also has anticoagulant functions via the blocking of platelet-activating factor. It also may act as a hormetin in that it can induce Nrf2 and reduce myocardial cell apoptosis [61].

Table 8.3 Treatment of cardiovascular disorders

Mode of therapeutic intervention	Examples	Comments
Determinants of health	Diet changes including: Increase in dietary antioxidants Decrease in polyunsaturated fatty acids from processed seed oils Moderation of saturated fats Optimal omega-3 fatty acid intake High dietary fiber	A variety of diets will accomplish this but all have: An abundance of plant foods Healthy sources of fatty acids from natural sources Limitation of excessive animal saturated fat Additional spices, beverages, and specialty foods that provide additional polyphenols and other antioxidants (grapes, red wine, turmeric, chili peppers, garlic, etc.)
Biochemical support	*Ginkgo biloba* *Crataegus oxycantha* and other species *Panax ginseng* *Allium sativum* and *Allium cepa* Coenzyme Q10 Magnesium Taurine Resveratrol	These agents work on all aspects of cardiac and vascular function. This includes mitochondrial function, vascular function, cell and organelle membrane stability, electrical conductance of the heart, coagulability, and collagen stabilization
Hormetic effects	Exercise *Ginkgo biloba* Beta-blockers	These have a preconditioning effect that maximizes tolerance to ischemia (exercise has many other intrinsic benefits such as improved blood flow and muscle strengthening)
Whole person approaches	Yoga Sauna therapy Homeopathic and dilute botanical medicines	Whole person approaches should not be overlooked given that many cardiovascular conditions are chronic and that improvements in function and quality of life are possible
Dampening maladaptive resources	Diuretics Statins	The sodium depletion of diuretics can reduce the ill effects of the renin release Statins have pleiotropic effects beyond lowering of cholesterol
Providing physiological regulation to restore homeostasis	Digitalis and other cardiac glycosides ACE inhibitors Antiarrhythmics	The use of synthetic antiarrhythmics requires advanced training Cardiac glycosides such as digoxin are very bioaccumulative and easily toxic ACE inhibitors reduce peripheral resistance

Crataegus oxyacantha and Other Species (Hawthorn)

Crataegus species are the ultimate heart tonic. They contain numerous proanthocyanins and flavonoids including vitexin rhamnoside and oligomeric proanthocyanidins. Clinically, *Crataegus* species (*oxyacantha*, *laevigata*, etc.) have been found to increase left ventricular output and increase exercise tolerance. Physiologically, *Crataegus* accomplishes a suite of effects that are all supporters of cardiac function [62]. There is the well-understood antioxidant effect which is common to proanthocyanidin oligomers. There is also an increase in eNOS activity which leads to increase nitric oxide production and arterial relaxation which delivers more blood flow to the heart. *Crataegus* also has properties of reducing neutrophil elastase which is important for reducing inflammation in the cardiac vessels (which is a long-term process that accelerates atherosclerosis), and some extracts may even increase calcium concentrations in the myocytes, leading to more forceful contractions. This is achieved by an inhibition of the enzyme phosphodiesterase, which reduces Na+/K+ ATPase. This effect is not as prolonged (nor potentially dangerous) as found with cardiac glycosides (i.e., *Digitalis* species), and *Crataegus* seems to increase the refractory period in cardiac myocytes, creating an antiarrhythmic effect.

Ginseng

Panax ginseng is well-known as an adaptogen—a herb that increases resistance to stress and restores homeostasis. Its anti-fatigue properties are helpful for those with decreased cardiac output. Some of the impact of ginseng appears to be hormetic in nature [63, 64].

Medicinal Mushrooms

Ergothioneine is an amino acid found in mushrooms and some other foods. It has been shown to have beneficial properties for the heart. It may inhibit monocyte binding to the endothelium of arteries which would work against plaque development. It also protects LDL from oxidation, which makes the LDL particle more atherogenic. The fungus *Cordyceps* has a compound cordycepin which has promising animal model evidence. It may inhibit doxorubicin damage during cancer treatment and, through MAPK inhibition, may reduce cardiac degenerative changes [65, 66].

Astragalus membranaceus

This herb has a long history of use in traditional Chinese medicine. It is used to increase the "qi" of the lung and spleen which can be done to increase the body's defensive abilities. In an excellent review of the actions of one fraction of *Astragalus*, the compound astragaloside IV, Zang et al. state that current data showed that AS-IV could protect myocardial ischemia, regulate sarcoplasmic reticulum Ca^{2+} pump, promote angiogenesis, improve energy metabolism, inhibit cardiac hypertrophy and fibrosis, and reduce myocardial cell apoptosis [67]. This is in vitro and rodent models of heart failure, so caution is needed in extrapolating this to human clinical settings. Given a long clinical history of *Astragalus membranaceus* as an adaptogen, the use of this herb in heart failure seems warranted, even if other therapies are the mainstay.

Resveratrol

This plant-derived substance (grapes are one source) performs many useful functions. It lowers oxidative stress in the artery. It also increases the production of nitric oxide which is essential for vasodilation. Resveratrol decreases levels of endothelin-1, which is a potent vasoconstrictor. Resveratrol decreased smooth muscle proliferation, a secondary but important phenomena that leads to atherosclerotic plaque growth. It has an effect on the immune system as well—with numerous immune cells having affinity for resveratrol. It inhibits the expression and binding activity of chemokine receptors on leukocytes and reduces expression of adhesion molecules on endothelial cells. This leads to less interaction between white blood cells and the endothelium and less plaque progression [68–70].

Generalized Support to the Whole Person

Blood Sugar and Macronutrient Support

Regulating blood sugar, and insulin levels, is important whole person support for the cardiovascular system. Hyperglycemia damages the proteins of the body and creates the conditions for atherosclerosis. Chronically high blood sugar and resultant high insulin levels increase inflammation levels in the body, and this also accelerates atherosclerosis.

Pulmonary Function

Pulmonary pathology will impact the heart. This is partly due to low oxygen levels in the bloodstream, as seen in chronic obstructive pulmonary disease. When oxygen saturation is poor, the heart has to increase its pumping action in order to provide oxygenated hemoglobin to the body—poor saturation means more cardiac output to compensate for it. Lung disease that has scar tissue formation may also impact the pulmonary vessels, which will increase pressure in the right ventricle. In some lung diseases, a right-sided heart failure can develop.

Autonomic Nervous System Function

The autonomic nervous system (ANS) is impacted by cardiovascular disease, particularly when the heart is damaged. Renin release will lead to more activation of the sympathetic branch of the ANS [52]. Nervine botanicals that help relieve stress and induce a more parasympathetic state can help restore this balance. Diaphragmatic breathing and relaxation exercises are also helpful in this regard.

Sauna Therapy

Sauna therapy has been found to reduce the symptoms of angina pectoris and to improve quality of life in heart failure. In Japanese studies, Waon therapy, a form of warm sauna, improves endothelial function and exercise tolerance. The renin-angiotensin-aldosterone system and natriuretic peptides may also be impacted by this type of therapy, leading to some inhibition of their release. A meta-analysis conducted in 2018 showed that exposure to an infrared sauna bath in 60 °C for 15 min, followed by a 30-min rest in warm environment, five times a week for 2 to 4 weeks, was associated with a significant reduction in B-type natriuretic peptide, cardiothoracic ratio, and an improvement in left ventricular ejection fraction. Sauna therapy has a blood pressure lowering effect and increases arterial compliance [71].

Yoga

Yoga has been shown to improve overall exercise tolerance and quality of life in those with heart failure. It has been helpful in lowering blood pressure, which in and of itself is an excellent non-pharmacologic management of hypertension. This could reduce the needed dose of or potentially (for milder cases) eliminate the need for drug therapy. In heart failure, hypertension is a function of adrenergic activation and sodium retention, with the hormone renin playing a major role. Physicians sometimes hit a limit to how much sodium they can deplete from a patient, as the changes might help relieve pulmonary edema but might not allow the kidneys adequate perfusion. A non-pharmacologic treatment such as yoga can alleviate this. Yoga also teaches people who practice it to breathe more deeply. The purposeful movement of yoga provide myofascial stretching and would seem to be good for allowing circulation through the extracellular matrix.

Hormetic Applications

Exercise, which makes oxygen demands on the cells of the heart, can exert a hormetic effect by both increasing mitochondrial numbers and pretreating myocardial cells to better tolerate ischemia (Table 8.3). The intensity and duration of exercise to achieve a hormetic effect must of course be tolerable and safe for patients with heart disease. Exercise is a form of preconditioning. It is a mild stressor and causes elevation of protective sestrin 2 proteins in the heart [72–75].

Panax ginseng, particularly the Rg1 ginsenoside, increases resistance of heart cells to stressors such as ischemia in a cell model of hormesis testing [64].

Nrf2 and preventing LDL oxidation are important factors for long-term health. The association between LDL levels and atherosclerosis risk is well-known. One mitigating factor in this association is the degree of oxidized LDL that becomes more dangerous. There are other mitigating factors as well, such as LDL particle size, general levels of inflammation, and total LDL presence. Nutrients that activate Nrf2 ("nuclear factor erythroid 2-related factor 2") cause it to be dissociated from a protein known as KEAP (Kelch-like ECH-associated protein). When Nrf2 is so liberated from KEAP, it can travel to the cell nucleus and bind to the DNA at a site known as the antioxidant response element (ARE). This binding causes transcription of genes that are responsible for proteins that acts as conjugates in detoxification reactions. This includes glutathione synthase. This also has an effect of strengthening antioxidant defenses. Compounds from Cruciferae family foods (broccoli, cauliflower, etc.) contain sulforaphane and other isothiocyanates. These are powerful binders to Nrf2-KEAP, and consumption of them leads to increased antioxidant product (intrinsically) [76].

Sauna therapy, in addition to the aforementioned physiological effects, is also a hormetin. It will elicit heat shock protein that leads to repair of folded proteins. Damage to the proteosome in cells leads to degenerative disease, including the cardiovascular system. Sauna and thermal therapy in general are also Nrf2 activators [71].

Symptom Dampening Effects

Mild Diuretics

Fluid retention is a regular issue in heart failure, and herbal diuretics can help with this to a small degree. In more advanced situations, a loop diuretic that causes more pronounced sodium depletion is going to be needed.

In mild hypertension, gentle diuretics such as *Taraxacum officinale* or *Equisetum arvense* combined with herbs that have a nervous system relaxing effect can be helpful.

In any of these situations, some degree of dietary sodium restriction is going to be needed for most people.

Hypertension due to release of the hormone renin can become a health risk. In the shorter term, very high pressure buildup can lead to extravasation of fluid from capillaries in the lung, resulting in fluid accumulation in the alveoli. This is termed pulmonary edema and it can be fatal. Longer-term hypertension can accelerate atherosclerosis and increase risk of stroke. Dietary sodium restriction of course is a good start. Some substances have natural calcium channel blocker effects. This can ease blood pressure, which reduces the burden on the heart. Natural substances that have this smooth muscle relaxing action will not create high magnitude effects and are not suitable for situations where aggressive disease management is the goal (such as acute pulmonary edema). However, as a longer-term influence on the cardiovascular system, they can be helpful.

Vinca Species

Catharanthus roseus (which was known as *Vinca roseus*) is a periwinkle plant originally from Madagascar. It has a traditional use in eclectic and naturopathic herbal medicine for treating hypertension. The *Vinca* alkaloids themselves have been turned into powerful oncology drugs, used with success for conditions such as Hodgkin's lymphoma. The monoterpene indole alkaloids of *Catharanthus roseus* have a calcium channel blocking effect. Low doses of this herb, such as 1 ml of the tincture, are generally safe. But this herb is contraindicated, that is, can never be used in pregnancy, because it has the ability to block mitosis which could be teratogenic or feticidal. Vinpocetine is a derivative of this herb and safer, but still contraindicated in pregnancy [77].

Leonurus cardiaca

Leonurus cardiaca (motherwort) has well-known vascular calming effects. It has been shown to have calcium channel blocking effects, which support its role in blood pressure and angina in traditional medicine. This plant contains major iridoid glucoside ferulic acid, chlorogenic acid, caffeic acid, cichoric acid, rutoside, lavandulifolioside, verbascoside, and isoquercitrin in *L. cardiaca* extract, as well as stachydrine in different parts of *L. cardiaca*, included, for the first time in literature, in the fruits (0.2%). The leaves' essential oil was found to contain caryophyllene, 39.8%; α-humulene, 34.8%; α-pinene, 5.6%; β-pinene, 0.5%; linalool, 0.7%; and limonene, 0.4%, while the ursolic acid present in the leaves was quantified to be 0.26%. Interestingly, essential oils, including monoterpene fractions, are well-known calcium channel blockers, which account for the ability of many carminative herbs to ease digestion and relax the bowel [78].

Olive Leaf Extract

Olive leaf extract from *Olea europaea* has been shown to have blood pressure lowering, LDL lowering, and endothelial inflammation reducing effects [79].

Reestablishing Physiological Constants

Cardiac Glycosides

Steroidal saponins from plants, such as *Digitalis lanata*, *Convallaria majalis*, and *Scilla maritima*, vary in their potency, but they have a common mechanism. These compounds can increase the force of left ventricular contractions. They do this by creating a higher concentration of calcium in the myocardial cell, where it can bind to troponin and create more forceful contractions [80]. It does so by inhibiting the Na+/K+ ATPase. When this occurs, *intra*cellular concentrations of sodium increase. This has an impact on another transmembrane protein in the cell. The sodium-calcium exchanger normally ejects a calcium ion by allowing a sodium ion into the cell. That motive force is created by the normal sodium gradient, which has *extra*cellular concentrations of sodium much greater than intracellular. But with the Na+/K+ ATPase inhibited to some degree, the sodium differential is changed, and the calcium exchanger loses its efficacy, and calcium builds up within the myocardial cell. This leads to more forceful contractions.

This may seem like a logical way to get more work out of the left ventricular pump. And until the 1970s, this was a first-line treatment for heart failure. It carries risks however, and sudden cardiac death is a real risk with high doses of these steroidal saponins. The problem with inhibiting the Na+/K+ ATPase is that all cells depend on this pump. The sodium and potassium differential across the cell membrane, with sodium being higher extracellularly and potassium being higher intracellularly, is a fundamental physiological equation. All excitable membranes, the heart and other muscles, nerves, and the brain, all depend on it for the proper electrical function. Depolarization and repolarization, which enable action potentials to occur and signals to be conducted down an excitable membrane, can't happen if this gradient is lost. So while a tiny amount of steroidal saponins can excite the heart, a slightly higher amount will create arrhythmias, and a higher amount than that will cause heart blocks and ventricular fibrillation.

Steroidal saponins build up in the body. The half-life for digitoxin, from the plant *Digitalis purpurea,* is over 2 days in length! In traditional herbal medicine, dilute preparations of these herbs were used. Observations by modern naturopathic physicians are that low doses of the botanical extracts are more tolerable than the typical drug prescription strength. The herbs *Convallaria majalis* (lily of the valley) tends to have less bioaccumulation and is more poorly absorbed. It is for this reason that any patient receiving digitalis glycosides ought to have their serum levels of digoxin or digitoxin measured regularly to ensure that the levels are not greater than 2.0 ng/mL. Clinical symptoms such as a bounding pulse and visual disturbances herald more serious issues.

In the 1970s, pioneering scientists at the University of Minnesota tested a new way to manage heart failure. Instead of stimulating the heart, they relaxed this arterial system, including the aorta, to a moderate degree. This relaxation led to decreased peripheral resistance, which allowed the ejected fraction of blood from the heart to move against less pushback. The kinetic energy created in a fluid system by the heart could move further. This seemed counterintuitive at first. Renin, released by the kidneys in response to poor cardiac output (and decreased intraglomerular pressure), causes sodium retention and a raising of blood pressure. Why soften the arterial muscular system in a case where the body's own compensation causes it to contract and when there is a risk that cardiac output might also "soften up"?

But the evidence showed that this worked. The early drugs used in this new approach of decreasing peripheral resistance were not the most specific—they used hydralazine and nitrates at first. Reducing peripheral resistance gave the heart the break it needed. An era of "pharmacologic" treatment of heart failure was ushered in. Eventually, ACE inhibitors (blockers of the angiotensin-converting enzyme) brought this approach to maturity.

ACE Inhibitors

Drugs that inhibit angiotensin-converting enzyme are mainstays for the treatment of heart failure. They are also used to treat hypertension, due to their interruption of one of the key pathways of high blood pressure. In patients with dysfunctional hearts, the ACE inhibitors allow for cardiac work to go further. ACE inhibitors are used in conjunction with diuretics, particularly loop diuretics, that deplete sodium from the body. This approach can reestablish homeostasis in the heart of the patient for some period of time, requiring occasional adjustments. The concomitant use of statins is meant to reduce atherosclerosis progression and plaque rupture [81].

Higher-Dose Statins

When used at very high doses, such as 60mg per day, statin drugs can suppress inflammation more strongly, stabilize plaques, and slow atheroma progression (Table 8.3). This is why these drugs do reduce mortality for those with established heart disease. Cardiologists know from experience as well as from research that these drugs can make a difference for their more advanced cardiac patients. At very high doses, the depletion of cholesterol can cause neuromuscular inhibition and possibly (but not conclusively established) elevated risk of dementia. This underscores the role of cholesterol in human cell membranes across the body [82].

Lung

The respiratory tract is designed to allow oxygen to come close enough to the capillaries to diffuse into the blood supply and to allow carbon dioxide (CO_2) to diffuse out. This respiratory activity is critical for cellular respiration, as aerobic metabolism depends upon available oxygen. This happens at the alveolar level. A precise structural arrangement of airways and vasculature in the lung enables this to happen efficiently. The right side of the heart moves its ejected blood to the pulmonary vasculature, providing pressure to ensure that pulmonary circulation returns to the left ventricle [83].

Each lung has a main bronchial tube, branching off from the trachea at the carina. These main stem bronchi branch off to different anatomical regions of the lung. These branch further, into bronchioles, and that leads to a further set of ramifications that become terminal bronchi. At that point, respiratory bronchioles branch off from a terminal bronchi. Each respiratory bronchiole has alveolar clusters surrounding it. The clusters are aggregations of alveoli, which are individually connected to venous- and arterial-derived capillaries. The higher-order veins and arteries are under control of the autonomic nervous system, allowing some degree of the shunting of blood flow to areas that are better oxygenated. Generally, upper poles of the lungs have higher oxygen concentrations (PO_2).

The alveolus has a respiratory membrane between its inner lumen (an air space) and its structural tissue and blood vessels, known as the respiratory membrane. Oxygen can diffuse from the air space to capillaries, and CO_2 can diffuse out. The lung has about 500 million alveoli, with variation between individuals.

The bronchial epithelium has mucus-secreting cells, which provide a trapping mechanism for particulate matter (carbon, dust, etc.) as well as bacteria. Mucus is moved up and out of the bronchial tree by the beating of cilia, flagellate-type projections. Secretory IgA is found in bronchial fluid, and resident macrophages in the lung parenchyma ingest particulate matter that cannot be coughed out.

Immune activation is partly dependent on macrophages (Fig. 8.2). Functionally, there are M1 and M2 populations [84–86]. M1 are similar to the overall Th1 immune functions, with attack of trespassing microorganisms as a major role. They respond to TNF-alpha, IF-gamma, and lipopolysaccharide. M2 can activate defenses against parasites, in the general manner of Th2 host defenses. M2 macrophages can be divided further into M2a, M2b, and M2c subsets. Of these subsets to M2, M2a are tasked with fighting parasites, M2b with handling immunoregulation, and M2b are tasked with remodeling and creation of extracellular matrix. Not surprisingly, M2b functions can be subverted by some neoplasms that are seeking to remodel the matrix to allow their own proliferation and spread. Anatomically, alveolar macrophages are equipped with rapid reaction defenses meant to squelch bacteria. They are derived during embryonic development. Parenchymal macrophages have a more regulatory role and are derived embryonically or from bone marrow, via conversion of monocytes. Monocyte-derived macrophages are quite polarizable depending on the cytokine input signal. That is, they can be shifted toward M1 or M2 depending on inputs.

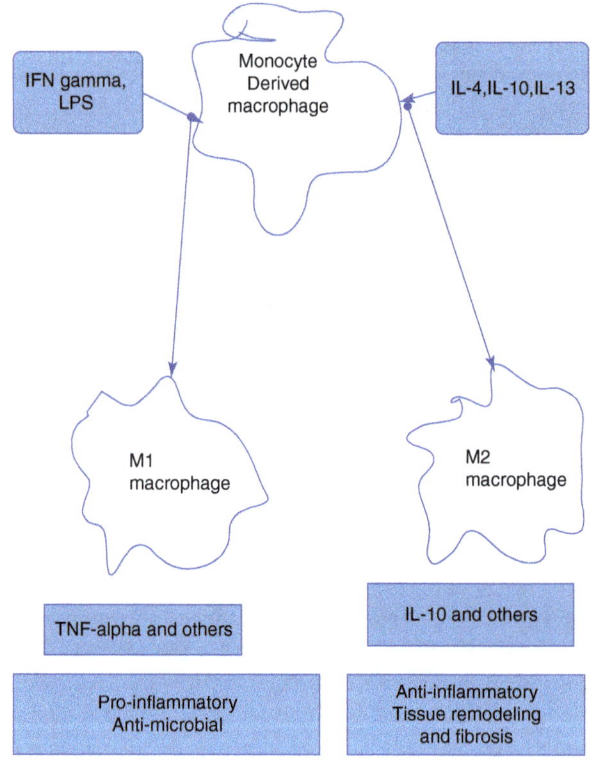

Fig. 8.2 M1 and M2 macrophages: both types of macrophages have an important role to play, but overactivation of one type can injure the lung

Hypofunction

Breathing happens automatically, and we are driven to do it. So it might seem improbable that breath would be a disturbed determinant of health, in the absence of a disease that impairs it. It is true that the ventilation with air and perfusion with blood, of alveolar units, and the rate of respiration tend toward efficiency from the time we are neonates. However, due to postural habits, hunched shoulders and tense anterior chest muscles due to computer work and reading, and acquired breathing habits, many people don't make enough use of their diaphragm. This reduces efficiency and also reduces the positive inputs to the brain, heart, and digestive system that occur with diaphragmatic breathing [87].

Hydration has a role to play in the health of the respiratory mucosa, and even mild dehydration can make the airways more sensitive. Sleep can be affected by sleep apnea, which causes shallow or even interrupted respiratory symptoms during the night. This can reduce growth hormone secretion and create a lack of proper rest. The hypoxia induced during apnea is a risk factor for heart disease [88].

The air we breathe of course has a major impact on the lungs. Air pollution, due to particulate matter, ozone, and sulfur dioxide can become deposited in the lungs or cause increased oxidative stress. Smog is a term for opaque air pollution formed from ultraviolet light reacting with automobile exhaust or coal emissions and some kind of volatile organic compound (VOC), such as gasoline or paints. Toxins in the air from the indoor growth of mold can be a detriment to the lungs and the nervous system [89].

Disordered Circulation and Communication

Blood circulation to the lung is critical for the lungs to carry out gas exchange. Heart failure, particularly right-sided, can impair circulation. A pulmonary embolism is a detached thrombus, often from the legs, that can block a pulmonary artery, with lethal consequences.

The circulation of air is a key factor in defining diseases of the lung. Restrictive lung diseases are those that make passage of sufficient airflow *into* the lungs difficult. Asthma is a very common restrictive lung disease. Airway edema and bronchoconstriction make filling the lungs less efficient (Table 8.4). Inflammation of the bronchioles will restrict air passage to terminal bronchioles and beyond. Exposure to asbestos or silica can lead to restrictive disease, as the lung parenchyma stiffens. Sarcoidosis, a granulomatous disease of the lung, can lead to decreases in volume.

Obstructive lung diseases can be due to a blockage, such as a tumor intruding into a large bronchi, or a foreign body. More commonly it is due to chronic obstructive pulmonary diseases, such as emphysema or chronic bronchitis [90]. This

Table 8.4 Levels of dysfunction in pulmonary disease

Levels of dysfunction	Tests to consider
Hypofunction: poor ventilation	Spirometry—possible decreased FVC
Impaired circulation and communication: restrictive or obstructive lung disease	Low FEV1 to FVC ratio (obstructive) or decreased FVC with decreased FEV1 but normal ratio (restrictive)
Inflammation	Sputum eosinophil test Culture and sensitivity Molecular rapid tests
Deeper inflammation and intrusion of the immune system	Sputum neutrophil test Bronchoscopy
Fibrosis and extreme compensations	Bronchoscopy Lung radiograph Lung CT
Deterioration of function	Bronchoscopy Lung radiograph Lung CT
Neoplasm	Above imaging and bronchoscopy with biopsy Consider that lung lesion may not be the primary tumor Referral to oncologist for comprehensive workup, genetic analysis, staging, etc.

decreases the rate at which air can be forced from the lungs, which interferes with the turnover of CO_2-dense air and its replacement with oxygen-rich air from inhalation. This will lower blood oxygen levels and raise CO_2 levels and acidity (Fig. 8.3).

Although the complications and disease progression are many, the disease cystic fibrosis has defective secretion as a hallmark. These patients cannot make normal mucus, and this leads to airway impairment, frequent infections, and later, lung fibrosis. This is due to a defect in the cystic fibrosis transmembrane conductance regulator (CFTR) gene, which makes the CFTR protein. This gene was discovered by Lap-Chee Tsui and his team at the Hospital for Sick Children in Toronto in 1989 [91]. Without this protein, there is a lack of the transmembrane channel of cells that produce mucus, perspiration, saliva, tears, and digestive enzymes (this condition will impact pancreatic exocrine function). Chloride membrane transport is impaired, and hydration of mucus decreases, making pulmonary mucus sticky and easily trapped in the lung—the opposite of mucus that can fulfill a protective and cleansing function.

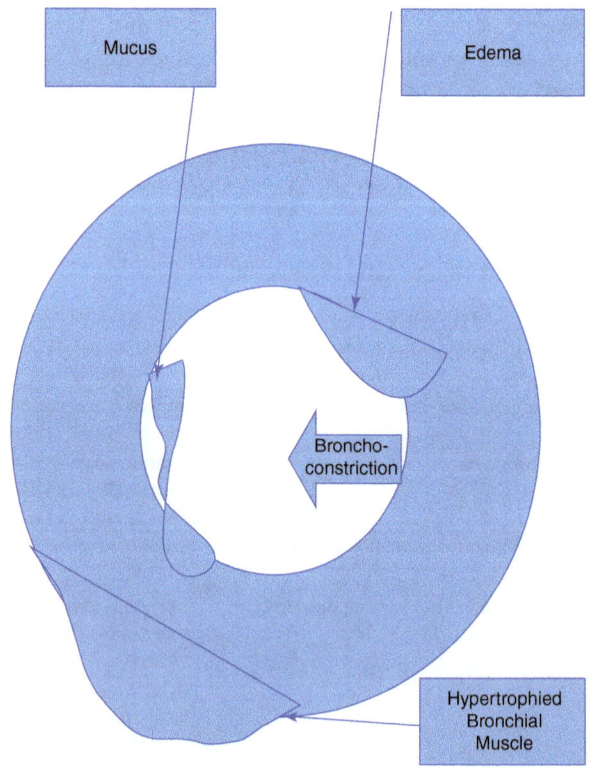

Fig. 8.3 Pulmonary obstruction: conditions such as chronic bronchitis create an obstructive lung disease through multiple factors, such as edema, excessive mucus, and bronchoconstriction with hypertrophied bronchial smooth muscle

Spirometry

Specific instrumentation that measures total air flow and its rate on expiration forms the basis of spirometry (Table 8.5). This information is captured and graphed in a report. Although the instruments and software behind this test are refined, a properly trained technician and a report by a pulmonologist are needed for accuracy [92].

In a spirometry test:

FEV1 = the forced expiratory volume at 1 s. This shows how much air the person can exhale within the 1st second of the test.

FVC = forced vital capacity. This is the maximum air that the patient exhales into the testing system.

FEV1/FVC ratio is the air exhaled in the 1st second over the total volume of air exhaled.

In restrictive lung disease, that patient might still be able to create a normal FEV1 with enough effort, but their lung volume is decreased. In obstructive disease, the FEV1 is by definition decreased—it's hard for them to force air out.

In restrictive lung disease, the FVC is decreased; it might still be normal in obstructive disease, but this will decline with continued parenchymal destruction.

In restrictive disease, the *ratio* of FEV1 to FVC is greater than normal. The amount of air that can pop out of the lung with effort is large compared to the air held in the lung as a whole. In obstructive disease, the FEV1 to FVC is decreased, as regardless of how much air is being held in the lung, the outflow of air in the first second is slow.

Table 8.5 Spirometry

Parameter of spirometry testing	Restrictive lung disease	Obstructive lung disease
FEV1	Normal or decreased	Decreased
FVC	Decreased	Normal or decreased
FEV1/FVC ratio	>Lower limit of normal range	<Lower limit of normal range

Inflammation

Acute inflammation is a natural response to infection, at which point both Th1 and Th2 responses will activate, with some infections requiring intense Th1 responses (Table 8.4). An example would be *Mycobacterium tuberculosis*. Infection seems to call upon both M1 and M2 macrophage response [86]. Cells such as macrophages, mast cells, and dendritic cells can detect an invading pathogen (Fig. 8.4). These

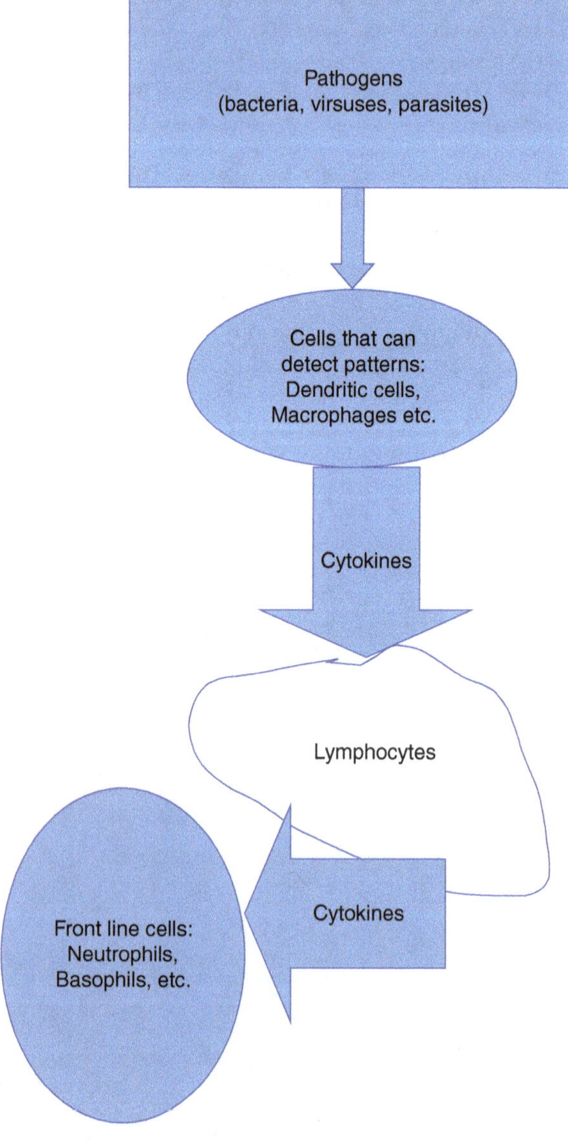

Fig. 8.4 Inflammation is a normal response to the presence of nonself antigens

cells can activate higher-level lymphocytes and natural killer cells. The lymphocytes including memory T cells will recruit effector cells such as neutrophils and basophils to fight the infection. Th2 mechanisms that can lead to antibody formation will also flow from this defense process.

Deeper Inflammation and Immune Involvement

Asthma is a chronic inflammation, with both M1 and M2 polarities present. The presence of much TNF-alpha activity and the large proportion of asthma that has an allergic component definitely implicate both Th2 and M2 populations. The remodeling of the lung tissue, which happens over time with asthma, also suggests M2 involvement [86].

But asthma can also involve M1 macrophages. These macrophage types will secret IL-23 which will induce Th1 and Th17 responses. This has an amplifying effect on asthmatic inflammation and explains aggressive neutrophil intrusion into lung tissue with asthma.

Inflammation in emphysema takes a different tack [93]. Neutrophils release elastases, in part due to oxidative injury and the degradation of alveolar membranes and endothelial surfaces due to toxins in cigarette smoke. This can overwhelm the control systems for elastases and damage tissues. Some people with genetic anti-alpha trypsin deficiency can develop emphysema even without having ever smoked.

Fibrosis and Extracellular Matrix Degeneration

As mentioned above, in COPD, the lung parenchyma is destroyed. The suppression of elastases, which are induced by lung damage, with anti-elastases, leads to degradation of alveolar walls and parenchyma (Table 8.4). This leads to too much autophagy of lung tissue. Lung macrophages get in on the act and secrete matrix metalloproteinase (MMP)-12, which further degrades elastin and lung parenchyma in general [94]. In response, matrix repair contains a lot of collagen, but not much elastin, and a stiff lung parenchyma replaces what was once an elastic organ that could return air on exhale through its own recoil [95]. Respiratory muscles will show overwork as COPD progresses as elasticity is lost, particularly in emphysema.

Fibrotic lung disease that is secondary to toxin exposure, such as silicosis, is hastened by M2 overactivation. As matrix is destroyed, as part of an overly exuberant reaction to alveolar damage, the repair response to this destruction is the laying down of excessive collagen.

In the variant of COPD called chronic bronchitis, the normal defenses of mucus secretion and coughing create more inflammatory responses and a thickening of the muscle layer and edema of the mucosa. This fills in with mucus and makes obstruction worse. Coughing and inflammation create more remodeling, and a vicious cycle ensues.

Dysfunction

As lung function decreases, due to impairment of gas exchange, the heart will have to work harder to move blood to the lungs and around the body. The poorer the oxygen saturation, the more circuits the heart must move the blood. Fibrosis also creates hypertension in the pulmonary blood vessels, which means that the right ventricle must work harder to push blood into that system. COPD patients often developed right ventricular failure. Generalized hypoxia has numerous effects on the body and will eventually be lethal.

Some lung damage is reversible, and the lung can compensate for damage but shunting circulation to viable areas. But various types of immune overactivation and remodeling can become out of control and spiral into lung failure.

Mitochondrial dysfunction is noted in patients with chronic lung deterioration [96]. This is due to increased oxidative stress and the release of damage-associated molecular patterns (DAMP), which can induce autophagy in mitochondria. Increased mitochondrial fission occurs as well. Although fission is a normal house cleaning process to remove senescent or damaged mitochondria, if this is driven too fast, the oxidative phosphorylation (and therefore aerobic) capacity of cells will decrease. These changes are going to appear in the airway epithelium, which will hasten degenerative processes.

Neoplasia

The toxins that can induce COPD, such as those found in tobacco smoke, are carcinogenic. Many people without any COPD or fibrosis develop lung cancer due to mutagenic compounds. Some lung cancers are metastases from other primary sites, such as the large intestine or breast. A particular type of lung cancer, known as mesothelioma, is a product of asbestos exposure [97]. This compound was used as a fire retardant and to wrap pipes in buildings in the past. Workers who mined it or handled it in manufacturing or construction developed this deadly cancer. These days, building codes will allow for leaving known asbestos containing materials alone if they do not contaminate the air, but rehabilitation of buildings that disturbs these materials requires very precise mitigation methods to safely remove asbestos.

Table 8.6 Improving indoor air quality

Measure to improve indoor air quality [99]	Benefit
Wash sheets, pillowcases, blankets in hot water	Destroy dust mites
Put special mattress covers and pillowcases on	Prevent dust mites from penetrating into non-washable mattress or foam pillow materials
Brush pets outside	Reduce indoor animal danger
Change filters on HVAC or room units	Even the best filters will clog with dust, dander, etc.
Maintain humidity levels at optimal	Too dry will irritate mucus membranes, too moist can encourage mold to grow
Eliminate sources of toxins such as volatile organic compounds, cigarette smoke, and radon	Reduce inflammation and cancer risk

Determinants of Health

Addressing adequate sleep and causes of sleep apnea might be necessary for proper round the clock breathing. Apnea can require investigation including a night spent at a lab getting a sleep study. Reducing caffeine, avoiding late night eating, eliminating devices such as smartphones and television from the bedroom, and keeping the sleeping environment comfortably cool might help. Some causes of apnea are obstructive and enlarged adenoids and collapse of the nasopharyngeal area in obese patients [86].

The indoor air quality of a home can help with breathing, which has high relevance for those with allergy (Table 8.6). Some homes have a HEPA (high-efficiency particulate-absorbing) filter built into their HVAC system. Others need to have HEPA-grade units into rooms. This removes dust, mold, animal danger, dust mite feces, dead skin cells, and air pollutants from the ambient air. This is particularly important in the sleeping area [98].

Hormetic Treatments

Some lung conditions are characterized by acute inflammation or chronic inflammation that is exacerbated by allergy or free radical stress. Nuclear factor erythroid 2-related factor 2 (Nrf2) is a protein that can migrate to the cell nucleus under conditions of increased oxidative stress. Nrf2 will bind to the antioxidant response element (ARE) and increase transcription of genes that encode for antioxidant/phase II proteins. An example is increasing production of glutathione synthase, which will increase the cell's supply of glutathione [100].

The dominance of proteases that destroy lung disease over the control anti-proteases discussed above is a major driving force in some lung conditions such as emphysema. Nrf2-deficient (knockout) mice developed emphysema in an experimental model. The elastase-dominant emphysema that smokers develop might be slowed by better Nrf2 activation. Various plant antioxidants such as Cruciferae, allium (garlic and onion), and turmeric can be potent Nrf2 activators.

Nrf2 activation can also elicit more production of sestrin 2. This is a protective protein that is elevated when cells and tissues are in danger. Increased sestrin 2 can decrease the excessive airway remodeling that happens in response to inflammation and which can progress to the point that it makes restrictive, or obstructive, lung disease worse [101].

Andrographis paniculata comes from several Asian medicine traditions including Ayurveda and traditional Chinese medicine. It contains a diterpenoid labdane called andrographolide. It has direct actions on activation of Nrf2 and increases antioxidant enzymes [102].

Biochemical Support

Antioxidants

In general, antioxidant support is valuable in a variety of pulmonary diseases (Table 8.7). In acute or chronic infection, antioxidants can support the immune system. In asthma, some antioxidants can decrease acute inflammation and protect the bronchial epithelium. In emphysema, antioxidants can lessen the activation of proteases. In chronic bronchitis, they can reduce inflammation and possibly slow the rate of bronchial remodeling. Antioxidants are not a cure-all for these conditions, but in terms of moving physiological responses to an adaptive versus a maladaptive state, they can be useful.

Table 8.7 Therapeutic approaches in pulmonary disorders

Mode of therapeutic intervention	Examples	Comments
Determinants of health	Address sleep apnea Indoor air quality Allergy proof home	Requires a careful history and patient education
Biochemical support	N-acetylcysteine, selenium, magnesium, ascorbic acid, and glutathione support Quercetin and other flavonoids *Ginkgo biloba* extract	Supplementation should be focused on particular processes
Hormetic effects	Increase antioxidant supply via Nrf2 activation Cruciferae, *Andrographis paniculata*	Some of these food sources have other benefits
Whole person approaches	Exercise Manual medicine Yoga Hydrotherapy including Steam inhalation	Movement and breath determinants are enhanced by many of these activities
Dampening maladaptive resources	Expectorants *Eriodictyon californicum* *Hedera helix*	These can be adjusted to patient tolerance or rotated if they become less effective over time
Providing physiological regulation to restore homeostasis	Bronchodilators Steroids Biologics Oxygen therapy	These are valuable and often necessary to prevent dyspnea

Cofactors for Intrinsic Antioxidants

Some of the most powerful oxidative stress control comes from enzymes that are made in the cell (Fig. 8.5). These include catalase, superoxide dismutase, and glutathione. Superoxide dismutase has several forms that use various metals to accept electrons. One form has copper and zinc, another has iron, and a third uses manganese. Once SOD has acted, it forms hydrogen peroxide, H_2O_2, which is less dangerous than superoxide radicals but rather unstable. At that point, the enzyme catalase and the protein glutathione can reduce H_2O_2 to stable oxygen (O_2) and water (H_2O) [103].

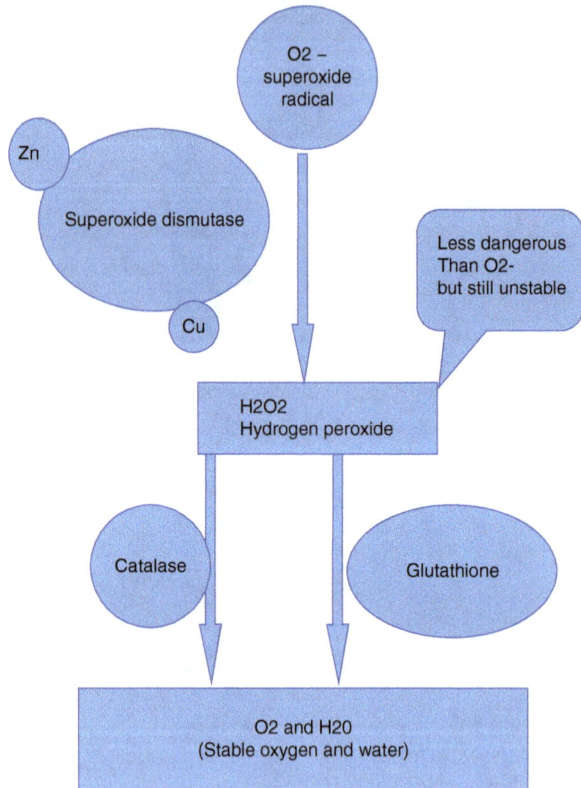

Fig. 8.5 Endogenous antioxidant systems: reactive oxygen species can be neutralized by superoxide dismutase, catalase, and glutathione

Glutathione

Glutathione is a central antioxidant protein [104]. It is formed by the combination of cysteine with glutamate to form gamma-glutamyl cysteine. This is catalyzed by the enzyme glutamate cysteine ligase. The next step is the conversion of gamma-glutamyl cysteine to glutathione which is catalyzed by glutathione synthetase. Magnesium is a cofactor for this reaction.

Glutathione can be spent, as in the above example of breaking hydrogen peroxide down to water (H_2O). This requires the enzyme glutathione peroxidase and is selenium dependent. Glutathione can be recharged by glutathione reductase, which is riboflavin dependent, and supported by vitamin C and alpha-lipoic acid.

The source of cysteine for this pathway can come from the diet (proteins) and *N*-acetylcysteine, a popular supplement. It can also come from homocysteine, an amino acid that comes from methionine.

Plant substances have direct antioxidant functions, and they can be sparing of glutathione by virtue of their maintenance of an optimal redox state in the cell. These include green tea, Cruciferae vegetables, milk thistle, and dandelion luteolin [104]. Overall, address oxidative stress is important in a variety of pulmonary conditions, be it chronic asthma or COPD [105].

Quercetin and Bioflavonoids

Flavonoids are naturally occurring phenols that can have remarkable tissue-specific effects. There are several variants of this group, including flavones, flavonols, etc. [106] (Table 8.8). Quercetin and kaempferol are two bioflavonoids that are found in many plant medicines. They have significant anti-inflammatory actions by reducing activity of the enzymes that lead to the product of inflammatory compounds. The enzymes include phospholipase A2 (via arachidonic acid), lipoxygenase, cyclooxygenase, and thromboxane. The flavonoids hesperidin, naringenin, and myricetin may also block enzyme phospholipase A2.

Patients with emphysema, where aggressive protease actions are destroying lung parenchyma, may benefit from these flavonoids. Myricetin, kaempferol, and quercetin have the ability to block elastase release. Many flavonoids can block histamine release, which makes them useful in asthma and seasonal allergies.

Due to the sometimes poor bioavailability of bioflavonoids, phytosome-bound forms, which combine the molecule with a phosphatidylcholine packaging, permit better absorption.

Table 8.8 Bioflavonoids

Type of flavonoid	Example	Sample herbal source
Flavanones	Eriodyctiol	*Eriodictyon californicum*
Flavanols	Kaempferol	*Anethum graveolens*
Flavones	Apigenin	*Thymus vulgaris*
Isoflavones	Genistein	*Glycine max*
Flavonols	Epigallocatechin gallate	*Camellia sinensis*
Anthocyanidins	Cyanidin	*Vaccinium myrtillus*

N-acetylcysteine

NAC or N-acetylcysteine can provide cysteine for glutathione production, which is helpful when there is excessive inflammation in the lung [107]. It has well-known mucolytic effects that make it useful in acute bronchitis, as well as chronic conditions such as cystic fibrosis and chronic bronchitis. Patients with pulmonary disease who live in large cities or are near industrial sources of emissions, are exposed to ozone from electrical discharges (such as subway cars), or who smoke or have cigarette smoke in home or work can benefit from this extra antioxidant support.

Ginkgo biloba

The maidenhair tree is a very ancient one and exceedingly hardy. The leaves of this tree are the source of the herbal medicine. Although simple dried herbs and tinctures exist, virtually all of the research on *Ginkgo biloba* is done with the standardized extract. This "*Ginkgo biloba* extract" (GBE) is 24% ginkgo flavone glycosides. *Ginkgo* also contains terpene glycosides. *Ginkgo* is a circulatory tonic and has uses in heart and blood vessel conditions. It is also an inhibitor of platelet-activating factor (PAF) which is why it can be anticoagulant. PAF is a primary inflammatory driver in the lung tissue. It is elevated in asthma and other inflammatory lung diseases. PAF production exacerbates lung injury, and continuous reinjury is a hallmark of circular inflammatory processes. *Ginkgo* has some potential, not yet fully investigated, for antiviral actions in the lung as well [108].

Whole Person Support

There is not one diet that makes lung conditions worse or one that heals them. In general terms, a diet that is prone to trigger inflammation needs to be adjusted. This can be due to specific allergic mechanisms or biochemical mechanisms that upregulate inflammatory gene expression.

The common denominators in generally pro-inflammatory foods are as follows:

- Excessively processed vegetable oils.
- Oils subjected to extreme heat such as deep-frying oils.
- Saturated fats in excessive amounts.
- Burnt foods.
- Polyaromatic amines from foods that dripped fat onto hot surfaces.
- Excessive amounts of refined sugars.

These examples raise the question of balance. Oils from a deep fryer are not needed by the body, and they increase oxidative stress, but a small amount in a diet high in plant foods can be a minor issue. A large amount of fried foods and omega-6 highly processed vegetable oils in a low plant food diet can increase inflammation.

This is due to oxidative stress, which can activate deeper inflammatory responses, and the push to eicosanoids (derived from fatty acids) that elicit inflammatory responses. They can also damage the intestinal epithelium, which creates more possibilities for hypersensitivity reactions to foods [109].

Likewise, burnt foods will contain cyclic aromatic compounds that increase oxidative stress. They also increase cancer risk, including lung cancer [110]. Excessive sugars will make the diet one of not only high glycemic index meals but high glycemic load, and the counterbalancing insulin secretion will increase inflammation.

Actual allergy is a different matter. Some people have immediate reactions to foods, such as milk protein, and express a type IV hypersensitivity reaction. This involves the allergen, a peptide of some kind, binding to specific IgE antibodies that are on the surface membrane of mast cells. This leads to degranulation of the mast cell, which releases histamine. This will cause edema, airway hypersensitivity, and bronchospasm [110].

Some food allergies seem to be a delayed hypersensitivity and work at the level of the gastrointestinal tract. These foods evoke immediate and delayed immune reactions at the level of the gastrointestinal epithelium. This can be reactions from local epithelial lymphocytes or cytotoxic T cell responses. Ideally, harmless food proteins are tolerated, and a certain influence by regulatory T cells in the lamina propria and lymphatic ensures that inflammation doesn't get out of hand. But sometimes these tolerance mechanisms fail. This can cause inflammation in the gut and loosening of intracellular adhesions. That allows more antigens to wash into the submucosal area, where antigen-presenting cells such as dendritic cells and macrophages will process them. This can lead to an upregulation of inflammation. It can also allow molecules that the patient has a small amount of type IV hypersensitivity for to find their way into the gut-associated lymphoid tissue. This can eventually lead to more activation in the body of inflammatory genes such as those that encode for NF-κB.

Diets rich in vitamins, antioxidants including polyphenolic compounds and terpenes, dietary fiber, omega-3 fatty acids, and trace minerals seem to decrease lung symptoms. Even in children with asthma, the closer their diets are to a Mediterranean diet plan, the less wheezing and other asthma symptoms they have [111].

Yoga and Qi Gong

Therapies that help people focus on breath are valuable in promoting good gas exchange and conditioning the person to diaphragmatically breathe. These very traditional practices have overall effects on energy level and feelings of well-being. Yoga has been found beneficial for both asthma and COPD [112, 113].

Hydrotherapy

The whole person effects of hydrotherapy are useful. Poor circulation of oxygen in more advanced lung conditions might be helped by contrast therapies that help stimulate circulation of blood. Immersion bath therapies have been found to be helpful. In a review of Khaltaev et al. [114], bathing in waters that have minerals, including sulfur, especially if warm and inhalation is practiced, can improve mucociliary clearance, reduce inflammatory cytokines production and inflammatory mucosal infiltration, reduce elastase secretion by neutrophils, preserve elastic properties of pulmonary interstitium, and thus facilitate expectoration. Infection frequency decreases with bathing, and sauna treatments reduce pneumonia risk. Repeated cold-water stimulations in COPD also reduce frequency of infections.

Manual Therapies

While not generally sufficient as a sole therapy, manual medicine is important in lung disease (Table 8.7). It might reduce muscle spasm in asthma. In COPD, manual medicine becomes very important. Mechanical changes to ventilation occur during long-term remodeling with COPD. The increase in AP chest diameter can disadvantage the diaphragm.

A 2017 study found that even one manual therapy treatment increased lung capacity and oxygenation. The treatment was comprised of the following [115]:

- Suboccipital release, 5 min
- Anterior thoracic myofascial and sternum release, 5 min
- Anterior cervical myofascial release, 5 min
- Costal ligament balance, 5 min
- Muscular energy technique to the following muscles:
  - Scalenes, 1 min and 40 s
  - Pectoralis minor, 1 min and 40 s
  - Latissimus dorsi and serratus anterior, 1 min and 40 s

Both diaphragmatic stretch techniques and diaphragmatic release techniques have been found effective to mobilize the diaphragm. With the diaphragm, accessory muscles, and postural muscles, the manual therapy reduces tightness and allows for more movement in expiration. The lengthening of muscles that are chronically tight and shortened is probably helpful too.

Exercise

Both strength exercises and daily movement have been found to improve clinical outcomes in patients with COPD. Any exercise program must keep the specific needs of the patient in mind: their heart fitness, the venue in which they exercise, the support and training they need to get to their goals, etc. Even patients with very severe COPD have improvements in exercise tolerance and quality of life if they do a tolerable (scaled to their current state) exercise regimen [116]. Combining exercise with respiratory muscle stretching can also yield benefits in COPD [117]. Exercise is also proven to be beneficial for patients with asthma [118].

Dampening Symptoms

Expectorants

Expectorant herbs work to clear mucus from the lungs. They do this by provoking the cough reflex via mild irrigation of the esophagus. The herbs that can do this usually have resins, saponins, or organic acids in them. Another mechanism is the loosening of mucus, which is aided by essential oils—found in many herbs that contain mono- and diterpenes.

Respiratory herbal medicines have nuanced differences.

Eriodictyon californicum (*Yerba santa*) is a plant that grows in semiarid regions, such as Southwestern California and Baja California region of Mexico. It contains an important flavonoid, eriodictyol, which has anti-inflammatory properties in the lung. It was used traditionally for coughs that have abundant secretions, to help expectorate mucus.

Tussilago farfara (coltsfoot) is a traditional herb with roots in Europe. It is expectorant and antitussive, by virtue of having antispasmodic qualities in the lung. Many strains of *Tussilago* species have pyrrolizidine alkaloids in them, which can be hepatotoxic. Moderate doses of *Tussilago farfara* can be used safely for a short time.

Trigonella foenum-graecum (fenugreek) is a well-known carminative used for gas and dyspepsia. It is also known as a galactagogue (increases breast milk supply). *Trigonella foenum-graecum* has antispasmodic properties and can be used in cases of asthma, to decrease bronchospasm [119].

Lobelia inflata is a very pharmacologically active herb that should be used in smaller doses. It contains piperidine alkaloids such as lobeline, which bind to ganglionic nicotinic receptors. At smaller doses, *Lobelia inflata* can decrease bronchospasm and loosen airway secretions. At higher doses it can cause nausea and emesis. And much higher doses can depress respiration.

Hedera helix

Ivy is a popular cough medicine in Europe, where the German Commission E has listed it as useful for respiratory tract infections. A 2021 systematic review indicated that ivy was a safe and effective treatment for cough and respiratory tract infections [120]. The benefit increased after several days of use, but patients did resolve their symptoms more quickly than placebo. These studies included a variety of etiologies of cough; it is likely that more aggressive lower respiratory tract infections that can progress to pneumonia will need more than ivy leaf. Specific conditions, such as pediatric asthma, have shown promise with this treatment, but the database is small. Some *Hedera helix* preparations are combined with *Thymus vulgaris* (thyme). This is an excellent pairing, as thyme is antimicrobial and mucolytic.

Reestablishing Homeostasis

As with many advanced pathologies, some measure of homeostasis has to be fixed in place by the use of pharmacotherapy, if self-healing is insufficient. There are very effective drugs to do this in asthma, COPD, and infections [121–123].

Bronchodilators

These medicines are useful across an array of pulmonary conditions (Table 8.7). They act via the autonomic nervous system to relax bronchial smooth muscle. This is helpful in asthma as well as obstructive lung conditions. Sympathomimetic medicines are beta-2-adrenergic agonists that bind to terminal sympathetic synapses in the bronchi. This includes bronchodilation. An alternate approach is to use selected muscarinic blockers, anticholinergic medicines with high affinity to parasympathetic terminal synapses in the bronchi. By acting as antagonists at these parasympathetic sites, they allow the sympathetic (adrenergic) input to dominate, leading to bronchodilation.

Steroids

Corticoidsteroids, usually inhaled but sometimes oral or intravenous, are a mainstay of many inflammatory diseases of the lung. They reduce inflammation, white blood cell infiltration, mucus production, airway hypersensitivity, and edema. They lead to improvements in symptoms and spirometry tests.

Biologics

Omalizumab (Xolair) is an example of an IgG antibody that targets IgE. This is particularly helpful for those with severe allergic asthma. It is a much more forceful approach than taking first- or second-generation antihistamines or even steroids. It has its risks, and anaphylactic reactions can occur in about 1 or 2 out of 1000 patients.

Antibiotics

As there are many lung infections, ranging from community-acquired pneumonia to rarer types of infection such as *Klebsiella* pneumonia, antimicrobial therapy is often used. It can be empirical (a frontline antibiotic is used for the presumed type of lung condition) or targeted based on a culture with sensitivity. Since the latter takes some time in the lab to produce information, physicians sometimes use an empirical prescription and order a culture and sensitivity should different therapy be needed.

Oxygen

For patients who have deteriorating lung function, supplemental oxygen is prescribed. A respiratory therapist will equip them and show them how to obtain the flow rate and concentration that their physician wants for them.

Neoplasm

Lung tumors require specialized treatment by oncology specialists. An integrative oncology approach that combines conventional medicine therapies and naturopathic physicians trained in providing supporting, adjuvant, and synergizing natural treatments is recommended.

Hepatic System

Key Functions

What does the liver do, and where do dysfunctions take place? What are the consequences?

The liver is the central metabolic clearinghouse for the body [124]. Nutrients that are absorbed in the gut find their way to the liver via the portal vein. The liver stores, repackages, and transforms these nutrients, dispersing them throughout the rest of the body. A branched drainage system for bile culminates in the hepatic duct, which drains to the small intestine. The hepatocytes have numerous endoplasmic reticula, in keeping with their role in protein synthesis. For example, the protein albumin, which is a major carrier of many proteins and nutrients and important for blood osmolarity, is synthesized in the liver.

Another unique aspect of the hepatocyte is its ability to biotransform an infinite number of chemical compounds, endogenous and exogenous. This is achieved through a two-step process. The first step is the use of a mixed function oxidase—a cytochrome enzyme. The cytochrome P450 system is a superfamily of isozymes. These are mixed function oxidases. When a chemical compound is processed by a P450 enzyme, it is in fact oxidized [125]. This would be counterproductive if the process stopped here. But the next step, which is the conjugation of a side chain to the now oxidized chemical intermediary, is crucial. This second conjugating step renders the chemical compound water soluble and harmless. This allows it to be excreted from the body. That excretion takes many forms, via the bile, urine, sweat, breath, or skin exfoliation.

The cytochrome P450 reaction is sometimes referred to as "phase I." The conjugation by side chains such as glutathione, acetyl and methyl groups, glucuronic acid, sulfur, and amino acids such as cysteine is termed "phase II." Free standing antioxidants protect the hepatocyte from collateral damage that might occur if electrophilic molecules or oxygen free radicals escape between phase I and phase II. These are sometimes synthesized by the cell, such as superoxide dismutase and glutathione [126]. Others are present through the diet, including ascorbic acid and various plant-derived antioxidants such as polyphenols and flavonoids.

The liver has clusters of cells known as lobules that are separated by connective tissue [124]. In between these lobule clusters are "triads" comprised of a small ramification of the portal vein (which derives from the portal circulation of the gut and contains nutrients and toxins), a branch of the hepatic artery with oxygenated hemoglobin that diffuses it further into the lobules through tiny capillaries, and a biliary canal that joins up with many other biliary canals to form the bile duct (Fig. 8.6). In the middle of the lobule is the hepatic vein, which is a conduit for the deoxygenated blood to return to circulation. It is also the place where products of the liver cells can reenter the circulation.

One conceptual schema for understanding the layout of the liver is to name the cells that are in closer proximity to the hepatic vein (in the central area of the triad), as zone 3. Zone 2 are cells more in proximity to the outer edge of the cluster of hepatic cells. Zone 1 is in proximity to the hepatic triads. This space has connective tissue and extracellular matrix. The geometric pattern of the structure is that of lobules having a hexagonal appearance (but they are three-dimensional).

When substances that are toxic enter the liver, they will first create damage in zone 1, where they leave portal circulation and enter the hepatic tissue. Any damage or necrosis from this kind of toxin will radiate from zone 1 outward. Toxins that

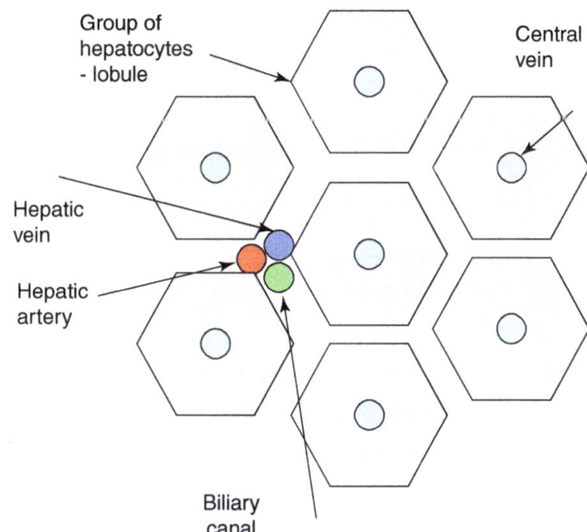

Fig. 8.6 Hepatic lobule: a precise and recursive pattern permeates the liver that allows for diffusion of venous blood from the portal vein system (gut) and arterial oxygenated blood. Bile is drained in proximity to hepatic cell clusters so as to allow for expulsion of waste products. The extracellular matrix serves as a zone of passage for all of these products

really become a problem *after* they are processed by the cytochrome P450 system will manifest necrosis in zones 2 and 3. Fortunately, many compounds that go through P450 processing cannot wreak havoc. They are neutralized by phase II enzymes, and those that escape are mopped up by various antioxidants present in the hepatocytes. But sometimes, the byproduct of a phase I (P450) reaction builds up so quickly leading to a cascade of oxidative stress that overwhelms phase II (conjugation). This is seen in many examples and a well-known one is an overdose with acetaminophen.

Other aspects of the liver include sinusoids, which are lower pressure areas of blood accumulation that are bordered by cells of the hepatic triad. Blood from the portal circulation mixes with arterial blood. Specialized macrophages that are stationary in the liver, known as Kupffer cells, are found in the sinusoidal lumen. These cells have toxin scavenging ability.

Hypofunction

The liver can hypofunction for several reasons including the following:

1. Cumulative damage that has weakened enough of the hepatocytes to make a noticeable decline in function.
2. Lack of nutrient cofactors that are required for the many enzymatic processes in the liver to proceed at a normal rate and scope.
3. Overexposure to multiple endogenous and exogenous toxins that saturated the hepatic detoxification capacity.

4. Genetic polymorphisms that selectively decrease the ability of the liver to process certain types of toxins [127].
5. Effects of drugs [128], ethanol, dietary supplements, and environmental toxins that might inhibit expression of certain phase I (cytochrome P450) enzymes. These influences might also saturate these enzymes as in example 3 above.

When this occurs, the patient will have feelings of malaise, nausea, and difficulty concentrating. The effects of certain bloodborne toxins will be better able to assert themselves, if hepatic clearance is suboptimal.

Defective Communication and Circulation

A progression, beyond hypofunction, is difficulty with the transit of hepatic byproducts back into the blood circulation or into the bile. This can be due to more advanced reasons, such as inflammation. It can also occur in the earlier phases of hepatic dysfunction. Triglyceride accumulation can start to congest the liver with fat accumulation in large intrahepatic vacuoles. An example is choline deficiency [127]. This nutrient can be synthesized, but it needs to be supplemented in the diet. It is important for controlling levels of homocysteine, which it can do when converted to betaine. Choline becomes phosphatidylcholine in the cell. It is essential for endoplasmic reticulum integrity and function, mitochondrial stability, and cell membrane function. If choline is lacking, the hepatocytes have difficulty packaging and secreting lipoproteins—fats cannot move out of the liver. So while most of the machinery of the liver remains intact, the circulation of fats starts to become impaired.

Inflammation

Toxic Injury

The liver has major responsibilities for processing both internally and externally derived compounds and preparing them for elimination from the body. This most often proceeds efficiently without creating too much damage. Not all substances can be safely handled by the liver, for example, the toxin of *Amanita phalloides*, the "death cap" mushroom, processed by the liver but simply overwhelms the normal defenses of the hepatocytes [129]. *Amanita phalloides* contains three main groups of toxins including amatoxins which do a lot of the damage in the human liver. The amatoxin—α-amanitin—inhibits RNA polymerase II, which impairs protein synthesis in the cell. This can lead to massive hepatotoxicity. This toxin becomes more potent after processing by cytochrome P450. Treatment involves strategies to increase glutathione such as N-acetylcysteine and (in Europe) intravenous silymarin. Another strategy is to give penicillin which competes with the amatoxin at the P450 stage. Other toxins, such as excessive iron intake, can be toxic independently of P450. Most toxins will find their way to P450 enzymes unless they cause such massive necrosis in the portal triad and canaliculi that they don't reach the hepatocytes in the hepatic lobules.

Some toxic reactions, such as the death cap mushroom, are so rapid that within 2 to 3 days the patient can go into acute liver failure. Toxicity from excessive consumption of acetaminophen can work this way as well [130]. Most of the acetaminophen a person consumes is eventually disposed of by direct conjugation to sulfate or glucuronic acid. About 10% of the acetaminophen is processed by P450 isozymes including CYP2E1. The byproduct is called N-acetyl-*p*-benzoquinone imine (NAPQI), which must be neutralized by glutathione. A small amount of acetaminophen will lead to this glutathione cleanup of a small fraction of the total dose, with mercaptans or cysteine conjugates showing up in the urine. But a large dose will produce so much NAPQI that it exhausts the supply of glutathione in the liver cell. This leads to mitogen-activated protein kinases MLK3 and ASK1, which activate JNK (c-Jun N-terminal kinases) in turn. JNK translocates into the mitochondria, creating even more oxidative stress. This has the unfortunate effect of rupturing the outer mitochondrial member. Occurrence of the mitochondrial permeability transition (MPT) and rupture of the outer membrane result in release of the endonucleases apoptosis-inducing factor (AIF) and endonuclease G (EndoG). This enzyme can cleave the bonds between nucleotides, and when they enter the nucleus of the cell, they can destroy the nuclear DNA. Thus a cytoplasmic free radical spillage leads to mitochondrial injury, with a cascade of destructive enzymes that target the cell's DNA.

Fatty Liver Disease

The infiltration of fatty acids into the liver, in levels that cannot be properly metabolized, is generally known as steatosis (Table 8.9). This follows certain stages. At first, the liver accumulates fatty acids and stores them in triglyceride form [131]. This gives the liver a swollen, yellowish appearance. On an ultrasound, this will appear more dense. Some people develop inflammation from this situation, and then they have steatohepatitis. Others go even further, and the inflammation becomes intense enough to disrupt liver function. If the liver undergoes a fibrotic reaction, the crosscutting collagen fibers that disrupt the precise architecture of the liver lead to cirrhosis. That in turn can lead to liver failure.

The two-hit model was a productive explanation for NAFLD for many years. This hypothesized that the fatty acid accumulation initially raised inflammation levels. Later, oxidative stress worsened the situation and led to hepatic necrosis. While these events are certainly well described, the evolution of NAFLD to NASH and beyond is multifactorial with immune responses, gut microbiota (through their impact on the immune system and the toxins they produce), mitochondrial function, and general nutrition status having complex interactions [132].

Table 8.9 Levels of dysfunction in hepatic disorders

Level of dysfunction	Evaluation
Hypofunction	Clearance tests Mild transaminase elevation (i.e., 3× normal upper limit)
Impaired circulation	Hyperbilirubinemia—often unconjugated Moderate transaminase elevation >3× normal range to 5× normal upper limit Elevated serum triglycerides
Inflammation	Transaminases elevated at any level but frequently more than 5× normal upper limit Elevated lactate dehydrogenase Elevated conjugated bilirubin Screening for autoimmune or infectious etiology
Deeper inflammation	Low normal or low serum albumin All findings as above
Fibrosis	Ultrasound and CT scans reveal fibrosis
Breakdown of function	Low albumin Portal hypertension High ammonia levels Hepatic encephalopathy
Neoplasia	Imaging and biopsy

Deeper Inflammation and More Aggressive Immune System Involvement

Infection, with viral agents such as hepatitis B or C, can lead to immune activation and damage to the liver. Th1 responses will target virally infected cells, which will lead to local inflammation and damage to healthy surrounding cells [133]. Over time, this leads to increased inflammation. As hepatocytes, both infected and innocent adjacent cells are destroyed; the levels of transaminase enzymes will increase in the blood (Table 8.10).

Some cases of fatty liver disease can progress to chronic inflammation, which can become severe enough to secretly damage the liver. Chronic use of some medications and some dietary supplements can also cause deeper inflammation. Once hepatocytes are damaged, this attracts more immune involvement, including immediate attention from regional and parenchymal macrophages. In any case of ongoing liver damage, steatohepatitis, alcoholic liver disease, and toxins other than ethanol, the long-term result can be hepatic fibrosis.

Table 8.10 Clinical phases of liver disease

Turning point	Threshold of progression measurement	Implications	Reversal
Lipid deposition in liver	Ultrasound scan	Will lead to dysfunction and inflammation	Clearance of triglyceride
Critical loss of hepatocytes	Albumin levels, ammonia levels, biopsy, ultrasound, decreased clotting	Will lead to progressive hepatic failure	Decrease in transaminases, increase in albumin, normal clotting tests
Chronic gallbladder dysfunction due to calculi	Increase transaminases, ultrasound or CT evidence of inflammation, clinical signs of colic and nausea	Increase likelihood of calculus blockage, cholestasis, and steatorrhea	Improvement in bile quality and flow Decrease in symptoms Gallbladder wall decreases in inflammatory signs

Fibrosis and Degeneration of the Extracellular Matrix

Stellate cells in the extracellular matrix of the liver elaborate a large amount of collagen, which disrupts hepatic architecture and function [134, 135]. TGF-β, platelet-derived growth factor, and epidermal growth factor activate the stellate cells. The strangulation of the liver with excessive collagen can disrupt the normal function. The liver is not only composed of productive cells; its structure helps with its overall function. There is a hepatic regenerative capacity, and some fibrosis can be undone. This dynamic feature may explain why those who are able to escape from a fibrosis-causing situation—hepatitis, alcoholism, and NALFD—can not only survive but gain considerable function under the right circumstances (certainly contingent on optimal nutrition). But as the extracellular matrix becomes stiffened and more dense with stellate cell-produced collagen, there will arrive a point of no return, where the architecture of the liver is too damaged.

Breakdown of Function

Liver Failure

When chronic inflammation of the liver or rapid damage due to infection, trauma, toxins, or autoimmune attack creates a secondary response, the functional capacity of the liver decreases (Table 8.9). This can lead to many acute and life-threatening issues [136]. This is due to three factors: the loss of total number of functioning hepatocytes, the decrease in function of hepatocytes due to intracellular aberrations such as mitochondrial dysfunction, and the breakdown of the normal architecture of the liver. This leads to lack of normal protein synthesis and biotransformation of toxins. As fibrotic tissue accumulates, the biliary system becomes strangulated (as portal triads lose their integrity). This leads to a kind of intrahepatic cholestasis and difficulty in disposing of conjugated toxins. Another serious issue is the lack of diffusion of the blood in the portal vein system. This creates a backpressure into the entire portal venous system. This congestion (along with decreased plasma oncotic pressure resulting from low albumin levels) can lead to ascites, which is the accumulation of fluid in the peritoneum due to leakage of water from the portal venous system. The swelling of the portal system can also cause serious and sometimes fatal problems such as esophageal varices-varicose veins in the esophagus that can rupture. Likewise, swelling of the hemorrhoidal plexus veins can lead to pain and bleeding from the rectal area.

As plasma oncotic pressure drops, the kidneys will release renin to maintain stable glomerular filtration. This leads to more sodium retention and therefore fluid retention, resulting in systemic hypertension. The liver will no longer efficiently dispose of nitrogen from the deamination of amino acids, and this will lead to ammonia levels in the systemic circulation rising. At the same time, various gut toxins, such as polyamines and lipopolysaccharides, will leak into the brain. A disrupted blood-brain barrier, due to insult from toxins and generalized inflammation, will permit more of these toxins to enter. This results in hepatic encephalopathy [137], with neurologic signs and symptoms, changes in mental status, and seizures, eventually leading to coma and death.

Neoplasia

The breakdown process described above, particularly the progression of fatty liver disease, can increase risk of hepatocellular carcinoma [138]. In the fatty liver disease process, a number of genetic expressions can facilitate progression to actual neoplasia [139]. Some of these genes are as follows:

- DNA methylation of histone cluster 2 H2B family member E (HIST2H2BE)
- Heat-shock protein family B (small) member 1 (HSPB1)
- Ribosomal protein L30 (RPL30)

- Aldolase, fructose-bisphosphate B (ALDOB)
- Regulation of miR-21 and miR-122

In patients with hepatitis B or C, the transformative, mutagenic effects of the virus, in addition to the inflammation, can increase risk of cancer.

Results of Disturbances to Determinants of Health

Without a doubt the highest impact disturbance is a nutritional one. The excessive intake of refined carbohydrates, including sucrose, glucose-fructose, and high-fructose corn syrup, contributes to the development of nonalcoholic fatty liver disease [140] (which can also be called metabolic fatty liver disease) (Table 8.11). In the past, excessive alcohol consumption was the most common cause of steatosis. It is still a significant cause. The overwhelming number of 2-carbon acetate units that flood the body when a person habitually consumes massive amounts of alcohol can lead to triglyceride accumulation in the liver. The injuries to the gut by ethanol can also lead to bacterial toxins entering the portal circulation and causing inflammation in the liver.

Table 8.11 Therapeutic approaches in hepatic disorders

Type of intervention	Treatment	Comments
Address determinants of health	Reduce sugar and refined carbohydrates in dietReduce omega-6 fats-seed oils Increase dietary fiber Increase plant foods	Improve hepatic function and helps with elimination; good sources of antioxidants and is less inflammatory (due to limitations of omega-6)
Address determinants of health	Sunlight (healthy and safe exposure)	Increase vitamin D levels Also helps with circadian regulation
Address determinants of health	Address sleep disturbance	Reduce risk of NAFLD Lower inflammation
Biochemical support	N-acetylcysteine	Support detoxification
Biochemical support	DIM, diindolylmethane	Support detoxification
Biochemical support	Silymarin (*Silybum marianum*)	Protect organelles and cell membranes, recharge glutathione, reduce transaminases
Biochemical support	*Schisandra chinensis*	Hepatoprotective

(continued)

Table 8.11 (continued)

Type of intervention	Treatment	Comments
Biochemical support	*Cynara scolymus*	Hepatoprotective, stimulates bile blow, antioxidant
Biochemical support	*Curcuma longa* (curcumin)	Use more absorbable forms (phytosome; with *Piper nigrum*; nanoparticle, etc.) Anti-inflammatory Anti-fibrotic Chemopreventive (may discourage the gene activation that is part of cancer process—promotes expression of protective genes)
Biochemical support	*Taraxacum officinale*	Hepatoprotective Encourages bile flow Contains luteolin—anti-inflammatory and chemopreventive
Biochemical support	Ascorbic acid (vitamin C)	Recharges glutathione Antioxidant in cytoplasm and serum Reduces risk of NAFLD
Biochemical support	Bile acid supplementation	Aids fat digestion May protect against NAFLD and speculatively neuroinflammation
Hormetic stimulation	Sauna and warm baths	Induce heat-shock protein—improve gut epithelial integrity which leads to less toxin challenge to the liver
Whole person support	Adequate protein	1.2 g of protein per kg body mass in liver failure—enough to preserve muscle mass but not add to ammonia burden
Whole person support	Fermented foods	Microbiome support and reduce toxin accumulation in the gut which can transit via the portal system to the liver and into the general circulation in chronic liver disease
Dampen symptoms	Antiviral drugs	Treat viral hepatitis
Dampen symptoms	Prednisone	Autoimmune hepatitis
Dampen symptoms	Metformin	Reduce insulin resistance in cases of NAFLD
Dampen symptoms	Branched chain amino acids	Protect the brain against ammonia toxicity
Create homeostatic balance by external means	Liver transplant	Sometimes the best option—but medical and naturopathic medical care can keep someone as healthy as possible and ready for their opportunity for a transplant

Excessive sugars, over time, can lead to insulin resistance [131]. This can occur independently of obesity but is often found in concert with it. The inflammation and triglyceride accumulation in the liver can direct connections to diet.

Sleep disturbance can be a contributing factor to the development of NAFLD [141], particularly, obstructive sleep apnea which can increase inflammation. Sleep apnea leads to intermittent episodes of hypoxia during the night which is associated with an increase in fasting glucose and insulin resistance. The activation of thc sympathetic nervous system may also accelerate liver inflammation.

Sunlight exposure and vitamin D levels might be disturbed in patients with not only NAFLD but also liver conditions in general [142]. This is best categorized as a determinant of health, although concerted higher-dose vitamin D supplementation is a promising therapy. For example, the evidence showing prolonged life and improved physiological parameters in chronic liver failure when treated with vitamin D is promising but not conclusive.

In rodent models, vitamin D reduced liver inflammation and was observed to decrease Toll-like receptors and increase nuclear factor erythroid 2-related factor 2 (Nrf2). Improved hepatic insulin sensitivity was noted in these studies.

In human studies, the greater the hepatic vitamin D receptor expression, the less severe the steatosis and inflammation. This benefit extends to the resident hepatic macrophages (Kupfer cells) which also elaborates less inflammation.

The fibrosis that hepatic stellate cells can create, which leads eventually to cirrhosis of the liver, is decreased by vitamin D. This involves the inhibition of platelet-derived growth factor and transforming growth factor beta and collagen expression in the liver.

Vitamin D reduces insulin sensitivity across the body and has a stabilizing effect on the gut and adipose tissue relative to the progression of their contribution to NAFLD. Glucose is taken up in muscle cells via increased expression of the insulin receptor and its associated glucose transporter (GLUT-4) in fat cells. The pancreas may even be protected by vitamin D, in that it is less likely to make exaggerated secretion of insulin in response to blood sugar levels.

The disruption to the gut can increase damage to the liver via degradation of tight junctions between intestinal epithelial cells and leakage of bacteria and toxins into the circulation (which is destined for the liver). Vitamin D appears to improve the tight junction integrity (barrier function) in the gut. It also improves activity of Treg subset of T cells, which is important in blunting inflammatory reactions in the gut [143].

Hormetic Remedies to Support Adaptive Resources

Exercise and improved blood flow lead to expression of heat-shock proteins that strengthen the integrity of the gut barrier [144]—the epithelial tight junctions and mucosa that prevent antigens from the trillions of gut bacteria, and broken down food particles, from pushing into the body (Fig. 8.7). This is important to the liver, as the portal circulation carries any such toxins to the liver, increasing its workload.

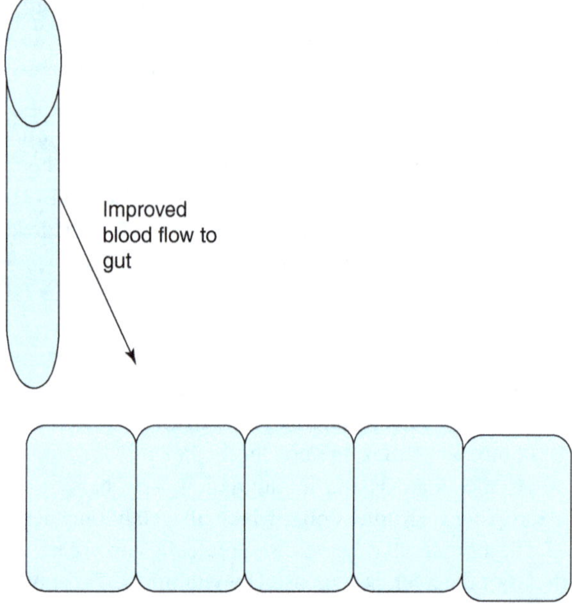

Fig. 8.7 Benefit of exercise on the gut: expression of heat-shock proteins leads to a more intact gut barrier

Relation to Specific Biochemical Support of Adaptive Responses

N-acetylcysteine

N-acetylcysteine provides a highly biologically available source of the amino acid cysteine. This can be used as a conjugation molecule in phase II of detoxification. It also has powerful stand-alone effects as an antioxidant. It can absorb free oxygen radicals and "spare" glutathione in the cell. This reduces hepatic damage in poisoning situations where glutathione stores are quickly exhausted [145].

DIM

3,3′-Diindolylmethane (DIM) is an important agent for the hepatic detoxification of hormones and for antioxidant functions throughout the body. It is a derivative of indole-3-carbinol, which is found in cruciferous vegetables. DIM appears to be able to limit fibrotic reactions in the liver in response to injury [145].

Silymarin

Silymarin is a flavonolignan, a phenol molecule derived from the milk thistle plant, *Silybum marianum*. Silymarin consists of flavonolignans (silybin, silibinin, isosilibinin, silychristin, isosilychristin, and silydianin) as well as a flavonoid (taxifolin). Silybin has two forms, silybin A and silybin B, and is the most prominent of the flavonolignans. It is only about 30 to 40% absorbed. Some supplements attach silymarin or simple silybin to phosphatidylcholine. This complex is better absorbed, with about 60% absorption. Additionally, phosphatidylcholine is a rebuilder of liver cell membranes.

Silybin is a powerful antioxidant and, in experimental models, has protected rats from liver destruction that would have been caused by the extreme hepatotoxin carbon tetrachloride [146]. Silybin can squelch nuclear factor-κB (NF-κB) activation, which is a pro-inflammatory signal that can lead to increased synthesis of cytokines. These include tumor necrosis factor-α (TNF-α) and Interleukins 1 and 6. There is strong evidence that silybin and silymarin, generally, suppresses hepatic fibrosis. When the liver has been acutely or repeatedly injured, the stellate cells of the liver can elaborate fibrotic tissue. While this is similar to classic remodeling responses after injury, it can induce hepatic fibrosis, which can progress to full-blown cirrhosis. Silybin can increase sensitivity to insulin, which is helpful in metabolic fatty liver disease. Silybin can increase GLUT-4 expression, which is important for maximum insulin effectiveness.

Silymarin is known to increase the glutathione content of cells, including reticulocytes. Silymarin can stabilize cell, organelle, and nuclear membranes. Evidence for silymarin in chronic viral infections shows that it does improve some histological parameters, but the impact on disease progression of chronic hepatitis B or C is unclear. On the other hand, the benefit in alcoholic liver damage is more pronounced. This benefit is far clearer in the inflammation and fibrosis that leads to cirrhosis versus the end stage where the entire liver is shot through with fibrotic tissue that strangles the portal and biliary circulation. Silymarin protects the mitochondria from ethanol toxicity. Ethanol is converted to acetaldehyde, and the excessive fatty acids engineered by ethanol are toxic to the mitochondria. A mitochondria with unstable membranes will generate, and leak, many free radicals. This damages the cell and the mitochondria even further. Silymarin has a mitochondrial sparing effect.

Although silymarin or other flavonolignans from *Silybum marianum* (the standardized extract which is 80% mixed flavonolignans or "silymarin" is often used in studies) do not shift the clinical course of established liver necrosis or fibrosis, it has other values. Its antioxidant use is valuable due to its nontoxic nature. In Germany, it is used as adjuvant therapy for *Amanita phalloides* poisoning, and this is in intravenous form. More recent research has looked at the value of silymarin in patients with nonalcoholic fatty liver disease. In these cases, it reduces transaminase levels. Given that much of the permanent damage is not yet done in this condition (which can progress to deeper inflammation and even cirrhosis), this presents a new use of silymarin [147].

Schisandra

Schisandra chinensis is an herb that has been used in traditional Chinese medicine for hundreds of years. It has multiple compounds, including schisandrin B, which have been studied extensively. One of the many effects of *Schisandra chinensis* is to protect the liver from injury, which it has proven able to do in experimental animal models using the benchmark carbon tetrachloride. This molecule (CCl4) is a potent inducer of hepatocellular necrosis [148]. Schisandrin B has been shown to have multiple effects that can protect against fatty liver disease. Some of the observed mechanisms that may be beneficial are inducing the activation of Nrf2 (which leads to an increase in production of antioxidants in the cell) and decreasing stress on the endoplasmic reticulum.

Curcuma longa

Curcuma longa is a tuberous plant in the same family as ginger (*Zingiber officinale*). It is found in South Asia and Africa and now is cultivated in many other warm climates. Curcuminoids are a group of similar compounds that account for the many biological actions of this plant. Curcumin is the most prominent, with much research attached to it and comprising the majority of the compound mixture. The total amount of curcuminoids in the turmeric root is quite high—about 4% [149].

Curcumin has affinity for a striking number of molecular targets. An effect well supported by research seems to be the reduction of NF-κB expression, which has a downregulating effect on inflammation. But curcumin has shown promise as a chemopreventive agent, inducing enzymes that are protective against the molecular cell and genetic processes that can lead to cancer development. It is important to note that curcumin performs well in binding to targets in vitro but is not as likely to find these cellular targets in vitro. Randomized controlled trials with curcumin have been mixed. Possibly, curcumin, and turmeric in general, should be considered more as a healing food that promotes homeostasis and decreases cellular damage. Moreover, the fact that curcumin does not behave precisely like a synthetic drug might also mean that it acts in a hormetic dose zone, as many phytochemicals do. In the liver, especially in cases of deeper inflammation, curcumin can decrease TGF-β and decrease collagen types I and III, as well as fibronectin formation. It will also reduce the apoptosis of hepatocytes.

Recent randomized controlled studies in a plethora of inflammatory conditions do show efficacy of curcumin in conditions such as vascular inflammation and insulin resistance. This bodes well for its role in NAFLD. Recent controlled trials did not show a superiority of curcumin supplementation over weight loss alone for NAFLD. However, a trial using a phytosome-bound curcumin product showed that short-term supplementation with curcumin improves liver fat and transaminase levels in patients with NAFLD [150]. Phytosome preparations of curcumin are much more bioavailable than regular extracts. For a substance that does not always hit the mark very forcefully, this increased bioavailability might be key.

Cynara scolymus

Globe artichoke is a popular food, and it has trophic and protective actions on the liver. It is very safe to eat, except for the spiny and hazardous part above the artichoke heart, aptly named the "choke". Cynara scolymus contains hydroxycinnamic acids such as chlorogenic acid, dicaffeoylquinic acids, caffeic acid and ferulic acid, caffeic acid derivative cynarine, and flavonoids such as luteolin and apigenin glycosides. The polyphenolic caffeic acid derivatives, such as chlorogenic acid, are powerful antioxidants. Luteolin has antioxidant, anti-inflammatory, and chemopreventive properties. It lowers hepatic enzyme levels [151]. Artichoke extracts, specifically the compound cynarine, have been known to relieve fatty liver disease since the 1970s in European studies. *Cynara scolymus* extracts have an effect on lowering LDL cholesterol (small effect) and reduce oxidation of LDL. In a 2018 randomized controlled trial for treating NAFLD with *Cynara scolymus*, the liver decreased in size, and the portal vein was less swollen. Bilirubin levels went down. Total cholesterol, low-density lipoprotein cholesterol, and other lipoproteins decreased. The levels of transaminases ALT and AST, indicators of hepatocellular damage, went down with this treatment [152].

Taraxacum officinale

Dandelion is much like globe artichoke. It has a very long history of medicinal use. Dandelion contains sesquiterpene lactones, which have bitter taste receptor affinity. It also contains caffeic acid derivatives that, like *Cynara scolymus*, have antioxidant effects. A good complement of vitamins and minerals certainly makes dandelion greens a very nutrient-dense food. As a concentrated herbal medicine, it has a traditional use for stimulating the flow of bile in the biliary tract and contraction of the gallbladder. It also has the capacity to protect the liver from damage. *Taraxacum officinale* is very high in luteolin, which has remarkable hepatoprotective, anti-inflammatory, and chemopreventive properties [153].

Vitamin C

Vitamin C is an important free-floating antioxidant, and it is used to reduce glutathione, making the latter capable of fulfilling its antioxidant role again (Table 8.11). Vitamin C deficiency, which can be found in up to 15% of the adult population, is implicated as a risk factor for NAFLD [154]. Increased inflammation in the vascular system and increased oxidative stress in the liver, both worsened in deficiency states of vitamin C (ascorbic acid), are part of the process of NAFLD development. It has reduced visceral obesity and NAFLD in an animal model [155]. In other liver pathologies, it seems logical to ensure that ascorbic acid status is optimal.

Bile Acid Supplementation

For patients with gallbladder issues such as calculi or who have had cholecystectomy or those who have had bariatric surgery, supplementation with bile acids is also possible. Conjugated bile acids are amphipathic molecules that emulsify the lipolysis product of dietary triglycerides and fat-soluble vitamins. An example is ursodeoxycholic acid (UDCA). Bile acid supplementation may protect against obesity [156]. The hypothalamus and other brain regions have been found to have bile acid receptors—the impact of bile acid agonists in this location is still under investigation.

Generalized Support: Whole Person and Multiorgan

The general diet for patients with liver disease has common denominators [157]: a wide selection of plant foods, controlled or low-refined carbohydrates, and adequate protein. For patients with chronic liver failure, usually those who have developed cirrhosis, there are specific dietary measures. One is a restriction of sodium. The patient with liver failure will begin to retain sodium. This is due to the release of renin by the kidney, in response to dropping oncotic pressure. While this adaptation is helpful for renal function, it can overcompensate and lead to worsening of ascites and to hypertension. Some patients in end-stage liver failure can develop hyponatremia, caused by excessive release of antidiuretic hormone by the pituitary, so this should always be considered.

Energy supply for metabolism has to be consistent throughout the day. Patients with liver failure will benefit from five smaller meals. They have difficulty with gluconeogenesis due to the loss of normal hepatic function. Their muscles might not properly receive glucose. Moreover, prolonged fasting will lead to catabolic consumption of proteins. This energy should still be balanced between fats, complex carbohydrates, simple carbohydrates (preferably from fruit, carrots, etc.), and protein. Patients need about 30 kcal per kg of body mass.

Protein is needed to prevent muscle wasting. As the metabolic functions of the liver decreases, muscles can be starved. Serum albumin will decrease, and amino acid delivery to muscles becomes impaired. Muscle breakdown is faster in these patients, and muscle synthesis is impaired. It used to be recommended that patients restrict protein to 0.6 g to 0.8 g of protein per kg of body mass. This was meant to ensure sufficient amino acid supply, without increasing the detoxification ammonia burden on the patient. It is now recommended that patients with liver failure consume 1.2 g of protein per kg of body mass to maintain as much muscle mass as possible [157]. The evidence indicates that this is safe. Those who have severe muscle wasting may be given 1.5 g per kg of body mass in order to rebuild some muscle.

Gut Health and the Microbiome

The microbiome can influence inflammation. Probiotics are useful for patients with a wide variety of presentations in liver disease. Establishing a healthy balance of species of bacteria can avoid higher levels of inflammation. The portal circulation leads directly to the liver. If an abundance of toxins such as lipopolysaccharides, polyamines, fungal cell wall components, etc. is reabsorbed into the portal circulation, they will easily bypass a liver that is barely functioning. This can contribute to systemic inflammation and irritate other organs, including the nervous system.

The dietary measures discussed above, which include adequate but not excessive protein, lots of plant foods, and a lack of deep fried, excessively sugary foods, will be a start toward good digestion and good bowel microbiota composition. If the patient has difficulty with digestion, then the use of supplemental digestive enzymes, HCl, and ox bile (or enzymes derived by *Aspergillus oryzae*) can do some of the work of digestion and allow for better absorption and fewer substrates entering the bowel.

A fermented milk containing probiotic *Lactobacillus casei Shirota* has been found to reduce inflammation in cirrhotic patients [158]. But it did not reduce intestinal permeability. It's unlikely that just one microbial species, given the complex ecosystem of the gut, is sufficient to adjust all aspects of a distressed liver

Role of Treatment to Dampen Maladaptive Resources

Metformin can help sensitive muscle cells to insulin and decrease some of the extremes of metabolic syndrome. While not a complete solution, it can be useful for patients with out of control metabolic syndrome [159].

Prednisone

Prednisone is going to be useful in patients with autoimmune hepatitis, who are having a flare-up, with hyperbilirubinemia, elevated transaminases, and declining homeostasis.

Antiviral Drugs

Pegylated interferon, ribavirin, and the newer (and costly) drugs ombitasvir/paritaprevir/ritonavir and dasabuvir can reduce viral load in cases of hepatitis C. The virus that causes hepatitis B is also inhibited by pegylated interferon, as well as drugs such as entecavir [160]. Ongoing hepatic inflammation and whatever degree of fibrosis has occurred are long-term issues, but these antiviral agents can help extinguish the viral destruction of the liver.

BCAA

Branched chain amino acids (BCAA) are leucine, isoleucine, and valine. They are very available to muscles, and one of the two key enzymatic pathways for their metabolism occurs extrahepatically. Branched chain amino acids may help support muscle mass in patients with liver failure (Table 8.11). BCAA also seem to stimulate cellular growth, via the mTOR pathway.

The evidence that they lead to improvement for patients with hepatic encephalopathy is quite good. BCAA seem to protect the brain from ammonia toxicity, which is a very dangerous feature of liver failure [161]. The Fisher ratio—of 3 branched chain amino acids to 2 aromatic amino acids: phenylalanine, tyrosine, and tryptophan—is important to prevent worsening of hepatic encephalopathy. BCAA may increase insulin levels, so while helpful in hepatic failure, these do not seem indicated in patients with metabolic syndrome and NAFLD.

Creation of Physiological Constants in Situations Where the Body System Cannot Do So Independently

Liver Transplant

There are many things that can be done to stop or slow the progression of liver pathology and to enhance liver regeneration. But if the liver becomes irreparably damaged, it is impossible to replicate its function, due to the diverse and massive amount of biochemical processing that takes place there. For some people, a liver transplant is their best option. Even in this case, medical and naturopathic medical support can help someone stay alive and as healthy as possible while they wait for a life-changing call [162].

Considerations in Chronic Disease

In most cases, naturopathic approaches can improve hepatic function and overall homeostasis. In situations such as NAFLD, a naturopathic approach can mitigate most of the inciting causes of this condition. But there are also excellent supportive therapies to reduce inflammation.

In chronic liver disease, there are numerous approaches that can help protect healthy hepatocytes from further damage and improve function. If a condition is very far advanced, it may not be clear if naturopathic intervention will ultimately postpone permanent disability or death from this condition. An example is cirrhosis of the liver. Although there is a lot to do to enable remaining cells to function, the massive disruptions to hepatic architecture seen in cirrhosis put constraints on how much regeneration can take place.

In chronic liver failure, alterations to diet, digestion, microbiota, and support and hepatic function can reduce the severity of illness. But again, if the cause is extensive necrosis of the liver, then the prolonging of life might be modest.

What is encouraging is that many hepatic conditions start out as gradual and accrue permanent damage over time. On that timeline, many naturopathic interventions can have benefits. Even in situations with measurable and (in imaging studies) observable liver damage, such as chronic alcoholism, there are many cases where the liver (or enough of the organ) can regenerate and the person can become high functioning. This is an attestation to the reserve function that is found in many body tissues and, of course, the adaptive, replacement, and remodeling responses that can be positive with the correct support and guidance.

Stomach, Small Intestine, and Exocrine Pancreas

The upper gastrointestinal tract, comprised of the stomach and duodenum, the exocrine functions of the pancreas, the jejunum and ileum segments of the small intestine, and the secretions of bile from the liver are the principal means by which we ingest, digestion, and absorb nutrients. These tissues are highly specialized in ways that make them able to perform all of those tasks. The intake and movement of food in a forward motion from proximal to distal require muscular contractions that are coordinated. The breaking down of food molecules into simpler, absorbable compounds and elements requires an entire spectrum of chemical enzymes and secretions [163]. The absorption of those smaller units into the bloodstream is accomplished by simple diffusion, facilitated diffusion, special transport molecules, and in the case of fats, direct absorption into the lymphatic system. The human experience of food is rewarding, and our interaction with food activates neurological and hormonal responses that optimize our digestion [164].

The act of swallowing itself is an amazing acrobatic act, with the involuntary phase occurring once a food bolus has passed the pharynx. Once the esophageal muscles contract and relax in a wave like motion to let food descend, the esophageal sphincter opens to allow the food bolus (masticated if needed and mixed with saliva and some salivary amylase and lipases) to enter the stomach. Any patient with esophageal issues such as achalasia can appreciate how much we depend on the esophagus to do its job.

Once in the stomach, food is subjected to intense chemical and mechanical actions. This has a pulverizing effect on food and a denaturing effect on proteins. This essentially creates more solubility and more surface area for the enzymatic treatment that is yet to come. The muscles of the stomach can pinch and roll the contents through squeezing motions. The cells of the stomach produce important digestive compounds. The parietal cells are found in the gastric glands, pit like structures within the mucosa. Parietal cells produce hydrochloric acid and can drop the gastric pH from a range of about 0.3–2.9 pH. Also in the gastric glands are chief cells that make pepsinogen, which is an inactive enzyme—a zymogen. When pepsinogen is exposed to hydrochloric acid, it converts to pepsin, which is a powerful cleaver of peptide bonds. These bonds are between amino acids. HCl is important to denature proteins, making them unfold, which opens them up to their secondary structures where larger stretches of their amino acid chains can be exposed to pepsin. Protein digestion is not completed in the stomach, but tertiary and some secondary structures are unraveled, amino acid chain length is decreased, and food is converted to a milky, watery mix that is ready to leave the stomach.

In the gastric gland, there are mucus-secreting cells. These are important for making a protective layer of mucus that prevents autodigestion of the stomach by its own acid and pepsin. The mucus layer has a layer of water with bicarbonate ions underneath the mucus, which acts as a second line of defense against the protons from HCl but still allows the pH of the stomach contents to remain low.

The stomach also produces intrinsic factor, which combines with vitamin B12, so that much later in the digestive flow, in the ileum, the B12 can be absorbed.

The pyloric valve is the gateway from the stomach antrum to the duodenum. The passage of food and liquids from the stomach to the small intestine is controlled in spurts. This is advantageous because regulating this transit provides the enzyme-rich environment of the duodenum with a limited volume of chyme (food mixture). This keeps the ratio of chyme to digestive juices in a productive range. This control of duodenal entry also presents a flooding of chemical particles into the duodenum, such as sugars, fats, and amino acids or proteins. That "dumping" of substances can cause, via osmosis, a flood of water into the duodenal lumen. This can cause blood pressure to drop suddenly, heart rate to rise, epinephrine to be released, and a watery diarrhea to ensue.

Once food is in the duodenum, it is subject to a barrage of enzymes from the pancreas. In order to neutralize the acidity of the chyme, the pancreas includes bicarbonate in its secretions. The enzymes work best in a more neutral pH range. Also entering the duodenum is bile from the gallbladder. Bile acts as an emulsifier of fats, breaking larger fat globules up into smaller micelles. This creates more access to triglycerides for pancreatic enzymes.

The enzymes at the pancreatic level include various proteases: trypsin and chymotrypsin. There are lipases which break down triglycerides into glycerol and free fatty acids. Amylases break down long-chain carbohydrates. These enzymes create shorter oligomers of amino acids and carbohydrates. At the border of the intestinal cell, enzymes that work to break down smaller peptides and disaccharides complete the process. Fatty acids are absorbed in their own process, diffusing into lymphatics and being carried to the venous system.

The small intestinal epithelium is sometimes called the brush border. It has villous (fingerlike) projections, which are covered in microvilli (smaller projections), which themselves have a colony of epithelial cells. These cells are highly specialized and can absorb nutrients through a variety of transport mechanisms. The epithelium has mucus-secreting cells, which lubricate the chyme, and it has the ability to release secretory IgA into the lumen for protection.

The small intestine also can sample the peptides and proteins that are in the gut lumen. Sometimes, mucosal cells take intact protein sequences directly into the lymphatic system. This provides antigen-presenting cells, such as dendritic cells, to process these proteins. This might be a cell wall component of a pathogenic organism. Or it could be a harmless food molecule. Immune processing by dendritic cells can lead to an amplified response. On the front line of the gut epithelium, there are also intraepithelial lymphocytes, which are prone to react to many challenges. In the background, in the gut-associated lymphatic tissue, there are regulatory T cells that can downregulate immune responses. This aspect of "tolerance" is extremely important for the avoidance of allergy and excessive inflammation.

The muscular layer around the small bowel has muscle fibers in different orientations. Some muscle fiber tracts are longitudinal, some wrap around the bowel, and some are circular. This is meant to push, roll, and chop food as a way to keep it moving forward and to continue to present food molecules to the epithelial surface. The innervation of the gut is via the autonomic nervous system. Nerve endings within the muscular layer and down into the mucosa transmit this information. The smooth muscle that wraps the gut shares calcium ions between muscle cells via a syncytium and facilitates wavelike depolarizations that coordinate contraction. This is known as peristalsis.

The vagus nerve and its branches also control secretions. A hormone, cholecystokinin, which increases after eating, can elicit stomach acid secretion, gallbladder contraction, and pancreatic secretion. This prepares the environment for the arrival of food. The acid-secreting cells of the stomach will increase their acid product when histamine is released by enterochromaffin-like cells, a neuroendocrine cell found in the gastrointestinal epithelium.

Hypofunction

Many gastric, pancreatic exocrine, and small bowel hypofunctional situations begin rather subtly. These tissues, being so vital to the acquisition of nutrients to sustain life, have a lot of redundancy. There is a lot of potential for loss built into the system.

A common finding is mild hypochlorhydria [165]. This can happen with age as the viability of the parietal cells begins to decline. This can progress to a more deteriorated state, but even with a relatively healthy mucosa, acid levels can decrease. This can be due to aging but also to chronic stress, with prolonged elevated cortisol levels (which also can make the stomach lining itself more vulnerable to the acid). Smoking will decrease gastric acidity (while it may seem counterintuitive, smoking may also increase the risk of peptic ulcers). Lack of nutrients such as zinc and B complex vitamins can decrease hydrochloric acid secretion.

The stomach can also be lax in its contractions, which is also an age-related phenomena. The small bowel seems to maintain peristalsis to a better degree. Some of this is actual tissue aging of the stomach and some of it is due to decreased innervation. There seems to be a decrease in gastric emptying by an average of 6 minutes for every 10 years in adults. Older adults will feel full longer due to this delayed gastric emptying. Medicines that have an anticholinergic function, such as those used for Parkinson's disease, impact gastric emptying. Many people use antacid drugs not to provide healing for peptic ulcers but to reduce symptoms of dyspepsia (indigestion). This will automatically lead to gastric hypofunction.

Impaired Communication and Circulation

More severe interruptions to normal gastric and small intestine activity can occur in the case of neurological damage. This can range from mild incoordination of the system to very impaired. The muscular contractions of these issues and the opening of the pyloric valve, as well as the release of pancreatic exocrine contents, are closely regulated and synchronized with other events. When this is no longer functioning normally, there can be symptoms such as pain, poor digestion, nausea, and difficulty digesting food and absorbing nutrients on account of poor breakdown.

Damage to the branches of the vagus nerve or to nerve plexuses of the sympathetic system can occur due to diabetes [166]. The combined effect of glycation of proteins and the buildup of sorbitol sugar in the Schwann cells that are there to support the nerves can cause permanent injury. In this case, gastric emptying can be delayed and the occurrence in excessive volumes of foods released into the duodenum. Diabetes is not the only way that gastric nerves get damaged; trauma, either directly to the nerve branches, or to the ganglionic neuron cell bodies, or even the nerves that synapse with them (preganglionic) that run down the spinal cord.

Pancreatic exocrine deficiency can have a major impact on digestion [167]. The lack of delivery of pancreatic enzymes into the duodenum will undermine an important phase of digestion where large proteins, carbohydrates, and globules of triglycerides ought to be broken down to smaller components. Pancreatitis is one cause of this. A past episode of pancreatitis can lead to a damaged organ parenchyma. A chronic pancreatitis will slowly use up the functioning exocrine cells. Although a gallstone can block the pancreatic duct, this will become a surgical emergency if it does not free itself. Non-pancreatitis causes of this condition can include lack of intervention, due to diabetes or other forms of nerve damage. Patients with cystic fibrosis will have deterioration of the pancreas and develop exocrine deficiency.

Although the cutoff for this diagnosis of pancreatic exocrine deficiency used to be <10% of normal secretions, this threshold is too absolute. A gradual decline of exocrine function will cause symptoms and will impair digestion. A person with less than 10% of his pancreatic proteases, lipases, and amylases will have very obvious malabsorption issues.

Bile flowing into the duodenum will decrease if the gallbladder contains thickened (initially referred to "sludge" when diagnostic ultrasound became commonly available) material and has a lack of bile acids [168, 169]. Some patients have their gallbladder removed due to cholecystitis which might progress to a calculus being impacted somewhere in the biliary ducts. Even after this removal, there is still a biliary flow from the liver into the common bile duct and to the duodenum. Although the larger volume release of bile from the gallbladder is reduced, the small volume of bile plus the pancreatic lipases can still accomplish some fat digestion.

Disordered motility, due to changes to the mucosa, microbiome, enteric plexus, vagal innervation, and overall nervous system (including CNS), contributed to irritable bowel syndrome. This noninflammatory disorder shows desynchronized slow wave and peristaltic activity. Some patients present with more spasm, others with atony, and many veer from one type of bowel electrical activity to another. Being multivariate in causes and presentations, it can be a challenging condition to treat [170].

Inflammation

Inflammation is a response to cellular injury. In the stomach and small intestine, this can be due to acid injury, infection, ischemic events, or autoimmune events. Sometimes this inflammation is transitory and recurring; other times it can progress to a more severe form. The chronicity and the severity have a bearing on the resolution of inflammation with a modest amount of tissue remodeling to put the affected area back to what it was—in structure and function.

The stomach is easily susceptible to inflammation in several ways. Its high acid environment will lead to mucosal damage should the normal defenses of that mucosa fail. Pathogens, such as food- or waterborne illness, can replicate and produce toxins in the stomach with nausea and vomiting occurring. *Helicobacter pylori* is a bacteria that lives in the gastric mucosa of many people, and in some of them, it can cause a degree of inflammation that damages the lining of the stomach [171]. It can act as a susceptibility factor for gastric ulcer. Some people have low-grade *H. pylori* infection and suffer no real ill effects. Others develop gastric or duodenal ulcers and, when given *H. pylori* eradication treatment, find that their ulcers heal.

When stress, smoking, or *H. pylori* decreases the mucus protection of the stomach, then HCl and pepsin can cause damage. The nonsteroidal anti-inflammatory drugs (NSAIDs), such as ibuprofen, aspirin, etc., will reduce the mucosal protection. This is due to the ability of these drugs to block the enzyme cyclooxygenase-1. This blockage will reduce pain and fever, hence the utility of these medications (they also have a COX-2 inhibition effect which decreases inflammation). Unfortunately, COX-1 inhibition also blocks gastric mucus production. Not surprisingly, patients with heavy long-term NSAID usage often have chronic inflammation.

The gastric mucosa can atrophy with age. Sometimes this atrophy is concomitant with low-grade inflammation. Atrophic gastritis is found in the majority of people over of the age of 70. The mucosa is inflamed and thinned out. Those with chronic *H. pylori* infection will have the most pronounced inflammation. Less commonly, an autoimmune component can cause this.

In the small bowel, there can be proximal infection with *H. pylori*. Across the small intestine, the number of bacteria is generally rather low. In the ileum, the terminal segment of the small intestine, the concentration of bacteria per mL of volume is 10^8. In the duodenum the concentration of bacteria per mL is only 10^3 [172]. When this is disturbed with abnormal species or if the bacteria from the large bowel infiltrate the small bowel to too large a degree, then the immune system will work to clear these bacteria, creating an inflammatory state.

The small intestine encounters a very wide array of proteins, from food, fungi, yeast, bacteria, virus, and damaged tissues. This area has an extensive complement of immune cells, both at the mucosal surface and in lymphatic tissues. But the gut learns to tolerate foods and to not overrespond to minor infections [173]. If it did not, the inflammation would be at a damaging level. This can happen in the case of food allergies. It can progress further with conditions such as celiac disease.

More Intense Inflammation and Involvement of the Immune System

If a peptic or duodenal ulcer is not resolved, the area of injury attracts white blood cells and becomes an area of active injury, inflammation, partial repair, and no complete resolution or remodeling (Table 8.12). This can grow into a larger ulcer crater that of course will permit more acid and pepsin to damage a wider diameter of tissue and dig deeper, perhaps penetrating into the submucosa. This might even progress to a penetration of the stomach muscular layer and serosa, allowing HCl and pepsin into the peritoneal cavity, with catastrophic results. Or it may find a branch of the gastric artery and create a hemorrhage.

In inflammatory bowel disease, with Crohn's disease being the most likely etiology of small bowel inflammation of this kind, although it does definitely impact the large intestine in many patients, a variety of phenotypes can have disease activity along the entire gastrointestinal tract [174]. Extraintestinal manifestations, such as iritis, vasculitis, polyarthritis, and even overlapped gastrointestinal issues such as cholangitis and celiac disease, can complicate Crohn's disease. Locally, white blood cell destruction of the small bowel wall leads to an ongoing destructive process. Granulomas are a consistent feature in Crohn's disease. The granulomatous inflammatory response is characterized by focal collections of macrophages, epithelioid cells, and multinucleated giant cells. These will cause inflammation that can eat into the wall of the bowel. The precise triggering event for this process is still under investigation. Gut microbiome composition seems to play a part.

Crohn's disease patients seem to have less microbiome diversity especially within the *Firmicutes* and *Bacteroidetes* phyla. This is one factor, and other susceptibility factors, such as genomic and proteomic states, interact with the shift to a narrow microbiome composition. Crohn's patients may have less effective Paneth cells. These specialist cells in the epithelium secrete antimicrobial peptide granules, one being the alpha-defensins, and can cultivate the composition of the microbiome to some extent.

Table 8.12 Levels of dysfunction of upper gastrointestinal disease (and diagnostic tests)

Level of dysfunction	Test	Finding	Comments
Hypofunction	Endoscopy with upper gastrointestinal tract view	Endoscopy extends into duodenum and jejunum—images and biopsy	Sedation but not general anesthesia required
Impaired circulation and communication	Stool analysis	Can detect signs of malabsorption	Undigested protein and putrefied protein, excessive fatty acids
Inflammation	*H. pylori* breath test	Carbon dioxide is exhaled after taking a urea-containing tablet	*H. pylori* has a urease enzyme
Inflammation	Stool test	*H. pylori* antigen	
Inflammation	Endoscopy	Visual inspection for gastric ulcer	Does not prove etiology but provides real-time information about state of gastric mucosa
Inflammation	Endoscopy	Biopsy and culture	Can be examined for signs of inflammation and *H. pylori*
Inflammation	Endoscopy	Rapid urea test	Uses urea and CO_2 detection to provide an in situ test for *H. pylori*
Inflammation	Endoscopy	*H. pylori* molecular test—DNA	Looks for *H. pylori* genetic material in a biopsy
Inflammation	Endoscopy with upper gastrointestinal tract view	Endoscopy extends into duodenum and jejunum—images and biopsy	Sedation but not general anesthesia required
Inflammation	Capsule endoscopy	Camera-enabled capsule swallowed to provide images of gut mucosa	Not directly controlled by surgeon
Deeper inflammation and immune involvement	Colonoscopy	Crohn's can extend to large intestine—images and biopsy can be obtained	General anesthesia and bowel prep required
Fibrosis and extracellular matrix degeneration	GI series	Radiographic findings of defects in mucosa, strictures, and fistulas	Barium required to create contrast
Fibrosis and extracellular matrix degeneration	MRI	Not universally used but can provide precise imaging and information about fistulas and inflammation depth	No radiation exposure Patient must wear hearing protection

(continued)

Table 8.12 (continued)

Level of dysfunction	Test	Finding	Comments
Decline of function	Blood work for malabsorption	Hemoglobin, electrolytes, albumen, carotenoids, B12, vitamin D	Wide spectrum of nutrient deficiency findings
Neoplasia	CT of intestine	Digital imaging from multiple levels	Can provide precise information about lesions

The antigens from the gut seem to provoke the immune system in Crohn's patients in ways that are far more drastic than normal. Innate immune cells in the gut epithelium and in the underlying lamina propria have specialized receptors to recognize antigenic patterns. These include Toll-like receptor and nucleotide-binding domain receptors (TLR and NOD). In the very dense gut-associated mucosal system, the dendritic cells can bind many different antigenic patterns. They do this not only by processing patterns that diffuse into the mucosa—dendritic cells have transepithelial dendrites that allow them to sample antigens in the gut lumen. Hypersensitivity to lipopolysaccharides emanating from gram-negative bacteria may have something to do with dendritic cell function.

In Crohn's disease, as in many immune-driven maladies, there is a disordered balance between cells that upregulate inflammation and those that induce immune tolerance. Effector T cells such as T helper [Th]1 or Th17 cells are there to protect against bacteria, fungi, and viruses, via releasing interferon-γ, TNF-α, and interleukins. Regulatory T cells secrete interleukin-10, transforming growth factor β, and can originate from the thymus or can be induced in the mucosa (i.e., Tr1) [175].

As the inflammation continues, it allows more antigens to cross into lymphatic areas where dendritic cells apprehend them. The damage to mucosal integrity will permit more antigenic challenges. The granulomas grow in size and number. It is well-known to gastroenterologists that total bowel rest will help the medicines they prescribe to work better and is used as a strategy to interrupt an intense flare-up.

During these more disease-active times, the inflammatory process can spiral out of control. Granulomas can start to progress in a transmural manner, burrowing into the mucosal layer and into the submucosa, then muscular layer. A fistula occurs when the lesions penetrate through the gut wall, breaking out of the serosal lining of the bowel (this can happen at any point and often in the proximal colon, not only the ileum or rest of the small bowel). This will release contents into the peritoneum if in the small or large intestine. Sometimes, two fistula lesions will meet between two loops of bowel [174].

Fibrosis and Extracellular Matrix Degeneration

In the stomach, with repeated ulcerations, a healing through fibrosis can occur. Due to necrosis, the stomach must heal the area like any wound healed by secondary intention. Fibrous tissue and a blood supply move in and create a nonspecialized collagen matrix. Over time, this becomes denser in collagen (as one would expect in the harsh environment of the stomach). This will eventually lose much of its circulation and even fibroblastic cells becoming a superdense scar. This will not have the glandular functions of the normal gastric epithelium, neither producing protective mucus nor releasing pepsinogen [176]. These scars can occur in the duodenum as well. Chronic esophageal reflux can also produce a recurring injury and reversion to a fibrotic state. The reflux of acid may also be aspirated and damage the lungs.

With the ongoing damage from inflammatory bowel disease, such as Crohn's, there is fibrous tissue healing in the ileum or other affected parts (Table 8.12). This of course will remove that area as a viable place for digestion and absorption. Strictures can occur, where the passage is narrowed, and this can lead to bowel obstruction.

Breakdown of Function

In the stomach, in addition to distorted architecture from healed ulcers, the viscus itself can age and become less able to generate secretions. This condition of atrophic gastritis is very common in the elderly and leads to less tolerance of larger meals and high-protein meals [177].

In the small bowel, ongoing inflammation can reduce the absorptive surface area and overall digestive capacity of the small bowel. If ileal disease is advanced and fibrosis can occur, then B12 deficiency is possible. The absorption of vitamin B12 is in the ileum, facilitated by binding to intrinsic factor that was made in the stomach. If the jejunum or duodenum are also involved, multiple nutrients will be difficult to absorb. Duodenal disease will greatly impact the absorption of fats and the fat-soluble vitamins (A, D, E, K) and iron. Malabsorption is a hallmark of Crohn's disease, and low serum albumin, anemia, and poor immune function (in spite of the overactive nature of the lesions) are found in the inflammatory stages and certainly in the permanently damaged phases of this disease [178, 179].

Malabsorption is also found in celiac disease. This enteropathy is driven by the immune system, in response to the presence of gluten and gliadin, two proteins found in wheat, rye, and other grains. Gluten is found as an additive in many foods (often used to enhance protein count on the nutrition facts label) and contamination

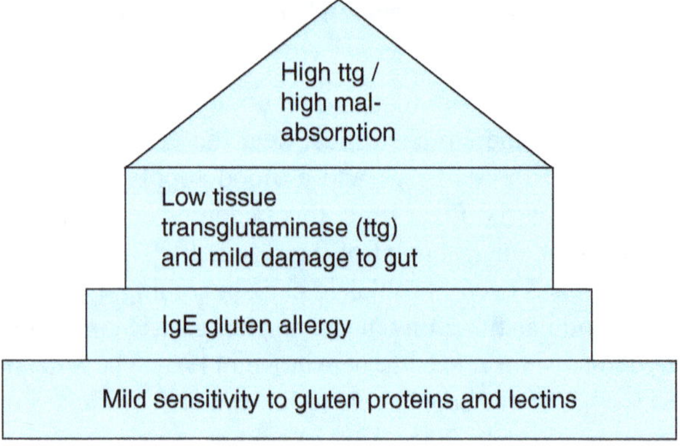

Fig. 8.8 Celiac allergy and sensitivity: adverse reactions to gluten and other grain components can be mild and persistent or extremely severe and acute

during food processing. Patients with celiac are at risk for other autoimmune conditions, and there is a strong genetic component. The patient will form antibodies against gluten and gliadin, and this will trigger, upon exposure, much more profound inflammation. The villi of the small intestine flatten out, and a widespread atrophy occurs. This obviously causes a major malabsorption syndrome. It was once thought that celiac was a juvenile condition (which it often is), and physicians recognized pure types in acute distress (loose stools, failure to thrive, vomiting). It is now known that many gradations of gluten intolerance, allergy, and milder forms of celiac are present (Fig. 8.8). The classic presentation is the "tip of the iceberg." In spite of the abundance of gluten-free products and cookbooks and perhaps an overattribution of many GI symptoms to "gluten intolerance," the problems caused by celiac are very real, and early diagnosis and strict gluten avoidance are key to avoiding extreme villous atrophy, bone density issues, and immune deficiency brought on by malnutrition [180].

Neoplasia

Helicobacter pylori is a class I carcinogen responsible for the initiation of mutations that lead to the majority of gastric cancers. Eradication of *H. pylori* early on can prevent this; late eradication is less preventive. The gastritis of *H. pylori* progresses into atrophic gastritis, intestinal metaplasia, dysplasia, and eventually to adenocarcinoma. Patients with atrophic gastritis have a greatly increased risk of gastric cancer, with an observed correlation of prevalence with severity of the atrophic gastritis [181]. This silent march to carcinoma in the stomach starting with *H. pylori* is known as Correa's cascade.

In the esophagus, if there is acid reflux, recurring damage will cause transition to a more dedifferentiated squamous epithelium known as Barrett's esophagus. This is a precancerous condition.

Crohn's disease itself doesn't cause cancer, but if a cell is mutated, the constant turnover of cells due to inflammation, damage, and repair on the gastrointestinal tract will cause all cells to be more active in dividing. High inflammation causes a proliferative effect [182]. Patients with Crohn's disease who lack nutrients may have a more difficult clinical course of treatment. It's unclear to what extent the damaged and fibrotic extracellular matrix in Crohn's disease permits cancer cells to spread. Some immune-suppressing drug regimens for Crohn's such as azathioprine (AZA)/6-mercaptopurine (6-MP) not only make the person more susceptible to infections with fungi and mycobacteria; they can also allow some types of cancer, such as lymphomas, to gain a better foothold in the body [183].

Supporting Adaptive Resources

Addressing the Determinants of Health

The upper gastrointestinal tract, plus the remainder of the small intestine, reflects the health of the individual including the emotional and mental state. Any undue stress can impact digestion, create dyspepsia, and increase the risk for peptic ulcer.

The stomach and small intestine are very attuned to the 24-h cycle of circadian rhythms. Special cells that initiate the migrating motor complex are found in the intestine between the longitudinal and circular muscle layers. These less intense motility mechanisms help clear the intestine of debris.

The larger spikes in motor activity that cause peristalsis in the gut are activated by several hormones: gastrin, ghrelin, cholecystokinin, and serotonin. There are also nervous inputs into the "gut clock" which is self-regulating but can recalibrate to the entire organism based on surges of melatonin and signal from the vagus nerve. Chronodisruption due to shift work, excessive light during the night, and insomnia can dysregulate motor activity and even hormonal balance of the gut [184]. Peptic ulcers, esophageal reflux disease, and inflammatory bowel disease are more likely in patients with disturbed circadian rhythms [185]. Melatonin increases blood vessel development to the gastric mucosa, increases gastric protective coating, and increases nitric oxide release. The lack of melatonin due to shift work, for example, can decrease the mucosal protections of the stomach. Trefoil protein (TFF2) is another protective factor for the mucosa of the gastrointestinal tract, and this tends to decrease in the elderly, in tandem with reductions in deeper sleep and shortened sleep cycles.

Inflammatory bowel disease incidence is lower in areas closer to the equator and higher in more temperate latitudes. Vitamin D status and sunshine exposure are lower in populations with higher incidence of Crohn's disease and other inflammatory bowel diseases [186]. The direct correlations have not been established—these conditions are multivariate. But it does suggest that in terms of earth and geological determinants of health, outdoor recreation, healthy and safe sun exposure, and adequate vitamin D are most important.

Stress is a general term for the chronic response to life events, circumstances, and beliefs that can activate the hypothalamic-pituitary axis. The general adaptation syndrome is the term created by Dr. Hans Selye, Nobel laureate in physiology and medicine for his work on the stress response. The gut and the brain have many hard connections via the nervous system as well as the endocrine system [187]. When stress levels are high and cortisol secretion is high and sustained, there are a number of adverse effects on the stomach, small intestine, and other gastrointestinal sites. Gastrointestinal motility can become erratic. The secretions from the stomach and pancreas decline and impact digestion. The intestine itself can lose the integrity of its intercellular tight junctions, which allow more transit of toxins and bacteria into the submucosal and the antigen processing systems there. Decrease blood flow to the gut can also reduce the healing abilities of that tissue. Strikingly, the microbial demographics of the gut can change under stress.

Hormetic Actions

Low-dose eugenol may have gastric healing effects that disappear with higher doses. Eugenol is from the clove plant (*Syzygium caryophyllatum*). It has local anesthetic effects and is antimicrobial. The impact on *H. pylori* could be an explanation for eugenol's effect. It also seems to increase the regeneration of the mucosa and reduce inflammation including expression of nuclear factor kappa beta [188]. Although microbial inhibition usually increases with higher concentrations of the antimicrobial, which would be a reason to use higher doses of clove extracts, the eliciting of hormetic responses is at a low dose. It is likely that eugenol acts in the low-dose zone in a different manner than higher doses, which is consistent with the U or J shaped dose response curve seen in hormetins (agents that act in a hormetic manner).

Capsaicin from *Capsicum frutescens*, or hot chili peppers, has beneficial effects on peptic ulcer. Patients were once told to avoid this spice and this plant as chili peppers can increase stomach acid and are irritants. But in fact capsaicin does not stimulate but inhibits acid secretion and stimulates alkali and the secretion of mucus. It is in part acting hormetically [188]. Capsaicin binds to the transient receptor potential vanilloid (TRPV), which leads to improved barrier function of the cells that line the stomach [189]. It reduces NSAID damage, lowers the inflammatory cytokine IL-8, and inhibits *H. pylori* [190, 191].

Biochemical Support

Healing of injured epithelium and moderating immune responses require biochemical support.

Glutamine

The amino acid glutamine is an energy source for upper gastrointestinal epithelium. It has been shown to increase healing rates [192]. It supports thc growth, healing, and metabolism of the gut lining after surgery or other traumas (Table 8.13). It can help restore the villi and therefore digestive function from damage to gut epithelium. It can be important to help patients with inflammation, ulcerations, granulomas, etc. and rebuild the intestinal lining. Too much glutamine all in one dose can cause nausea, probably due to a hypertonic effect. A dose of 1 to 2 g at a time up to 6 g a day is the best way to use this amino acid.

Table 8.13 Treatment considerations for upper gastrointestinal disorders

Level of therapy	Treatment	Comments
Address determinants of health	Stress mitigation	Remove pro-inflammatory and mucosa weakening influences Changes to behavior and circumstances will naturally vary between individuals
Address determinants of health	Sleep improvement	Restore circadian regularity
Biochemical support	Bioflavonoids	Strengthen mucosa and modulate inflammation Example: 500 mg rutin per day
Biochemical support	Glutamine	Promote healing of upper GI—important energy source 1 g of glutamine 3× day
Biochemical support	Probiotics	Modulate inflammation, suppress pathogenic species, induce gut protective secretions Example: Ten billion CFU of *Lactobacillus* spp., *Bifidus* spp. *Saccharomyces boulardii* three billion CFU *Bacillus coagulans* and *Bacillus subtilis* 4 CFU
Biochemical support	Cabbage	Provide glutamine and methionine for stomach ulcer healing (might exacerbate some small intestine disorders) 1 serving a day Cabbage juice 1/2 cup per day
Biochemical support	*Tripterygium wilfordii*	Decrease expression of pro-inflammatory genes; reduce apoptosis of intestinal epithelial cells 300 mg 20:1 extract
Biochemical support	Demulcents	Provide protective mucilage *Ulmus fulva* 2 g per day powered

(continued)

Table 8.13 (continued)

Level of therapy	Treatment	Comments
Biochemical support	Astringents	Mild hemostatic effects 3 mL of *Geranium maculatum* 2×/day
Biochemical support	*Glycyrrhiza*	Support epithelial repair, decrease inflammation, protect epithelium DGL powder 1/8 teaspoon 3 times day (equivalent to 300 mg tid)
Biochemical support	Pycnogenol	Antioxidant effects, assist with epithelial repair 1 g per day
Biochemical support	*Nigella sativa*	Suppress oncogene activation due to *H. pylori* infection 1 g per day or 5 mL of tincture 2×/day
Biochemical support	I.V. vitamin C	Anti-inflammatory/antioxidant support/collagen repair 5 g in I.V. drip 1 g in I.V. push
Hormetic stimulation	Use of *Capsicum frutescens*	Capsaicin in small amounts can bind to select receptors and promote healing
Whole person therapy	Dietary treatment-specific carbohydrate or FODMAP diet	Avoid foods that trigger rapid increase in inflammation Reduce bacterial overgrowth Nutritional plan with sample menu and foods to avoid list
Dampen symptoms	Medical beverages—hypoallergenic multinutrient antioxidant—anti-inflammatory	Provides basic sustenance during elimination of suspected dietary triggers/can provide antioxidants, glutamine, anti-inflammatory substances Follow directions—typically 4 to 8 scoops per day of standard medical beverages. Food introduction per physician direction
Dampen symptoms	H2 blockers/ATPase inhibitors	Reduce HCl in stomach
Induce homeostasis with external means	Total bowel rest—parenteral nutrition	Provide basic sustenance during total bowel rest As prescribed by hospital or infusion center based on patient's age, sex, and body mass
Induce homeostasis with external means	Antibiotic therapy	Eradicate *H. pylori* Treat infections associated with IBD
Induce homeostasis with external means	Anti-inflammatory therapy	Arrest destruction of the intestine by IBD

Cabbage and Vitamin U

In the 1950s, before the arrival of H2 blocking drugs, one of the experimental treatments for stomach ulcer was cabbage juice (*Brassica oleracea* var. *capitata*). The researchers of the time postulated a "vitamin U" that had the healing properties [193]. This "U" are various metabolites of methionine that are high in cabbage and other *Brassica* species, such as kale, broccoli, collards, brussels sprouts, etc. Cabbage is also very high in glutamine, which is important in restoring energy and supporting healing to the upper gastrointestinal epithelium.

Ganoderma lucidum

Ganoderma lucidum, or reishi mushroom, has multiple uses including general immune support and regulation of metabolism and insulin levels [194]. It may help with Crohn's disease. The cytokine tumor necrosis factor-alpha is implicated in disease activity in Crohn's. *Ganoderma lucidum*, although it raises levels of other cytokines, suppresses TNF-alpha. This doesn't eliminate the need for medical intervention, especially during flare-ups of Crohn's. But it can help encourage a less active immune state relative to the gut.

Curcumin

Curcuma longa, the turmeric spice plant, yields a group of compounds known as curcuminoids. Curcumin is the most plentiful. It has well-known effects on blocking inflammation and has affinity for multiple molecular targets. In inflammatory bowel disease, it has been shown to reduce oxidative stress in the bowel, decrease neutrophil chemotaxis, and support epithelial healing [195]. This effect in IBD suggests that curcumin might be anti-inflammatory to duodenal and gastric mucosa. Curcumin may demonstrate many actions in vitro, but its ability to migrate to targets in the body and bind in a forceful enough manner is in question. The use of standardized extracts, phytosome standardized extracts, or nanocapsule-delivered curcuminoids is perhaps the way to overcome the absorption and delivery shortcomings of this amazing substance. In spite of its promise, curcumin should not be overrelied on at the expense of other synergistic treatments.

Other Antioxidants

Melatonin

Melatonin, produced by the pineal gland and retina to some extent, has been shown to reverse colitis in a murine model [196], as does n-acetylcysteine. In a human study with colitis, it improved the disease activity index [197]. Melatonin has some general anti-inflammatory effects including for the gastrointestinal tract [198]. It can be useful in helping reset the circadian clock for those with sleep interruption.

Pycnogenol

Pycnogenol, from *Pinus maritima*, is a proanthocyanidin oligomer, with free radical scavenging abilities. It has been shown to reduce oxidative stress markers in children with Crohn's disease in a small clinical trial. In another human trial, pycnogenol administration reduced thromboxane levels in children with Crohn's disease, which can reduce inflammation and thrombosis [199].

Tripterygium

Tripterygium wilfordii Hook is an herb with a use in traditional Chinese medicine [200]. It has multiple anti-inflammatory targets. Compounds, such as (+)-medioresinol-di-O-beta-D-glucopyranoside, kaempferol, beta-sitosterol, triptolide, nobiletin, zhebeiresinol, (3,4-dihydro-4-hydroxy-6-methoxy)-2H-1-benzopyran, and wilforlide A, are able to influence inflammo-regulatory genes. Moreover, mitogen-activated protein kinase (MAPK) can be affected by kaempferol, nobiletin, and triptolide which might be beneficial. Overactivation of protein kinases is found in the inflamed mucosa of Crohn's patients. Apoptosis, via the caspase-3 pathway in the intestinal epithelium, can impair the integrity of that mucosal surface, allow antigens to push in, and trigger more immune response in an already inflamed environment. Caspase-3 can be affected by kaempferol, beta-sitosterol, and triptolide.

Digestive Enzymes

When a patient has malabsorption due to destruction of the enzymes of the small bowel due to Crohn's disease or celiac or has pancreatic exocrine deficiency, then they may need supplementation. This replacement therapy might be a temporary measure to get them renourished or might have to persist for a long time. Enzymes from animal source, bovine or porcine, are literally taken from the pancreas of these animals. These might be combined with HCl to provide extra protein degradation but can easily be found without HCl. In terms of any actual amount for a patient, Creon (pancrelipase) [201], one of six FDA-approved pancreatin products, contains 3000/9500/15,000 units of lipase, protease, and amylase, respectively, at the lower dose. The highest dose of Creon has 36,000/114,000/180,000 units of lipase/protease/amylase. Pancreatic enzymes are commonly available as a dietary supplement in addition to prescription formulations. In that case, it is advisable to use only products from trusted and upper tier, in terms of quality processes and transparency, manufacturers. The products can be used for digestive assistance and even show efficacy for those with serious pancreatic disease in terms of digestive support [202].

For patients who do not want porcine- or bovine-derived products or simply don't feel well taking them (which could be allergy), there are fungal-derived enzymes from *Aspergillus oryzae* [203]. These are manufactured to leave out the yeast source and be enzymes only, but it's conceivable that some patients with allergies to fungi and yeast might have to be careful with some preparations. These enzymes are prepared with various balances, some being lipase focused, for patients with biliary issues or general fat malabsorption, and others being higher in proteases.

Demulcent Herbs

Demulcent herbs are those that contain mucilaginous substances. Mucilage is composed of polar polysaccharides which contain hexose and pentose sugars and uronic acids. It Plants aggregate these in their roots. *Althea officinalis* and *Ulmus fulva* (marshmallow plant and slippery elm, respectively) are good sources of these. Mucilage is sticky and adheres to mucosal surfaces. This can provide a protective coating in gastritis, peptic ulcer, and inflamed small intestine of inflammatory bowel disease. Under these conditions, the cell membranes of the epithelial cells appear to gather more phosphatidylcholine, and neutrophil migration and inflammation decrease. Demulcents are not a complete solution for these inflammatory conditions, but they do provide some protection from damage and can aid in the healing process. They are also useful in irritable bowel syndrome [204].

Astringent Herbs

Tannins come in two forms, condensed and hydrolyzable. Gallic acid and ellagic acid are building blocks along with glucose or another sugar. Hydrolyzable tannins include gallotannins and ellagitannins. Gallotannins are typically found in berries and grapes (and therefore red wine). These create an astringent taste experience.

Astringents can temporarily cross-link collagen, due to their many hydroxyl residues. This has a tissue-binding effect. Topically, astringents are used as "styptics"; they stop pinprick bleeding or mild abrasions that occur when shaving or due to some kind of chafing. Internally, astringents, if they come into contact with a mucus membrane, will have a small antihemorrhagic effect by pulling together the surface proteins. This can be helpful when there are small amounts of bleeding to the stomach. This won't solve the underlying problem that is causing the gastritis or early ulceration, but it can, along with demulcents, provide some support for healing. Tannins can draw together tissues, suppress *H. pylori* and provide antioxidant support [205]. This gives herbs such as *Geranium maculatum* (a source of tannins) a useful role in treating gastric ulcer.

Vitamin C

Vitamin C levels in the diet are inversely associated with peptic ulcer. It is now known that *H. pylori*-induced gastritis inhibits active intragastric secretion of ascorbic acid in the stomach. The *H. pylori* infection reduces the total vitamin C concentration in the gastric mucosa by converting the majority of the vitamin to dehydroascorbic acid. This form of ascorbic acid is further oxidized to irreversible metabolites such as 2,3-diketo-L-gulonic acid. Patients with lower gastric pH tend to have higher ascorbic acid levels, and those with higher pH—achlorhydria—have lower ascorbic acid levels. Vitamin C decreases bleeding and speeds healing (Table 8.13). Adequate body stores of ascorbic acid reduce the risk of gastric cancer [206, 207].

Glycyrrhiza glabra

Licorice herb, or *Glycyrrhiza glabra*, has been used for gastritis and peptic ulcer (Table 8.13). It is a demulcent and has those basic protective properties. It also has some degree of healing support for the gastric mucosa. Deglycyrrhizinated licorice is a dietary supplement that avoids the potential aldosterone-raising effect of prolonged, higher-dose use of licorice. *Glycyrrhiza glabra* has been found to enhance eradication of *H. pylori* when used as a synergist with conventional treatment [208]. Through the induction of RNA-binding protein human antigen, licorice also seems to restore intestinal homeostasis after antibiotic treatment [209]. Antibiotics, such as clindamycin, can slow down intestinal cell growth and repair. This is offset with licorice treatment.

Nigella sativa

Black seed is a traditional medicine with many uses. It contains thymoquinone and thymol. These appear to suppress the oncogenic (cancer promoting) proteins from *H. pylori*. Although eradication of *H. pylori* is a good goal, the fact that it can reassert itself and increase stomach cancer risk indicates that black seed would be an important dietary supplement for patients with recurrent and chronic *H. pylori* infection [210].

Rutin

Quercetin is a bioflavonoid that is helpful to the stomach and has anti-allergy properties. The glycoside of quercetin, known as rutin, is found in many foods including citrus. It has been shown to decrease inflammation in animal inflammatory bowel disease models [211].

Whole Person Support

The day-to-day diet for patients with Crohn's disease has an impact on disease activity. The specific carbohydrate diet was used as far back as the 1920s by Dr. Hass and later popularized by Elaine Gottschall, in books (based on extensive experience, beginning with her own daughter) such as *Breaking the Vicious Cycle*. This diet eliminates many complex grains, especially those that are a source of gluten. This protein can provoke inflammation and loosen intracellular tight junctions in the gut epithelium, which can drive up Crohn's disease activity [212].

Not surprisingly, many Crohn's patients improve on the Mediterranean diet, with its high omega-3, polyphenol-rich, and high fruit and vegetable content [213]. It is important to keep in mind that just because a Crohn's patient is not classically celiac doesn't mean that gluten and gliadin will not provoke their inflammatory state [180]. Hybridized wheat as it is now consumed has an abundance of these proteins, and avoidance is going to benefit many Crohn's patients, even if it is not a factor for all patients.

Diets that restrict fermentable oligosaccharides, such as the FODMAP diet, also eliminate many Cruciferae and sweet foods and legumes [213]. This has shown some benefit for Crohn's patients, and interestingly, this same diet is used as part of the treatment for patients with small intestine bacterial overgrowth. In that condition, the bacterial count in the small bowel begins to rise to levels beyond the normal, and species of this flora are altered. Perhaps in the Crohn's patients who benefit from FODMAP, in addition to the basic autoimmune mechanism, the presence of particularly pro-inflammatory bacteria may be a driver of the disease process.

Anxiety and Depression

Anxiety can worsen the progression of peptic ulcer, and psychological stress in general is known to be a powerful etiological factor. Crohn's disease and the disruptions to daily life and the suffering it can cause can exacerbate anxiety and depression.

A 2020 systematic review and meta-analysis sought to look at non-pharmacologic interventions for patients with inflammatory bowel disease, such as cognitive-behavioral therapy, mindfulness-based therapy, Breath-Body-Mind workshop, guided imagery with relaxation, solution-focused therapy, yoga, and multicomponent interventions. The researchers' pooled evidence from all non-pharmacologic interventions showed that these interventions significantly helped to reduce anxiety, depression, and disease-specific quality of life (QOL) in adults with inflammatory disease compared to control groups [214].

Probiotics

Probiotics and a healthy gut microbiota are important for the gastrointestinal tract, including the stomach and small intestine [215]. Combination of *Saccharomyces boulardii* and *Lactobacillus* is helpful for Crohn's. They help with gut healing and immune tolerance [216, 217]. There are a plethora of ways in which probiotics might help with *H. pylori* infection and these same physiological changes. Beneficial bacteria will compete with *H. pylori* for adhesion receptors. They can elaborate short-chain fatty acids such as lactic and butyric acids, which lowers pH and inhibits *H. pylori*. *Lactobacillus plantarum* and *L. rhamnosus* have this ability. Other protective substances are the bacteriocins which are proteins that inhibit *H. pylori*, and this may also inhibit urease, an alkalinizing product of the pathogen. Mucosal surfaces have protective strategies to defend against noxious substances and pathogens found within the intestinal lumen. Mucins are large complex glycoproteins that protect intestinal mucosal surfaces from microbial pathogens by limiting access of environmental matter to their epithelial cells [218]. Several mucins have been identified. *H. pylori* is known to suppress MUCI and MUC5 gene expression in a human gastric cell line [219]. It has been shown that in vitro studies with probiotics such as *L. plantarum* and *L. rhamnosus* increase the expression of MUC2 and MUC3 genes, and therefore extracellular secretion of mucin by colon cell cultures can inhibit the adherence of pathogenic bacteria. This ability of these strains restores the mucosal permeability of gastric mucosa and inhibits the adherence of pathogenic bacteria such as *H. pylori*.

Current research is showing that probiotics are helpful alongside more targeted therapies for gastrointestinal diseases. Fermented foods, which have many benefits for the body, can provide these probiotics.

Acupuncture

Acupuncture is a whole person therapy that is customized to the patient based on an analysis of their current signs and symptoms. Current trials, at the very least, indi cate an improvement in quality of life in patients with inflammatory bowel disease [220].

Dampening Maladaptive Responses

Methotrexate is an anti-inflammatory drug that reduces immune activity. Prednisone is a powerful corticosteroid drug that can reduce inflammation and works quickly. These are both used for Crohn's disease and other autoimmune conditions.

High-dose *Curcuma longa* in a standardized extract delivered in a nanoparticle form might also help to quickly relieve inflammation, as would intravenous vitamin C [221].

In the stomach, sucralfate is a synthetic coating that can be used for acute ulcers. A common palliative measure for ulcers are antacids. These are proton-accepting molecules that can neutralize stomach acid, such as aluminum hydroxide or calcium carbonate. These buffering agents can relieve symptoms but do not put many ulcer patients into a state of healing. This is not suppressing as the causes of this condition—NSAIDs, stress, smoking, and *H. pylori* infection—will continue to weaken the gastric and duodenal mucosa. Excessive uses of antacids can create a type of alkalosis by neutralization of so many protons in the body and, of course, decrease digestive function.

From a naturopathic perspective, very small doses of tincture of *Atropa belladonna* will have an anticholinergic effect. The alkaloids in *Atropa belladonna* such as atropine bind to muscarinic receptors that the vagus nerve synapses with. This can block the vagal input for stomach acid secretion, which does have an impact on total acid levels. This should be thought of as a short-term solution, to permit healing to take place while causes are addressed [222, 223]. These anticholinergic alkaloids were being used for gastric ulcer prior to the appearance of H2 blocking agents [224].

ATPase Blocker or H2 Blocker

Once a gastric ulcer has taken root, the presence of gastric acid and pepsin will frustrate efforts to heal. A granuloma of sorts will set in, and it may widen and deepen. Some duodenal or gastric ulcers can progress to the point of hemorrhage. Some gastric ulcers will cause a perforation, allowing gastric contents to leak out into the peritoneum creating a medical emergency. A breakthrough in treatment was the development of histamine 2 receptor antagonists in the 1960s. When ingesting food, a hormone called gastrin causes the enterochromaffin-like cells to release the chemical histamine. There are histamine receptors (H2) on gastric parietal cells, and then bound, this leads to acid release. H2 blockers act as reversible antagonists to this receptor. Examples include ranitidine and cimetidine [225].

Newer and even more powerful drugs are the ATPase inhibitors (Table 8.13). These drugs act on the parietal cells to inhibit their release of protons into the gastric lumen. They can reduce gastric ulcer by up to 90%. This clearly allows some healing time, but like other measures, recurrence of ulcer is highly likely if causes are not addressed [225].

Imposing Homeostasis by Physiological Control

For *H. pylori* treatment, a current approach to antibiotic therapy, is quadruple therapy that includes an ATPase inhibitor, esomeprazole, metronidazole, and amoxicillin, for 7 days, with another 7-day period where Levofloxacin is given instead of amoxicillin (Table 8.13). Another common protocol is a bismuth-based therapy with bismuth tripotassium dicitrate, tetracycline, esomeprazole, and metronidazole [226]. This can disrupt the gut microbiome and even cause a decrease in serum levels of the appetite-enhancing hormone ghrelin [227]. Some increased use of fermented foods or probiotic supplementation is needed after such a therapy [158].

Very powerful therapies for Crohn's disease block the actions of the immune system at a fundamental level. Tumor necrosis factor (TNF) inhibitors, such as adalimumab, keep disease activity at a lower level. The risks of these drugs include susceptibility to infections where the main line of defense is cellular-mediated immune response (Th1). An example is *Mycobacterium tuberculosis* [228].

Total Bowel Rest: TPN

As a way to break the inflammatory cycle, sometimes patients with Crohn's are put on total bowel rest. They are fitted with an intravenous catheter and receive an intravenous drip of a total parenteral nutrition preparation each day. This has all the required nutrients, including amino acids, lipids, dextrose, and vitamins and minerals [229].

Surgeries are a step beyond this, and sometimes a portion of the small intestine, particularly the ileum, is so damaged that a segment of it is surgically resected. Surgeons may also perform an ileal bypass procedure. This surgery will connect the proximal ileum or jejunum to the large intestine, with the bypassed portion of ileum being stapled off to prevent leakage. This removes the exposure of food antigens to the ileum. These can be reversed at a time when the disease is less active.

Management concepts:

- Address disturbed or inadequately supported determining factors of health.
- Address immediate pathological drivers such as *H. pylori.*

Table 8.14 Crohn's disease activity index

Variable	Description	Scoring	Multiplier
Number of liquid stools	Sum of 7 days		×2
Abdominal pain	Sum of 7 days' rating	0 = none 1 = mild 2 = moderate 3 = severe	×5
General well-being	Sum of 7 days' rating	0 = generally well 1 = slightly under par 2 = poor 3 = very poor 4 = terrible	×7
Extraintestinal complications	Number of complications listed	Arthritis/arthralgia, iritis/uveitis, erythema nodosum, pyoderma gangrenosum, aphthous stomatitis, anal fissure/fistula/abscess, fever >37.8 °C	×20
Antidiarrheal drugs	Use in the previous 7 days	0 = no 1 = yes	×30
Abdominal mass		0 = no 2 = questionable 5 = definite	×10
Hematocrit	Expected observed hematocrit	Men: 47 observed Women: 42 observed	×6
Body weight	Ideal/observed ratio	[1 − (ideal/observed)] × 100	×1 (not < −10)

- Support the function and healing of the mucosa.
- Employ more powerful anti-inflammatory/symptom-dampening strategies if needed.
- Carefully monitor progress and be alert for medical emergencies.
- Use benchmarks such as laboratory tests, imaging, and Crohn's disease activity index (Table 8.14) in addition to clinical signs and symptoms to measure progress.

Lower Gastrointestinal Tract

The lower gastrointestinal tract is the large intestine with the ileocecal value/cecum on the proximal end and the rectum and anal area on the distal. The colon functions to reabsorb water from the contents moving out of the small intestine. That mixture is very hydrated with gastric and pancreatic secretions, plus whatever water enters the lumen of the small intestine via the mucosa.

The large intestine also carries an enormous amount of bacteria, about 10 times the number of the cells in the human host. These further break down unabsorbed food, manufacture some vitamins, and in health, resist many pathogenic species. The large intestine microbiota (an extremely important aspect but not the only piece of the human microbial puzzle) has a complex and important relationship with the immune system, nervous system, and organs [230].

The colon has a mucosa that has mucus-secreting properties, but its main purpose is to absorb water. The portal circulation extends to the large intestine, and this is carried back to the liver. This allows the liver to process any gut-derived toxins. The colon, like the small intestine, has a strong wave of peristaltic activity that occurs with the arrival of food and liquids. This stretches the colonic walls and further stimulates contraction. There are migrating motor complexes that sweep the colon as well [231]. Located within muscle layers are mesenchymal cells known as the cells of Cajal. These connect the muscle complex with the autonomic nervous system and provide a pacemaker function.

Functional disorders such as constipation and so-called irritable bowel syndrome, infections, microbial imbalances, inflammation, and neoplasm are the key issues that arise clinically.

Hypofunction

Constipation is a commonly encountered hypofunction that occurs in the colon. This can be due to multiple causes, ranging from simple dehydration to more complex neurological damage to the cells of Cajal and the autonomic nervous system. Lack of dietary fiber will contribute to constipation. The bulking and water-retaining aspects of fiber lead to stretching on the colon and encourage muscle contraction [242]. The breakdown of dietary fiber by gut bacteria also provides energy to the colon in the form of short-chain fatty acids such as acetate, butyrate, propionate, etc. Constipation is found with difficulty passing stool, decreased frequency of stool (less than 3 bowel movements per week per the Rome criteria [232], which is a very low standard for what should be a daily function), sense of retention, hard or lumpy consistency, and need for laxatives [233].

A colon that does not, literally, have a proper fermentation process occurring and that does not have adequate dietary fiber and an appropriate balance of microbial genera and species will impact the body in multiple ways. Immune and neurological functions will be altered. Nutritional products such as biotin and vitamin K will decrease.

Impaired Motility, Circulation, and Secretion

Irritable bowel syndrome [170] is a common spectrum of functional disturbances that create cramping and alterations in bowel activity. The motility of the colon appears to be erratic. The cause of this dysregulation of coordination between smooth muscle, enteric plexus, cells of Cajal, and autonomic nerves seems to differ between patients.

For some patients, stress and changes of function in the autonomic nervous system lead to the erratic behavior of the bowel. For others, it seems that the microbiome is altered. Both of these facts might be exacerbated by excess fermentation of carbohydrates in the gut, such as oligosaccharides, and refined sucrose, dextrose, etc.

Barrier function between epithelial cells in the colon might be impaired, which can lead to immune activation. This somewhat contradicts the concept of a purely "functional" and not organic problem, as this introduces a degree of inflammation. Hypersensitivity of the intrinsic nervous tissue in the gut may be a factor, and for some patients (perhaps 20%), the gut is irritated by bile acids.

The Rome criteria is used to categorize IBS, and this incorporates the Bristol stool scale [233] (Table 8.15). IBS-D patients are patients with pain and predominantly diarrhea or very mushy stools. IBS-C is predominantly constipated. IBS-M is both at different times, at least 25% of the stools being constipation and at least 25% being diarrhea. IBS-U is undefined which is so erratic that over time there is no consistent pattern.

Diarrhea is an increase in frequency and volume of stools, with a watery or even liquid consistency. It might be accompanied with nausea and abdominal pain [234]. Long-term functional diarrhea can occur due to oversecretion of hormones such as vasoactive intestinal polypeptide. Many diarrhea causes are of an infectious and inflammatory nature. Some are associated with the abovementioned irritable bowel syndrome. Another cause is osmotic diarrhea. This happens when too many particles or molecules are in the large intestine. The osmotic draw on water causes a flooding of the colon and diarrhea. Taking too many foods with sugar alcohol sweeteners such as sorbitol can create this osmotic event, as can taking supplemental magnesium (a beneficial practice for some people) in too high a dose. Malabsorption of sugars, such as lactose, can create osmotic issues. When a patient receives a colonoscopy, they must do a colon preparation the day before to clean out all stool from the colon. This is often PEG—polyethylene glycol—solution, which causes a massive osmotic effect and numerous liquid stools.

Laxatives can induce diarrhea [235]. Some, like "milk of magnesia," are intentionally osmotic. Others, such as cascara sagrada (*Rhamnus purshiana*), work through a chemical mechanism to induce chloride secretion into the lumen, causing

Table 8.15 Bristol stool scale

Types	Description	Category
Type 1	Separate hard lumps, nutlike	Constipation
Type 2	Sausage-shaped but lumpy	Constipation
Type 3	Sausage like with cracks on surface	Normal
Type 4	Like a sausage or snake, smooth on surface	Normal
Type 5	Soft blobs with clear-cut edges	Lack of fiber
Type 6	Fluffy pieces with ragged edges, mushy	Mild diarrhea
Type 7	Watery, no solid pieces, entirely liquid	Diarrhea

a flow of water into the colon with a similar net effect. These plant-based laxatives, the anthraquinone laxatives, also have the effect of stimulating nerve endings in the colon.

The problem with chronic or extreme laxative use is the dehydration and loss of electrolytes. Some people use these chronically as treatment for constipation. Others use them as part of a behavioral disorder. The electrolyte depletion, including potassium, sodium, and chloride, caused by overuse of these medicines can be dangerous, leading to cardiac arrhythmias.

The blood supply to the colon is from the superior mesenteric artery (SMA), inferior mesenteric artery (IMA), and internal iliac arteries. These can undergo infarction due to atherosclerosis. This is a medical emergency, as a portion of the colon can undergo ischemic necrosis, and secondary bacterial infection can cause a massive and fatal infection of the peritoneum.

Inflammation

Transient inflammation in the colon and rectal area can occur because of infection. This can settle into chronic low-grade infection or become a more serious pathologic issue. Individuals who have a lack of immunoglobulin A and who consume too many dietary sugars and fermentable carbohydrates can end up with an overgrowth of the yeast *Candida albicans* [236] in the gut. For people who are not severely immunocompromised (to whom *Candida* spp. can pose a serious threat), this chronic low-grade infection can decrease quality of life (mental and physical fatigue, gastrointestinal symptoms such as IBS, and exacerbation of some allergies).

In a sense, the lower gastrointestinal tract is always in a low-grade state of inflammation. The lymphocytes residing in the gut-associated lymphoid tissue (GALT) [237] and intraepithelial lymphocytes must respond to challenges from trillions of gut microorganisms. Their success in controlling the microbiota (cultivating it and creating some boundaries—notwithstanding the fact that the microbiota influences the human organism in turn) keeps the inflammation from becoming more intense. The presence of regulatory T cells and mechanisms of tolerance keeps the antigen challenge in the gut from becoming too serious an issue when no actual invasion across the epithelium is occurring.

Autoimmune conditions, such as Crohn's disease, with its penetrating granulomas, often affects the colon [238]. The inflammatory bowel disease, ulcerative colitis, will (in addition to extraintestinal manifestations such as uveitis) cause inflammation of the colonic mucosa (Table 8.16). In this autoimmune disease, the surface of the colon becomes inflamed and sloughs off. This leads to bloody diarrhea and very often anemia due to so much daily blood and iron loss. The recurring defects in the colon epithelium can give rise to opportunistic infections, simply due to the many fecal bacteria that are present. When the veins of the hemorrhoidal plexus become dilated, often due to chronic constipation, low fiber in the diet, and straining at stool, these can become permanently prolapse. This leads to internal or

Table 8.16 Levels of dysfunction in lower gastrointestinal disease

Levels of dysfunction	Test	Comments
Hypofunction	Stool classification	Observation
Hypofunction	Stool analysis	Findings can range from identifying a pattern of microorganisms to deeper issues such as evidence of malabsorption
Disordered circulation and communication	Rome criteria for IBS classification	Observation and symptoms
Electrolytes	Part of chem screen panel	May show concentrated sodium levels and depletion of potassium
Inflammation	Histological specimen	Obtained on biopsy
Inflammation	Complete blood count	Anemia, most likely microcytic
Deeper inflammation	Colonoscopy	Shows inflammation and destruction of colonic mucosal lining
Fibrosis	Barium radiograph	Stricture found in colon
Degeneration of Function	CT scan	May show more detailed areas of prolapsed, dilated, scarred colonic tissue
Neoplasia	Colonoscopy with biopsy	Gold standard for lesion identification and staging
Neoplasia	CT scan	Identifies lymph node involvement

even external hemorrhoids that can become inflamed and infected. The same set of conditions can give rise to bulges in the wall of the distal sigmoid colon and rectum, known as diverticulosis. These saclike or fingerlike projections, the diverticula, can trap fecal material and become inflamed. This can progress to bacterial infection—diverticulitis.

Deeper Inflammation

Ulcerative colitis can and often does progress to be a life-changing and dangerous disease. It can present as right- or left-sided or even proctitis. It can start with damage to the barrier created by colonic epithelium [238]. Once there is a crack in the dam so to speak, the microbes in the colon can start to ramp up a very intense inflammatory response. The inflammatory cells, TH9, have been implicated in damaging the frontline epithelial cells and interfering with healing, aided by IL-13. The resident lymphoid cells, which are important to push back sudden infections, can become constantly activated, and they will keep intense inflammation going. Extraintestinal manifestations can be found in both ulcerative colitis and Crohn's disease (Table 8.17).

Clostridium difficile is a very aggressive microbe that can be acquired in hospitals, nursing homes, and other care facilities [239]. It takes advantage of an already disrupted microbiome, since many existing species in the human gastrointestinal

Table 8.17 Extraintestinal manifestations of ulcerative colitis

Tissue/ region	Extraintestinal manifestation
Eyes	Uveitis, episcleritis
Lungs	Bronchiectasis, cryptogenic organizing pneumonia
Skin	Erythema nodosum, pyoderma gangrenosum, psoriasis, Sweet's syndrome
Joints	Peripheral arthritis (type 1—pauciarticular, mirrors active IBD; type 2—polyarticular, independent of IBD activity), ankylosing spondylitis
Mouth	Aphthous stomatitis

tract will suppress it. People who have recently used antibiotics are at risk as well. A milder case will have watery diarrhea, and a more severe case presents with very intense abdominal pains, high volume diarrhea, and fever. *Clostridium difficile* can lead to bowel perforations or to such extensive necrosis of the colon that the bowel becomes dilated and necrotic. If the person recovers, it can leave the bowel without normal nerve function, weak, dilated, and prone to constipation. Patients can also develop renal failure from such severe dehydration.

Fibrosis and Extracellular Matrix Degeneration

Long-term inflammation can lead to strictures in the bowel, due to adhesions from scar tissue. A type of fibrosis that can occur is radiation colitis [240]. This is damage to the large intestine due to radiation therapy for cancer. This can be local lymph nodes that may have colon cancer cells in them that are being irradiated as part of treatment. Or it can be collateral damage from radiation treatment for prostate cancer. Damage to nerves and scarring can be caused by the powerful radiation energy. These types of treatments are more precise than they used to be, but this condition still occurs.

Deterioration of Function

With continued inflammation, loss of nerve input, and even with fibrosis secondary to a necrotizing event, the colon can lose its ability to reabsorb water. In some cases, either due to extreme inflammatory bowel disease, or extensive damage due to infection, or cancer spread, the colon, or part of it, is resected. This might lead to an anastomosis with the rectum or the creation of an ostomy for a colostomy bag to capture feces.

Neoplasia

Colonic (and rectal) adenocarcinoma accounts for about 95% of all colon cancers [241]. It can develop from dysplastic polyps that hang like grapes or more condensed tumors. The right and left colon can develop this, as can the rectum (Table 8.16). Colorectal cancer can also be caused by the human papilloma virus. The screening test, colonoscopy, is considered the most reliable and also allows the surgeon to take a biopsy of any mass and to resect polyps. Some patients develop colon cancer before they are old enough to be sent for routine screening tests. While the death rate of people ages 45 to 54 from colon cancer is less than those above 75 years of age, the death rate in that 45–54 cohort has risen since 1999. A newer form of screening is to use computerized tomography (CT) scans of the colon to look for masses. CT scans of the colon do detect polyps and tumors, but are not quite as accurate as the colonoscopy. CT scans cannot yield an actual tissue biopsy, or allow a surgeon to excise a suspicious mass.

Determinants of Health

The consumption of adequate fiber is extremely important for the colon to function properly. Dietary fiber helps with water retention, decreases transit time, and provides some stretch to the colonic walls which encourages peristalsis (Table 8.18). It supports beneficial microflora [242]. Humans need at least 14 or more grams of dietary fiber a day, and 25 g is probably optimal. Many people get much less. The breakdown of fiber, as mentioned above, yields short-chain fatty acids, which are important energy sources for the lower gastrointestinal epithelium. Fiber can also absorb toxins and trap cholesterol.

Abundant plant foods are helpful to prevent colon cancer. These foods have natural antioxidants and anti-inflammatory compounds. Many vegetables and spices have compounds that help encourage expression of genes that either protect against mutation or help to induce naturally protective apoptosis of cells that are beginning the process of transformation into cancer.

Avoiding burnt foods and overconsumption of broiled and heat-injured foods, as well as decreasing nitrates and nitrites from preserved foods, reduces colon cancer risk [243].

Functional issues such as irritable bowel syndrome are highly influenced by stress levels and sleep. These determinants of health can make a significant difference when the quality of life in functional bowel diseases is considered [244].

As simple as it sounds, adequate hydration is important to prevent constipation. Dietary fiber really requires hydration, and a diet with the fiber that is needed for health will also require lots of water. People who postpone defecation due to work habits or avoidance of pain (e.g., due to hemorrhoids) can also become constipated [245].

Table 8.18 Mayo score/disease activity index (DAI) for ulcerative colitis

Symptom or region	Finding	Points	Net score
Stool frequency	Normal for patient	0	
	1–2 stools > normal	1	
	3–4 stools > normal	2	
	5 or more stools > normal	3	
Rectal bleeding	No blood	0	
	Streaks of blood in stool less than half of the time	1	
	Obvious blood in stool most of the time	2	
	Blood alone passed	3	
Appearance of mucosa on endoscopy	Normal/no disease activity	0	
	Mild (erythema, decreased vascular pattern, mild friability)	1	
	Moderate (marked erythema, absent vascular pattern, friability, erosions)	2	
	Severe (spontaneous bleeding, ulceration)	3	
Physician's rating based on symptoms including abdominal discomfort, quality of life, and physical exam findings	Normal	0	
	Mild disease	1	
	Moderate disease	2	
	Severe disease	3	
		Total >>>>>>>	

A commonly used scoring system that is mentioned in the medical literature

Hormesis

Dietary polyphenols can act both as antioxidants and have a hormetic effect that induces protective enzymes produced by the cell's protein machinery. In the colon, polyphenols work to absorb oxidative stress and thereby reduce lipid peroxidation, generation, and absorption of AGEs/ALEs (advanced glycation end products/ advanced lipid oxidation end products). In the bloodstream, they seem to induce powerful antioxidant enzymes via the antioxidant response element [246].

Green tea, a polyphenol-containing plant, contains (–)-epigallocatechin-3-gallate (EGCG). This acts hormetically to increase cell resistance against chemical or oxidative stress, with the benefit being greater at lower concentrations. EGCG has been shown to have a genetic-stabilizing effect on normal colonic cells in the experimental model but have the opposite effect on adenocarcinoma cells [247].

Biochemical Support

Carminatives

The term carminative refers to a broad range of plants that can relax the smooth muscle of the bowel (Table 8.19). In a symptomatic sense, they can relieve a feeling of retained gas. If that's a sense of tightness in the stomach, then carminatives will ease that. If there is cramping and bloating in the colon, these herbs and the compounds they contain will help. They have an ability to gently relax the smooth muscle of the gut, not to the degree that they slow peristalsis down but the resting tone decreases. This is due to the terpenes in the herbs, which act as weak calcium channel blockers in the gut smooth muscle.

Relaxing the colon alone is not always the answer to cramping. Digestion of food, and the choices of food itself of course, will impact the gut. If protein digestion is poor due to low stomach acid, low pancreatic exocrine function, or small bowel issues, then excess protein is in the gut and will be putrefied by enteric bacteria. Unabsorbed fats, due to pancreatic or biliary problems, will cause loose stools that are foul smelling due to rancidification. Excess carbohydrates, in the form of sugars, will cause fermentation in the colon. Symptomatic relief of these symptoms might help, but an approach to the gut that does not address digestion is only palliative.

Table 8.19 Treatment considerations for lower gastrointestinal disorders

Mode of treatment	Therapy	Comments
Address determinants of health	Stress reduction, social determinants of health	Some cases of IBS are affected by stress
Address determinants of health	Increase dietary fiber, plant foods, and hydration	All needed for colonic function
Hormesis	Polyphenols, green tea	Amounts of green tea can be on the lower end versus higher amounts
Biochemical support	*Scutellaria baicalensis* or Chinese skullcap	Decreases inflammation
Biochemical support	Astringents	Bind together inflamed tissues, reduce secretions
Biochemical support	Demulcents	Coat and soothe inflamed tissue
Biochemical support	High amounts of probiotic supplementation	Particularly important after a course of antibiotics
Biochemical support	*Saccharomyces boulardii*	Competes against *Clostridium difficile*; helps repair intestinal epithelium
Biochemical support	*Piper nigrum*	Decreases inflammation in colonic mucosa

(continued)

Table 8.19 (continued)

Mode of treatment	Therapy	Comments
Biochemical support	Fiber supplementation	Needs to be accompanied by plentiful water intake
Biochemical support	*Foeniculum vulgare*	Reduces spasms in gut
Whole person support	Fermented foods, i.e., natural live yogurt, kefir, tempeh, sauerkraut, etc.	Provides a blend of probiotics and their own nutritional substrate
Dampening symptoms	Colon hydrotherapy	Can be effective in removing impacted feces, some benefits for constipation
Dampening symptoms	Laxatives	Provide short-term relief from constipation, use as part of plan to restore normal function, avoid long-term use if possible
Dampening symptoms	Enteric-coated peppermint oil	Target bowel relaxation medicine
Dampening symptoms	Bentonite clay	Absorbs fluids and toxins
Maintain homeostatic balance	Anti-inflammatory medicines for colon	5-ASA
Maintain homeostatic balance	Immune modulation medicines	Tumor necrosis factor antagonists

Foeniculum vulgare

Fennel is a flavorful carrot family (Apiaceae) flowering plant that is widely consumed as food, such as roasted fennel. It is very useful for cramping of the bowel, in addition to treating dyspepsia. Fennel contains anethol, a phenylpropanoyl derivative, and various terpenes such as pinene and limonene [248]. Fennel decreases spasm in the gut and has some digestive supporting actions because of its flavor. Fennel has antioxidant effects that are active in the gut, and in experimental modes, it inhibits necrotizing colitis.

Scutellaria

Scutellaria baicalensis, or Chinese skullcap, is found in the traditional Chinese medicine system. It is used for intestinal inflammations and infections. Constituent flavones such as baicalin and baicalein are among the compounds found in this plant, and they have antibacterial and hepatic protective effects.

Piper nigrum

Piper nigrum, or black pepper, is a very popular condiment. It is consumed worldwide (as are other *Piper* species). It is rich in terpenes, in particular beta caryophyllene. The pepper in shakers that has sat out exposed to the air for weeks or months loses its potency through oxidation [249]. Peppercorns that are kept in a sealed container and then ground in a pepper mill are going to be the most potent. Beta-caryophyllene has strong anti-inflammatory properties and, in an experimental colitis model, has reduced disease. Beta-caryophyllene reduces tumor necrosis factor-alpha (TNF-α), interleukin-1β (IL-1β), interleukin-6 (IL-6), and nuclear factor kappa-light-chain-enhancer of activated B cells (NF-κB). This is helpful in other inflammatory conditions in addition to colitis. There is also some binding to cannabinoid receptors (CB2).

Saccharomyces boulardii

Saccharomyces boulardii is a spore forming yeast that is used therapeutically [217]. It gained popularity in the 1990s as clinical experience and research supported its use for *Clostridium difficile* intestinal infection. It can be useful in other intestinal issues where inflammation has degraded the epithelium, such as inflammatory bowel disease. *S. boulardii* has some remarkable functions, the mechanisms for which are still being determined. It seems to act as a decoy binding site for certain pathogenic bacteria, leading them away from the true gut epithelial cells. It creates some antibacterial compounds, but how specific that is for pathogens is unclear. It also has a trophic or healing effect on the intestinal epithelium. This is of importance, as in inflammatory and allergy diseases, the tight junctions between colonic epithelial cells lose integrity. That permits excess antigens to flow into the antigen processing mechanisms and immune cells that lie below the mucosal layer. That immune activation can perpetuate and accelerate inflammation.

Fiber Supplementation

In both functional-motility issues of the large intestine and inflammatory ones, such as ulcerative colitis and postinfectious damage to the colon, supplementing fiber is warranted. A popular type of product to accomplish this that many patients know is psyllium supplements. This is a good water-soluble fiber. This has a bulking action and a healing action by leading short-chain fatty acids (SCFA) by enteric bacteria [242]. The SCFAs are important energy sources for the colonic epithelium. More specialized fiber supplements are a way to add to dietary (food) sources [250]. Some of these byproducts, such as butyrate, appear to have direct anti-inflammatory actions on the gut. "Prebiotics," oligosaccharides, and dietary fibers that act as a substrate for enteric bacteria seem to be helpful in irritable bowel syndrome. Some fiber supplements combine insoluble and soluble carbohydrate dietary fiber, including shorter molecules such as pectins. Lignans, which are not actual carbohydrates, are found in flax seeds, and these have similar benefits to dietary fiber from carbohydrate molecules. Dietary fiber supports the gut microbiome, which has an influence on the nervous system [251]. This is relevant to lower gastrointestinal conditions such as irritable bowel syndrome and constipation.

Demulcent Herbs

These herbs have mucilaginous characteristics, containing glycoproteins that form an adherent, soothing, and healing layer on the colonic mucosa. These are going to be of particular benefit where there is irritation or inflammation. For example, several scoops a day of *Ulmus fulva* (slippery elm) will help coat and sooth a colon that is irritated from inflammation, including many of the causes of diarrhea [204].

Astringent Herbs

Astringents, such as *Geranium maculatum* (cranesbill) or *Ceanothus americanus* (New Jersey Tea), have gallic acid derivatives that can pull proteins together. They do this by cross-linking the proteins with many hydroxyl groups. It can be useful in secretory diarrhea, where too much fluid is being lost, but it doesn't mean that rehydration and electrolyte replenishment aren't needed.

Astringents can be helpful when there are dilated hemorrhoids. These veins in the anal area can become dilated, inflamed, and painful. Witch hazel (*Hamamelis virginiana)* is available in medicated pads that can be used to dab the area [252]. Or witch hazel water, an extract that is easily available, can be added to a shallow bath where the patient can soak and relieve pain.

Whole Person Support

Fermented foods [158] are an important part of any diet (Table 8.19). Traditional cuisines mostly have some form of them. They provide probiotics in a food matrix that allows them to thrive. They are whole person support in the sense that these foods condition the immune system, produce nutrients, sometimes produce neurotransmitters, protect against microbial aggression, improve the integration of the epithelium of the gut, and even help with normal motility and neurological function of the gut.

A traditional fermented food such as sauerkraut contains the following organisms: *Enterobacter cloacae*, *Bifidobacterium dentium*, *Enterococcus faecalis*, *Lactobacillus casei*, *Lactobacillus delbrueckii*, *Staphylococcus epidermidis*, *Lactobacillus curvatus*, *Lactobacillus brevis*, *Weissella confusa*, *Lactococcus lactis*, *Enterobacteriaceae*, *Leuconostoc* spp., *Yarrowia brassicae.*

Tempeh, a fermented soy food from Indonesia, contains the following: *Enterococcus faecium*, *Rhizopus oryzae*, *Rhizopus oligosporus*, *Mucor indicus*, *Mucor circinelloides*, *Geotrichum candidum*, *Aureobasidium pullulans*, Alternaria alternata, *Cladosporium oxysporum*, *Trichosporon beigelii*, *Clavispora lusitaniae*, *Candida maltosa*, *Candida intermedia*, *Yarrowia lipolytica*, *Lodderomyces elongisporus*, *Rhodotorula mucilaginosa*, *Candida sake*, *Hansenula fabianii*, *Candida tropicalis*, *Candida parapsilosis*, *Pichia membranifaciens*, *Rhodotorula rubra*, *Candida rugosa*, *Candida curvata*, *Hansenula anomala.*

Miso, a fermented soy paste from Japan, contains the following: *Enterococcus faecium*, *Rhizopus oryzae*, *Rhizopus oligosporus*, *Mucor indicus*, *Mucor circinelloides*, *Geotrichum candidum*, *Aureobasidium pullulans*, *Alternaria alternata*, *Cladosporium oxysporum*, *Trichosporon beigelii*, *Clavispora lusitaniae*, *Candida maltosa*, *Candida intermedia*, *Yarrowia lipolytica*, *Lodderomyces elongisporus*, *Rhodotorula mucilaginosa*, *Candida sake*, *Hansenula fabianii*, *Candida tropicalis*, *Candida parapsilosis*, *Pichia membranifaciens*, *Rhodotorula rubra*, *Candida rugosa*, *Candida curvata*, *Hansenula anomala.*

Kimchi, a fermented vegetable food from Korea, has the following: *Leuconostoc gasicomitatum*, *Leuconostoc gelidum*, *Leuconostoc mesenteroides*, *Weissella koreensis*, *Weissella confusa*, *Lactobacillus sakei*, *Lactobacillus plantarum*, *Lactobacillus curvatus*, *Trichosporon domesticum*, *Trichosporon loubieri*, *Saccharomyces unisporus*, *Pichia kluyveri.*

Kefir is a fermented milk from the Caucasus region and has the following: *Lactobacillus kefiri*, *Lactobacillus paracasei*, *Lactobacillus parabuchneri*, *Lactobacillus casei*, *Lactobacillus lactis*, *Lactococcus lactis*, *Acetobacter lovaniensis*, *Kluyveromyces lactis*, *Saccharomyces cerevisiae.*

Kombucha, a fermented tea from China, contains the following: *Komagataeibacter xylinus*, *Saccharomyces cerevisiae*, *Zygosaccharomyces bailii. Brettanomyces bruxellensis*, *Acetobacter pasteurianus*, *Acetobacter aceti*, *Saccharomyces cerevisiae*, *Zygosaccharomyces bailii*, *Brettanomyces bruxellensis*, *Acetobacter xylinum*, *Zygosaccharomyces* spp., *Acetobacter*, *Gluconacetobacter.*

This multitude of microbes has unique properties in each food. For instance, kefir has been found to inhibit *Candida albicans*, *Salmonella typhi*, *Shigella sonnei*, *Staphylococcus aureus*, and *Escherichia coli*. The foods have their own unique, nonmicrobial uses as well. The sulfur-containing compounds from sauerkraut improve detoxification systems in the liver. Soy contains phytoestrogens, such as daidzein and genistein.

Dampening Symptoms

Enteric-Coated Peppermint Oil

Mentha piperita, or peppermint, contains numerous terpenes, with a large proportion of that fraction being the monoterpene menthol. Like other carminatives, peppermint helps relax the smooth muscle of the gut (Table 8.19). It also has antibacterial effects. The idea of enteric coating peppermint oil is twofold. On the one hand, it releases its contents further down in the gastrointestinal tract where it can directly affect the gut mucosa, nervous system, and muscle. The coating also prevents immediate release of the peppermint oil in the stomach, which can irritate the gastric mucosa (in these amounts), and relaxes the lower esophageal sphincter which will allow reflux of gastric contents into the esophagus.

There is solid evidence that enteric-coated peppermint oil is helpful in irritable bowel syndrome [253]. The IBS-D (diarrhea) variant might need a different approach than overreliance on enteric-coated peppermint oil [254]. It is advisable to consider drawing on the considerable variety of carminatives: ginger, cardamom, fennel, anise, cilantro, pepper, cumin, and many more options that help regulate digestion and colon activity.

Colon Hydrotherapy

There are two indications for irrigating the colon. One is to remove hardened stool to alleviate constipation. The other is to remove putrefied matter, including hardened fecal material that does not join the fecal stream (is adherent to the mucosa), and help support discharge of waste matter from the body. Irrigating this area can be done in a clinical setting with a flow-based colon hydrotherapy machine. This must involve a trained individual who will not over fill the colon to some dangerous level of pressure. It must be 100% sterile to avoid spread of microbial or viral disease. Enemas, which are self-contained units that can deliver a smaller volume, such as 250 mL of water, to the rectum, are a lower intensity way to achieve some irrigation especially if constipation is the problem. In a recent study, the reported success rate of irrigation for functional constipation is about 50%, comparable to or better than the response seen in trials of pharmacologic therapies. Colonic irrigation is a safe treatment benefitting some patients with functional constipation, which is a chronic refractory condition. There are variations in reported results and overall weaker trials.

Laxatives

Laxatives increase the volume, liquidity, and frequency of stools. Botanically derived laxatives are typically of the anthraquinone type [255]. These herbal medicines contain compounds such as anthracene-type core with a sugar molecule attached, the so-called anthraquinone glycosides. When these are consumed, enteric bacteria cleave the sugar residue and release the aglycone. This molecule, a quinone-containing substance such as emodin, is free to act on the large intestine. This causes chloride to be released into the gut lumen, and water follows. The anthraquinones also irritate nerve endings in the mucosa. The influx of water causes expansion of the colon and more peristalsis (Fig. 8.9).

These medicines are useful to break a cycle of constipation but shouldn't be used to the point of dependence. Overuse can cause dehydration and electrolyte depletion, including potassium. There is some speculation that they can increase colon cancer risk, perhaps due to the similarity of the anthraquinones to anthracene from coal tar, a known mutagen. A short-term use of these medicines, perhaps for 2 weeks, when combined, with increased hydration, fiber, core exercise, and regular stool habits, can help to reset a pattern. They should not be used chronically, although many people use them that way as they are readily available at any pharmacy. Laxative herbal species include *Rhamnus purshiana*, *Aloe vera*, *Rheum palmatum*, and *Cassia senna* (cascara sagrada, aloe, turkey rhubarb, and senna, respectively). *Rheum palmatum* (rhubarb) also increases mucin production [256]. A form of rhubarb used in traditional Chinese medicine, combined with *Paeonia lactiflora*, appears to help balance T17 and Treg leading to less inflammation in inflammatory colitis [257].

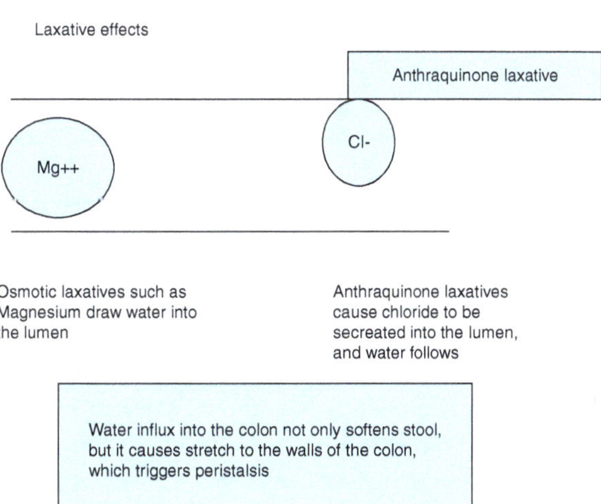

Fig. 8.9 Laxative effects: anthraquinone laxatives and magnesium salts both cause influx of water into the colon but through different mechanisms

Bentonite Clay

Bentonite is absorbent aluminum phyllosilicate clay which has a volcanic origin. The name comes from Fort Benton, Wyoming, which has plentiful amounts [258]. It is also called montmorillonite clay, as it can be found in the region of France called Montmorillon. This clay is safe to eat in small amounts (it is found in powder that can be added to water or in capsules), and it will absorb many toxins. In the gastrointestinal tract, it will absorb excess water. This is a safer naturopathic approach to excess secretion than more aggressive medicines that block peristalsis, as those can be quite dangerous for some of the conditions discussed in this chapter, such as active ulcerative colitis. Bentonite will absorb many microbial toxins, as well as fungal and industrial toxins (such as polychlorinated compounds). It may encourage microbial growth of normal enteric bacteria, but its precise impact on the complex microflora is not known. An adsorbent material can potentially bind minerals. Bentonite would not be a permanent supplement but something to be used shorter term for excess secretions or detoxification. This could be in IBS-D or simple secretory diarrhea.

Homeostatic Maintenance

Anticholinergic Botanicals

Atropa belladonna is also known as the deadly nightshade plant. It has been used as a medicine for thousands of years and also used as a poison, with case reports going back to the Roman Empire. It is a small herbaceous plant from the nightshade (Solanaceae) family, which also includes potatoes, peppers, and tomatoes. It contains powerful tropane alkaloids such as atropine and scopolamine. These alkaloids have some structural similarity to acetylcholine, and they can bind to the acetylcholine receptor. They have an affinity for the postganglionic receptors in the parasympathetic nervous system. These are muscarinic receptors. At these sites, atropine and scopolamine act as antagonists. This will reduce parasympathetic input into the gut muscle, and slow peristalsis. These have antispasmodic actions on the gut and so have a use in intense irritable bowel syndrome. The doses are very small, 1ml or less. Overuse can lead to some very serious side effects, such as mania, hallucinations, tachycardia, arrhythmias, and death. Scopolamine is also used as an anti-nausea drug, and drop doses of *Atropa belladonna* might be useful for some stomach complaints [223, 224]. In emergency medicine, atropine is used to increase heart rate in cases of extreme bradycardia. The military has atropine injectors as an antidote against certain nerve agents. This is because atropine has affinity for the neuromuscular junction, and *overstimulation* of that junction will lead to diaphragmatic paralysis and laryngospasm when people are exposed to nerve agents such as sarin. Using *Atropa belladonna* to reduce spasm in IBS is a palliative measure and must be done with caution. Less serious but troublesome side effects are dry mouth, slow gastric emptying, constipation, and poorer digestion. Contraindications include pregnancy, autonomic neuropathy of the gastrointestinal tract (as *Atropa* will further reduce vagal input, leading to food retention), and narrow angle glaucoma. Mydriasis is a well-known effect of these substances including synthetic anticholinergics used to reduce muscle rigidity and tremor in Parkinson's disease. That pupillary dilation can induce an attack of extreme ocular hypertension in someone with narrow angle glaucoma.

Pharmacologic Anti-Inflammatories

These are the reliable and long-standing first-line medical treatments for ulcerative colitis. These include oral sulfasalazine, diazo-bonded 5-aminosalicylates (5-ASA), and mesalamine [259] (Table 8.19).

These are often combined, during flare-ups, with prednisone to get inflammation under control and induce a state of remission. Immune-modulating pharmaceutical treatment are a class of agents that were introduced in the late 1990s and have become mainstay treatments for inflammatory bowel disease.

Patients with ulcerative colitis often respond to the newer immune-modulating drugs. One class is tumor necrosis factor antagonist antibodies, such as infliximab (which appears to be excellent for patients new to these drugs), ustekinumab, and tofacitinib [260, 261].

The Renal System

The renal system consists of the kidney, ureters, bladder, and urethra. This is not only a system of elimination. The kidney is a major organ of metabolism, and it has distinct endocrine functions. It receives a major supply of aortic blood, up to 25%, and filters about 200 L of fluid a day [262]. This blood is dispersed into small arterioles and either nourishes the connective tissue or becomes capillaries in the glomerular apparatus. These glomeruli are very dense capillary structures that are found bundled within Bowman's capsule, and clusters of these capsules make up a nephron; the kidneys have about 1 to 1.5 million of these each. Bowman's space is the area between the capsule and the capillaries.

Proteins typically will not pass out of the capillaries, because the somewhat permeable capillary walls have negatively charged proteins that form "fenestrations," a sort of net to hold albumin and other proteins in. But glucose, electrolytes, urea, and other substances do leave. This drains into a proximal tubule. In the proximal tubule, potassium and hydrogen ions are secreted. Water and glucose are reabsorbed, and by cotransportation, sodium enters the cells that line this tubule. Urea is excreted but some is later reabsorbed. In the distal convoluted tubule, more sodium and water are reabsorbed, as well as magnesium, chloride, calcium, and potassium. Additional water is reabsorbed in the loop of Henle. In the proximal tubule, urate, oxalate,

Table 8.20 Glomerular filtration rate

Estimated glomerular filtration rate	Interpretation
90 or higher	Normal range (varies with age with patients in their early 20s being 115 and up)
60–89	Possible early renal disease
15–59	Renal disease
Less than 15	Renal failure

some vitamins such as ascorbate, creatine, and other natural substances, as well as many drugs, are excreted.

The mechanism for creating various osmolarities in this system—allowing for reabsorption of wanted substances and continued excretion of unwanted—is a remarkable sequenced process of chemical reactions. All of this flow eventually traverses a connecting duct and then goes into a collecting duct to eventually drain into the ureter [262, 263].

The glomerular filtration rate is the rate at which the blood supply is processed through the nephrons of the kidney. In an experimental and more accurate sense, certain test substances such as inulin are administered to a patient and then measured in the urine over time. Far more common, and inexpensive, is the measurement of creatine, which is a byproduct of normal muscle turnover (Table 8.20). Creatinine clearance is calculated as follows [264]:

$$\text{Creatinine clearance} = \text{urinary creatinine} ? \text{urinary flow rate} / \text{plasma creatine}$$

In an even more practical sense, just a serum creatinine can be used to estimate creatinine clearance.

$$\text{The estimated creatinine clearance} = \frac{\left(140 ? \text{patient}^{?}\text{s age}\right) ? \text{Mass}(\text{kg}) ? \left[0.85 \text{ if female}\right]}{72 ? \left[\text{Serum Creatinine}(\text{mg/dL})\right]}$$

The creatinine clearance overestimates the GFR by about 10 to 20%.

The GFR decreases slowly but steadily from age 30 on. This happens along with a decrease in the renal plasma flow (RPF), although at age 80, the GFR starts to decline more slowly than the RPF. These changes don't lead to renal failure in older age in the healthy, although they will impact the excretion of drugs. A 20-year-old male has a GFR of about 110 (mL/min/1.73 m^2) and by age 65 may be down to 60. Those with hypertension or diabetes are at risk of ending up with serious kidney defects before they die of other causes.

The kidneys are susceptible to injuries like other organs. They can be damaged by toxins such as heavy metals or drugs such as cisplatin. Atherosclerosis can impinge blood flow, and arterial fibrosis and stiffening can also impact the flow rate into the kidney. Heart failure that leads to decreased cardiac output will drop the pressure in the kidney, which can lead to renal failure.

The kidney has powerful endocrine functions that create far-acting effects on the body. One hormone is renin, which has sodium-retaining and adrenergic effects on the blood system [265]. It is converted to angiotensin I and II which also lead to increased blood pressure. Renin secretion is a way that the kidney can continue to function in the face of poor left ventricular output. Kallikreins are serine proteases that act on blood proteins to produce bradykinin, which will relax blood vessels. Kidneys are crucial to the hematological system. Erythropoietin activates erythrocyte production in the blood vessel. In the proximal tubule, vitamin D3 (1,25(OH)2) creates the action of the enzyme 1alpha-hydroxylase on D2.

Urine enters the ureter at the renal pelvis and travels to the bladder. In the bladder, it is held back by the bladder sphincter, which can be voluntarily controlled. The bladder has a muscular wall, and the inner epithelium is able to secrete IgA and a layer of mucin that discourages bacteria from adhering to it.

Hypofunction

There is a gradual decline of kidney function over the life span [264]. Plasma flow into the kidney decreases, and the ability of the kidney to put the blood flow it receives through the glomeruli declines. The reabsorption of electrolytes, vitamins, and even water can become less efficient.

The bladder may become less tolerant of overfilling with age or due to neurogenic pain patterns, as seen in some conditions such as interstitial cystitis. The bladder sphincter may also lose its tone, leading to incontinence. This can be minor, or it can be severe or progressive enough to impact the quality of life.

Lack of Circulation and Communication

Vascular issues in the kidney can constrain blood flow. One intense form of this is renal artery stenosis [264]. This is often simply a manifestation of atherosclerosis in these arteries. The patient usually has atherosclerotic plaques in other arteries, but the renal artery can be unluckily a focal point of blockages. A small percentage of renal artery stenosis patients, perhaps 2%, suffer from fibromuscular dysplasia.

When the renal artery cannot deliver adequate blood flow to the kidney, this leads to decreased plasma flow and then decreased glomerular filtration rate (Table 8.21). This can lead to renal failure. But the kidney will counter this situation by releasing renin. This powerful hormone is key to activating the fundamental control system, the renin-angiotensin-aldosterone pathway. This will lead to an increase in blood pressure by sympathetic nervous system activation. The blood pressure will rise. With regard to the kidney, the efferent arterial circulation (away from the kidney) will become more pressurized than the afferent circulation (into the kidney, toward the glomeruli). That raises the intrarenal, intraglomerular pressure and thus restores an adequate glomerular filtration rate. The secondary activation of aldosterone will raise blood pressure by leading tubular reabsorption of sodium and water. This adaptation prevents renal failure, but it comes with a price-systemic hypertension. This adaptation is not only caused by renal artery stenosis. Poor cardiac output due to weak left ventricular muscle or restrictive cardiomyopathy and poor left ventricular filling can have the effect of inadequate afferent arterial pressure to the kidney.

The kidney has an extrinsic autoregulatory system. The tubuloglomerular feedback system is the principal mechanism that can sense fluctuations in GFR and the flow of blood into the kidney [266]. The macula densa are clusters of sensing tubular epithelial cells in the thick ascending loop of Henle (downstream from the proximal tubules). The macula densa can detect drops in fluid pressure in the loop. This sends a signal to the juxtaglomerular cells, which are in the smooth muscle of the afferent arterioles. They can directly cause vasodilation of these arteries, and an additional way they have to increase GFR is that they can secrete renin.

Kidney innervation consists of both afferent and efferent nerves, of which the efferent is strictly sympathetic [267]. These nerves make up the renal plexus and receive inputs from the celiac and aorticorenal plexuses as well as the so called "least" splanchnic nerve, which originates from the T12 level. The least splanchnic nerve is primarily responsible for the afferent signaling from the kidney to the brain. The least splanchnic nerve also carries visceral efferent fibers.

Sympathetic input to the organ is via visceral efferent fibers, traveling from spinal cord, and ganglia, to the kidney. These nerves stimulate beta-1-adrenergic receptors in the juxtaglomerular cells of the kidney. Much like the effect of the kidney's intrinsic autoregulation, this input will activate the renin-angiotensin-aldosterone system.

Communication to the bladder can be impaired due to neurologic deficits [268]. These can arise from trauma, radiation (for treating cancer), toxins, multiple sclerosis, diabetes, infection, and other insults to the visceral nerves and the smooth muscle of the bladder. This can progress to the point, and it often does in the case of spinal cord injuries, where the patient needs continual catheterization.

Urine flow is from the kidney down the ureters, to the bladder, and then out through the urethra. This can be reversed to a degree, when a lack of outflow causes a pressure build up, such as that caused by bladder outlet obstruction. This can happen because of a renalith, a stone, in the bladder. It can also happen in urethral obstruction due to prostatic enlargement in males [269] and in narrowing of the ureters (there is a congenital form of this). The increase in hydrostatic pressure in the ureters and then the pelvis of the kidney is known as hydronephrosis [270]. It can begin to cause necrosis of the kidney eventually and is a condition that must be treated.

Inflammation

An example of an inflammatory response is acute kidney injury (AKI) [271]. This is when some physiological state or external agent leads to sudden kidney damage, which might progress to a rapid-onset kidney failure. Events that cause a sudden drop in blood pressure can shock the kidney and surpass the regulatory systems that the organ would normally use to maintain its own perfusion, pressure, and filtration rate.

This could include the following:

- Allergic reactions that lead to edema—such as a bee sting.
- Heart failure with a sudden exacerbation and lower than usual left ventricular output.
- Vascular collapse due to infection—toxic shock.
- Burns that lead to sudden extravasation of fluids and hypovolemic shock.

Acute kidney injury can also occur due to the aforementioned blockage of urinary flow, due to the following:

- Calculi (stones).
- Prostatic urethral compression.
- Neurogenic bladder (i.e., due to trauma to nerves or a flare-up of a demyelinating disease such as multiple sclerosis).

Deeper Inflammation and Immune Involvement

Renal infection can occur when a bladder infection ascends to the level of the kidneys. When this progresses, it will lead to edema of the kidney, which causes stretch of the renal capsule [271]. The patient will have very tender kidneys and pain that is reported in the flank. A high fever with chills is usually seen. Patients with weakened immune systems, those who are catheterized, and those with any kind of obstruction or hydronephrosis are at risk.

Bacteria that cause infection are many and include *Streptococcus pyogenes*, *Staphylococcus aureus*, *Escherichia coli*, and *Mycobacterium tuberculosis*. Viruses can also infect the kidney including dengue fever virus, hepatitis B and C, and hantavirus. Fungi can also impact the kidney, arising from a bladder infection, especially in immunocompromised individuals. The species that are most likely to make the leap from bladder to kidney are *Candida*, *Aspergillus*, *Mucor*, *Cryptococcus*, and *Histoplasma*.

Table 8.21 Levels of dysfunction in renal disease

Level of dysfunction	Tests to consider
Hypofunction	Urinary dipstick
Hypofunction	Serum electrolytes
Hypofunction	Microalbuminuria
Impaired circulation and communication	Creatinine clearance test (24-h urine and blood creatinine)
Impaired circulation and communication	Renal ultrasound Doppler
Impaired circulation and communication	Voiding cystourethrography
Impaired circulation and communication	Serum albumin
Impaired circulation and communication	Urinary albumin direct measurement
Inflammation	Autoimmune markers
Inflammation	Urine culture and sensitivity
Inflammation and increased immune activity	Antineutrophil cytoplasmic antibodies
Fibrosis and matrix deposition	Computerized tomography
Fibrosis and matrix deposition	Kidney biopsy
Decline of function	Blood urea nitrogen
Decline of function	Many of the above tests

Kidneys can be caught in the cross fire of acute illnesses, such as kidney injury simply due to the toxins made during bacterial sepsis, such as lipopolysaccharide from gram-negative bacteria. Neoplasms within white blood cells can create proteins that have damage to organs including the kidneys. For instance, the amyloid proteins created by some lymphomas and multiple myeloma can deposit in the kidneys. Autoimmune vasculitis can lead to sudden kidney injury [272]. Some inflammations in the kidney due to autoimmune attack will have antibody signatures (Table 8.21). The neutrophil-produced myeloperoxidase will be elevated, showing white blood cell destruction of the kidney. Anti-glomerular basement membrane (anti-GBM) disease also impacts the lungs. Another manifestation of deeper inflammation in the kidney is tubular necrosis due to a drug reaction, or some of the above injuries to the kidney, including any etiology that leads to poor perfusion.

IgA nephropathy can result from aberrant IgA structures that attract the attention of the immune system as a whole [273]. When IgG or IgM antibodies bind to this unusual IgA, it forms immune complexes. These can become lodged in glomeruli and attract more immune attention, leading to acute kidney injury and rapidly progressing glomerulonephritis. It can also lead to chronic kidney disease.

Fibrosis and Extracellular Matrix Degeneration

Scleroderma is a form of reactive collagen formation where some injury (poorly understood) to the intima of blood vessels causes a reactive overproduction of collagen. This can lead to blocked blood vessels, lesions on the skin, solid tumors of collagen within organs, and in about 10% of patients with this condition, a degree of kidney injury that can lead to acute renal failure [273]. This can present with hypertension, as the kidney attempts to maintain its perfusion. But left untreated, renal failure can result. The problem seems to begin with damage to the endothelium, the layer of cells that line the intima of the arterioles in the kidney. An exaggerated response to injury can lead to intimal proliferation and a narrowing of renal arterioles.

Stone Formation

Calculi form in the kidney when minerals come out of solution and crystalize [274] (Table 8.21). This is more likely to happen under certain conditions, such as dehydration (chronically) and excretion of elevated amounts of the minerals.

Calcium oxalate stones are formed by those who are excretors of oxalate and those who consume excessive foods such as rhubarb, nuts, soy beverage, buckwheat, etc. Ascorbic acid consumption in excess of 1 g a day can contribute to this but can be offset with supplementing magnesium. Citrate, phosphate, and purines can also form calcium stones. Struvite stones are less common and result from infections with bacteria such as *Proteus* species or *Klebsiella* species. These stones contain magnesium ammonium phosphate.

Renal calculi can cause obstructions, depending on their size and location. They can also dislodge and become trapped in the duct system. The resulting stretch on the main ducts of the kidney or ureters is one of the most painful presentations. The Greek physician Hippocrates even mentions surgery to alleviate it.

Polycystic kidney disease is a hereditary disease. There is an autosomal dominant and recessive type [275]. Cysts form in the epithelium of the kidney, and excessive growth factors, such as epidermal growth factor, initiate the initial cysts. Epithelial cells will start to proliferate, and then extracellular matrix is deposited in ways that begins to crowd out or destroy normal cells and the architecture of the nephrons. Inflammation increases, and macrophages contribute to the epithelial destruction and excessive repair. Eventually, the kidney is overtaken with cystic tissue and involuted nephrons that no longer function.

Diabetes, if chronic and not properly controlled, can lead to renal failure. Cells are damaged by glycosylation which damages protein structure [276]. There is also the accumulation of sorbitol which saps the kidney epithelial cells of needed energy. The vascular disease that accompanies diabetes can begin to erode the arteriole function of the kidney. The blood pressure inside the glomerulus will rise in part due to hyperproliferation of the extracellular matrix. This is found in the mesangial area, which is the structure matrix of the tufts of arterioles that make up glomeruli. This matrix hyperproliferation leads to a thickening of the basement membrane of the glomeruli, which can lead to proteinuria. The elevated pressures in the kidney contribute to this fibrotic reaction (Fig. 8.10). The tubule system of the kidney can also suffer the fate of matrix proliferation, undergoing hypertrophy but later sclerosis,

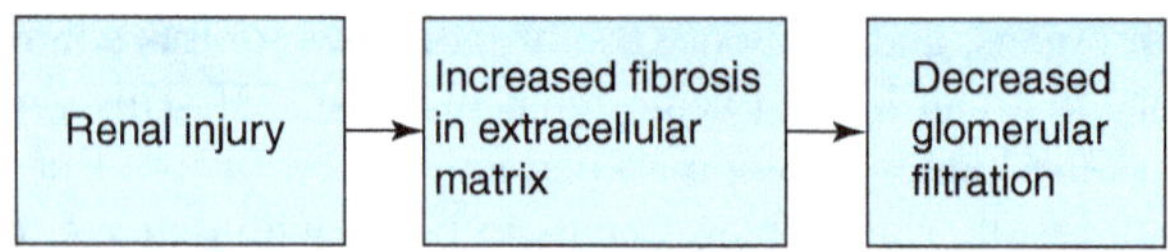

Fig. 8.10 Extracellular matrix degeneration and the kidney: decreased glomerular filtration and proteinuria result from hyperproliferation of matrix in the basement membrane of the glomeruli

with inflammation, and matrix deposition. Hypertension can also lead to fibrosis and chronic kidney disease, as can autoimmune attack, obstructive conditions, and toxin exposure.

Decline of Function

Chronic kidney disease will result from loss of functioning glomeruli, destruction of renal tubules, or degradation of blood supply to the kidney including the arterioles that feed the nephrons. As the glomerular filtration rate decreases, it becomes harder for the kidney to function [277]. Hypertension will result from renin activation, but that will only help for so long. Patients will have azotemia—buildup of urea in the bloodstream. This can cause inflammation of the pericardium and encephalitis. Kidney failure also leads to hyperkalemia and hypocalcemia. This can be detrimental to the heart and lead to serious arrhythmias and cardiac arrest.

The nephrotic spectrum refers to levels of renal dysfunction, particularly with proteinuria. Protein will leak through glomeruli that have lost their fenestrations [278]. Protein loss in urine might be greater than 3.5 g/day, which will start depleting levels of albumin in the blood and even lead to lipid dysfunction and accumulation. Edema will occur because of loss of osmotic pressure in the blood due to the relative absence of protein.

Kidney failure will necessitate dialysis, in order to clean the blood of urea [279]. Patients will lose protein during the process, which involves a semipermeable membrane that filters the blood, so posttreatment meals are meant to return the patient to positive nitrogen status. Kidney transplants are often a last resort, and many people are alive and healthy today because of this. The general precepts of supporting the kidney discussed below are helpful for many of these patients, but, given the nuances of pre- and posttransplant, consultation with a kidney specialist and using clinical recommendations from naturopathic physicians who have worked with this population and their surgeons are strongly advised.

Neoplasm

Renal cell carcinoma can emerge as a primary site, and it can present with symptoms at first that seem like kidney infection. It can spread to other sites, such as the bone [280]. Will's tumor is a nephroblastoma that is found in children [281]. The kidney can also be a site of metastasis of cancer from a primary site, such as the prostate.

Treatment

Determinants of Health

Hydration is important for kidney health (Table 8.22). Heat stress (exposure to heat that excessively challenges the body's bioregulatory responses) and dehydration can lead to compensatory mechanisms that, if extreme, lead to acute kidney injury [282]. Humans can perspire up to 2 L per hour under some conditions. Without compensations, the loss of water from all compartments and the loss of sodium would be lethal. Blood volume drops in dehydration, and the decrease in filtration in the kidney leads to renin secretion due to its intrinsic balancing systems. Additionally, baroreceptors in the systemic vasculature result in increased renal sympathetic nerve activity and renin secretion. This will keep someone functioning, but ongoing dehydration can overwhelm these compensations. Elevated blood pressure will also damage the kidney longer term. Patients who take diuretics must be careful to hydrate adequately, as do those who are exposed to heat due to climate, occupation, sports, etc.

Sleep is impacted by chronic kidney disease, with apnea being worse due to swelling of tissues. It appears that sleep restriction has an adverse effect on kidney disease for reasons still under investigation [283, 284]. The chemoreflexes that detect low oxygen and high carbon dioxide in the blood seem to be more dysregulated in those with chronic kidney disease. But these patients are more likely to have diabetes, morbid obesity, and high levels of inflammation and oxidative stress.

Sunlight is a health-giving need for humans, not to the point of radiation burning, but daily moderate exposures will maintain circadian rhythms and promote vitamin D synthesis. In chronic kidney disease, there is a lack of active vitamin D3 in the bloodstream, due to defects in conversion of D2 to D3 [285]. Supplementing the active form, D3, is probably needed, but proper sun exposure to at least optimize precursor levels in the bloodstream can help, especially before kidney failure is very far advanced.

Table 8.22 Treatment considerations in renal disorders

Mode of therapeutic intervention	Examples	Comments
Determinants of health	Hydration	Thirst loses its accuracy with age; some patients on diuretic or who are heat exposed are dehydrated
Determinants of health	Sleep	Impacted by and may impact chronic kidney disease
Determinants of health	Sunlight	Vitamin D production
Determinants of health	Prenatal health and nutrition	Can have long-term effects on kidney development
Biochemical support	*Ginkgo biloba*	Reduce inflammation, protect kidney tissue from toxins, reduce matrix deposition
Biochemical support	*Centella asiatica*	Anti-fibrotic
Biochemical support	*Tripterygium wilfordii*	Decrease BUN
Biochemical support	*Hibiscus sabdariffa*	Mitochondrial protection
Biochemical support	*Glycyrrhiza glabra*	Protection from toxins
Biochemical support	*Nigella sativa*	Pretreatment against ischemia, protection against heavy metals, antioxidant, and anti-inflammatory
Biochemical support	*Agathosma betulina* and *A. crenulata*	Monoterpenes, traditional bladder medicine
Biochemical support	*Arctostaphylos uva-ursi*	Bacteriostatic, best in alkaline environment
Biochemical support	*Vaccinium macrocarpon*	Decrease bacterial adherence to bladder, disrupt biofilm
Biochemical support	Serratiopeptidase and other enzymes	Disrupt biofilms
Hormetic action	*Erigeron breviscapus* and *Scutellaria lateriflora*	Increase NRF activation
Whole person support	Dietary changes to control hyperglycemia	Diabetes support
Whole person support	Probiotics and fermented foods; limitation of tryptophan sources	Trimethylamine N-oxide and indole reduction
Whole person support	Hydrotherapy and aquatic exercise	Improve circulation, remove uremic material from blood
Whole person support	Avoid renal-damaging drugs	Might have to use such medications and offset damage to kidneys with natural therapy

Table 8.22 (continued)

Mode of therapeutic intervention	Examples	Comments
Dampening maladaptive responses	Urinary antibiotics	Treat renal or bladder infections
Dampening maladaptive responses	Low PRAL foods	Reduce acid formation
Dampening maladaptive responses	Vitamin D supplementation	Treat hypophosphatemia, vitamin D deficiency
Induce homeostasis	Hospitalization	Fluids, electrolytes, glycemic levels, and acid-base balance will need to be monitored and adjusted if necessary
Induce homeostasis	ACE inhibitors, ARB	Reduce exercise blood pressure and sodium retention—but must not overtreat
Induce homeostasis	Surgery and lithotripsy	Calculi removal
Induce homeostasis	Dialysis	Remove waste products from blood
Induce homeostasis	Renal transplant	Must prevent rejection

Prenatal health has connections to renal development and disease later in life. Under conditions of toxin exposure, stress, and especially malnutrition, it is hypothesized that the brain receives developmental priority in the developing human. While too late for those adults and children with kidney disease, it is a reminder that prenatal health determining factors have a profound and long-term impact [286].

Biochemical Support

Ginkgo biloba

Ginkgo is generally vascular protective, and since inflammation of the arterioles, hypertension, atherosclerosis, and vasoconstriction all work against the kidney, it would seem to be a helpful treatment. EGb 761or "EGb" is a heavily researched standardized extract of *Ginkgo biloba*. It was developed and put on market in the early 1970s by IPSEN in France and Dr. Willmar Schwabe Pharmaceuticals in Germany. EGb contains 24% flavonol glycosides and 6% terpene lactones [287, 288]. Flavonoids include quercetin, kaempferol, and isorhamnetin. Terpenoids are the ginkgolides A, B, C, J, and M and bilobalide. EGb is well-known as an antioxidant, vasodilatory, and vascular protective. It has specific nephroprotective actions.

In studying kidney toxin injury, rats and mice were used as an experimental model. While not at the level of evidence of a clinical trial, let alone a group of randomized clinical trials, the nutritional value and the potential biochemical effects of an herbal extract can be studied this way. In this type of research, EGb 761 reduced damage to the kidney tubular system and reduced the matrix proliferation that can lead to declining kidney function [289, 290]. Not only is there less thickening of the matrix, but it appears that the epithelium (crucial to the function of the tubule system and the glomerular system in the nephrons) did not revert to undifferentiated matrix.

One studied toxin is the drug methotrexate [291]. This is an anticancer drug used to treat multiple myeloma. It is also used in autoimmune diseases such as rheumatoid arthritis, to decrease inflammation via suppressing white blood cell activity. The kidney has to excrete toxins and methotrexate can injure the kidney tubules. Creatinine and blood urea nitrogen will rise, and there are expanded glomeruli, damaged tubules, and involuted glomerular tufts. EGb 761 prevented these changes. Other studies looking at kidney restriction due to diabetic neuropathy also showed ameliorating effects of EGb 761. These benefits also apply to those undergoing dialysis, reducing inflammation [292]. The anticancer drug cisplatin can damage the kidneys, and it has been known since the 1990s, based on research done in Japan, that EGb 761 can be protective in experimental models [293]. This appears to extend to the damage from Adriamycin as well.

These protective benefits are probably due to the incredible antioxidant effects of GBE. But the flavonoids and terpenes in this remarkable plant also have anti-inflammatory effects and are protective of mitochondria. Ginkgo biloba extract lowers TGF-beta levels, and suppressess PI3K/Akt/mTOR. This pathway is an important cell cycling axis that leads to repair, but overexpression can increase cancer progression, and it appears to be overexpressed after injury with drugs such as methotrexate and cisplatin. This is an unclear action of *Ginkgo biloba*, but perhaps it helps restore bioregulation, where a situation of imbalance exists.

Centella asiatica

Centella asiatica has anti-fibrotic effects on the kidney (Table 8.22). This can slow the extracellular matrix proliferation that accompanies glomerular expansion in chronic kidney disease. While there are no clinical trials of *Centella asiatica* in polycystic kidney disease, it could in theory be helpful in slowing down the process, through an anti-inflammatory action, as it could be in diabetic kidney disease [294].

Tripterygium wilfordii

Tripterygium wilfordii has a long history in Chinese medicine. It has been shown in human trials of renal disease to decrease blood urea nitrogen and decrease urinary albumin. It can cause gastrointestinal upset and may have potential toxicity to the ovary and cause some liver damage. It can be used safely and, in combination with other treatments for chronic kidney disease, could improve the clinical status of patients [295].

Hibiscus sabdariffa

Extracts of this herb can improve defensive enzymes that protect mitochondria and cell membranes—catalase and glutathione. In a diabetic renal disease model, *Hibiscus sabdariffa* extracts reduce oxidative damage to the kidney and improve some functions of the proximal tubule [296].

Glycyrrhiza glabra and Isoliquiritigenin

Isoliquiritigenin is a flavonoid found in licorice (*Glycyrrhiza glabra*). It has antioxidant properties, like many flavonoids. But it also can induce stress in the endoplasmic reticulum. This is a transient and low-intensity enough effect to lead to a cytoprotective compensatory response. In an experimental model, isoliquiritigenin conferred protection against nephrotoxicity from cisplatin, a powerful chemotherapeutic drug. Kidney cells that were pretreated with isoliquiritigenin and then exposed to cisplatin have less oxidative stress and less cellular death. They maintained their glutathione peroxidase levels. *Glycyrrhiza glabra*-treated mice in an experimental model of gentamicin (an antibiotic)-induced renal damage showed normal kidney architecture on a cellular level in the *Glycyrrhiza*-treated group as opposed to signs of damage and inflammation in controls [297].

Nigella sativa

This is also known as black cumin seed. It contains a compound thymoquinone that may protect against kidney injury due to toxins such as pesticides, chemotherapeutic drugs such as those mentioned above, and some heavy metals (lithium, cadmium, lead, arsenic, mercury, and platinum). Much like *Ginkgo biloba*, *Nigella* extracts may pretreat the kidney to tolerate disruptions in blood flow. It increases antioxidant defenses such as glutathione levels. It has anti-inflammatory actions such as lowering TNF-alpha and IL-6. It has anti-fibrotic effects via inhibition of TGF-β1. It reduces kidney cell apoptosis by inhibition of caspase 9 [297, 298]. It has been found to lower serum creatinine, blood urea, and urinary protein, and raise glomerular filtration rate.

Urinary Antiseptics

These are herbs that have known bacteriostatic actions that can assist the immune system in clearing bacterial infections.

Arctostaphylos uva-ursi is also known as bearberry (Table 8.22). This is an herb that has traditional uses for bladder infection; it contains arbutin which is metabolized to hydroquinone in the liver. This compound is excreted in the urine. The herb was used traditionally for enuresis and difficulty producing a urinary stream due to bladder infection. It works better in a more alkaline urine. It appears to be safe for the kidney, although in the most ill of kidney patients it would be wise to avoid quinone excretion [299].

Agathosma betulina and *A. crenulata* (formerly known as *Barosma crenulata*) are plants native to South Africa and they have a long history of use for the bladder. European physicians learned about them, and they became part of compendiums across Europe and the United States. As antibiotics and sulfonamides became standard of care, they fell out of use in mainstream medicine. Both species contain volatile oils, with many terpenes such as limonene, isomenthone, pulegone, and others. The *betulina* species seems to have more of these compounds. It does not have modern clinical trials, but it does have cell, animal, and in vitro preclinical research [300]. More importantly, it has a very long history of use in African medicine and, later, the medicine of other areas of the world.

Biofilm Disruption

Patients with recurring bladder infections may have biofilm formation on the bladder epithelium. A biofilm is a type of extracellular matrix that bacteria and fungi can create. It has fibrin and other proteins and polysaccharides such as alginate. Biofilms are not just a hangout for bacteria although they are important for bacteria to adhere to the epithelium [301]. They also help bacteria to hide from immune cells and to some degree to communicate with each other via autoinducers that encourage the bacteria in the area to jointly secrete a biopolymer. Just as plaque on teeth allows bacteria to gain a foothold, a biofilm in the bladder can make infections stubborn and recurrent (interestingly, the inventor of the microscope, Antonie van Leeuwenhoek, first described biofilms from his own teeth in 1683). Enzyme therapy, which helps with biofilms in the gut and will help with the bladder to some extent, can work to break bonds in the biofilm. Serratiopeptidase and other proteases are used to help weaken the biofilm bonds. *Vaccinium macrocarpon* (cranberry) is consumed as juice or food or in capsules to weaken the biofilm. It contains D-mannose, which is also taken on its own for this purpose. *Allium sativum* (garlic) is also a good biofilm disruptor [302, 303]. The various monoterpenes such as thymol and rosmarinic acid can be helpful too [304].

Hormesis

Hormetic agents may increase levels of the prostaglandin (anti-inflammatory generally) PGC1α and the adaptive protein SIRT1. This may protect kidney tissue including the tubular system and reduce fibrosis. *Erigeron breviscapus* is a member of the daisy family and is used in the system of traditional Chinese medicine. It contains a flavonoid scutellarin. It has blood sugar-stabilizing effects but also may reduce oxidative stress and inflammation in the kidney via activation of increased protective enzymes via the Nrf2 pathway [305]. Scutellarin is also found in *Scutellaria lateriflora*, an herb used as a nervine. Levels of superoxide dismutase are also increased by this herb. It appears that diabetic complications, including renal ones, are caused by a force feeding of the electron transport chain by too much pyruvate. This leads to an overrunning of the electron transport chain, a relative lack of ATP utilization, and increased oxidative stress. The aforementioned *Nigella sativa* works to protect kidney cells via a hormetic mechanism, among its other effects, via preconditioning effects on the endoplasmic reticulum [298].

Whole Person

Diabetes prevention and proper management are important for the prevention of kidney disease for millions of people. This means tight control of blood sugar achieved by careful daily monitoring of blood glucose levels. For IDDM, that includes the most efficient insulin regimen they can carry out, including ultrafast-acting insulin at meal times, as well as a very healthy diet. For many NIDDM diabetics, the diet of choice is quasi-Mediterranean [306–308]. Some patients respond to lower carbohydrate intakes than the Mediterranean diet, and some do well with a specific carbohydrate diet. The standard nutritional recommendation includes making half of the "plate" as it were fruits and vegetables.

These plant foods will:

- Create satiety.
- Slow down gastric emptying thus lowering the net glycemic index of a meal.
- Provide fiber which supports gut health and lowers serum cholesterol.
- Displace high-sugar foods, nutrient-poor foods.
- Provide many vitamins and minerals.
- Provide phytonutrients that protect the body, including the kidneys from glycation end products.
- Decrease inflammation.

Although IDDM patients have to think about the balance of food versus insulin dose, many of the same principles of healthy eating apply.

For those in generally good health, a diet that meets requirements and provides anti-inflammatory actions is sufficient. Optimal hydration is a part of that.

For people with existing kidney disease, they may have to obtain sufficient but not excessive protein, to keep blood nitrogen and urea under control. Potassium must be limited in renal failure, due to the inability to excrete it [309].

For those who are stone formers, low oxalate foods, purine restriction, supplemental magnesium, and very good hydration are important [310].

Drug Toxicity

Nephrotoxic drugs have to be avoided when possible, and if they can't be avoided, then some of the nephroprotective plants mentioned above should be included [311].

Examples of drugs that can injure the kidneys are as follows:

Lowering glomerular filtration rate: blood pressure drugs can do this too well, which of course can cause reactive kidney injury. NSAIDs, such as ibuprofen, can also lower GFR.

Damage the kidney parenchyma: NSAIDs, rifampin, many anticancer drugs, lithium.

Damage renal tubule: aminoglycosides, foscarnet, amphotericin B, adefovir, cisplatin.

Crystal and calculus formation: acyclovir, ampicillin.

Microbiota

Trimethylamine N-oxide or TMAO is produced by gut bacteria, from dietary protein, particularly animal-derived protein, and carnitine, phosphatidylcholine, betaine, and choline (which are generally very useful substances). In the liver it becomes monooxygenase, which is secreted by the kidneys. Systemically, TMAO is a risk factor for atherosclerosis, and it will upregulate inflammation [312]. Plant-focused diets do reduce TMAO levels. Patients with chronic kidney disease have increased TMAO (perhaps due to decreased GFR), most likely because they cannot adequately excrete it, and those with higher TMAO have been shown to have higher 5-year all-cause mortality. In animal models, TMAO appears to increase renal fibrosis. Therefore, TMAO is both more likely to be elevated in chronic kidney disease and is capable of damaging the kidneys further.

Indole is formed when gut bacteria break down. In the liver it undergoes phase I processing and becomes the form 3-hydroxyindole, and in phase II becomes indoxyl sulfate. Although a small amount of indoxyl sulfate is normal and tolerable, in someone with kidney disease, it causes increased damage by increasing NF-κB and cell death, as well as fibrotic reactions via expression of genes that create transforming growth factor beta. The kidney tubular cells have trouble repairing the damage and fibrotic reactions predominate.

Simple probiotic supplementation does not seem to reduce TMAO, but it is likely that nonsymbiotic species of bacteria will be more of a problem. For patients with kidney disease, choosing more plant protein options and keeping an eye on tryptophan sources (pork, poultry, eggs, dairy, some nuts) are wise. Eating some fermented foods as probiotic sources can possibly help. The anti-inflammatory actions discussed elsewhere in this chapter and book may be the best insurance against uremic toxins such as TMAO.

Physical Medicine

Hydrotherapy, using a wet sheet pack application, might help remove urea from skin in the chronic kidney disease patient. Exercise in the water is also a good idea. In a 10-year observational study of chronic kidney disease patients, all patients in a small group of 7 regular aquatic exercises were alive and not on dialysis versus mortality (3) or dialysis (2) for 55% of the non-exercisers [313]. While far too little to be statistically useful, it raises some interesting questions about movement and water and how this might be detoxifying for such patients.

Patients with chronic pain in the bladder, are often diagnosed with interstitial cystitis (some patients so diagnosed have occult infections that have evaded detection, such as yeast infection that has been missed). Various manual therapies, such as spinal manipulation, might ameliorate nervous system dysfunction from tissue to the spinal cord and to the brain and so might local microcurrent therapy, TENS therapy, or acupuncture.

Dampen Symptoms

In the case of bladder or kidney infections, antibiotics have been the mainstay for years. Overuse has negative health consequences, and many bladder issues can be solved without resorting to very intensive antibiotic therapy [314]. However, in the elderly, bedridden, immunocompromised, catheterized, and for those with renal infections versus bladder only, antibiotics are extremely important. Fluoroquinolones such as ofloxacin and ciprofloxacin are powerful antibacterials (Table 8.22). These drugs can have adverse effects such as gastrointestinal upset, dizziness, elevated transaminases, eosinophilia, and some strange effects such as Achilles heel rupture. The older drugs such as sulfamethoxazole and trimethoprim (Bactrim) are still used and can still be very effective.

For patients with chronic disease and metabolic acidosis, an alkali diet might be helpful. The potential renal acid load (PRAL) is known for most foods, with meat, wheat, cheese, and fish being very high and acid forming (a positive PRAL). Vegetables, fruit, and fruit juices are alkalizing (a negative PRAL score). Citric acid can become bicarbonate in the body; hence fruit juices can be good. Fats are neutral and this is helpful to keep in mind in terms of energy requirements [315].

Vitamin D supplementation can help with deficiency and as a treatment for hypophosphatemia, which can destroy bone tissue. Actual phosphate supplements are used as well [316].

Induce Homeostasis

Acute kidney injury, if it is severe, requires hospitalization. Fluids, electrolytes, glycemic levels, and acid-base balance will need to be monitored and adjusted if necessary. For patients taking many medications, their levels will have to be adjusted in some cases due to changes in pharmacokinetics and elimination via the kidney [317].

Blood pressure control using angiotensin-converting enzyme (ACE) inhibitors or angiotensin II receptor blockers (ARBs) are used to control hypertension (Table 8.22). These cannot be used too aggressively however. If the compensations made by the kidney via the renin-angiotensin-aldosterone system are completely suppressed, then GFR may plummet [318].

Nephrolithiasis is sometimes self-limiting, although extremely painful. For impacted stones, surgery or lithotripsy (pulverizing calculi using acoustic energy) are needed. Ureteral stents sometimes are put in to ensure flow.

For those with kidney failure, dialysis is necessary [279]. There are several forms (including peritoneal dialysis), but commonly a dialysis machine, that filters the patient's blood through a semipermeable membrane, is used. This removes urea, excess sodium, and fluids and moderates potassium and bicarbonate.

Some patients might receive a kidney transplant. One kidney allograft can keep a patient alive and healthy, and the donor can live with one. Compatibility and rejection prevention are vital considerations in this remarkable life-saving procedure [319]. There are naturopathic physicians who, integratively and in harmony with the nephrologist team, contribute to the care of patients pre- and posttransplant.

Central Nervous System

The central nervous system stands astride many control systems of the body and is a massive processor of information from sensory inputs and has many outputs into the motor and autonomic systems. The brain can filter and interpret incoming information and synchronize activities of various brain regions. Of course, the capacity of the human brain for higher-order reasoning, memory, and synthesis and the expression of personality, emotions, love, and spiritual experiences involve the brain in different ways.

The central nervous system maintains a certain autonomy, with the microvasculature of the brain possessing the blood-brain barrier [320]. This exerts tight control on what can enter and leave the brain. The endothelium of the small blood vessels in the brain is constructed to be difficult to penetrate, with tight junctions in between intimal epithelial cells increasing that integrity. Special transporters that allow molecules in, and out, of the brain are another control. Pericytes, specialized contractile cells, can exert pressure on nearby capillaries, squeezing them more shut. Thus the brain can protect itself against toxins but still receive glucose, oxygen, amino acids, etc.

More recently, a "glymphatic system" was discovered by anatomists [321]. Before the microvascular gets down to the capillary level, there are penetrating arteries that feed the capillaries. These penetrating arteries are boxed in by the "end feet" of astrocytes, but there is a small space in between both structures. This area of fluid between artery and astrocytic feet is called the Virchow-Robin space. This has a small amount of fluid, which drains into the greater cerebral spinal fluid compartments. Circulation of this area is pulsatile and influenced by cardiac contraction. It is an area where waste products can be discarded, including amyloid protein. There is also immunologic activity here, including the presence of macrophages. Although the brain maintains integrity, the blood-brain barrier is more of a boundary, than a tightly sealed membrane. Cerebrospinal fluid drains ultimately into the lymphatic system, a process that depends on gravity. Prolonged space flight can lead to neuro-ocular syndrome, a degenerative change due to lack of CSF clearance in zero gravity conditions.

Neuroplasticity is a process by which brain function can restore itself but physically and functionally remodeling [322]. While a certain amount of "rewiring" occurs with everyday learning, neuroplasticity can extend to the movement of neuronal relay systems to new brain tissue areas. This is evidenced in recovery after stroke, when tissue attrition is overcome and speech, gait, or digital movement is remapped onto new areas of the brain. There are limits to this process, and too much damage can destroy so many neuronal relay bridges that the brain cannot keep up. This is seen after massive trauma but also in neurodegenerative diseases such as Alzheimer's.

Neurotrophins are the chemical side of neuroplasticity. Brain-derived neurotrophic factor (BDNF) is one of them. Brain repair accelerates with accentuation of protein transcription in the neuron and in the synapse. The specific synaptic effect seems to be driven by microRNA, which can influence the expression of genes post-transcript. So the proteasome of the synapse changes, and in some cases, this leads to more sprouting of synaptic connections. BDNF could be said to grow the network.

The brain is an extremely complex structure made of tissue and nerves that control everything we do, from voluntary actions such as walking to involuntary actions such as breathing. The brain is responsible for communicating moment by moment with all other parts of the body through the central nervous system and the peripheral nervous system. The brain is also responsible for managing our emotions and thoughts and for nurturing our short-term and long-term memory. Scientists are slowly discovering its secrets, but in many ways, the brain is still a new frontier.

Aging-related diseases are no less complex and continue to challenge neurologists to fully understand them.

There are about 100 billion cells in the human brain. The way to count brain cells and to accurately count neurons and non-neuron cells (such as glial cells) has continued to become more accurate [323]. Each cell has about anywhere from 10 to 100 thousand connections to other cells. This leads to trillions of possible circuits, an astonishing level of complexity. Network neuroscience [324] is an intensively active field of research in attempting to understand the dynamics of this universe in itself we call the brain. Neurons have excitable membranes, which allow an electrical current to be transmitted by ion flux across a semipermeable membrane. At the terminal end of an axon is a synaptic area. At this point, specially packaged chemicals that have affinity for receptor sites on other neurons are waiting. The depolarizing signal that arrives causes these neurotransmitters to migrate to and fuse with the presynaptic (secreting cell) membrane, where they go into a synaptic space and can bind to receptors on the postsynaptic cell. This can cause a change in the membrane potential of that other neuron and, at a certain threshold, trigger a depolarizing signal on that neuron. Or it can lower the potential and make it less likely to fire (inhibition).

Anatomy of the Brain

The major structures and substructures of the brain are well-known. Neuroimaging and the accumulated knowledge of the BrainMap database (that links structures to mental processes) have led to continued refinements in mapping [325]. The brain is made of three main parts: the forebrain, midbrain, and hindbrain. The forebrain consists of the cerebrum, thalamus, and hypothalamus (part of the limbic system). The midbrain consists of the tectum and tegmentum. The hindbrain is made of the cerebellum, pons, and medulla. Often the midbrain, pons, and medulla are referred to together as the brain stem.

Although there are discrete tasks, the brain is an integrated whole.

Forebrain

In embryonic development, the most anterior of the three regions that become the brain differentiates into the telencephalon and diencephalon. The forebrain is composed of the following:

Cerebral cortex (which is divided into 4 lobes)
Cingulate gyrus
Corpus callosum
Thalamus
Hypothalamus

Amygdala
Hippocampus

The cerebral cortex (also known as the cerebrum or neocortex) is two thirds of the total brain mass. It is the seat of reasoning but also motor and sensory processing. The cerebral cortex is composed of two hemispheres, right and left, that are connected by the corpus callosum.

The four lobes of the cerebral cortex are as follows:

Frontal lobe: reasoning, executive function, movement, emotional regulation.
Parietal lobe: movement, perception of stimuli.
Occipital lobe: visual processing.
Temporal lobe: perception of auditory stimuli, speech.

Thalamus

The thalamus intercepts sensory information, including pain signals.

Hypothalamus

The hypothalamus regulates hormonal functions, including commanding many secretions of the pituitary gland.

Limbic System

The limbic system is comprised of the thalamus, hypothalamus, amygdala, and hippocampus. Emotional functioning and anxiety and alarm reactions heavily involve this system.

The hippocampus has special importance in the encoding of memories. People with hippocampal lesions can suffer anterograde amnesia; they can't form many new memories.

Midbrain

The midbrain includes the colliculi, tectum, and tegmentum. This region also contains the substantia nigra where the neurotransmitter dopamine regulates and refines motor signals to the body. The midbrain is heavily involved in visual and auditory processing and overall alertness.

Hindbrain

Cerebellum

The cerebellum (or hindbrain) has two hemispheres and has a highly folded surface or cortex. The learning and execution of motor skills are highly dependent on cerebellar function. It also seems to help to coordinate tasks in general.

The pons and medulla, which mark the end of the brain and beginning of spina core thereafter, have nuclei for many cranial nerves. The medulla controls many basic homeostatic functions via the autonomic nervous system.

The Brain Extracellular Matrix

The brain has an extracellular matrix, just like other tissues. It accounts for about 20% of brain mass. In a current working model of the synapse, the quadripartite model, the synapse is actually composed of four entities. The pre- and postsynaptic neurons, the astrocytes, and the extracellular matrix form this [326, 327]. The matrix encloses the synapse, and particularly perineuronal nets, which have matrix proteins, encase the synapse, especially of inhibitory synapses. This prevents leakage of neurotransmitters from the synaptic area. The extracellular matrix in the brain has similar types of proteins: glycosaminoglycans (including protein-bound proteoglycans) and structural proteins such as collagen, elastin, fibronectin, and laminin. The brain ECM seems to have an effect on neuroplasticity. Moreover, in brain aging, the brain vascular endothelial glycocalyx is an important component of the blood-brain barrier (BBB) [328]. If the glycocalyx is disturbed, it can lead to loss of integrity of the BBB.

Engrams

Engrams are the hypothesized physical location of memory, vis-a-vis designated neurons. A brilliant work in progress that has gained enormous ground is by the work of Sheena Josselyn at Hospital for Sick Children, her team, and others around the world [329]. Using cutting-edge cell marking, fluorescing, and visualization techniques, they have shown that specific neurons are developed by CREB (cyclic adenosine monophosphate response element-binding protein) into designated neurons that correspond to learning (and are missing in the absence of learning). It is difficult to summarize such elegant science in a short space, but this is bound to be an area of continued scientific progress. Memory is not only ongoing electrical impulses but can be encoded by designated neurons or ensembles of neurons that have somehow structurally retained information and may communicate with our engram neurons and engram neuron ensembles.

Disease Origination

Disturbed Determinants and Hypofunction

Sleep

The brain has intense needs for energy, and it has a vast circulatory perfusion network to deliver oxygen and nutrients. The preferred energy source is glucose, but the brain can accept ketone bodies when glucose levels decrease due to fasting or inability to use glucose in insulin deficiency.

Sleep has fundamental importance for brain health. Sleep progresses from light stage 1 through progressively deeper stages 2, 3, and finally 4. Beyond stage 4 are bursts of rapid eye movement (REM) sleep. During stage 4 and REM sleep, a number of neurotransmitter and hormone effects occur. These changes seem to be critical to brain development, growth, and repair. Disturbances to these hormonal secretions and gene expression seems closely linked with cognitive impairment and exacerbation of dementia. The suprachiasmatic nucleus (SCN) is important to set regular sleep patterns, and yet it seems to receive damage in chronic sleep deprivation.

Systemic inflammation and vascular aging will worsen with sleep deprivation, which long term can impact the central nervous system. In a shorter-term sense, chronic sleep deprivation impairs blood circulation within the brain. It may also slow the outflow of lymph and toxins via the glymphatic system, which is a risk factor for brain aging and cognitive decline.

The synaptic spaces in the brain, including the memory critical hippocampal region, widen in sleep deprivation. Cortisol levels rise, and growth hormone levels fall. This seems to decrease hippocampal activity and repair. In animal models, learning decreases under these conditions [330].

The many ways in which sleep deprivation hurts the brain, and the hippocampal region of it, are still unraveled. Damage and learning impairment via a p38MAPK pathway is one hypothesis. Decreases in brain-derived growth factor are known to occur in sleep deprivation, and this is probably linked to change in other gene systems, including the lowering of phosphorylated cyclic adenosine monophosphate (cAMP) response element-binding protein (CREB). Depressed CREB levels might lower BDNF levels, which leads to decay of neuronal network resilience [331].

Hydration

Obviously, drinking enough water is needed to be optimally healthy; dehydration does affect brain function. People who take diuretics to lower blood pressure can become dehydrated. Warm weather and outdoor exercise can lead to water and electrolyte loss. With aging, the sense of thirst becomes less fine-tuned, and someone can be dehydrated before they realize it. The elderly are more susceptible to cognitive changes with dehydration; with younger subjects in studies, alertness is impacted by dehydration, but cognitive change is not as clear (such as speed of mental processing, word recall, etc.) [332].

Social Support and Activity

A 2017 systematic review looking at social engagement and support relative to cognitive function, across 39 studies, found that these determining factors of human health had an impact on cognition [333]. Executive function and working memory were improved as well as visual spatial processing speed. Other reviews have concluded that people who avoid social isolation by having larger social networks and socializing had better late-life cognitive function.

Exposure to Nature

Cognitive decline may not slow down with exposure to nature, although quality of life would seem to be improved. However, mood disorders, particularly depression, are helped when a person is spending time in natural settings. That implies that in mood issues, not spending any time outdoors, especially in environments that are not "human-scaped," can lower resilience.

A time-honored practice in naturopathic medicine is a literal return to nature. So it comes as no surprise that getting people into a truly natural setting is salutatory [46].

Day and Night Cycles

Closely allied to sleep quality are properly functioning day and night cycles. The circadian clock is tuned by daytime exposure to light and nighttime darkness. Light is detected by specialized retinal photoreceptors. This sends a signal down the retinohypothalamic tract to a circadian pacemaker in the hypothalamic suprachiasmatic nuclei. From there, nerves to the pineal gland will lead to normal night-focused melatonin production. If a person's eyes receive nighttime light exposure, it reduces melatonin production. Because nerves from the superior cervical ganglion are involved in the final signaling to the pineal gland, patients who have had upper spinal cord or ganglionic damage will develop melatonin/circadian problems.

If circadian rhythms begin to drift, then the nighttime repair activities, including lymphatic outflow from the brain, will be compromised [334]. Urban light pollution, but also room devices that emit light, can disrupt these cycles. To some extent noise pollution can do this as well. The well-known effects of shift work have this effect, and more recently, those with extreme visual impairment due to retinal or nervous system damage who don't have light perception (versus a blurred vision that does have it) can develop circadian desynchrony.

Impaired Circulation and Communication

Cerebral blood flow is provided by the carotid arteries and the vertebral arteries. When they are compromised, there can be generally reduced perfusion [335] (Table 8.23). Some patients with partially blocked carotid arteries will develop a transient blockage due to a thrombus due to an unstable plaque. This can lead to a transient ischemic attack, which can present like an incipient stroke. Vertebral arteries can become calcified and can dissect, which can be extremely dangerous.

Poor or erratic cerebral blood flow is a common cause of mild cognitive impairment. This problem is not always focused on the larger arteries in the neck, circle of Willis, and major cerebral arteries. The ramifying blood vessels can become obstructed due to inflammation. As the vast network of cerebral arterioles, capillaries, and the larger arterial branches that feed them becomes attenuated, irregular

Table 8.23 Levels of dysfunction in neurological disease

Levels of dysfunction	Tests to consider
Hypofunction	Cognitive assessments EEG (electroencephalogram) DNA tests for hereditary conditions Neurological physical examination with mapping of dermatome or myotome deficits Patient history can help guide testing and determine possible locations of lesions
Impaired circulation and communication	Carotid artery ultrasound or CT Evoked potential study (sensory signal transmission speed) • Auditory • Visual • Somatosensory Angiography (arteriogram of brain)
Inflammation	Blood tests for infection C-reactive protein (inflammation) Cerebrospinal fluid analysis Laboratory testing for Lyme disease
Deeper inflammation	MRI (weighted depending on suspected lesion) CT scan Single-photon emission computed tomography (SPECT) Positron emission tomography (PET) Heavy metal blood testing
Fibrosis	Biopsy PET scan
Loss of function	Disease scales such as: • Alzheimer's Disease Assessment Scale-Cognitive • Multiple Sclerosis Impact Scale (MSIS-29) subscale • Unified Parkinson's Disease Rating Scale
Neoplasm	MRI CT Biopsy

flow through the larger arteries will have a more dramatic impact. Tissues have less collateral circulation and are already at risk of ischemia.

Circulation of cerebrospinal fluid (CSF) is important; if impaired, it can lead to increased intracranial pressure which can be life-threatening. A less acute but increasingly important phenomena is the inability of perivascular fluids to flow out into the CSF and eventually into the lymphatic system. This can be impaired due to poor cardiac output and also due to a lack of deeper sleep. Dysregulation of circadian rhythms is important in this event. Without adequate discharge by the glymphatic system, amyloid and other waste products can accumulate in the brain.

Pericytes are specialized cells that surround the blood vessels of the brain at their terminal aspects. Pericytes coordinate with glial cells and the endothelium of blood vessels to maintain the blood-brain barrier [336]. They also work to dispose of waste and to prevent excessive immune infiltration into brain tissue by leukocytes (or called immune privilege). When communication and coordination among pericytes, glial cells, and vascular endothelium break down, it can contribute to toxin accumulation, inflammation, and leukocyte infiltration.

Communication between different brain regions can change, in ways that are not yet pathological but can cause changes in function. For example, in attention deficit hyperactivity disorder, signaling between executive functions of the brain, reward centers, and emotional centers is established in ways that sustained attention on tasks that others might find relatively easy to maintain becomes a challenge [337]. There are, of course, certain values ascribed to a neurotypical brain versus someone (and this category of people has tremendous diversity within it) who is neurodiverse. Children and adults with sensory processing disorder may have challenges in integrating multichannel sensory and motor outputs [338].

Inflammation

Microglial cells are a specialized, macrophage-like cell that live within the immune privileged compartment of the central nervous system [339]. They are present from embryological development. When inflammation is prolonged, the microglial cells will begin to revert to glycolysis instead of aerobic metabolism. This produces lactate as a byproduct. Microglial cells will also show mitochondrial fission under these circumstances [340].

Melatonin has immune downregulating effects in the brain, a reason why proper circadian rhythms are important [341]. C-reactive protein is elevated in patients with major depression, a sign that systemic inflammation is contributing [342]. Likewise, patients with post-COVID syndrome exhibit changes to cognition and mood [343].

The blood-brain barrier (BBB) is an important source of integrity. While not an absolute boundary, it does regulate passage of proteins into the brain and in that way can module or control inflammation [344]. With brain aging, oxidative stress, or toxin injury, the endothelial glycocalyx of the brain blood vessels is damaged, and this is the beginning of a loss of microstructure and integrity of the BBB. That allows more inflammatory cells, as well as proteins that those cells might mount a reaction to, to penetrate the brain.

Deeper Inflammation and Immune Involvement

Inflammation can progress to more robust and sustained microglial cell activation, with increased oxidative stress and damage to neurons. In conditions such as multiple sclerosis, direct immune system intrusion into the CNS can create acute inflammatory lesions, when myelin protein becomes the target.

When neurons are stricken with excessive amyloid protein and other injuries, they can be pushed toward necroptosis instead of apoptosis [345]. When tumor necrosis factor levels are high, such as in systemic inflammation, this can also push cellular death in the brain toward necroptosis. This is triggered by receptor-interacting protein kinase 1 (RIPK1) and similar kinases. Necroptosis promotes further cell death and neuroinflammation in diseases such as multiple sclerosis, sclerosis, amyotrophic lateral sclerosis, Parkinson's disease, and Alzheimer's disease.

A downside of necroptosis is that it releases damage-associated molecular patterns (DAMP). Instead of neurons simply fragmenting into smaller, nonviable units as in apoptosis (which remodeling cells such as microglia can prune away), the DAMP can activate more forceful immune responses by binding to Toll-like receptors on white blood cells. This can accelerate a cycle of injury.

Inflammation is meant to come to an end, and inflammation terminating signals such as resolvins (specialized pro-resolving mediators or SMP) can achieve this. These are produced from long-chain essential fatty acids such as the 20-carbon eicosapentaenoic acid and the 22-carbon docosahexaenoic acid [346, 347]. In chronic or severe acute inflammatory conditions in the CNS, the SMP are not able to control the inflammation, sometimes due to the inciting damaging event still being in operation. A brain abscess is an extreme example.

CNS infections can be acute and chronic [348]. In the pre-antibiotic era, chronic CNS infections such as latent and tertiary syphilis occurred because of *Treponema pallidum* infection. This still occurs in the United States and globally, but not at the scale that it once did. Fungal infections are more likely to strike those who are immunocompromised. Aggressive bacterial infections, whether of the meninges or as a brain abscess, can occur in those subjected to overwhelming exposure, immunocompromised including those taking biologic drugs that block deep immune reactions, and due to traumatic events that physically break the blood-brain barrier.

Viruses can cause encephalitis and there are many instances. More recently, SARS-CoV-2 has been shown to create microhemorrhages in the brain as well as to induce neuron apoptosis. Herpes viruses have long been known to lead to CNS infection, as has measles (*Morbillivirus*).

From the late twentieth century until now, medicine has struggled to prevent and treat various tick-borne illnesses. Lyme disease due to the bacteria *Borrelia burgdorferi* is a prime example, and it can cause long-term symptoms that are clearly a transection of latent or occult infection, immune activation, various cell death pathways, and the ill effects of cytokine levels that perpetuate inflammation and ongoing, dysfunctional immune involvement in the CNS [349]. These are often complex issues that are difficult for a drug orientation approach to address, with serological issues that require expertise. This underscores a fact about many neurological disorders that they can require particularly astute detective work to ascertain a diagnosis.

An interesting hypothesis is that chronic fungal infections can accelerate Alzheimer's disease. This is one possible etiology that can amplify the damage process. There are many gut and brain relationships that are still being investigated, including translocation of microorganisms from the gut to the brain [350].

In traumatic injury to the brain, astrocytes sometimes create ongoing damage as a secondary response to the initial injury. Microglial cells, much like macrophages elsewhere in the body, have an M1/M2 dualism. The M1 microglial cells are pro-inflammatory and can be destructive. The M2 type of microglial cells is pro-repair [351, 352]. Activation of aggressive astrocyte responses (or too prolonged response) and M1/M2 microglia imbalance may account for some of the differences in degree of repair and degeneration in people who have suffered traumatic brain injury.

Multiple sclerosis is an autoimmune disease where self-directed T helper (Th)1 and Th17 cells turn their guns on the brain and myelinated cells in the spinal cord [353]. Antigens, quite possibly gut originated, ramp up cytokines such as interleukin (IL)-1 and interferon (IFN)-γ by Th1 cells and IL-17 by Th17 cells. This has a cascading effect on immune activation, and with the further recruitment of matrix metalloproteinases, there is damage to the blood-brain barrier. That breach of the barrier for immune privilege allows cytotoxic T cells to get into the CNS.

Glutamate excitotoxicity is a mechanism of rapid damage that is under investigation as a contributing factor and perhaps inciting cause for neurodegenerative diseases such as amyotrophic lateral sclerosis [354]. N-methyl-3,4-methylenedioxyamphetamine (MDMA) is known as "ecstasy" and is used as a drug of abuse. It can cause excessive release of glutamate in the hippocampus and serotonin release in the brain. This is contributing to the feelings of well-being and excitement the drug induces. In mouse and rat models, MDMA can damage the hippocampus and the substantia nigra. While translation to human effects is less clear, it is a reminder that substances that cause extreme elevations in neurotransmitters (beyond what is typically considered a therapeutic effect), such as MDMA, cocaine, methamphetamine, etc., may have long-term sequelae. Likewise, agricultural workers who are exposed to pesticides appear to have a higher incidence of neurodegeneration [355].

Of importance in our society of high omega-6 consumption from heavily processed seed oils is the pathway of cellular death known as ferroptosis [356]. This is an iron catalyzed pathway to cell death. It can occur when the hydroxyl radical is formed in the presence of iron. An amplified form of this damage can occur in neurons involving polyunsaturated fatty acids. Reactive oxygen species from mitochondrial activity can cause a propagating reaction (a chain reaction) of oxidation of lipids. Iron can accelerate this process, and create a necrosis reaction. Much like the aforementioned necroptosis, the damage-associated molecular patterns can bind to Toll-like receptors on immune cells and activate immune responses that can cause more damage. Ferroptosis-induced inflammation will also cause a rise in expression of NF-κB which has an association with cancer.

Fibrosis and Extracellular Matrix Degeneration

As neurological degeneration proceeds, signs of permanent reaction to injury will accumulate. Tau protein and amyloid will accrue. Tau protein is evidence of disintegration of microtubules in the neuron [357]. This is sometimes described as neurofibrillary tangles. This is true of both Azlherimer's disease and other sources of dementia. Cerebrovascular disease will lead to dementia, and blood vessels will eventually show signs of atherosclerotic plaque accumulation and stiffening due to calcium deposition (Table 8.23). Amyloid will develop after acute injury, such as from a brain abscess or radiation therapy for cancer. White matter may be disrupted and show sclerosis.

In brains that are aging rapidly, those beset with dementia, and those with inflammatory conditions, there are changes to the extracellular matrix. Hyaluronic acid might decrease and have a negative effect on neuroplasticity and repair. The perineuronal (and perisynaptic) nets, which depend on the matrix, are damaged by overactivation of microglial cells [358, 359]. These defensive cells can be triggered by BBB disruptions, the intrusion of lipopolysaccharide due to bacterial infections, and the presence of pro-inflammatory cytokines. When the perisynaptic nets disappear, neurons are vulnerable and can be destroyed. Like the foundation of a house, the extracellular matrix plays a critical role in brain integrity.

In multiple sclerosis, in time, a fibrosis and loss of function occur instead of healing and remyelination [360]. This leads to a worsening of the clinical course of the disease, with disability and loss of motor and sensory functions. Oligodendrocyte cells ought to "patch up" the demyelinated areas but they fail to do so. The extracellular matrix in this situation begins to change, with a different composition of proteins, including chondroitin sulfate. In that sense, the matrix did not initially cause the damage, but it permits more inflammation to continue and block proper repair. A matrix dysfunction is strongly associated with the fibrotic and permanently damaged state in multiple sclerosis. Likewise, matrix dysfunction is associated with dementia progression, as well as some neuropsychiatric disorders such as bipolar disorder and schizophrenia.

Decline of Function

Imaging, including vascular perfusion studies, shows that there are losses to gray matter in neurodegeneration [361]. Cortical atrophy coincides with enlargement of ventricles [362]. This outstrips the adaptive resources of the brain, such as neuroplastic movement of memories and functions, over to the remaining healthy areas. In people suffering from post-traumatic brain injury, this can progress to encephalitis. Not only is there cortical shrinkage, but synaptic density is reduced, and the same kind of plaques that characterize other dementia causes is present.

Dementia and states like it are evidenced by loss of executive function, memory, learning ability, and eventually motor skills and sensory processing (Table 8.24). Diseases like multiple sclerosis may start with white matter damage with motor and

Table 8.24 Alzheimer's disease assessment scale-cognitive subscale

1. Word recall task: you are given three chances to recall as many words as possible from a list of 10 words that you were shown. This tests short-term memory
2. Naming objects and fingers: several real objects are shown to you, such as a flower, pencil, and a comb, and you are asked to name them. You then have to state the name of each of the fingers on the hand, such as pinky, thumb, etc. This is similar to the Boston Naming Test in that it tests for naming ability, although the BNT uses pictures instead of real objects to prompt a reply
3. Following commands: you are asked to follow a series of simple but sometimes multistep directions, such as "make a fist" and "place the pencil on top of the card"
4. Constructional praxis: this task involves showing you four different shapes, progressively more difficult such as overlapping rectangles, and then you will be asked to draw each one. Visuospatial abilities become impaired as dementia progresses, and this task can help measure these skills
5. Ideational praxis: in this section, the test administrator asks you to pretend you have written a letter to yourself, fold it, place it in the envelope, seal the envelope, address it, and demonstrate where to place the stamp. (While this task is still appropriate now, this could become less relevant as people write and send fewer letters through the mail.)
6. Orientation: your orientation is measured by asking you what your first and last name are, the day of the week, date, month, year, season, time of day, and location. This will determine whether you are oriented x 1, 2, 3, or 4
7. Word recognition task: in this section, you are asked to read and try to remember a list of 12 words. You are then presented with those words along with several other words and asked if each word is one that you saw earlier or not. This task is similar to the first task, with the exception that it measures your ability to recognize information, instead of recall it
8. Remembering test directions: your ability to remember directions without reminders or with a limited amount of reminders is assessed
9. Spoken language: the ability to use language to make yourself understood is evaluated throughout the duration of the test
10. Comprehension: your ability to understand the meaning of words and language over the course of the test is assessed by the test administrator
11. Word-finding difficulty: throughout the test, the test administrator assesses your word-finding ability throughout spontaneous conversation [417]

sensory implications, but continued inflammation can eventually lead to cognitive changes for some patients.

Regardless of the etiology, chronic neuroinflammation, toxin accumulation, and attrition of cells will lead to severe consequences and profound neurological deficits.

Neoplasia

Many neurodegenerative issues are not direct causes of cancer in the central nervous system. Various types of brain tumors can arise, including the glioblastoma, including unfortunately in children. Metastases, from lung, breast, colon, and other cancers, can travel to the brain.

Some recent research suggests that melanoma may spread to the brain making amyloid protein similar to that found in Alzheimer's patients [363]. Melanoma cells make a protein known as amyloid-beta. This protein can activate the astrocytes in the brain and create a neuroinflammation that encourages metastasis. While this is not a causal relationship between the two diseases, it is noteworthy that amyloid can create this cancer-enabling environment.

Therapy

Neurological diseases vary greatly in their presentation and the regions of the central nervous system that they impact. Some neurological conditions only directly impact the peripheral nervous system. Even though specific attention must be given to diagnosis, etiology, and treatment, there are some common themes that underlie many CNS conditions. The treatment progression that follows is aimed at reducing damaging factors and processes and increasing resilience.

Address Determinants of Health

Sleep has a major impact on health and the function of the brain [330, 331]. For reasons outlined above, it is important to have deeper (stage 3 and 4) sleep, as well as REM sleep (Table 8.25). In order to do that, sleep must be deep and prolonged enough so that a cycle of sufficient duration (at least 90 min) can play out. Sleep hygiene is a term for creating the conditions for sleep such as: being relaxed, having a quiet cool room, blocking out artificial light from outside or devices in the house, restricting caffeine later in the day, not eating too close to bedtime, and addressing muscle tension and pain. Patients with central or obstructive apnea will need to have those issues addressed. Sometimes weight loss is helpful, but chronic sleep apnea ought to be evaluated by a sleep specialist.

Table 8.25 Therapeutic considerations in neurological disorders

Mode of therapeutic intervention	Examples	Comments
Address determinants of health	Sleep	May be deficient due to apnea, lifestyle, light exposure, pain, and stress—solution depends on finding cause
Address determinants of health	Socialization/support	Individuals have different needs; isolation and mental deterioration are major risks for the elderly
Address determinants of health	Hydration	Can impair condition performance. Thirst may not be a sufficient indicator of hydration
Biochemical support	Mitochondrial antioxidant support: zinc, copper, vitamin C, vitamin E	Plant food-rich diets can achieve this although zinc status may need additional support
Biochemical support	*Bacopa monnieri*	Improved memory and learning, decrease amyloid accumulation
Biochemical support	*Salvia officinalis*	Improved memory and learning
Biochemical support	N-acetylcysteine	Support acetylcholine production
Biochemical support	Vitamin B12	Methylation support
Biochemical support	*Panax ginseng*	Neural repair, cognitive enhancing, anti-inflammatory, reduce amyloid and Tau accumulation
Biochemical support	*Ginkgo biloba*	Cognitive enhancement, hippocampal protective, preconditioning against ischemia, improve function in dementia (mild)
Biochemical support	*Withania somnifera*	Neuroregenerative, antioxidant support, neuroprotective
Biochemical support	*Hericium erinaceus*	Neuroregenerative, increase BDNF, antidepressive
Biochemical support	*Rhodiola rosea*	Increase catecholamine activity, increase resistance to stress
Biochemical support	*Curcuma longa*	Reduces neuroinflammation, neuroprotective; nanoparticle delivery shows promise
Biochemical support	*Cannabis sativa*	Reduces pain, spasticity, and anxiety. Can also reduce inflammation. THC doses should be small. CBD has a U-shaped dose-response curve
Biochemical support	Vitamin D	Address deficiency, reduce neuroinflammation
Biochemical support	Alpha-lipoic acid	Versatile antioxidant, decrease loss of brain mass (early disease)

Table 8.25 (continued)

Mode of therapeutic intervention	Examples	Comments
Hormetic effects	Very low-dose THC	Increase in cognitive function but only at very low doses
Hormetic effects	Exercise	AMPK, SIRT3, neurogenesis
Hormetic effects	Caloric restriction	Metabolic switch, PGC1α, BDNF activation
Hormetic effects	Dietary sources of NRF activators	Increase protection from oxidative stress (ARE activation)
Whole person therapies	Fermented foods, probiotics	SCFA production, improved gut integrity, lowered inflammation
Whole person therapies	Wahls/modified Paleolithic diet	Decrease autoimmune activity and brain destruction
Whole person therapies	Omega-3 supplementation or rich food sources	Decrease inflammation, brain structure (cod liver oil was an omega-3 source prescribed by MS treatment researcher Dr. Swank)
Whole person therapies	Movement therapy and Feldenkrais	Neuromuscular activity increases sensory input to the brain; better brain and body communication; improved proprioception; alternate or more efficient ways to move
Whole person therapy	Physical therapy	Increase strength and coordination
Whole person therapy	Occupational therapy	Learn new skills for daily activities, sensory processing and sensory, brain, and muscular integration
Whole person therapy	Detoxification	Decrease blood-brain barrier damage, decrease damage to the brain extracellular matrix (improve integrity of quadripartite synapse)
Dampen maladaptive responses	Prednisone	Decrease inflammation rapidly, limit damage in autoimmune or post-trauma situations
Dampen maladaptive responses	Antispasmodics: baclofen (drug); *Valeriana officinalis*, *Scutellaria lateriflora* (botanical medicines)	Decrease pain and stiffness
Maintain homeostasis with external control	Ketamine and NMDA antagonists	Decrease depression
Maintain homeostasis with external control	Psilocybin	Serotonin activity
Maintain homeostasis with external control	L-dopa	Provide dopamine for movement regulation

(continued)

Table 8.25 (continued)

Mode of therapeutic intervention	Examples	Comments
Maintain homeostasis with external control	Anticholinergics	Decrease rigidity (Parkinson's)
Maintain homeostasis with external control	Recombinant antibodies (i.e., natalizumab)	Deactivate immune signals
Maintain homeostasis with external control	TNF blockers	Suppress inflammation that would target the brain
Maintain homeostasis with external control	Aricept and acetylcholinesterase	Increase memory and cognition

Socialization and mental stimulation are paramount. Humans are social beings, and if support and interaction with others is cut short, actual cognitive changes will start occurring. Taking on mental challenges, such as learning new skills, new languages, exploring neighborhoods, and solving puzzles, is important for neuroplasticity to stay optimized [333]. The brain, including the hippocampus, responds to demands made upon it. Likewise, if someone, especially later in life, simply repeats the same routines and doesn't learn new things or take on new challenges, they begin to lose global intellectual capacity [364]. The challenges that can spur hippocampal activation do not have to be the same in one's eighth decade as in one's third decade. But novelty and the creation of new neural pathways are the key.

Adequate hydration, which might mean drinking somewhat beyond thirst, and a diet that supplies steady energy are an improvement for many patients. The brain may prefer glucose, but sudden extreme spikes in blood sugar followed by insulin-driven crashes do not make for steady concentration and peak mental performance. That's why a glycemically balanced menu, with more complex carbohydrate sources, healthy fats, and adequate protein, is needed.

Biochemical Support

Mitochondrial Support

Mitochondrial dysfunction or death can be a source of necroptosis of neurons. This leads to loss of functioning neurons but also inflammatory reactions that can lead to further damage [365]. Superoxide (oxygen with an unpaired electron) is very destructive of all aspects of the cell: DNA, organelles including mitochondria, cell membrane, etc. Mitochondria contain many fatty acids which are there for beta oxidation. Free radical damage to one fatty acid can cause a propagation reaction and massive fatty acid oxidation within the mitochondria. Superoxide dismutase (SOD) is an important step in removing the superoxide anion, although catalase and glutathione are important to take the product of SOD, which is hydrogen peroxide, into water and stable oxygen. The sirtuin-3 protein will increase SOD activity. When polyunsaturated fatty acids are oxidized, one of the byproducts is the aldehyde 4-hydroxynonenal (HNE). This reaction compound can covalently modify cysteine, lysine, and histidine residues of proteins and alter to degrade their function. Zinc, copper, and manganese are cofactors of SOD. Vitamin C and vitamin E are important for regenerating glutathione [366]. *N*-acetylcarnitine can be a source of fuel for the mitochondria, which is well absorbed by the body. It can also enter the brain and provide acetyl groups for the making of acetylcholine. This is an important neurotransmitter for memory and attention.

Bacopa monnieri

Bacopa monnieri is a plant with a long use in Ayurvedic medicine for improving mental abilities and sleep and to enhance the sensory organs. Biochemically, it has antioxidant and anti-inflammatory effects, and it can block amyloid production (Table 8.25). It also improves memory and mental processing.

In shorter-term boosts to memory, *Bacopa* does increase synthesis and persistence (via inhibition acetylcholinesterase) of the neurotransmitter acetylcholine [367]. Some of the active constituents which are linked most directly to CNS effects are the triterpenoid saponins. These are the bacosides, a family of about 12 compounds. These compounds reduce markers of DNA damage and increase antioxidant enzymes.

In small trials with *Bacopa*, improvements in the following have been noted:

- General recall.
- Orientation to stimuli.
- Executive function.
- Digit forward and backward counting.
- Visual reproduction (drawing a picture based on a picture viewed seconds ago) [368–370].

Salvia officinalis

Commonly known as sage, there are several varieties, with *S. officinalis* being used in herbal medicine most commonly. *Salvia* has many compounds in it, both phenolics, terpenes, and flavonoids.

Phenolic compounds include the following:

- Caffeic acid
- Vanillic acid
- Ferulic acid

- Rosmarinic acid
- Salvianolic acid
- Lithospermic acid
- Sagerinic acid
- Yunnaneic acid

Flavonoids include the following:

- Luteolin
- Apigenin
- Hispidulin
- Kaempferol
- Quercetin

Terpenes include the following:

- Alpha-thujone
- Beta-thujone
- Cineole
- Alpha-humulene
- Beta-caryophyllene
- Carnosic acid
- Ursolic acid

The flavonoids, and the phenolic compounds seem to limit oxidative stress and injury to neurons. Much of this oxidative stress originates from the respiratory mechanisms of the mitochondria. The flavonoids such as luteolin and quercetin can increase BDNF. Terpenes have numerous CNS effects, including interaction with the endocannabinoid system. Rosmarinic acid and ursolic acid have hippocampal protective activities [371].

B12

Vitamin B12 is an important factor in methylation reactions. Populations of both children and the elderly who have adequate B12 status perform better on cognitive tests than those who are deficient. Deficiency can occur because of lack of dietary intake and also due to gastrointestinal changes, such as inflammatory bowel disease resulting in ileitis (B12 is absorbed in the ileum), ileal bypass surgery, atrophic gastritis, pernicious anemia, gastric bypass surgery (the intrinsic factor from the stomach needs to bind properly with B12 for optimal absorption), and various polymorphisms that lead to relative lack of enzymes (i.e., methylene tetrahydrofolate reductase (MTHFR), transcobalamin 2 receptor (TCN2)) [372]. These polymorphisms are not always severe enough to cause deficiency, but they can be, or they can combine to result in B12 deficiency. In these situations, intramuscular B12 or even sublingual B12 supplementation would be indicated.

Panax ginseng

Ginseng has a long history of use in traditional Chinese medicine as a whole person tonic, with many applications for fatigue, aging, and poor immune function. It is a widely used herb across the world, with the United States being a major cultivator and exporter of the herb. It is considered an adaptogen, in that it can increase resistance to stress and endurance. It has numerous compounds that have a positive effect on cognition [370] (Table 8.25).

Beta amyloid (Aβ) is formed in the body from Aβ precursor protein (APP). As has been mentioned, it creates cellular debris that leads to some of the plaquing observed in the brains of those with dementia, including Alzheimer's. It is inhibited by extracts of ginseng [373, 374].

Some of the many compounds isolated and studied from *Panax ginseng* include the following:

20S-protopanaxadiol
Panaxadiol
Ginsenoside a1
Ginsenoside a2
Ginsenoside Rb1
Ginsenoside Rb2
Ginsenoside Rb3
Ginsenoside Rg2
Ginsenoside Rg3
Ginsenoside Rh3
Ginsenoside Rg 4
Panaxoside Rg4
Panaxoside Rg1
Panaxoside R4
Panaxoside Re
Panaxoside Rh1
Panaxoside a1
Panaxoside a2
Panaxoside Rh1
Panaxoside R1
Notoginsenoside ST4

The research on *Panax ginseng* ranges from rodent models to clinical trials. In terms of biochemical actions, it appears that the above compounds, to varying degrees, can:

Reduce amyloid accumulation.
Reduce neurofibrillary tangles.
Decrease neuronal apoptosis.
Decrease neuroinflammation via NF-κB.
Inhibit acetylcholinesterase and boost acetylcholine levels in the brain.

Increase expression of BDNF (which may be an effect secondary to above actions).

Panax ginseng has some neuroprotective and recovery benefits from those with acute CNS injury from stroke [375]. Ginsenoside Rb1 appears to be particularly suited for this task. Ischemic stroke (versus hemorrhagic) is where a thrombus has formed leading to blockage of blood flow and ischemia in the brain. A standard and helpful medical treatment is recombinant tissue plasminogen activator (rt-PA). This treatment can cause brain bleeds, but co-administration of GRb1 may reduce this risk.

In addition to cognitive and neurorehabilitative effects of ginseng, it may also be useful for patients with depression if neuroinflammation is prominent, and it has proven its usefulness as an adaptogen for those under stress [376, 377].

Ginkgo biloba

Ginkgo biloba, the maidenhair tree, is used extensively for circulatory support, including cerebral circulation. It has protective actions on the hippocampus (Table 8.25). It also seems to have pretreatment effects on the brain, to protect it from future ischemic events [378, 379].

A 2019 publication in *CNS Neuroscience and Therapeutics* by the Asian Clinical Expert Group on Neurocognitive Disorders created evidence-based consensus recommendations regarding the use of EGb 761® in neurocognitive disorders with/without cerebrovascular disease [380]. EGb 761 is a standardized extract of *Ginkgo biloba* that has a set amount of terpenoids such as bilobide. (Many commercial products also standardize to flavone glycosides (24%).)

The Asian Expert Group stated that key randomized trials and robust meta-analyses have demonstrated significant improvement in cognitive function, neuropsychiatric symptoms, activities of daily living (ADL), and quality of life with EGb 761® versus placebo in patients with mild-to-moderate dementia. The group also stated that those with mild cognitive impairment showed improvement.

Ginkgo biloba decreases platelet-activating factor. For those taking anticoagulants, they may have to avoid this herb. Many surgical centers will not operate if the patient has used *Ginkgo biloba* in the preceding 10 days. But for the average patient, *Ginkgo* does not seem to be a problem in terms of bleeding.

It is also important to note that *Ginkgo* will not prevent Alzheimer's disease from occurring, nor will it work as effectively in making improvements in those with very advanced dementia.

Withania somnifera

Withania somnifera is also known as ashwagandha, another adaptogenic herb with a traditional use in Ayurvedic medicine for thousands of years. It has been used in that system of medicine for calming the mind but also as an anthelmintic, astringent, and aphrodisiac. Compounds include a series of similar withanosides and withanolides. There are also the compounds denosomin and sominone. In experimental models, these compounds can protect neurons from injury and help to degrade beta amyloid proteins in the neuron that can become senile plaques [370, 381]. They also support neurite outgrowth in vitro, axonal regeneration in vitro, and synaptic reconstruction in vitro and in vivo. Memory improvement is another observation in animal research models. In animal models, *Withania* hastened recovery from injuries (such as contusions) to the spinal cord.

In experimental models of Parkison's disease, with induction from toxins that resemble pesticides used in agriculture, *Withania* was protective. It reduced cell death and increased glutathione levels in the substantia nigra. This might be helpful in reducing the attrition of dopaminergic cells, although data from human studies is lacking. *Withania* compounds are lipid protecting and relieve oxidative stress, and this might be central to their ability to prevent neuronal damage and the damaging effects of calcium influx that can follow from such damage.

Hericium erinaceus

Hericium erinaceus, or lion's mane mushroom, has gained popularity as a dietary supplement. It has a broad array of compounds that goes beyond the common immunomodulating beta-glucans found in many medicinal mushrooms. It contains β-glucans, erinacines, hericenones, alkaloids, sterols, and volatile aromatic compounds [382]. Ergothioneine is a sulfur-containing derivative of the amino acid, histidine. It is a remarkable compound in this mushroom that may protect neural tissue from hypoxia-inducing factors. Its ability to enter the brain is superior to some other substances due to the ERGO-specific transporter OCTN1/SLC22A4. It seems to be a neuron-specific antioxidant. This is not only important for preventing aging but helpful for those patients attempting to recover from neurologic damage and neuroinflammation. This could include patients suffering a relapse of multiple sclerosis and those with ongoing neuroinflammation due to viral infections or autoimmune disorders. It has antidepressive function and may increase BDNF levels.

Rhodiola rosea

Rhodiola rosea is a cognitive support herb, often used for those with fatigue and under stress. It may support neurotransmitter levels, especially in those with depression, or cognitive impairment (Table 8.25). It may also increase neuron viability. It can boost monoamines (serotonin, norepinephrine, and dopamine) and acetylcholine (memory) in the presynaptic terminals of neurons. It may even increase the number of serotonin receptors in some parts of the brain. It seems to have an anti-inflammatory effect on the brain. It has well-known positive effects on stress and in lowering feelings of aggression [371, 383, 384]. *Rhodiola* can, like other adaptogens, help patients adapt to stress. It seems to do that by acting as a corticotropin-releasing factor antagonist, which lowers total cortisol release. This is important in helping level off stress responses, so that these responses are present but not excessive.

Curcuma longa

Turmeric is a dietary spice made from the root of *Curcuma longa*. Curcuminoids are one fraction of the compounds in this plant, and curcumin is the most plentiful of the curcuminoids. It has been studied extensively and found to have anti-inflammatory and chemopreventive properties. It reduces microglial responses [385, 386]. The problem with curcumin is that it has impressive pharmacodynamics but poor pharmacokinetics. It is difficult to absorb, it is rapidly metabolized and excreted, and it does not always even make it to the cellular target in question. Absorption is increased by packing the curcumin with phosphatidylcholine or taking it with *Piper nigrum* (black pepper).

A newer technology is that of using curcumin nanoparticles. These are well absorbed and may deliver more curcumin to the actual targets [387].

As an anti-inflammatory for multiple sclerosis, it seems to have benefits. Nanoparticle curcumin, when administered to patients with multiple sclerosis, has changed gene expression of pro-inflammatory cytokines, evidenced by real-time polymerase chain reaction testing [388]. The mRNA expression of genes for IL-1B, TNF-α, NF-κB, and other cytokines that can lead to poor MD progression was reduced by curcumin (in nanoparticles). This delivery form of curcumin also has been shown to decrease the levels of Th17 lymphocytes, which are implicated in more disease activity. Myelin basic protein increased in patients treated with curcumin in nanoparticles, which suggests that it may increase healing and restoration of nerve function in those with relapsing-remitting MS.

In research involving the mechanisms of Parkinson's disease (molecule models, not human studies), curcumin nanoparticles seemed to reduce the oxidative stress and inflammation of the kind that destroys dopaminergic cells in the brain. An experimental delivery system uses nanoparticles to deliver L-dopa and curcumin [389]. It's doubtful that curcumin will become a mainstay for Alzheimer's disease. In all likelihood, a combination of anti-inflammatory and circulatory-stimulating measures are more important. Curcumin seems to be effective in animal models of experimental autoimmune encephalomyelitis (EAE) which is used to study MS pathogenesis. By extension, other neuroinflammatory diseases, such as chronic Lyme disease or some presentations of post-COVID syndrome, might be the more specific situations where curcumin can do the most good. It does appear that particular attention must be paid to pharmacokinetics if curcumin is to live up to its potential based on earlier explorations of its molecular targets.

Cannabinoids

Cannabis sativa is a widely used medicinal plant that also has well-known recreational uses. It is used safely by some and overused and abused by others and occasionally, like most psychoactive substances, can cause adverse reactions. Too much, following the typically pattern of a U-shaped dose-response curve, can suppress attention and memory. Recent research indicates that substantial use of cannabis over time can lead to impaired cognitive performance.

Cannabis has developed into innumerable cultivars, which has created variable combinations of compound ratios across them. The three most studied compounds in *Cannabis* are tetrahydrocannabinol (THC), cannabidiol (CBD), and the terpenes. There are several isomers of THC and of CBD. The terpenes are ones that are commonly seen in other plants: pinene, linalool, caryophyllene, humulene, myrcene, and many others. These compounds all have different affinities for receptors and different clinical or physiological effects (differences which are less distinct within these categories) [390].

The compounds in *Cannabis* bind to the receptors of the endocannabinoid system [391]. This is a response to injury/adaptive protection system found throughout the body. The natural agonists are *N*-arachidonoyl-ethanolamine (AEA; anandamide) and 2-arachidonoylglycerol (2-AG). Activation of this system decreased inflammation, pain, spasticity, and anxiety. There are two types of receptors in this system. The CB1 receptors are congregated in the central nervous system but have extra CNS presence. The CB2 receptors are located outside of the CNS, particularly on cells of the immune system, but there are CB2 receptors there.

THC binds to CB1, leading to reductions in pain, spasticity, and anxiety. It is also psychoactive and can cause euphoria, sensory changes, and for some people dissociative and even hallucinatory symptoms. Cannabidiol (CBD) acts as a partial antagonist to the CB1 receptor, which might offset some of the psychoactive effects, when patients take products that have a mix of these compounds [392, 393].

CBD binds to the CB2 receptors, and this has an anti-inflammatory, antispasmodic, and anodyne effect. Although much of this activity is in the extra CNS and immune cells, some CBD do bind to microglial cells in the brain and have an anti-inflammatory effect. Terpenes bind to cannabinoid receptors and may also modulate them—changing the receptor's behavior when it encounters natural or exogenous ligands that bind to it. Terpenes also have action on cellular membrane proteins that are called transient receptor potential cation channels (TRP). These are involved in the modulation of pain signals. The actual endocannabinoid system and the greater TRP population may have interactions that regulate pain.

There are many variables in treatment when considering two distinct receptors (CB1 and CB2), dozens of active compounds, and interrelated systems (immune, TRP, etc.) [394]. Moreover, different cultivars of *Cannabis sativa* have different signature levels of compounds, depending on their genetics but also the soil, harvesting time, climate, etc. To add to this complexity, dispensary preparations have different compound levels due to manipulation of these factors. This makes for a different level of complexity in studying these medicines versus looking at a single agent. There are single agents in use. The natural product cannabidiol (CBD) is used as an often self-prescribed over the counter supplement but also doctor recommended. This is distilled however to create a CBD isolate. There are synthetic THC-like and CBD-like products on the market. Some are FDA-approved for seizures or spasticity. Other products place THC to CBD compounds in a 1:20 (for instance) ratio. A full-spectrum cannabis product has the full gamut of compounds. A broad-spectrum product is effectively "THC free" but has dozens of other compounds. As mentioned, CBD isolate is supposed to have just cannabidiol.

The synergy that occurs between these compounds can be part of their power. This has been referred to as the "entourage effect." Herbal synergy is not a new concept. Physicians and healers that use plants as medicines have been aware of this clinically for centuries. Recent research has described instances of synergy using modern pharmaceutical chemistry techniques of extraction, isolation, and identification of compounds and testing them using cell assay methods to detect changes in effect. For instance, Wagner et al. found that numerous compounds in Saint John's wort extract (*Hypericum perforatum*) could impact multiple receptor sites at neurons [395].

Cannabis preparations can be used to treat spasticity [396]. This occurs when damage to upper motor neurons leads to loss of regulation and inhibition of lower motor neurons. Multiple sclerosis, cerebral vascular events, or amyotrophic lateral sclerosis can cause this upper motor neuron damage.

Pain relief is possible with cannabis products [397]. Neuropathic pain can result from impingement of nerve roots or even pressure on the spinal cord due to spinal stenosis. Diabetic neuropathy can lead to neuritis. Some patients have a central pain syndrome and complex regional pain syndrome, which might be somewhat downregulated by the use of a full-spectrum product. Even using CBD isolate can help with sleep in the case of this chronic pain syndrome or fibromyalgia.

Neuroinflammation might be alleviated by cannabis products. This can be chronic, such as some cases of depression, or episodic, such as in relapsing-remitting multiple sclerosis. Even though the brain is more CB1 dominant, the activation of CB2 receptors there can downregulate inflammation.

Vitamin D

Vitamin D starts as calciferol in the skin which serves as a precursor but must be activated by ultraviolet light. It is hydroxylated in the liver to 25-hydroxyvitamin D [25(OH)D] and then hydroxylated again in the kidney to its physiologically active form 1,25-dihydroxyvitamin D [1,25(OH)2D], also known as "calcitriol." Vitamin D is also consumed dietarily. Fish and fish liver contain it. Fortified food, such as milk and dairy products, and fortified orange juices are another source.

Vitamin D has a high prevalence of suboptimal levels or even frank deficiency. About one in five adults in the United States does not have recommended serum ranges of vitamin D. It can have anti-inflammatory effects, and when deficient, inflammation may be harder to control. Multiple sclerosis patients may have fewer relapses if they take supplemental D or consume D-rich foods [398].

Alpha-Lipoic Acid

Alpha-lipoic acid is a powerful antioxidant that can operate in both water- and fat-soluble compartments. It has been shown to decrease the rate of brain mass loss in Alzheimer's disease. In experimental models of multiple sclerosis (autoimmune encephalitis), it can decrease T cell intrusion into the brain [370, 399].

Hormetic Support

Certain stimuli can elicit adaptive responses from the central nervous system, and this is observed to be in a typically U-shaped dose (or exposure)-response curve. These are basically hormetic responses, although there is often some overlap and difficulty in differentiation where a biologically protective food or plant is a true hormetin. Aside from the predominant feature of stimulation in the low-dose zone, there is also the feature of direct stimulation and genetic expression versus a strong interplay of agonist and receptor in larger amounts or versus a metabolic/nutritional pathway. That is to say, a secondary response elicited from the brain tissue accounts for the benefit [400].

In a recent discussion of hormesis and cognition, Calabrese describes how the impact of tetrahydrocannabinol (THC) from *Cannabis sativa* (marijuana) has a biphasic dose-response relationship with cognition. Higher amounts of THC may decrease acetylcholine in the brain, but small amounts can increase hippocampal neurogenesis [401]. This appears to be hormetic in nature, with histone acetylation as a positive byproduct of low-dose stimulation. In a mouse model, prolonged oral cannabinoid administration prevents neuroinflammation, lowered β-amyloid levels, and improved cognitive performance. Cannabidiol (CBD), which is found in the plant and has agonist affinity for CBD2 receptors (and some antagonism for CBD1 receptors, which THC is an agonist for), seems to offset cognitive impacts of THC. Perhaps further clinical investigation will show that low THC doses or high CBD-low THC (i.e., a 20:1 ratio) products might have cognitive enhancement effects and possible neural repair impacts on the elderly.

Peroxisome proliferator-activated receptor-gamma coactivator (PGC)-1alpha is a stimulant of mitochondrial biogenesis. Neurons can only create a small amount of the substantial energy they require through glycolysis; about 90% of their energy needs is via oxidative phosphorylation. According to Mattson, dietary restriction and exercise stimulate increased levels of PGC1α and circulating ketones (such as 3-β-hydroxybutyrate), which then induce the expression of BDNF to help maintain dendritic spines [402].

Sirtuins are protective (preserve cell viability, decrease apoptosis, necroptosis) proteins. They are often elicited in response to stressors on the cell. SIRT3 is a sirtuin found in the CNS. Exercise may also induce neuronal expression of SIRT3, which is known to mediate hormetic responses to oxidative, excitotoxic, and bioenergetic stressors through the hyperacetylation of mitochondrial superoxide dismutase 2 and cyclophilin D [403, 404].

The mild and transient increase in cellular oxidative stress (due to upregulation of oxidative phosphorylation) that occurs in exercise can activate the Nrf2-KEAP1 mechanism. This leads to translocation to the nucleus of the Nrf2 protein (nuclear factor erythroid 2-related factor 2). That in turn activates the antioxidant response element which is actually a number of chromosome regions that, when activated, lead to enhanced transcription of antioxidant-detoxification genes. This leads to more of these protective enzymes and proteins, such as superoxide dismutase and glutathione.

Exercise, such as running, stimulates the genesis of new neurons, and intermittent fasting supports their survival and maturation (Fig. 8.11). These activities may

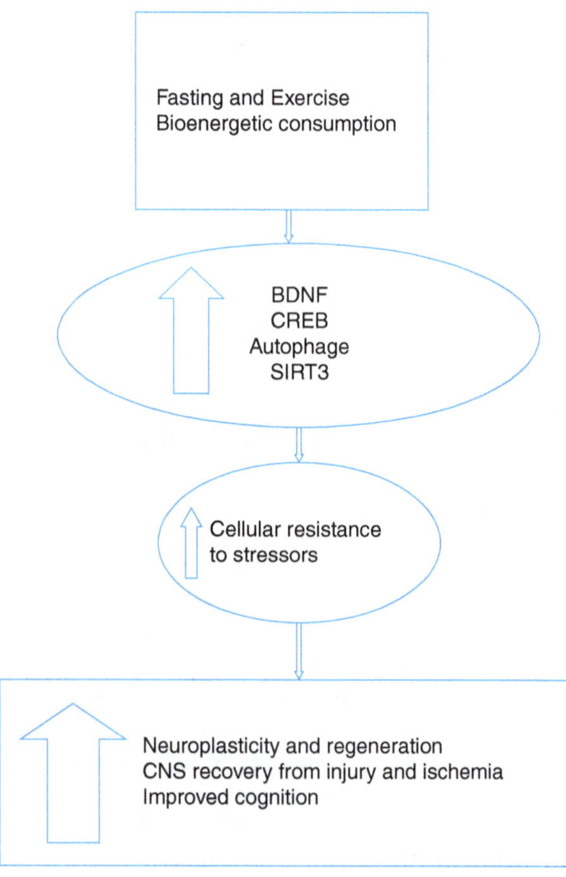

Fig. 8.11 Neuroprotective effects of exercise: as Mattson [405] and others have described, exercise (and caloric restriction) can lead the expression of proteins that protect, repair, and regenerate neural tissues

also positively benefit autophagy (removing deleterious, unneeded proteins in the neuron) (Table 8.25). They also strengthen synaptic plasticity and cognition. AMPK (AMP-activated protein kinase) is a cellular energy status responsive enzyme (activated when the ratio of ATP to AMP and/or ADP decreases which will of course be activated under exercise stress). This enzyme leads to more cleanup of junk proteins via autophagy. Too much AMPK can start to warp and destroy neurons, so the periods of recovery from exercise are important—not only to rest muscles but to allow mitochondria and cellular antioxidant systems to repair and renew themselves [404, 406, 407].

Whole Person Therapy

Gut Brain Pathways

It is well established that the actions of bacterial and other microorganisms in the gut influence the brain. This is accomplished via neurotransmitter production, changes to the immune system, increased or changed transit of gut proteins into the bloodstream, inflammasome complex formation, and neural signals. The brain, via the autonomic nervous system, and the immune system itself can regulate much of the activity in the gut.

The specific microbial profiles in different neurological conditions vary. The pathogenesis of inflammasome activation and its relation to inflammation within the CNS are still an area of investigation. Some common denominators across neuroinflammatory and neurodegenerative diseases have been noted. These include the following:

- Short-chain fatty acid production: decreased SCFA production in the gut, which depends on healthy microflora and the consumption of dietary fiber, appears to be decreased in many neurological condition.
- Decreased diversity of microflora species: in many diseases, the breadth of different species becomes narrowed.
- Increased immune activation due to degradation of tight junctions in between gut epithelial cells: the barrier to protein entry becomes weakened.
- Inflammatory upregulation: gut-associated T lymphocytes, gut innate immune responses, and inflammasomes (special receptors, trigger proteins, and caspase-1) are more populous and active in these neurological conditions [350, 408].

It would be advisable for patients with these conditions to be evaluated for bacterial, fungal, or protozoal overgrowth. They should consume more fiber and eat fermented foods. They might use supplemental probiotic preparations for some period of time, especially if they have been using antibiotics. They should avoid foods to which they are allergic or those that can damage gut integrity, such as excessive sugar alcohols (sorbitol), excessive ethanol, and various food additives such as carrageenan.

Wahls/Modified Paleolithic Diet

The original modified Paleolithic (Wahls™) diet was different than a paleo diet in that it called for nine cups of vegetables a day (including leafy greens, Cruciferae, seaweed, and nutritional yeast). Some gluten-free grains are allowed but no gluten, nightshades, or legumes [408]. This diet has reduced MS-related fatigue, and it is different than a much older diet, the Swank diet, that has low saturated fat and adequate omega-3 [409]. There are current clinical trials for this modified Paleolithic diet underway.

Omega-3 Fatty Acids

These are fatty acids with a carbon-carbon double bond at the omega-3 carbon. They are not synthesized by humans and they are metabolically needed. Generally, omega-3 fats are obtained from eating certain plant foods, such as walnuts and flaxseeds, and eating fish or meat from animals that graze on grass (pastured not lot fed) or were fed high omega-3 feed. Some omega-3 DHA (docosapentaenoic acid) supplements are fungal sources [410].

Not only do these fatty acids make some inflammation-regulating products in the body, but the human brain mass contains many of them. Some modern diets are deficient. The ratio of these fats to the type of omega-6 fats from seed oils (corn, canola, soy, cottonseed, etc.) is quite low. This imbalance can be pro-inflammatory. Moreover, the resolvins that can quell inflammation in the brain are derived from omega-3 fats.

Movement Therapy and Feldenkrais

Movement therapies can be helpful to people with neurological conditions. They send various kinds of sensory input to the brain, which helps with remodeling and repair. Movement therapies, such as yoga, Pilates, dance, water-based exercise, and the Feldenkrais method, can help patients become more efficient in their movements. They relieve tight fascia and can even help patients learn better movement patterns.

Physical Therapy and Occupational Therapy

Physical therapy is extremely important for patients undergoing rehabilitation for stroke [411].

Incredible progress can be made by patients. Those with spinal cord injuries and traumatic brain injuries and those who have been treated for cerebral or spinal neoplasms can benefit from not only strengthening but the motor skills that come with intensive physical therapy. Stiffness and spasticity can be helped by physical therapy, and this is important for those with Parkinson's disease, multiple sclerosis, and other types of upper motor neuron pathology. The physical therapy needed for patients with neurological conditions is more specialized. Smaller centers for therapy that focus on treating sports injury or arthritis-related pains may not have the expertise.

Occupational therapy looks at daily activities, in both efficiency and overcoming obstacles. This is important for those with cognitive impairment. It is also very important for those with some residual deficit, where learning new motor patterns and strategies is needed. Occupational therapists have therapeutic activities that help the brain integrate sensory information, executive function, and motor coordination. This can be helpful for those who have lost function or are having trouble adapting to a changing set of circumstances as they navigate a chronic neurologic disease or recover from a severe episode of accident [412, 413].

Detoxification

Toxins can enter the brain extracellular matrix and cause it to dysfunction. In ways that are being discovered in recent and current research, these matrix changes can impact neural function and response to injury. Synaptic plasticity can be impaired in these circumstances. Mercury and aluminum can accumulate in the brain and can damage the extracellular matrix. Nickel can deplete ascorbic acid, making oxidative stress damage and formation of hydroxylated proteins in the matrix more difficult. While there is no direct way to pull heavy metals, chlorinated compounds, etc. out of the brain, the basic principles of reducing toxin load apply here. That involves the following:

- Reducing exposure.
- Providing nutrients that can act to chelate or bind toxins in the actual tissues.
- Providing the cofactors for the operation of hepatic detoxification enzymes.
- Ensuring that antioxidant levels are adequate.
- Encouraging normal local removal of toxins or toxin-thiol or toxin-protein complexes.
- Opening up eliminative pathways in the body.

In the case of the brain, proper deep sleep and thus activation of the glymphatic system are needed. At the same time, control of inflammation and a high-functioning endothelial environment in the vascular system are needed to protect BBB integrity.

Dampening Pathological Reactions/Maladaptive Responses

In acute neuroinflammatory situations, prednisone is often used in the short term. Patients who have optic neuritis due to MS will be given a high dose of this.

Antispasmodic medicines can help with spasticity. Some herbal medicines can fulfill this purpose, including *Valeriana officinalis*. Benzodiazepines and drugs such as baclofen are used as prescriptions for muscle spasticity. Patients with Parkinson's disease often take anticholinergic medicines to reduce rigidity and tremor.

Maintain Homeostasis by Pharmaceutical Intervention

Biological medicines that strongly control the immune system, such as blocking tumor necrosis factor, are often used as long-term medicines in autoimmune neurological diseases. Newer treatments also include recombinant antibody treatments to block inflammatory cytokines of the immune system.

Neurotransmitter levels are adjusted by some medicines. For example, selective serotonin reuptake inhibitors can raise the level of serotonin in the synapse (Table 8.25). This has been shown to improve depressive symptoms and sometimes anxiety symptoms. Norepinephrine reuptake inhibitors have similar effects. This is the so-called monoamine hypothesis. Newer pathways include drugs that are antagonists to the N-methyl-D-aspartate (NMDA). This is a glutamate-binding receptor. Infusions of ketamine have been shown to cause rapid (in hours) improvements in severely depressed patients. Ketamine can however cause dissociative experiences and is hard to tolerate for some [414]. Research on this class of drugs for depression is ongoing. For patients with Parkinson's disease that lack dopaminergic input, they may take L-dopa in order to provide this catecholamine.

The N-methyl-D-aspartate (NMDA) antagonist drugs are being used to treat Alzheimer's and Parkinson's disease. Glutamate excitotoxicity is one pathway of neural loss due to necroptosis and exuberant inflammatory responses to damage-associated molecular patterns that arise when cells literally fragment. Alzheimer's treatment also continues to involve drugs that boost acetylcholine in the brain, such as Aricept. Drugs that target Tau protein are under investigation for Alzheimer's disease.

Psilocybin is an indolealkylamine that is found in mushrooms [415]. It is being explored for depression treatment and has in studies performed as well as escitalopram, a common antidepressant. Psilocybin has very strong action on the serotonin system. The use of actual mushrooms versus an extracted single agent is, of course, under investigation and in clinical use.

Patients with multiple sclerosis have more options than in the past. Prednisone is still used. Interferon beta-1 has been used since the 1990s for MS. Newer treatments involve monoclonal antibodies that block selective signaling molecules in the immune system. Natalizumab blocks alpha integrins [416]. There are many more and this type of therapy continues to evolve. It is a form of control of immune function. It is not without risks; for patients with progressive multiple sclerosis, these are powerful new tools to prevent disability.

Musculoskeletal System

The musculoskeletal system includes the axial and articular skeleton, ligaments, muscles, tendons, fascia, and—by proximity—peripheral nerves. This is a high-relevance area to naturopathic medicine. Pain is one of the most common office complaints [418]. In developed countries, back pain is the fourth most common office complaint, and arthritis is the sixth most common. There is a commitment in health care as a whole to find non-opioid solutions to pain. Naturopathic approaches work to improve the function of this system and to relieve inflammation and pain. Naturopathic physicians are trained to recognize that physical therapy, pharmacologic intervention, and surgery all have their necessary roles to play in patient management.

There are other aspects of treatment of this system that are relevant to naturopathic medicine. Healing is a phenomenon that can proceed when the conditions for health are met and the physician has facilitated the process of healing. As Zeff and Snider pointed out, structural correction is an important step in the therapeutic approach of naturopathic medicine [419]. Structure does not completely determine function, but it does influence it, and collapse of structure will have serious consequences. For example, patients with emphysema, a form of COPD, have changes to their diaphragmatic function. In obstructive respiratory diseases such as emphysema, the anterior-posterior chest diameter increases. Accessory muscles of breathing are recruited to help push trapped air out of stiff lungs. The change to the dimensions of the thorax leads to less efficient diaphragmatic muscle contraction [87]. This is problematic for the act of breathing itself. Physical therapies involving mobilization to turn breathing back to normal diaphragmatic breathing have been shown to increase blood oxygen levels and slow respiratory rate in COPD patients.

Another example would be the tensile nature and flexibility of the fascial system. Fascia wraps muscles, has innervation, and provides structural support. It has a memory of sorts, in that postural patterns have a way of settling in and the fascia contracts or mobilizes along those lines. If a person has a chronic muscular pain pattern, working to shift their fascial tightness and flexibility seems like an intuitively useful thing to do to make any pain relief they obtain more profound and long-lasting [420].

The articular surfaces of the skeletal system contain different planes of movement and discrete muscular orientation of muscles that synergize or brake (oppose) each other. The surface of joints contains various types of cartilage, which is an avascular, collagen, structure that provides low friction movement. Cartilage is a solidified type of matrix, and it has collagen-producing cells called chondrocytes [421]. Hyaline cartilage is the type found in most appendicular joints. It has type II collagen and is also found in non-joint areas such as the nose and the larynx. Isogenous groups are clusters of chondrocytes (up to 8) that create their own belt of matrix that surrounds them. Fibrous cartilage is found in the joints of the spine, the symphysis pubis, the jaw, and the menisci of the knees. It has more type I collagen, and the chondrocytes are arrayed in rows.

Fibrous joints are found in fixed areas that normally have very little movement, such as sutures in the cranium, and syndesmosis areas such as the radioulnar joint. More common and movable are the synovial joints [422]. These have six general patterns, depending on their planes of motion and configurations, such as "ball and socket." A synovial joint has a joint capsule surrounding it and, on the inner lining of that capsule, a special membrane that secretes a lubricating and protective fluid (Fig. 8.12). These joints will swell when the joint is damaged and inflamed.

The musculoskeletal system has some unique properties in that it has contractile tissue and the scaffolding that allows that contractile tissue to create motion in a purposeful manner [423, 424]. It performs an important role in maintaining blood sugar in that muscles are a major target for the hormone insulin and major glucose consumer. It has communication via the nervous system, and this follows several pathways. Sensory nerves send information to the thalamus via the spinothalamic pathway. Proprioceptive information goes to the brain via the posterior columns and originates in special Golgi bodies in tendons, where muscles attach to bone. Fascia has innervation and blood and lymph flow. For good reasons, fascia and muscle together can be considered as the myofascial system, which has a variety of tissue types with different densities. The brain controls movement, and the CNS receives much sensory data from the body. Not all movement requires conscious control, such as walking or repetitive tasks. Movement is learned and refined using various brain centers, including the cerebellum.

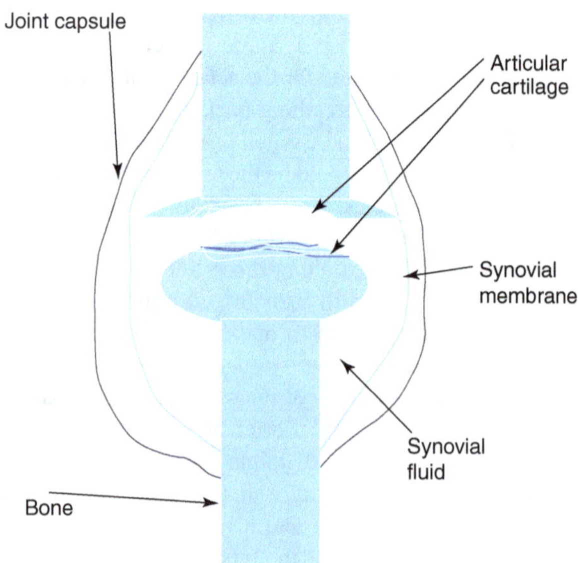

Fig. 8.12 Synovial joint: the synovial membrane and fluid provide lubrication and nourishment for the articular aspects of the joint

Nerves that supply direct afferent inputs to the muscles originate from the anterior horn cells of the spinal cord. Motor tracks that travel down the spinal cord synapse with the secondary motor cells in the anterior horn of the spinal cord. Destruction of the upper motor neurons leads to spasticity and hyperlexia due to lack of inhibition of muscular tone and deep reflexes. Destruction of lower motor neurons leads to flaccid paralysis, atonia, and muscle wasting, due to lack of motor input and loss of trophic factors from nerve to muscle. Peripheral nerves can become damaged from trauma and inflamed in diabetes and other illnesses. Sometimes it is difficult to discern if pain originates from local factors such as tissue ischemia or toxicity, peripheral nerve dysfunction, or even the brain itself. Fibromyalgia is an example where "central" CNS pain is present, but clinical findings and research also point to "local" or tissue-based pain. The communication between all of these tissues is so continuous and pervasive that while it is necessary to look at anatomical and functional distinctions (upper vs. lower, central versus peripheral, nerve versus tissue, muscle versus fascia), it pays to remember that they influence each other.

Bone acts as the scaffolding or framework of the body [425]. It is an active tissue with constant cell turnover. As a protein matrix infused with minerals (hydroxyapatite), it is dependent on nutritional and metabolic states of the body just as any other tissue. Bone acts as a reservoir for calcium, which allows parathyroid hormone and calcitonin hormones to maintain calcium homeostasis in the blood. As part of the greater musculoskeletal system, it has nervous, vascular, and lymphatic flow, and it reflects what is happening in local tissues. For example, degenerated synovial joints will display microfractures on the end plates of bone.

Hypofunction

Loss of function can happen due to lack of movement, incorrect or inefficient movement patterns, and lack of strength and flexibility. These issues can of course reduce the freedom of movement and performance that someone might have in life. It's natural to have faster and freer movement at a young age than much later in life. But lack of or dysfunctional movement sets the stage for more actual painful and later degenerative changes in the musculoskeletal system.

People settle into postural and movement patterns [426, 427]. That can include the following:

- Carrying the head forward with the shoulders slumped.
- Overly pronating the feet and putting excessive stress on the medial aspect of the knee [427].
- Tightening up in the chest muscles due to hours a day of keyboarding and phone work.
- Jerking the head around during shoulder checks while driving instead of unlocking the joints in the upper spine (occipito-atlanto-axial complex).

So not only are these habits not very efficient, but they move tissues in vectors and in ways that are not really what they are set up for. At first, this is easy to compensate for or ignore. Later, it will lead to pain. If that pain is suppressed or ignored, without treating the biomechanical and structural issues that cause it, it will lead to bona fide degenerative changes.

Physical deconditioning will also lead to less muscle strength and less agility than a person who is moderately active should have [428]. This is a loss of opportunities to strengthen the cardiovascular system. The brain also benefits from exercise, in increased circulation but also BDNF production, and the sheer sensory input that occurs. Bone density increases especially with weight-bearing-type exercise. Injuries in general might be less likely if reflexes, proprioception, and joint stability are improved by a person's choice of exercise.

Strength, reflexes, joint health, and other aspects of the musculoskeletal system decline with age. It is known that those who remain active are more likely to stay active. People at advanced ages benefit from adopting an exercise regimen, and rehabilitative treatments and exercises can help those who are older. The type of exercise that one does, and the conditioning to do it, is a matter of personal choice. For some patients with chronic pain, aqua exercise—aerobic, strength, and flexibility focused—is ideal. For others, rapid movement and elevated heart rate such as exercise classes or running are what relieves their stress or focuses their attention. For the very old, walking, Tai Chi, gardening, etc. are excellent exercises that confer many benefits. And we see athletes of many ages that show that the human body can be conditioned and maintained to engage in higher levels of performance into a very long life span.

Disordered Communication and Circulation

For joints, circulation of blood and lymph allows nutrients and oxygen to nourish the joint tissues. The synovial membrane and the synovial fluid have a vital role in the health of the articular surfaces. Supporting fibrous tissues, ligaments, and cartilage depend on circulation of this fluid for nutrition and gas exchange. Cartilage is an avascular tissue and must obtain oxygen and nutrients via diffusion [429].

Muscle tissue has a high need for vascular supply. The myoglobin in the muscle needs an oxygen supply. Muscle tissue can burn glucose, the carbohydrate skeleton of amino acids (via the Krebs cycle), and fats [430]. Muscles are capable of high amounts of aerobic metabolism but also carry out anaerobic metabolism. This produces lactic acid as a waste product, and this must be carried off with CO_2 and other metabolic waste products such as phosphates and sulfates. If a muscle lacks a vascular supply, the patient will have ischemic pains upon exertion (Fig. 8.13). Muscle will atrophy at a certain point to reflect the upper limits of metabolic capacity that have decreased due to a constrained blood supply.

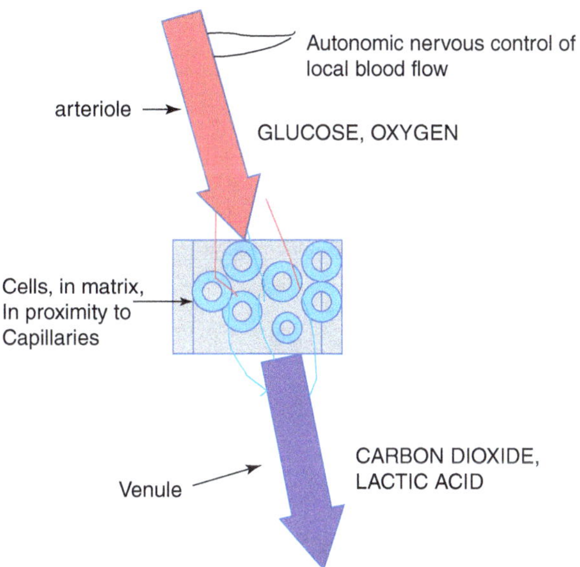

Fig. 8.13 Circulation and gas exchange: work performed by muscle tissue requires the inflow and outflow of blood to move oxygen and glucose in and carbon dioxide and lactate out

In advanced vascular diseases, due to atherosclerosis and diabetes mellitus (which often occur together), the circulation to peripheral nerves degrades their function and health [431]. Other exacerbating factors in diabetes will damage these nerves. Normal fracture repair requires adequate circulation, and insufficient vascular supply will hamper healing post-fracture or acceptance and rehabilitation from joint prostheses especially in smaller joints, such as the ankle.

As nerve function decreases, the autonomic nervous control of vascular beds becomes less finely tuned (Table 8.26). Sensory information and proprioceptive information decay, which leads to injury and poor healing. An extreme example of this phenomenon is the Charcot joint [432]. This is a deterioration of foot structure in patients with long-standing neuropathy, usually diabetic. Similar clinical pictures Charcot arthropathy can occur elsewhere in the body, but the foot is a common target. The lack of nervous input can lead to repetitive tendon strains and leads to lack of intrinsic coordination of motor, sensory, and autonomic nerves. The foot becomes swollen, weak, and very prone to reinjury and infection.

Patients that have demyelination of nerves due to multiple sclerosis will have interrupted sensory and motor communication to the central nervous system [360]. Sensory processing disorder is a complex phenomenon in children where the integration of sensory and motor information lacks coordination at the brain level [338]. This underscores that nervous coordination issues in the musculoskeletal system can be due to local lesions but also involve, ultimately, higher processing centers in the nervous system.

Table 8.26 Levels of dysfunction in musculoskeletal disease

Level of dysfunction	Test
Hypofunction	Range of motion testing
Hypofunction	Resisted strength and coordination testing
Hypofunction	Postural assessment
Impaired circulation and communication	Sensory nerve testing on physical examination
Impaired circulation and communication	Nerve conduction velocity test
Impaired circulation and communication	Multidimensional health assessment questionnaire
Inflammation	Widespread pain index
Inflammation	C-reactive protein
Inflammation	Erythrocyte sedimentation rate
Inflammation	Joint and bone radiographs
Inflammation	Diagnostic ultrasound
Inflammation	Radiographs (osteomyelitis)
Deeper inflammation and immune involvement	Rheumatoid arthritis score
Deeper inflammation and immune involvement	CT scan of joints, bone
Deeper inflammation and immune involvement	MRI of muscle, joints
Deeper inflammation and immune involvement	Arthroscopy
Deeper inflammation and immune involvement	Fluorescence-aided tomography
Decline of function	Physical examination
Fibrosis and matrix degeneration	Muscle or joint biopsy
Fibrosis and matrix degeneration	Imaging studies
Fibrosis and matrix degeneration	Bone density studies (DEXA)
Neoplasia	Radiographs, biopsy, nuclear imaging

Inflammation

Inflammatory changes to joints occur due to trauma, infection, osteoarthritis, and autoimmune events. Inflammation has four phases: acute nonspecific responses, more invasive cell-mediated responses, resolution, and post-response remodeling. In a structure such as a muscle, bone, or joint, these are normal responses. Mechanical and physical forces take their toll on the musculoskeletal system. Injury and infection normally impact these tissues. The inflammatory acute responses pave the way for healing. An example is a simple fracture of a bone. Provided that it is set properly, a callus will form, and fibroblastic activity and then mineralization will occur after an acute phase. If the tissue is young and vital, this process will cycle very quickly.

Even in the absence of infection, when joint or muscle tissue is traumatized or simply breaks down under use, there is release of damage-associated molecular

Table 8.27 Variations in joint disease

Arthritis/joint disease	Physical finding
Osteoarthritis	Distal interphalangeal joints, knee, ankle, hip
Ostcoarthritis	Mono- or polyarticular
Osteoarthritis	Inflammation subtle or very low
Rheumatoid arthritis	Inflammation is high
Rheumatoid arthritis	Polyarticular (more than 5 joints)
Rheumatoid arthritis	Metacarpophalangeal, carpal
SLE	Polyarticular, metacarpophalangeal, carpal, inflammation high
Gout	First metatarsal or phalangeal, inflammatory, monoarticular
Inflammatory bowel disease	Locations vary, oligoarticular (2 to 4 joints), inflammatory

patterns (DAMPS) [433]. Damage to the extracellular matrix will release DAMPS as well. There is an actual receptor on various antigen-presenting cells, called Toll-like receptors that detect the presence of DAMPS. When Toll-like receptors are bound on the target cells, they in turn release cytokines that attract other immune cells. Neutrophils arrive early, as they are frontline leukocytes that can attack bacteria.

This inflammation will eventually resolve, although other immune cells may get involved along the way. Muscles with inflammation will be tender and painful upon contraction. Joints will show swelling and tenderness. Inflamed fascia and tendons lead to movement restriction and pain.

In osteoarthritis, there is a lack of the more dramatic and destructive inflammation that is seen in infection and various autoimmune joint diseases particularly rheumatoid arthritis [434] (Table 8.27). There is really no neutrophil engagement of the joint. However, mechanical damage and DAMPS can lead to synovitis, albeit at a lower level of activity than actual rheumatic conditions. This often involves the arrival of monocytes, which can convert into M1 macrophages, that will cause more extensive damage. Arthralgia can manifest in inflammatory bowel disease, which shows that immune activity against tissues is now extraintestinal and impacting joint tissue.

Damage to hyaline cartilage that is extensive can lead to a blood clot, and the defect will be filled in with fibrocartilage. This is not as good as the original cartilage, but it will allow the function of the joint to resume. We see in some rehabilitated injuries an onset of arthritis later in life, and this sufficient but not ideal cartilage repair mechanism for large tears and avulsions is certainly one reason.

Inflammation is even present in fibromyalgia, a condition that is noted for a non-inflammatory presentation [435]. In this case, mast cells appear to have a special role. Thalamic, mast cell overactivation in the brain may oversensitize the central nervous system to afferent pain signals. In the actual peripheral tissues, mast cells are often in proximity to sensory nerves, and they might impact those nerves through secretion of pro-inflammatory IL-31 and secretory granules that contain pain-triggering substances such as bradykinin. Mast cells have been reported to be more numerous in skin samples from fibromyalgia patients.

Complex regional pain syndrome (CRPS) is a chronic pain condition where patients have recurring pain, even after an injury is resolved [436]. The patient can become hypersensitive to all pain sources and easily develop new pain foci. Those with underlying pain, inflammation, and stress are more at risk. It appears to be a central pain phenomenon, but often a focal peripheral issue is the trigger.

Deeper Inflammation and Immune Involvement

Under normal conditions, with a cessation of injury or elimination of infection, the normal control systems on inflammation lead to resolution and usually some extracellular matrix (ECM) remodeling. In more advanced damage to muscles, fascia, joints, or even bone, a chronic inflammatory process will set in.

The clinical condition of synovitis in rheumatoid arthritis is an example of a more aggressive inflammation (Table 8.27) and so are of osteomyelitis and autoimmune rhabdomyolysis. Even in later stages of osteoarthritis, there are inflammatory pathways that accelerate destruction of support tissues and cartilage, which can release IL-1. Neutrophils are attracted to damaged tissues, and their release of IL-17 will bring in more cellular immune responses [437].

Dendritic cells are more active in rheumatoid arthritis, and special dendritic cells actually migrate to the area of synovitis [438]. These in turn attract Th1 responses. Th1 lymphocytes secrete IL-2, IFN-γ, and TNF-β which upregulate the immune response. Increased joint damage will accelerate the inflammation.

Other sources of deep inflammation include systemic lupus erythematosus which can lead to tendonitis and myositis (Table 8.26) [439]. Arthritis can result from joint attack in diseases like ulcerative colitis, as a more severe extraintestinal manifestation of the disease. Rhabdomyolysis, due to muscle ischemia, crush injuries, extreme exercise, dehydration, and toxic drug reactions, leads to myonecrosis [440]. Excessive calcium builds up in muscle cells due to failure of energy production and failure of the ATPase that could push calcium out via a cotransporter. The muscle cell dies, and the release of myoglobin can injure the kidneys. Gout is a type of inflammatory tissue and joint pain due to the crystallization of uric acid in the great toe or other distal joints. Polymorphonuclear cells attempt to scavenge the uric acid crystal, rupture in the process, and trigger a very painful and noticeable inflammatory cascade.

Deep infection of bones can happen for a number of reasons including postsurgical. But *Mycobacteria tuberculosis* infection of bone (Pott's disease when it infects the spine) are still reported [441]. In the past, there were far more primary, secondary, and tertiary cases of syphilis (*Treponema pallidum*) bone infection and destruction. Gonococcal arthritis occurs due to an actual septic arthritis in the joint. Psoriatic arthritis, on the other hand, is immune related.

Extracellular Matrix Degeneration and Fibrosis

Matrix breakdown leads to different end results, depending on which part of the musculoskeletal system is affected. In osteoarthritis, cytokines, prostaglandins, and reactive oxygen species can lead to apoptosis of the chondrocytes, the cartilage-creating cells. This seems to be accomplished by apoptosis of the mitochondria in those cells. In rheumatoid arthritis, the synovial membrane begins to activate angiogenesis, which might seem beneficial as a provider of nutrients to cartilage, but ends up being destructive [442].

In the chondrocytes, there are receptors for ECM components, such as fibronectin or type II collagen [443, 444]. This binding can cause release of matrix metalloproteinases (MMP), which can cleave and disassemble matrices. While important for remodeling and repair, excessive MMP can start to degrade the extracellular matrix. Over time, there is less fibroblast and chondroblast activity and more lysis of collagen including the specialized cartilage structure. Bone will also undergo erosion along with destruction of joint structures (Table 8.26). Bones in general lose matrix as one ages, and the well-known conditions of osteopenia and more advanced osteoporosis result from a poorly mineralized matrix.

Muscles can structurally deteriorate. Shrinkage in size due to aging or lack of use and decreased mitochondria are tolerable to a point. In more advanced muscle degeneration, total mitochondrial populations decrease. The basement membrane of muscle fibers disintegrates. This is more noticeable in situations where muscles have weakened quickly or after tendon rupture, as opposed to simply disuse atrophy. It can occur in muscle fibrosis due to degenerative conditions, such as a muscular dystrophy [445]. Autoimmune effects, toxins, and some pharmaceutical drugs can lead to muscle degeneration.

Decline of Function

When physical changes to the musculoskeletal system become long term due to remodeling of ECM, changes to mitochondria, and destruction of some tissues, there is an unavoidable change in function. Joints that are degenerated will have trouble bearing weight or acting as levers under high stress. In some advanced rheumatic diseases, the joint will lose its basic alignment, with deviation and loss of stability. This can go so far as to be a true subluxation where the tendons slip off of the normal track they ought to be on (this can occur in the cervical spine as well in rheumatoid arthritis) [446]. This leads to a weakened and sometimes barely usable joint, such as loss of grip strength in advanced rheumatoid arthritis.

Muscle wasting due to infection, atrophy, necrosis, etc. can lead to weakness. In the past, many patients had loss of substantial muscle mass in some parts of the body due to poliomyelitis, a virus which attacks the anterior horn cells of the cord. The degeneration that resulted led to flaccid paralysis but also a loss of muscle viability due to a shutoff of nervous input and trophic factors. Some patients recovered function but later have had post-polio syndrome, a fatigue/wear and tear syndrome due to a net loss of enough nervous input to put undue stress on the surviving nerves and the motor units that they control. In many cases of muscle atrophy, the mitochondria are found to be decreased having undergone fission or fusion [447].

If joints, fascia, muscle, and peripheral nerves degenerate, the central nervous system will lose some degree of control over these areas. The CNS may still have the potential for proper control, but without the sensory input and the ongoing communication and execution of motor pathways, the coordinating functions deteriorate. This is why movement, and physical therapy in some cases, is vital even when people have lost some structure and function. What they do with what they have left is paramount.

Neoplasm

Bone and joint cancer, in the sense of neoplasia that originates from these tissues, impacts several thousand people a year in the United States. Osteosarcoma is most common in teenagers and children [448]. Ewing sarcoma is most common in teenagers and young adults. There are also metastases of cancers that originate from other tissues that travel to bone, with prostate, breast, and lung cancers. Multiple myeloma is a white blood cell neoplasm that can spread to bone. These cancers all tend to be osteolytic, although prostate metastases can be osteoblastic (bone forming). Soft tissue sarcomas and rhabdomyosarcoma (muscle) are other neoplasms of this system.

Determinants of Health

Movement is an important determining factor of health, and patients with pain conditions, arthritis, and even myofascial tightness need to incorporate this into their life. The CDC has reported that the national average for physical inactivity is 25.3% [449]. Additionally, the majority of adults does not get enough exercise, and a solid quarter are basically not moving. Many people spend more time in their desk chair than their actual bed.

This has deleterious effects on pain, joint function, proprioception, agility, and strength. A completely sedentary life not only sets the stage for many disturbances of function in the musculoskeletal system. It also works to keep the system from repairing itself.

Hydration

Dehydration will limit exercise performance. If dehydration proceeds because of heat, exercise, and perspiration, this can lower blood volume. Skeletal muscles are susceptible to this change, as their oxygen reserve is limited. Joint pain is made worse by dehydration [450]. It has been found recently that hydration attained by daily water consumption of more than 2.5 L has a robust impact on reducing the symptoms of disabling claudication and rest pain caused by peripheral vascular disease. The fascial system needs to be pliable and lubricated which is more difficult if water compartments are low.

Stress

A generalized and prolonged stress response, typified by elevated or prolonged daily cortisol secretion, will have an amplifying effect on pain. It has been suggested that there may be a link between post-traumatic stress disorder (PTSD) and complex regional pain syndrome. The cortisol that is elevated in many people with chronic stress reactions might reduce inflammation and pain at first, but over time, as adaptation fails, pain and inflammation will return [451].

Nutrition

In order for any body system to function properly, the essential nutrients must be present (Table 8.28). In preserving the integrity of bone, for example, dietary calcium, vitamins D and K, boron, magnesium, and zinc must be adequate [452]. Poor daily intake of omega-3 fatty acids; vitamins B1, B3, B6, B12, and D; magnesium; zinc; and β-carotene is also associated with chronic neuropathic or inflammatory pain.

Biochemical Support

Chondroitin Sulfate, Glucosamine Sulfate, Methylsulfonylmethane

These substances provide structural components of cartilage and have been reported to reduce pain symptoms in arthritis [453] (Table 8.28). Chondroitin sulfate is notable in that it is closest to actual ECM fragments of cartilage, but as a larger molecule, it is unclear how digestible and absorbable it is. For many years, clinical trials involving these supplements have varied. One study will show reduction in pain,

Table 8.28 Treatment considerations in musculoskeletal disorders

Level of intervention	Treatment	Comments
Determinants of health	Hydration	Joint hydration and pain levels relate to hydration status
Determinants of health	Nutrition	Bone density and neuromuscular function are impacted by nutritional deficiency
Determinants of health	Address stress	Stress that is prolonged or intense can elevate pain levels
Biochemical support	Chondroitin sulfate, glucosamine sulfate, methylsulfonylmethane	Provide sulfur and some lubricating effects to joints, reduces pain symptoms
Biochemical support	*Arnica* gel	Anti-inflammatory, anodyne
Biochemical support	Vitamin C, cherries, and strawberries	Antioxidant, tissue strengthening
Biochemical support	*Boswellia serrata*	Anti-inflammatory
Biochemical support	Vitamin D	Bone mineralization, anti-inflammatory
Biochemical support	*Harpagophytum procumbens*	Anti-inflammatory
Biochemical support	*Cannabis sativa*	Immunomodulation, anti-inflammatory, anodyne
Biochemical support	*Tripterygium wilfordii*	Pain relief
Biochemical support	*Cinnamomum cassia*	Anti-inflammatory
Biochemical support	*Curcuma longa*	Anti-inflammatory; nanoparticles might have best delivery
Biochemical support	Omega-3 fatty acids	Shift eicosanoid/prostanoid balance to an inflammatory one/offset omega-6 to omega-3 imbalances
Hormetic effects	2LARTH and ultradilute pro-inflammatory cytokines	Downregulate inflammatory activity secondary to a direct stimulatory effect
Hormetic effects	Traumeel and microdoses of pro-inflammatory botanicals	Downregulate inflammation
Whole person support	Acupuncture	Reduce pain
Whole person support	Gut microbiome	Reduce immune activation and systemic inflammation
Whole person support	Dynamic neuromuscular stabilization	Facilitate integration of function of neuromuscular system
Whole person support	Rolfing/structural integration	Reintegrate the fascial system
Whole person support	Elimination diet	Provide respite and identify most provocative foods
Whole person support	Anti-inflammatory diet	May provide reduction in symptoms; other important health benefits

Table 8.28 (continued)

Level of intervention	Treatment	Comments
Whole person support	Hydrotherapy	Provide circulatory support, lymph drainage, improved cellular activity, pain relief
Whole person support	Aquatic exercise	Leverage benefits of water (support of joints, improved proprioception, hydrostatic effects, resistance, myofascial loosening) to permit movement and exercise
Dampening symptoms	NSAIDs	Decrease in pain and inflammation
Dampening symptoms	Amitriptyline	Decrease neuropathic fibromyalgia symptoms
Dampening symptoms	Corticosteroids, prednisone	Decrease inflammation and tissue destruction
Dampening symptoms	Opioids	Pain relief—cautions against premature use, tolerance dependance
Dampening symptoms	Topical capsaicin: low intensity (OTC creams); high intensity (physician-administered capsaicin treatment)	Defunctionalize afferent sensory nerves carrying information from nociceptive receptors
Induce homeostasis	Autoimmune antibodies	Block inflammation at a fundamental level
Induce homeostasis	Methotrexate	Block cellular immune functions; limit joint destruction
Induce homeostasis	TNF blockers	Decrease inflammation at a fundamental level—immunosuppression
Induce homeostasis	Surgery: reparative, reconstructive, fusion	Repair or reconstruct joints where damage is advanced; in some cases arthrodesis is needed as last resort

another not. The trend would be that these substances don't really reverse degeneration but might increase joint lubrication and reduce pain. As naturopathic physician and nutrition expert Dr. Michael Murray has observed, these substances are sources of sulfur, in particular, methylsulfonylmethane (MSM), a physiological form of sulfur, which is a critical component of cartilage matrix [454].

Topical *Arnica*

Arnica montana is a traditional herbal medicine. It is not safe to take in large amounts. A gel or ointment that contains *Arnica montana* is anodyne, and it has anti-inflammatory effects. These are topical applications [455].

Vitamin C, Cherries, and Strawberries

Vitamin C is important for tissue integrity and as an antioxidant and is often supplemented in pain and inflammatory conditions. Cherries are high in vitamin C and in polyphenols and have been found to be beneficial in reducing inflammation in gout. Strawberries have been shown to reduce pain and inflammation in obese adults with osteoarthritis. Diets that emphasize plant foods will provide these sorts of benefits, although focused consumption of these foods or extracts of them can also be recommended in times of increased pain and disease activity [456].

Vitamin D

Vitamin D is well-known for its critical role in calcium homeostasis. But it also has effects on pain. Nociceptors are found in the skin and are important in the initial transduction of signals that denote pain. Receptors for vitamin D are found in the skin, dorsal root ganglia, and brain. Epidermal growth factor receptor and glial cell line-derived neurotrophic factor are able to upregulate the development of nociceptors in the skin, too many of these nociceptors can increase pain levels. Vitamin D regulates the expression of these growth factors. Vitamin D has improved vascular functions in patients with diabetes and vitamin D deficiency. Since about 20% of the adult population is deficient in D and vascular degeneration goes hand in hand with diabetic neuropathy, this is an important potential treatment. The fact that supplementing vitamin D to all patients with one type of presentation does not yield consistent results is more indicative of the fact that studying a nutrient and prohormone in the same manner as an NSAID is not a well-thought-out research model. Rather, the task is to identify pain syndrome individuals with low serum levels of vitamin D and ensure that they have the sufficient amount of D for normal inflammation and nociceptive regulation [457]. Vitamin D receptors are found in various immune cells, and NOD-like receptors appear to receive vitamin D, which reduces expression of mTOR [458, 459]. It is also needed to prevent muscle wasting [460]. Given the potential effects on pain and sensitivity, inflammation activation, muscle health, and the need to support bone density in many arthritis conditions, at the very least, ensuring that patients with musculoskeletal conditions have adequate vitamin D is important in naturopathic care.

Boswellia spp.

Boswellia serrata

This plant has powerful anti-inflammatory substances that are helpful for joint or muscle inflammation. A double-blind, placebo-controlled human trial was conducted to evaluate the safety and efficacy of a standardized oral supplementation of

Boswellin®, a novel extract of *Boswellia serrata* extract (BSE) containing 3-acetyl-11-keto-β-boswellic acid (AKBBA) with β-boswellic acid (BBA). Knee pain improved, and blood levels of the inflammatory marker C-reactive protein decreased [461]. It can also be combined with *Curcuma longa* [462].

Cannabis sativa

This plant and its many cultivars have a broad range of anti-inflammatory and anodyne actions. There are three major categories of compounds in it: tetrahydrocannabinol (THC), cannabidiol (CBD), and terpenes. There are varieties of each of these compounds. It can be used in a variety of rheumatic conditions [463].

Cannabidiol, which is consumed as an oil and an isolate, has anti-inflammatory properties. It binds to endocannabinoid 2 receptors on immune cells. Rheumatoid arthritis synovial fibroblasts, which are overactive collagen producing cells that destroy joints from within, are downregulated by CBD. Topical CBD can relieve joint pain and is a non-NSAID way to provide relief for those with osteoarthritis.

Broader-spectrum cannabis products decrease disease activity in rheumatoid arthritis.

Cannabis products can be very helpful to those with fibromyalgia. This includes CBD oils but also 1:20 THC to CBD preparation and many other forms. Improvement in sleep quality is one immediate benefit. In a 2019 clinical trial of cannabis for patients with fibromyalgia, pain intensity (scale 0–10) reduced from a median of 9.0 at baseline to 5.0 ($p < 0.001$).

Harpagophytum procumbens

Harpagophytum procumbens is a popular arthritis remedy (Table 8.28). It has been used for this purpose for a long time by the Khoisan people of Southern Africa. It contains iridoid glycosides, the harpagosides. It has a good human research basis to conclude that it will lower arthritis pain [464, 465]. It can lead to some gastric upset, which might be in part due to the cyclooxygenase inhibition of the iridoid glycosides. A recent clinical trial using Teltonal (a standardized extract of *Harpagophytum procumbens*) and a meloxicam (an NSAID) showed that both were equally effective, with Teltonal being a good option for those who cannot tolerate NSAIDs. Iridoid-containing plants are under investigation for their anti-inflammatory effects, which extends beyond osteoarthritis to muscle and joint inflammation. These effects range beyond COX-1 or COX-2 inhibition to the lowering of TNF, for example. *Cornus officinalis* is one example. It is a medicine for dispersing swelling and pain in traditional Chinese medicine and is being investigated as an anti-inflammatory.

Tripterygium wilfordii

Tripterygium wilfordii contains sesquiterpenes, diterpenes (triptolide, triptolide, and triptonide), triterpenes (celastrol, pristimerin, and wilforlide A), lignans, glycosides, and alkaloids. It has been found to be similar to methotrexate in reducing the symptoms of rheumatoid arthritis in a 2-year study [466].

Curcuma longa

Curcuma longa is well-known for its anti-inflammatory effects. Because it is poorly absorbed and it does not always travel to its cellular targets in vivo, there are phytosome and nanoparticle forms of curcumin (one of the most active compounds in turmeric). In vitro, curcumin reduces the production of IL-1β, TNF-α, MCP-1, and MIP-1α. A systematic review found that *Curcuma longa* and extracts that were enriched with curcumin (one of the active molecules) were effective in reducing pain in arthritis [467].

Omega-3

The use of supplementation with omega-3 fatty acids can lead to clinical improvement of inflammatory conditions of the musculoskeletal system. Reports of clinical improvement in systemic lupus erythematosus and rheumatoid arthritis support this [468]. This includes fish oil supplementation, krill oil, and flaxseed oil. These fats shift the production of prostanoids from pro-inflammatory to anti-inflammatory. Many diets are imbalanced with too few omega-3 fats relative to omega-6. When omega-3 is supplemented for patients with pain where inflammation is less prominent feature, such as osteoarthritis or fibromyalgia, the results are lacking. This does not mean that these patients have optimal omega-3 nor does it mean that some of these patients won't benefit. But this kind of supplementation should be an adjunctive therapy. Consuming sources of these omega-3 fats, including cod liver oil (also a source of vitamin D and A), is probably a better start.

Whole Person Support

Gut Microbiome and Pain

Gut microbiome constituents and immune relationships with them can influence pain and inflammation. Changing the microbiome with diet and fermented foods doesn't necessary cure all widespread or localized pain phenomenon, but it can help. *Coprococcus* comes as a bacteria that produces butyric acid. This has a nutrition and anti-inflammatory effect on the gut. When the gut is well nourished and maintains good intraepithelial tight junctions, there is less slippage of excess antigens into the underlying immune networks. It is not the actual sampling of antigens from the gut by the immune system that is the problem; it is the influx of those proteins in a way that provokes immune reactions and does not allow for tolerance mechanisms to kick in. Moreover, some gut-derived toxins such as lipopolysaccharide can go systemic and provoke immune reactions in different sites across the body.

Pro-inflammatory cytokines and postanoids, such as tumor necrosis factor-alpha and chemokine, are released by immune cells when they are activated by antigen. These pro-inflammatory compounds can sensitize nociceptors in the tissues. This will make a person more likely to have a pain response, and that response may propagate itself in people with central pain phenomena (such as complex regional pain syndrome). As has been well-known for years, the *Bifidobacterium* spp., *Lactobacillus* spp., and *Lactococcus* and *Pediococcus* species can be anti-inflammatory. Gut bacteria can make regulating compounds that reduce pain signals [469–472]. In a randomized, controlled trial, rheumatoid arthritis patients who received a different type of microbe—*Bacillus coagulans*—had less pain and disability [473]. The trillions of microbes of the gut produce neurotransmitters and stimulate the vagus nerve sending communication to the brain. This has implications for central pain phenomena, as well as peripheral pain sensitization.

Fascial System: Rolfing

Direct work with the fascial system can be important for integrating and strengthening the musculoskeletal system. Some forms of physical therapy, some traditional osteopathic manipulative therapies, and various advanced bodywork methods can not only relax but unwind and retune the fascia. Pioneering work on this was done by Ida Rolf in the twentieth century, and the method that she taught is known as Rolfing [474]. It is also known as structural integration [475].

Dynamic Neuromuscular Stabilization (DNS)

DNS is a rehabilitative system based on the work of the Prague School of physical therapy (Prague School of Manual Medicine, including Karel Lewit, Vladimir Janda, Vaclav Vojta and Frantisek Vele). Professor Pavel Kolar, PT, PhD, a Czech physiotherapist, is the foremost developer of DNS in the twenty-first century [476]. It incorporates modern neurophysiology and neuroanatomy findings, including developmental concepts, particularly developmental kinesiology. Practitioners work to help the body relearn optimal function by integrated movements, working with the core stabilization systems of the body and recapitulating primal but fundamental motor postures and scripts. Dynamic neuromuscular stabilization, or "DNS" as it is commonly referred to, is a manual and rehabilitative approach to optimize the movement system based upon the scientific principles of DK. The developer of DNS is rapidly gaining attention and acceptance in the sports rehabilitation and performance arena for both the recovery from musculoskeletal overuse injuries and in injury prevention.

The integrated spinal stabilizing system (ISSS) as described by Kolar, is comprised of balanced coactivation between the deep cervical flexors and spinal extensors in the cervical and upper thoracic region, as well as the diaphragm, pelvic floor, all sections of the abdominals, and spinal extensors in the lower thoracic and lumbar region. This is just one example of fundamental principles, but the ISSS is an important balancing point to work around. Infants that successfully develop motor skills are balanced in the ISSS. Adults with arthritis, pain, poor posture, and spinal issues tend to have a weak or imbalanced ISSS.

Acupuncture

Acupuncture is part of a wider system, and while it can be used locally for specific pain areas, it is in fact one modality in the system of traditional Chinese medicine. That means that while specific points can elicit certain benefits, the selection of points according to the principles of Chinese medicine and used within a treatment plan congruent with those principles is the best use of this modality. Current reviews of the evidence of acupuncture in chronic pain, and generally musculoskeletal pain, show benefits [477, 478].

Elimination Diets

An elimination diet is a way to identify foods that can activate certain symptoms: pain, muscle weakness, inflammation, etc. It does not identify the precise mechanism. Patients undergo a restrictive diet that excludes foods most commonly associated with allergy. This includes wheat and gluten-containing foods, dairy, soy, beef, citrus, and corn, with some diets adding more. Typically, processed foods that tend to contain many additives and allergens (such as "hydrolyzed vegetable protein" from soy or wheat) are avoided. The patient does this regimen for 2 or 3 weeks until their symptoms (joint pain, inflammation, widespread pain) decrease. Then they reintroduce one food group every 3 days. They introduce the food, put it back on the shelf, and wait 3 days. If symptoms return, that food is considered a possible aggravating factor or allergen. Elimination diets can give people an overview of what sets off their symptoms, and they do often get a respite from inflammation or other symptoms during the washout period. For some patients, just eliminating gluten, or monosodium glutamate, or intermittent fasting can lower pain levels [479].

Anti-Inflammatory Diet

Going beyond avoidance, there are anti-inflammatory diets, which stress foods that downregulate inflammation, as well as avoid promoters of inflammation. There are variations on the theme of what constitutes an anti-inflammatory diet. Patients with acute flare-ups of autoimmune diseases sometimes find respite in a medicinal beverage that has rice protein, medium-chain triglycerides, a modest amount of carbohydrates, and the essential nutrients (vitamins, minerals). These are sometimes fortified with antioxidant polyphenolic molecules from grapes, rosemary, milk thistle, etc.

In a 2020 very thorough investigation into the use of an anti-inflammatory diet for individuals who suffered from rheumatoid arthritis, there were benefits seen. Patients were worked intensively to monitor what they ate, and their various health measurements before and after the study were recorded. The treatment group did not do overall better on DAS28-ESR (Disease Activity Score in 28 joints—erythrocyte sedimentation rate). But they did have improvement in components of that score, including reduction of swelling in some joints [480].

The diet included the following:

Fish (mainly salmon) 3–4 times/week.
Vegetarian dishes with legumes 1–2 times/week.
Potatoes.
Whole grain cereals.
Vegetables.
Yogurt for sauces.
Spices and other flavorings.
Fruits.
Breakfast of low-fat dairy, whole grain cereals, pomegranate and blueberries, nuts, and juice shots with probiotics.
The probiotic shot used contained *Lactobacillus plantarum* 299v and was provided to the participants 5 days/week
Meat consumption was limited to no more than three servings per week.

This was a Swedish study comparing the participants to the controls who were on an average Swedish diet. The use of diets that focus on health promoting foods probably has a much bigger impact in other countries, including the United States. The obesity rate, although rising in Sweden, is about 10%; in the United States, it sits at 30%.

In a 2021 systematic review, the Mediterranean diet showed improvement in some aspects of rheumatoid arthritis. It found that the Mediterranean diet demonstrated improvements in patient pain scores. These are not the same as seeing radiographic evidence of joint repair, but they have significance for quality of life [481].

This is a reminder that in naturopathic practice, although biochemical knowledge of a diet and its performance in clinical trials is important, there is also a place for trial working with patients to compare two or more dietary approaches. Given the complexity of the human genome and the microbiome that interacts with diet, it is not surprising that diversity of responses to food are consistently seen in research and most certainly in practice.

Hydrotherapy

The use of water to improve health and reduce pain is an ancient facet of medicine. The use of water as a modality traverses many traditions and cultures. In terms of the historical forerunners of naturopathic medicine, Hippocrates recommended medicinal baths, using waters from different sources with different mineral contents, and he described the effects of hot and cold treatments. Naturopathic hydrotherapy can include whole body wraps, sauna, steam treatment, and alternating hot and cold applications [482].

Aquatic Exercise

Exercise in the water is a highly beneficial treatment for patients with all manner of musculoskeletal issues (Table 8.28). Water provides support and relieves the joints of much of the force of gravity. Water provides resistance to movement, which makes for a good resistance exercise, but also slows the movement of joints and reduces injury. The buoyancy experience of being in water can be stimulating, and the hydrostatic pressure on the body can move body fluids toward the core through a gentle squeezing action. Studies on fibromyalgia and aquatic exercise show reduction in tender points. For patients with joint damage due to rheumatoid arthritis, the stabilizing effects of water can make exercise possible where it was not before. Many neuromuscular rehabilitation processes can benefit from water. Multiple sclerosis patients may aggravate from the warm nature of the therapy pool. But in many conditions of painful muscles, fascia, tendons, and joints, the warmth helps to loosen up and soften tissues, and patients seemingly come alive in terms of movement [483].

Hormesis

Traumeel and similar products, such as T-Relief, contain dilutions of botanical and mineral substances that are in higher amounts pro-inflammatory (Table 8.28). Dilutions of these substances, such as the Traumeel medicine, have demonstrated anti-inflammatory effects. This medicine also appears to increase the production of inflammation resolving substances [484].

The herbs in these formulations are in "X" dilutions which means a 1 in 10 dilution. In an ampule of Traumeel, which is used for injection therapy, there are as follows:

- *Aconitum napellus* 2X 1.32 μL 5.22X
- *Arnica montana*, radix 2X 2.20 μL 5.00X
- *Bellis perennis* 2X 1.10 μL 5.30X
- *Belladonna* 2X 2.20 μL 5.00X
- *Calendula officinalis* 2X 2.20 μL 5.00X
- *Chamomilla* 3X 2.20 μL 6.00X
- *Echinacea* 2X 0.55 μL 5.60X
- *Echinacea purpurea* 2X 0.55 μL 5.60X
- *Hamamelis virginiana* 1X 0.22 μL 5.00X
- Hepar Sulphuris Calcareum 6X 2.20 μL 9.00X
- *Hypericum perforatum* 2X 0.66 μL 5.52X
- Mercurius solubilis 6X 1.10 μL 9.30X
- *Millefolium* 3X 2.20 μL 6.00X
- *Symphytum officinale* 6X 2.20 μL 9.00X

These sterile ampoules are injected into painful sites, such as aggregation of tight myofascial tissue.

Traumeel, T-Relief, and similar products are very commonly used by patients as gels or creams. These are also very dilute. Herbal substances such as *Aconitum napellus* are only safe in very small amounts. *Aconitum napellus* is considered a plant poison as it causes sodium channels in excitable membranes to stay in an open position, effectively blocking depolarization. This has a numbing effect, and aconite has a traditional usage for pain. However, crude amounts can cause death due to cardiac arrhythmias or paralysis of muscles of respiration.

2LARTH is a dilute medicine that contains pro-inflammatory cytokines. Ultradilutions of these cytokines, such as the very pro-inflammatory tumor necrosis factor-alpha, have shown benefit in rheumatoid arthritis. Micro-immunotherapy in this sense is used as an ultralow-dose stimulation to have a net effect of downregulating a process [485, 486].

2LARTH®

Ingredients:

- IL-1—10
- IL-2—10
- TNF-α—10
- SNA®-ARTH
- SNA®-HLA-I
- SNA®-HLA-II

Dampening Symptoms

Nonsteroidal anti-inflammatory drugs (NSAIDs) are a primary therapy for reducing pain and inflammation [487]. They are used across the entire spectrum of neuromuscular pain and inflammation conditions including osteoarthritis and rheumatoid arthritis. These drugs can lead to gastrointestinal bleeding and are not tolerated by all. Misoprostol is sometimes added to these drugs to help protect the gastric mucosa.

Some of the more common NSAIDs are as follows:

- Ketorolac
- Diclofenac
- Naproxen
- Meloxicam
- Diclofenac
- Ibuprofen
- Acetaminophen
- Acetylsalicylic acid

The tricyclic antidepressant amitriptyline is used as a main therapy to reduce fibromyalgia pain. It is also used for diabetic neuropathy [488].

In myositis or acute flare-ups of rheumatoid arthritis, prednisone and other corticosteroids are used to reduce inflammation and reduce damage.

Opioid pain control is used across different musculoskeletal pain disorders. In the past several years, the use of non-opioid pain control or, at the least, minimalist approaches to the use of opioids has gained traction due to the many incidences of opioid abuse and overdose in the past two decades. Guidelines for osteoarthritis typically recommend using an NSAID or some other pain relief first and even then prescribing opioids for a short time [489].

Topical capsaicin in the form of very powerful 8% capsaicin patches has been shown to be beneficial in diabetic neuropathic and other forms of chronic pain. Capsaicin is the counterirritant and circulatory stimulant found in *Capsicum frutescens*. An 8% application is left on the patient for an hour, with the patient and physician using masks, gloves, and draping to prevent eye, respiratory tract, and skin irritation. The effect of reduced pain lasts for several weeks. Capsaicin appears to defunctionalize afferent neurons through interaction with TRPV1 receptors that carry pain signals to the brain [490].

Far less concentrated capsaicin-containing creams and ointments are available over the counter, usually with 0.025% or 0.05% capsaicin. These are most effective for pain near the surface of the skin, such as osteoarthritis of the fingers.

Imposing a Homeostatic Balance with Pharmaceuticals

Longer-term control comes from methotrexate and antibodies that block components of the immune signaling pathway. There are tumor necrosis factor blockers that include antibody products as well as etanercept. These drugs can significantly lower disease activity. They are in general referred to as DMARDS—disease-modifying antirheumatic drugs [491] (Table 8.28).

Stronger pain suppression is sometimes found with infusions of, or nasal delivery of, ketamine. This drug has a history as a dissociative anesthetic. It is an *N*-methyl-D-aspartate (NMDA) antagonist. Fibromyalgia patients have found this helpful [414].

Surgical releases and reconstruction are important modalities but should be used only when there is a clear structural component to correct that does in fact produce pain. Other approaches to reduce pain ought to be tried first, as surgery, no matter how beneficial, cannot be undone.

References

1. Oberman R, Bhardwaj A. Physiology, Cardiac. In: StatPearls [Internet]. Treasure Island, FL: StatPearls; 2022. Accessed 21 Jul 2021.
2. Steven S, Frenis K, Oelze M, Kalinovic S, Kuntic M, Bayo Jimenez MT, et al. Vascular inflammation and oxidative stress: major triggers for cardiovascular disease. Oxid Med Cell Longev. 2019;2019:7092151.
3. Bachschmid MM, Schildknecht S, Matsui R, Zee R, Haeussler D, Cohen RA, et al. Vascular aging: chronic oxidative stress and impairment of redox signaling-consequences for vascular homeostasis and disease. Ann Med. 2013;45(1):17–36.
4. Daiber A, Hahad O, Andreadou I, Steven S, Daub S, Münzel T. Redox-related biomarkers in human cardiovascular disease—classical footprints and beyond. Redox Biol. 2021;42:101875. https://pubmed.ncbi.nlm.nih.gov/33541847.
5. Di Nicolantonio JJ, O'Keefe JH, Wilson W. Subclinical magnesium deficiency: a principal driver of cardiovascular disease and a public health crisis. Open Heart. 2018;5:e000668.
6. Ridker PM. The JUPITER trial: Results, controversies, and implications for prevention. Circulation. 2009;2:279–85.
7. Del Buono MG, Montone RA, Camilli M, Carbone S, Narula J, Lavie CJ, et al. Coronary microvascular dysfunction across the spectrum of cardiovascular diseases: JACC state-of-the-art review. J Am Coll Cardiol. 2021;78(13):1352–71.
8. Guijarro C, Cosín-Sales J. LDL cholesterol and atherosclerosis: the evidence. Clin e Investig en Arterioscler Publ Of la Soc Esp Arterioscler. 2021;33(Suppl 1):25–32.
9. Kvietys PR, Granger DN. Role of reactive oxygen and nitrogen species in the vascular responses to inflammation. Free Radic Biol Med. 2012;52(3):556–92.
10. Kim Y-W, West XZ, Byzova TV. Inflammation and oxidative stress in angiogenesis and vascular disease. J Mol Med (Berl). 2013;91(3):323–8.

11. Fioranelli M, Bottaccioli AG, Bottaccioli F, Bianchi M, Rovesti M, Roccia MG. Stress and inflammation in coronary artery disease: a review psychoneuroendocrineimmunology-based. Front Immunol. 2018;9:2031.
12. Ferrucci L, Fabbri E. Inflammageing: chronic inflammation in ageing, cardiovascular disease, and frailty. Nat Rev Cardiol. 2018;15(9):505–22.
13. Zhu Y, Xian X, Wang Z, Bi Y, Chen Q, Han X, et al. Research progress on the relationship between atherosclerosis and inflammation. Biomolecules. 2018;8(3):80.
14. Rosin NL, Sopel MJ, Falkenham A, Lee TDG, Légaré J-F. Disruption of collagen homeostasis can reverse established age-related myocardial fibrosis. Am J Pathol. 2015;185(3):631–42.
15. Jin H-Y, Weir-McCall JR, Leipsic JA, Son J-W, Sellers SL, Shao M, et al. The relationship between coronary calcification and the natural history of coronary artery disease. JACC Cardiovasc Imaging. 2021;14(1):233–42.
16. Frangogiannis NG, Kovacic JC. Extracellular matrix in ischemic heart disease, part 4/4: JACC focus seminar. J Am Coll Cardiol. 2020;75(17):2219–35.
17. Díez J, González A, Kovacic JC. Myocardial interstitial fibrosis in nonischemic heart disease, part 3/4: JACC focus seminar. J Am Coll Cardiol. 2020;75(17):2204–18.
18. Martín-Fernández B, Gredilla R. Mitochondria and oxidative stress in heart aging. Age (Dordr). 2016;38(4):225–38.
19. Oka T, Hikoso S, Yamaguchi O, Taneike M, Takeda T, Tamai T, et al. Mitochondrial DNA that escapes from autophagy causes inflammation and heart failure. Nature. 2012;485(7397):251–5.
20. National Sleep Foundation. Sleep by Numbers—Basics of Sleep [Internet]. https://www.thensf.org/sleep-facts-and-statistics/. Accessed 27 May 2022.
21. Domínguez F, Fuster V, Fernández-Alvira JM, Fernández-Friera L, López-Melgar B, Blanco-Rojo R, et al. Association of sleep duration and quality with subclinical atherosclerosis. J Am Coll Cardiol. 2019;73(2):134–44.
22. Covassin N, Singh P. Sleep duration and cardiovascular disease risk. Sleep Med Clin. 2016;11(1):81–9. https://linkinghub.elsevier.com/retrieve/pii/S1556407X15001381.
23. National Sleep Foundation. Understanding circadian rhythms [Internet]. https://www.thensf.org/what-is-a-circadian-rhythm/. Accessed 27 May 2022.
24. Javeed N, Matveyenko AV. Circadian etiology of type 2 diabetes mellitus. Physiology (Bethesda). 2018;33(2):138–50.
25. Wright L, Simpson W, Van Lieshout RJ, Steiner M. Depression and cardiovascular disease in women: is there a common immunological basis? A theoretical synthesis. Ther Adv Cardiovasc Dis. 2014;8(2):56–69.
26. Bucciarelli V, Caterino AL, Bianco F, Caputi CG, Salerni S, Sciomer S, et al. Depression and cardiovascular disease: The deep blue sea of women's heart. Trends Cardiovasc Med. 2020;30(3):170–6.
27. Celano CM, Huffman JC. Depression and cardiac disease: a review. Cardiol Rev. 2011;19(3):130–42.
28. Fiorentini D, Cappadone C, Farruggia G, Prata C. Magnesium: biochemistry, nutrition, detection, and social impact of diseases linked to its deficiency. Nutrients. 2021;13(4):1136.
29. Xia N, Li H. Loneliness, social isolation, and cardiovascular health. Antioxid Redox Signal. 2018;28(9):837–51.
30. Freak-Poli R, Ryan J, Neumann JT, Tonkin A, Reid CM, Woods RL, et al. Social isolation, social support and loneliness as predictors of cardiovascular disease incidence and mortality. BMC Geriatr. 2021;21(1):711.
31. Ghaemi Kerahrodi J, Michal M. The fear-defense system, emotions, and oxidative stress. Redox Biol. 2020;37:101588.
32. Ginty AT, Kraynak TE, Fisher JP, Gianaros PJ. Cardiovascular and autonomic reactivity to psychological stress: neurophysiological substrates and links to cardiovascular disease. Auton Neurosci. 2017;207:2–9.
33. Cohen BE, Edmondson D, Kronish IM. State of the art review: depression, stress, anxiety, and cardiovascular disease. Am J Hypertens. 2015;28(11):1295–302.

34. Román GC, Jackson RE, Gadhia R, Román AN, Reis J. Mediterranean diet: the role of long-chain ω-3 fatty acids in fish; polyphenols in fruits, vegetables, cereals, coffee, tea, cacao and wine; probiotics and vitamins in prevention of stroke, age-related cognitive decline, and Alzheimer disease. Rev Neurol (Paris). 2019;175(10):724–41.
35. Tang C, Wang X, Qin L-Q, Dong J-Y. Mediterranean diet and mortality in people with cardiovascular disease: a meta-analysis of prospective cohort studies. Nutrients. 2021;13(8):2623.
36. Rees K, Takeda A, Martin N, Ellis L, Wijesekara D, Vepa A, et al. Mediterranean-style diet for the primary and secondary prevention of cardiovascular disease. Cochrane Database Syst Rev. 2019;3(3):CD009825.
37. Fitó M, Estruch R, Salas-Salvadó J, Martínez-Gonzalez MA, Arós F, Vila J, et al. Effect of the Mediterranean diet on heart failure biomarkers: a randomized sample from the PREDIMED trial. Eur J Heart Fail. 2014;16(5):543–50.
38. Filippou CD, Tsioufis CP, Thomopoulos CG, Mihas CC, Dimitriadis KS, Sotiropoulou LI, et al. Dietary approaches to stop hypertension (DASH) diet and blood pressure reduction in adults with and without hypertension: a systematic review and meta-analysis of randomized controlled trials. Adv Nutr. 2020;11(5):1150–60.
39. Salomé M, Arrazat L, Wang J, Dufour A, Dubuisson C, Volatier J-L, et al. Contrary to ultra-processed foods, the consumption of unprocessed or minimally processed foods is associated with favorable patterns of protein intake, diet quality and lower cardiometabolic risk in French adults (INCA3). Eur J Nutr. 2021;60(7):4055–67.
40. Highly processed foods form bulk of U.S. youths' diets [Internet]. https://www.nih.gov/news-events/nih-research-matters/highly-processed-foods-form-bulk-us-youths-diets.
41. Ramsden CE, Zamora D, Majchrzak-Hong S, Faurot KR, Broste SK, Frantz RP, et al. Re-evaluation of the traditional diet-heart hypothesis: analysis of recovered data from Minnesota Coronary Experiment (1968-73). BMJ. 2016;353:i1246.
42. Lawrence GD. Perspective: the saturated fat-unsaturated oil dilemma: relations of dietary fatty acids and serum cholesterol, atherosclerosis, inflammation, cancer, and all-cause mortality. Adv Nutr. 2021;12(3):647–56.
43. Estruch R, Ros E, Salas-Salvadó J, Covas M-I, Corella D, Arós F, et al. Primary prevention of cardiovascular disease with a mediterranean diet supplemented with extra-virgin olive oil or nuts. N Engl J Med. 2018;378(25):e34.
44. Thosar SS, Butler MP, Shea SA. Role of the circadian system in cardiovascular disease. J Clin Invest. 2018;128(6):2157–67.
45. de la Guía-Galipienso F, Martínez-Ferran M, Vallecillo N, Lavie CJ, Sanchis-Gomar F, Pareja-Galeano H. Vitamin D and cardiovascular health. Clin Nutr. 2021;40(5):2946–57.
46. Evans GW. The built environment and mental health. J Urban Health. 2003;80(4):536–55.
47. Casas R, Sacanella E, Urpí-Sardà M, Chiva-Blanch G, Ros E, Martínez-González M-A, et al. The effects of the mediterranean diet on biomarkers of vascular wall inflammation and plaque vulnerability in subjects with high risk for cardiovascular disease. A randomized trial. PLoS One. 2014;9(6):e100084.
48. Smith F, Faydenko J. Use of cardiac risk biomarker testing in a naturopathic medicine teaching center: Lessons on standard of care. Eur J Integr Med. 2020;36:101135. https://www.sciencedirect.com/science/article/pii/S1876382019304470.
49. Sarriá B, Martínez-López S, Sierra-Cinos JL, García-Diz L, Mateos R, Bravo L. Regular consumption of a cocoa product improves the cardiometabolic profile in healthy and moderately hypercholesterolaemic adults. Br J Nutr. 2014;111(1):122–34.
50. Schwedhelm E, Maas R, Freese R, Jung D, Lukacs Z, Jambrecina A, et al. Pharmacokinetic and pharmacodynamic properties of oral L-citrulline and L-arginine: impact on nitric oxide metabolism. Br J Clin Pharmacol. 2008;65(1):51–9.
51. Ma H, Johnson SL, Liu W, DaSilva NA, Meschwitz S, Dain JA, et al. Evaluation of polyphenol anthocyanin-enriched extracts of blackberry, black raspberry, blueberry, cranberry, red raspberry, and strawberry for free radical scavenging, reactive carbonyl species trapping, anti-glycation, anti-β-amyloid aggregation, and mic. Int J Mol Sci. 2018;19(2):461. https://pubmed.ncbi.nlm.nih.gov/29401686.

52. McMurray JJV, Packer M, Desai AS, Gong J, Lefkowitz MP, Rizkala AR, et al. Dual angiotensin receptor and neprilysin inhibition as an alternative to angiotensin-converting enzyme inhibition in patients with chronic systolic heart failure: rationale for and design of the prospective comparison of ARNI with ACEI to determine impact on global mortality and morbidity in heart failure trial (PARADIGM-HF). Eur J Heart Fail. 2013;15(9):1062–73.
53. Peoples JN, Saraf A, Ghazal N, Pham TT, Kwong JQ. Mitochondrial dysfunction and oxidative stress in heart disease. Exp Mol Med. 2019;51(12):1–13.
54. Brown DA, Perry JB, Allen ME, Sabbah HN, Stauffer BL, Shaikh SR, et al. Expert consensus document: mitochondrial function as a therapeutic target in heart failure. Nat Rev Cardiol. 2017;14(4):238–50.
55. Di Lorenzo A, Iannuzzo G, Parlato A, Cuomo G, Testa C, Coppola M, et al. Clinical evidence for Q10 coenzyme supplementation in heart failure: from energetics to functional improvement. J Clin Med. 2020;9(5):1266.
56. Garrido-Maraver J, Cordero MD, Oropesa-Avila M, Vega AF, de la Mata M, Pavon AD, et al. Clinical applications of coenzyme Q10. Front Biosci. 2014;19:619–33.
57. Zozina VI, Covantev S, Goroshko OA, Krasnykh LM, Kukes VG. Coenzyme Q10 in cardiovascular and metabolic diseases: current state of the problem. Curr Cardiol Rev. 2018;14(3):164–74.
58. Li S, Wang J, Xiao Y, Zhang L, Fang J, Yang N, et al. D-ribose: potential clinical applications in congestive heart failure and diabetes, and its complications (Review). Exp Ther Med. 2021;21(5):496.
59. Bkaily G, Jazzar A, Normand A, Simon Y, Al-Khoury J, Jacques D. Taurine and cardiac disease: state of the art and perspectives. Can J Physiol Pharmacol. 2020;98(2):67–73.
60. Chrysant SG, Chrysant GS. Association of hypomagnesemia with cardiovascular diseases and hypertension. Int J Cardiol Hypertens. 2019;1:100005.
61. Tian J, Liu Y, Chen K. Ginkgo biloba extract in vascular protection: molecular mechanisms and clinical applications. Curr Vasc Pharmacol. 2017;15(6):532–48.
62. Tassell MC, Kingston R, Gilroy D, Lehane M, Furey A. Hawthorn (Crataegus spp.) in the treatment of cardiovascular disease. Pharmacogn Rev. 2010;4(7):32–41.
63. Kim H-G, Cho J-H, Yoo S-R, Lee J-S, Han J-M, Lee N-H, et al. Antifatigue effects of Panax ginseng C.A. Meyer: a randomised, double-blind, placebo-controlled trial. PLoS One. 2013;8(4):e61271.
64. Calabrese EJ. Hormesis and ginseng: ginseng mixtures and individual constituents commonly display hormesis dose responses, especially for neuroprotective effects. Molecules. 2020;25(11):2719.
65. Wang H-B, Duan M-X, Xu M, Huang S-H, Yang J, Yang J, et al. Cordycepin ameliorates cardiac hypertrophy via activating the AMPKα pathway. J Cell Mol Med. 2019;23(8):5715–27.
66. Wu R, Yao P-A, Wang H-L, Gao Y, Yu H-L, Wang L, et al. Effect of fermented Cordyceps sinensis on doxorubicin-induced cardiotoxicity in rats. Mol Med Rep. 2018;18(3):3229–41.
67. Zang Y, Wan J, Zhang Z, Huang S, Liu X, Zhang W. An updated role of astragaloside IV in heart failure. Biomed Pharmacother. 2020;126:110012.
68. Xu L, Wang R, Liu H, Wang J, Mang J, Xu Z. Resveratrol treatment is associated with lipid regulation and inhibition of lipoprotein-associated phospholipase A2 (Lp-PLA2) in rabbits fed a high-fat diet. Evid Based Complement Alternat Med. 2020;2020:9641582.
69. Li H, Xia N, Hasselwander S, Daiber A. Resveratrol and vascular function. Int J Mol Sci. 2019;20(9):2155.
70. Huang Y, Zhu X, Chen K, Lang H, Zhang Y, Hou P, et al. Resveratrol prevents sarcopenic obesity by reversing mitochondrial dysfunction and oxidative stress via the PKA/LKB1/AMPK pathway. Aging. 2019;11(8):2217–40.
71. Källström M, Soveri I, Oldgren J, Laukkanen J, Ichiki T, Tei C, et al. Effects of sauna bath on heart failure: a systematic review and meta-analysis. Clin Cardiol. 2018;41(11):1491–501.
72. Gomes-Neto M, Rodrigues ESJ, Silva WMJ, Carvalho VO. Effects of yoga in patients with chronic heart failure: a meta-analysis. Arq Bras Cardiol. 2014;103(5):433–9.

73. Calabrese EJ. Preconditioning is hormesis part II: how the conditioning dose mediates protection: dose optimization within temporal and mechanistic frameworks. Pharmacol Res. 2016;110:265–75.
74. Liu Y, Li M, Du X, Huang Z, Quan N. Sestrin 2, a potential star of antioxidant stress in cardiovascular diseases. Free Radic Biol Med. 2021;163:56–68.
75. Liu Y, Du X, Huang Z, Zheng Y, Quan N. Sestrin 2 controls the cardiovascular aging process via an integrated network of signaling pathways. Ageing Res Rev. 2020;62:101096.
76. Zhang Q, Liu J, Duan H, Li R, Peng W, Wu C. Activation of Nrf2/HO-1 signaling: an important molecular mechanism of herbal medicine in the treatment of atherosclerosis via the protection of vascular endothelial cells from oxidative stress. J Adv Res. 2021;34:43–63.
77. Thieme M, Sivritas SH, Mergia E, Potthoff SA, Yang G, Hering L, et al. Phosphodiesterase 5 inhibition ameliorates angiotensin II-dependent hypertension and renal vascular dysfunction. Am J Physiol Renal Physiol. 2017;312(3):F474–81.
78. Fierascu RC, Fierascu I, Ortan A, Fierascu IC, Anuta V, Velescu BS, et al. Leonurus cardiaca L. as a source of bioactive compounds: an update of the European Medicines Agency Assessment Report (2010). Biomed Res Int. 2019;2019:4303215.
79. Ismail MA, Norhayati MN, Mohamad N. Olive leaf extract effect on cardiometabolic profile among adults with prehypertension and hypertension: a systematic review and meta-analysis. PeerJ. 2021;9:e11173.
80. Kreis W. The Foxgloves (Digitalis) revisited. Planta Med. 2017;83(12–13):962–76.
81. Riegger AJ. ACE inhibitors in congestive heart failure. Cardiology. 1989;76(Suppl 2):42–9.
82. Vinci P, Panizon E, Tosoni LM, Cerrato C, Pellicori F, Mearelli F, et al. Statin-associated myopathy: emphasis on mechanisms and targeted therapy. Int J Mol Sci. 2021;22(21):11687.
83. Verhoeff K, Mitchell JR. Cardiopulmonary physiology: why the heart and lungs are inextricably linked. Adv Physiol Educ. 2017;41(3):348–53.
84. Byrne AJ, Mathie SA, Gregory LG, Lloyd CM. Pulmonary macrophages: key players in the innate defence of the airways. Thorax. 2015;70(12):1189–96. http://thorax.bmj.com/content/70/12/1189.abstract.
85. Kosyreva A, Dzhalilova D, Lokhonina A, Vishnyakova P, Fatkhudinov T. The role of macrophages in the pathogenesis of SARS-CoV-2-associated acute respiratory distress syndrome. Front Immunol. 2021;10:682871. https://pubmed.ncbi.nlm.nih.gov/34040616.
86. Kadomoto S, Izumi K, Mizokami A. Macrophage polarity and disease control. Int J Mol Sci. 2021;23(1):144.
87. Ricoy J, Rodríguez-Núñez N, Álvarez-Dobaño JM, Toubes ME, Riveiro V, Valdés L. Diaphragmatic dysfunction. Pulmonology. 2019;25(4):223–35.
88. Javaheri S, Barbe F, Campos-Rodriguez F, Dempsey JA, Khayat R, Javaheri S, et al. Sleep apnea: types, mechanisms, and clinical cardiovascular consequences. J Am Coll Cardiol. 2017;69(7):841–58.
89. Manisalidis I, Stavropoulou E, Stavropoulos A, Bezirtzoglou E. Environmental and health impacts of air pollution: a review. Front Public Health. 2020;8:14.
90. Bagdonas E, Raudoniute J, Bruzauskaite I, Aldonyte R. Novel aspects of pathogenesis and regeneration mechanisms in COPD. Int J Chron Obstruct Pulmon Dis. 2015;10:995–1013.
91. CFTR gene [Internet]. Medline Plus. https://medlineplus.gov/genetics/gene/cftr/.
92. Haynes JM. Basic spirometry testing and interpretation for the primary care provider. Can J Respir Ther. 2018;54(4). https://pubmed.ncbi.nlm.nih.gov/31164790. https://doi.org/10.29390/cjrt-2018-017.
93. Barnes PJ. Cellular and molecular mechanisms of asthma and COPD. Clin Sci (Lond). 2017;131(13):1541–58.
94. Gharib SA, Manicone AM, Parks WC. Matrix metalloproteinases in emphysema. Matrix Biol. 2018;73:34–51.
95. Kulkarni T, O'Reilly P, Antony VB, Gaggar A, Thannickal VJ. Matrix remodeling in pulmonary fibrosis and emphysema. Am J Respir Cell Mol Biol. 2016;54(6):751–60.

96. Yao R-Q, Ren C, Xia Z-F, Yao Y-M. Organelle-specific autophagy in inflammatory diseases: a potential therapeutic target underlying the quality control of multiple organelles. Autophagy. 2021;17(2):385–401.
97. Beasley MB, Galateau-Salle F, Dacic S. Pleural mesothelioma classification update. Virchows Arch. 2021;478(1):59–72.
98. James C, Bernstein DI, Cox J, Ryan P, Wolfe C, Jandarov R, et al. HEPA filtration improves asthma control in children exposed to traffic-related airborne particles. Indoor Air. 2020;30(2):235–43.
99. Environmental Protection Agency. Care for your air: a guide to indoor air quality [Internet]. https://www.epa.gov/indoor-air-quality-iaq/care-your-air-guide-indoor-air-quality. Accessed 28 May 2022.
100. Pall ML, Levine S. Nrf2, a master regulator of detoxification and also antioxidant, anti-inflammatory and other cytoprotective mechanisms, is raised by health promoting factors. Sheng Li Xue Bao. 2015;67(1):1–18.
101. Kim M, Kowalsky AH, Lee JH. Sestrins in physiological stress responses. Annu Rev Physiol. 2021;83:381–403.
102. Liao W, Lim AYH, Tan WSD, Abisheganaden J, Wong WSF. Restoration of HDAC2 and Nrf2 by andrographolide overcomes corticosteroid resistance in chronic obstructive pulmonary disease. Br J Pharmacol. 2020;177(16):3662–73.
103. Younus H. Therapeutic potentials of superoxide dismutase. Int J Health Sci. 2018;12(3):88–93. https://pubmed.ncbi.nlm.nih.gov/29896077.
104. Minich DM, Brown BI. A review of dietary (phyto)nutrients for glutathione support. Nutrients. 2019;11(9):2073. https://pubmed.ncbi.nlm.nih.gov/31484368.
105. Barnes PJ. Oxidative stress-based therapeutics in COPD. Redox Biol. 2020;33:101544.
106. Lago JHG, Toledo-Arruda AC, Mernak M, Barrosa KH, Martins MA, Tibério IFLC, et al. Structure-activity association of flavonoids in lung diseases. Molecules. 2014;19(3):3570–95.
107. De Flora S, Balansky R, La Maestra S. Rationale for the use of N-acetylcysteine in both prevention and adjuvant therapy of COVID-19. FASEB J. 2020;34(10):13185–93.
108. Ibrahim MA, Ramadan HH, Mohammed RN. Evidence that Ginkgo Biloba could use in the influenza and coronavirus COVID-19 infections. J Basic Clin Physiol Pharmacol. 2021;32(3):131–43.
109. Li X, Nian B-B, Tan C-P, Liu Y-F, Xu Y-J. Deep-frying oil induces cytotoxicity, inflammation and apoptosis on intestinal epithelial cells. J Sci Food Agric. 2022;102(8):3160–8.
110. Moorthy B, Chu C, Carlin DJ. Polycyclic aromatic hydrocarbons: from metabolism to lung cancer. Toxicol Sci. 2015;145(1):5–15.
111. Amazouz H, Roda C, Beydon N, Lezmi G, Bourgoin-Heck M, Just J, et al. Mediterranean diet and lung function, sensitization, and asthma at school age: the PARIS cohort. Pediatr Allergy Immunol. 2021;32(7):1437–44.
112. Yang Z-Y, Zhong H-B, Mao C, Yuan J-Q, Huang Y-F, Wu X-Y, et al. Yoga for asthma. Cochrane Database Syst Rev. 2016;4(4):CD010346.
113. Holland AE, Hill CJ, Jones AY, McDonald CF. Breathing exercises for chronic obstructive pulmonary disease. Cochrane Database Syst Rev. 2012;10:CD008250.
114. Khaltaev N, Solimene U, Vitale F, Zanasi A. Balneotherapy and hydrotherapy in chronic respiratory disease. J Thorac Dis. 2020;12(8):4459–68.
115. Cruz-Montecinos C, Godoy-Olave D, Contreras-Briceño FA, Gutiérrez P, Torres-Castro R, Miret-Venegas L, et al. The immediate effect of soft tissue manual therapy intervention on lung function in severe chronic obstructive pulmonary disease. Int J Chron Obstruct Pulmon Dis. 2017;12:691–6.
116. Paneroni M, Simonelli C, Vitacca M, Ambrosino N. Aerobic exercise training in very severe chronic obstructive pulmonary disease: a systematic review and meta-analysis. Am J Phys Med Rehabil. 2017;96(8):541–8.
117. Wada JT, Borges-Santos E, Porras DC, Paisani DM, Cukier A, Lunardi AC, et al. Effects of aerobic training combined with respiratory muscle stretching on the functional exercise

capacity and thoracoabdominal kinematics in patients with COPD: a randomized and controlled trial. Int J Chron Obstruct Pulmon Dis. 2016;11:2691–700.
118. Ding S, Zhong C. Exercise and asthma. Adv Exp Med Biol. 2020;1228:369–80.
119. Godfrey A, Saunder P. Principles and Practices of Naturopathic Botanical Medicine. Toronto, Ontario: CCNM Press; 2010.
120. Baharara H, Moghadam AT, Sahebkar A, Emami SA, Tayebi T, Mohammadpour AH. The effects of Ivy (Hedera helix) on respiratory problems and cough in humans: a review. Adv Exp Med Biol. 2021;1328:361–76.
121. Duffy SP, Criner GJ. Chronic obstructive pulmonary disease: evaluation and management. Med Clin North Am. 2019;103(3):453–61.
122. Mauer Y, Taliercio RM. Managing adult asthma: the 2019 GINA guidelines. Cleve Clin J Med. 2020;87(9):569–75.
123. Pakhale S, Mulpuru S, Verheij TJM, Kochen MM, Rohde GGU, Bjerre LM. Antibiotics for community-acquired pneumonia in adult outpatients. Cochrane Database Syst Rev. 2014;2014(10):CD002109.
124. Trefts E, Gannon M, Wasserman DH. The liver. Curr Biol. 2017;27(21):R1147–51.
125. Manikandan P, Nagini S. Cytochrome P450 structure, function and clinical significance: a review. Curr Drug Targets. 2018;19(1):38–54.
126. Prysyazhnyuk V, Sydorchuk L, Sydorchuk R, Prysiazhniuk I, Bobkovych K, Buzdugan I, et al. Glutathione-S-transferases genes-promising predictors of hepatic dysfunction. World J Hepatol. 2021;13(6):620–33.
127. Corbin KD, Zeisel SH. Choline metabolism provides novel insights into nonalcoholic fatty liver disease and its progression. Curr Opin Gastroenterol. 2012;28(2):159–65. https://pubmed.ncbi.nlm.nih.gov/22134222.
128. Montané E, Santesmases J. Adverse drug reactions. Med Clin. 2020;154(5):178–84.
129. Garcia J, Costa VM, Carvalho A, Baptista P, de Pinho PG, de Lourdes BM, et al. Amanita phalloides poisoning: mechanisms of toxicity and treatment. Food Chem Toxicol. 2015;86:41–55.
130. Park BK, Dear JW, Antoine DJ. Paracetamol (acetaminophen) poisoning. BMJ Clin Evid. 2015;2015:2101.
131. Byrne CD, Targher G. NAFLD: a multisystem disease. J Hepatol. 2015;62(1 Suppl):S47–64.
132. Del Campo JA, Gallego-Durán R, Gallego P, Grande L. Genetic and epigenetic regulation in nonalcoholic fatty liver disease (NAFLD). Int J Mol Sci. 2018;19(3):911.
133. Mysore KR, Leung DH. Hepatitis B and C. Clin Liver Dis. 2018;22(4):703–22.
134. Toosi AEK. Liver fibrosis: causes and methods of assessment, a review. Rom J Intern Med. 2015;53(4):304–14.
135. Parola M, Pinzani M. Liver fibrosis: pathophysiology, pathogenetic targets and clinical issues. Mol Aspects Med. 2019;65:37–55.
136. Arroyo V, Moreau R, Kamath PS, Jalan R, Ginès P, Nevens F, et al. Acute-on-chronic liver failure in cirrhosis. Nat Rev Dis Primers. 2016;2:16041.
137. Weissenborn K. Hepatic encephalopathy: definition, clinical grading and diagnostic principles. Drugs. 2019;79(Suppl 1):5–9.
138. Llovet JM, Kelley RK, Villanueva A, Singal AG, Pikarsky E, Roayaie S, et al. Hepatocellular carcinoma. Nat Rev Dis Primers. 2021;7(1):6.
139. Khemlina G, Ikeda S, Kurzrock R. The biology of hepatocellular carcinoma: implications for genomic and immune therapies. Mol Cancer. 2017;16(1):149.
140. Mundi MS, Velapati S, Patel J, Kellogg TA, Abu Dayyeh BK, Hurt RT. Evolution of NAFLD and its management. Nutr Clin Pract. 2020;35(1):72–84.
141. Marjot T, Ray DW, Williams FR, Tomlinson JW, Armstrong MJ. Sleep and liver disease: a bidirectional relationship. lancet. Gastroenterol Hepatol. 2021;6(10):850–63.
142. Barchetta I, Cimini FA, Cavallo MG. Vitamin D and metabolic dysfunction-associated fatty liver disease (MAFLD): an update. Nutrients. 2020;12(11):3302.
143. Fakhoury HMA, Kvietys PR, AlKattan W, Anouti F, Al Elahi MA, Karras SN, et al. Vitamin D and intestinal homeostasis: barrier, microbiota, and immune modulation. J Steroid Biochem Mol Biol. 2020;200:105663.

144. Keirns BH, Koemel NA, Sciarrillo CM, Anderson KL, Emerson SR. Exercise and intestinal permeability: another form of exercise-induced hormesis? Am J Physiol Gastrointest Liver Physiol. 2020;319(4):G512–8.
145. Nabi T, Nabi S, Rafiq N, Shah A. Role of N-acetylcysteine treatment in non-acetaminophen-induced acute liver failure: a prospective study. Saudi J Gastroenterol. 2017;23(3):169–75. https://pubmed.ncbi.nlm.nih.gov/28611340.
146. Abenavoli L, Izzo AA, Milić N, Cicala C, Santini A, Capasso R. Milk thistle (Silybum marianum): a concise overview on its chemistry, pharmacological, and nutraceutical uses in liver diseases. Phytother Res. 2018;32(11):2202–13.
147. Kalopitas G, Antza C, Doundoulakis I, Siargkas A, Kouroumalis E, Germanidis G, et al. Impact of Silymarin in individuals with nonalcoholic fatty liver disease: a systematic review and meta-analysis. Nutrition. 2021;83:111092.
148. Wang H, Che J, Cui K, Zhuang W, Li H, Sun J, et al. Schisantherin A ameliorates liver fibrosis through TGF-β1mediated activation of TAK1/MAPK and NF-κB pathways in vitro and in vivo. Phytomedicine. 2021;88:153609.
149. Nelson KM, Dahlin JL, Bisson J, Graham J, Pauli GF, Walters MA. The essential medicinal chemistry of curcumin. J Med Chem. 2017;60(5):1620–37.
150. Panahi Y, Kianpour P, Mohtashami R, Jafari R, Simental-Mendía LE, Sahebkar A. Efficacy and safety of phytosomal curcumin in non-alcoholic fatty liver disease: a randomized controlled trial. Drug Res. 2017;67(4):244–51.
151. Moradi S, Shokri-Mashhadi N, Saraf Bank S, Mohammadi H, Zobeiri M, Clark CCT, et al. The effects of Cynara scolymus L. supplementation on liver enzymes: a systematic review and meta-analysis. Int J Clin Pract. 2021;75:e14726.
152. Panahi Y, Kianpour P, Mohtashami R, Atkin SL, Butler AE, Jafari R, et al. Efficacy of artichoke leaf extract in non-alcoholic fatty liver disease: a pilot double-blind randomized controlled trial. Phytother Res. 2018;32(7):1382–7.
153. Pfingstgraf IO, Taulescu M, Pop RM, Orăsan R, Vlase L, Uifalean A, et al. Protective effects of Taraxacum officinale L. (Dandelion) root extract in experimental acute on chronic liver failure. Antioxidants. 2021;10(4):504.
154. Ipsen DH, Tveden-Nyborg P, Lykkesfeldt J. Does vitamin C deficiency promote fatty liver disease development? Nutrients. 2014;6(12):5473–99.
155. Lee H, Ahn J, Shin SS, Yoon M. Ascorbic acid inhibits visceral obesity and nonalcoholic fatty liver disease by activating peroxisome proliferator-activated receptor α in high-fat-diet-fed C57BL/6J mice. Int J Obes (Lond). 2019;43(8):1620–30.
156. Castellanos-Jankiewicz A, Guzmán-Quevedo O, Fénelon VS, Zizzari P, Quarta C, Bellocchio L, et al. Hypothalamic bile acid-TGR5 signaling protects from obesity. Cell Metab. 2021;33(7):1483–1492.e10.
157. Yao CK, Fung J, Chu NHS, Tan VPY. Dietary interventions in liver cirrhosis. J Clin Gastroenterol. 2018;52(8):663–73.
158. Dimidi E, Cox SR, Rossi M, Whelan K. Fermented foods: definitions and characteristics, impact on the gut microbiota and effects on gastrointestinal health and disease. Nutrients. 2019;11(8):1806. https://pubmed.ncbi.nlm.nih.gov/31387262.
159. Zhou J, Massey S, Story D, Li L. Metformin: an old drug with new applications. Int J Mol Sci. 2018;19(10):2863.
160. González-Grande R, Jiménez-Pérez M, González Arjona C, Mostazo TJ. New approaches in the treatment of hepatitis C. World J Gastroenterol. 2016;22(4):1421–32.
161. Gluud LL, Dam G, Les I, Marchesini G, Borre M, Aagaard NK, et al. Branched-chain amino acids for people with hepatic encephalopathy. Cochrane Database Syst Rev. 2017;5(5):CD001939.
162. Bodzin AS, Baker TB. Liver transplantation today: where we are now and where we are going. Liver Transpl. 2018;24(10):1470–5.
163. Goodman BE. Insights into digestion and absorption of major nutrients in humans. Adv Physiol Educ. 2010;34(2):44–53.

164. Livovsky DM, Pribic T, Azpiroz F. Food, eating, and the gastrointestinal tract. Nutrients. 2020;12(4):986.
165. Guilliams TG, Drake LE. Meal-time supplementation with betaine hcl for functional hypochlorhydria: what is the evidence? Integr Med (Encinitas). 2020;19(1):32–6.
166. Goldberger JJ, Arora R, Buckley U, Shivkumar K. Autonomic nervous system dysfunction: JACC focus seminar. J Am Coll Cardiol. 2019;73(10):1189–206. https://pubmed.ncbi.nlm.nih.gov/30871703.
167. Perbtani Y, Forsmark CE. Update on the diagnosis and management of exocrine pancreatic insufficiency. F1000Research. 2019;8.
168. Boyer JL. Bile formation and secretion. Compr Physiol. 2013;3(3):1035–78.
169. Miyamoto T, Ebihara T, Kozaki K. The association between eating difficulties and biliary sludge in the gallbladder in older adults with advanced dementia, at end of life. PLoS One. 2019;14(7):e0219538.
170. Ford AC, Sperber AD, Corsetti M, Camilleri M. Irritable bowel syndrome. Lancet. 2020;396(10263):1675–88.
171. Yang J-C, Lu C-W, Lin C-J. Treatment of Helicobacter pylori infection: current status and future concepts. World J Gastroenterol. 2014;20(18):5283–93.
172. Sender R, Fuchs S, Milo R. Revised estimates for the number of human and bacteria cells in the body. PLoS Biol. 2016;14(8):e1002533. https://pubmed.ncbi.nlm.nih.gov/27541692.
173. Ghavami SB, Yadegar A, Aghdaei HA, Sorrentino D, Farmani M, Mir AS, et al. Immunomodulation and generation of tolerogenic dendritic cells by probiotic bacteria in patients with inflammatory bowel disease. Int J Mol Sci. 2020;21(17):6266.
174. Baumgart DC, Sandborn WJ. Crohn's disease. Lancet. 2012;380(9853):1590–605.
175. Petagna L, Antonelli A, Ganini C, Bellato V, Campanelli M, Divizia A, et al. Pathophysiology of Crohn's disease inflammation and recurrence. Biol Direct. 2020;15(1):23.
176. Arakawa T, Watanabe T, Tanigawa T, Tominaga K, Fujiwara Y, Morimoto K. Quality of ulcer healing in gastrointestinal tract: its pathophysiology and clinical relevance. World J Gastroenterol. 2012;18(35):4811–22.
177. Li Y, Xia R, Zhang B, Li C. Chronic atrophic gastritis: a review. J Environ Pathol Toxicol Oncol. 2018;37(3):241–59.
178. Celiac disease. Am Fam Physician. 2014;89(2):Online.
179. Malamut G, Cording S, Cerf-Bensussan N. Recent advances in celiac disease and refractory celiac disease. F1000Research. 2019;8.
180. Roszkowska A, Pawlicka M, Mroczek A, Bałabuszek K, Nieradko-Iwanicka B. Non-celiac gluten sensitivity: a review. Medicina (Kaunas). 2019;55(6):222.
181. Holleczek B, Schöttker B, Brenner H. Helicobacter pylori infection, chronic atrophic gastritis and risk of stomach and esophagus cancer: results from the prospective population-based ESTHER cohort study. Int J Cancer. 2020;146(10):2773–83.
182. Dulai PS, Sandborn WJ, Gupta S. Colorectal cancer and dysplasia in inflammatory bowel disease: a review of disease epidemiology, pathophysiology, and management. Cancer Prev Res (Phila). 2016;9(12):887–94.
183. Pasternak B, Svanström H, Schmiegelow K, Jess T, Hviid A. Use of azathioprine and the risk of cancer in inflammatory bowel disease. Am J Epidemiol. 2013;177(11):1296–305.
184. Duboc H, Coffin B, Siproudhis L. Disruption of circadian rhythms and gut motility: an overview of underlying mechanisms and associated pathologies. J Clin Gastroenterol. 2020;54(5):405–14.
185. Chrobak AA, Nowakowski J, Zwolińska-Wcisło M, Cibor D, Przybylska-Feluś M, Ochyra K, et al. Associations between chronotype, sleep disturbances and seasonality with fatigue and inflammatory bowel disease symptoms. Chronobiol Int. 2018;35(8):1142–52.
186. Tabatabaeizadeh S-A, Tafazoli N, Ferns GA, Avan A, Ghayour-Mobarhan M. Vitamin D, the gut microbiome and inflammatory bowel disease. J Res Med Sci. 2018;23:75.
187. Konturek PC, Brzozowski T, Konturek SJ. Stress and the gut: pathophysiology, clinical consequences, diagnostic approach and treatment options. J Physiol Pharmacol. 2011;62(6):591–9.

188. Mahmoud MF, Nabil M, Abdo W, Abdelfattah MAO, El-Shazly AM, El Kharrassi Y, et al. Syzygium samarangense leaf extract mitigates indomethacin-induced gastropathy via the NF-κB signaling pathway in rats. Biomed Pharmacother. 2021;139:111675.
189. Seebohm G, Schreiber JA. Beyond Hot and spicy: TRPV channels and their pharmacological modulation. Cell Physiol Biochem. 2021;55(S3):108–30.
190. Fattori V, Hohmann MSN, Rossaneis AC, Pinho-Ribeiro FA, Verri WA. Capsaicin: current understanding of its mechanisms and therapy of pain and other pre-clinical and clinical uses. Molecules. 2016;21(7):844.
191. Satyanarayana MN. Capsaicin and gastric ulcers. Crit Rev Food Sci Nutr. 2006;46(4):275–328.
192. Coëffier M, Claeyssens S, Hecketsweiler B, Lavoinne A, Ducrotté P, Déchelotte P. Enteral glutamine stimulates protein synthesis and decreases ubiquitin mRNA level in human gut mucosa. Am J Physiol Gastrointest Liver Physiol. 2003;285(2):G266–73.
193. Cheney G. Vitamin U therapy of peptic ulcer. Calif Med. 1952;77(4):248–52.
194. Liu C, Dunkin D, Lai J, Song Y, Ceballos C, Benkov K, et al. Anti-inflammatory effects of ganoderma lucidum triterpenoid in human Crohn's disease associated with downregulation of NF-κB signaling. Inflamm Bowel Dis. 2015;21(8):1918–25.
195. Hassanalilou T, Ghavamzadeh S, Khalili L. Curcumin and gastric cancer: a review on mechanisms of action. J Gastrointest Cancer. 2019;50(2):185–92.
196. Terry PD, Villinger F, Bubenik GA, Sitaraman SV. Melatonin and ulcerative colitis: evidence, biological mechanisms, and future research. Inflamm Bowel Dis. 2009;15(1):134–40.
197. Shahrokh S, Qobadighadikolaei R, Abbasinazari M, Haghazali M, Asadzadeh Aghdaei H, Abdi S, et al. Efficacy and safety of melatonin as an adjunctive therapy on clinical, biochemical, and quality of life in patients with ulcerative colitis. Iran J Pharm Res. 2021;20(2):197–205.
198. Carrascal L, Nunez-Abades P, Ayala A, Cano M. Role of melatonin in the inflammatory process and its therapeutic potential. Curr Pharm Des. 2018;24(14):1563–88.
199. Kolacek M, Paduchova Z, Dvorakova M, Zitnanova I, Cierna I, Durackova Z, et al. Effect of natural polyphenols on thromboxane levels in children with Crohn's disease. Bratisl Lek Listy. 2019;120(12):924–8.
200. Zhang J, Huang Q, Zhao R, Ma Z. A network pharmacology study on the Tripteryguim wilfordii Hook for treatment of Crohn's disease. BMC Complement Med Ther. 2020;20(1):95.
201. WebMD. Pancreatin tablet—uses, side effects, and more [Internet]. https://www.webmd.com/drugs/2/drug-1457/pancreatin-oral/details. Accessed 30 May 2022.
202. Thorat V, Reddy N, Bhatia S, Bapaye A, Rajkumar JS, Kini DD, et al. Randomised clinical trial: the efficacy and safety of pancreatin enteric-coated minimicrospheres (Creon 40000 MMS) in patients with pancreatic exocrine insufficiency due to chronic pancreatitis—a double-blind, placebo-controlled study. Aliment Pharmacol Ther. 2012;36(5):426–36.
203. Ido H, Matsubara H, Kuroda M, Takahashi A, Kojima Y, Koikeda S, et al. Combination of gluten-digesting enzymes improved symptoms of non-celiac gluten sensitivity: a randomized single-blind, placebo-controlled crossover study. Clin Transl Gastroenterol. 2018;9(9):181.
204. Ried K, Travica N, Dorairaj R, Sali A. Herbal formula improves upper and lower gastrointestinal symptoms and gut health in Australian adults with digestive disorders. Nutr Res. 2020;76:37–51.
205. de Jesus NZT, de Souza FH, Gomes IF, de Almeida Leite TJ, de Morais Lima GR, Barbosa-Filho JM, et al. Tannins, peptic ulcers and related mechanisms. Int J Mol Sci. 2012;13(3):3203–28.
206. Aditi A, Graham DY. Vitamin C, gastritis, and gastric disease: a historical review and update. Dig Dis Sci. 2012;57(10):2504–15.
207. Toh JWT, Wilson RB. Pathways of gastric carcinogenesis, helicobacter pylori virulence and interactions with antioxidant systems, vitamin C and phytochemicals. Int J Mol Sci. 2020;21(17):6451.
208. Chen G, Bei B, Feng Y, Li X, Jiang Z, Si J-Y, et al. Glycyrrhetinic acid maintains intestinal homeostasis via HuR. Front Pharmacol. 2019;10:535.

209. Hajiaghamohammadi AA, Zargar A, Oveisi S, Samimi R, Reisian S. To evaluate of the effect of adding licorice to the standard treatment regimen of Helicobacter pylori. Braz J Infect Dis. 2016;20(6):534–8.
210. Shakeri F, Gholamnezhad Z, Mégarbane B, Rezaee R, Boskabady MH. Gastrointestinal effects of Nigella sativa and its main constituent, thymoquinone: a review. Avicenna J Phytomed. 2016;6(1):9–20.
211. Habtemariam S, Belai A. Natural therapies of the inflammatory bowel disease: the case of Rutin and its Aglycone, Quercetin. Mini Rev Med Chem. 2018;18(3):234–43.
212. Suskind DL, Lee D, Kim Y-M, Wahbeh G, Singh N, Braly K, et al. The specific carbohydrate diet and diet modification as induction therapy for pediatric Crohn's disease: a randomized diet controlled trial. Nutrients. 2020;12(12):3749.
213. Jiang Y, Jarr K, Layton C, Gardner CD, Ashouri JF, Abreu MT, et al. Therapeutic implications of diet in inflammatory bowel disease and related immune-mediated inflammatory diseases. Nutrients. 2021;13(3):890.
214. Davis SP, Bolin LP, Crane PB, Crandell J. Non-pharmacological interventions for anxiety and depression in adults with inflammatory bowel disease: a systematic review and meta-analysis. Front Psychol. 2020;11:538741.
215. Zhang J, Wu HM, Wang X, Xie J, Li X, Ma J, et al. Efficacy of prebiotics and probiotics for functional dyspepsia: a systematic review and meta-analysis. Medicine. 2020;99(7):e19107.
216. Vitetta L, Vitetta G, Hall S. Immunological tolerance and function: associations between intestinal bacteria, probiotics, prebiotics, and phages. Front Immunol. 2018;9:2240.
217. Pais P, Almeida V, Yılmaz M, Teixeira MC. Saccharomyces boulardii: what makes it tick as successful probiotic? J Fungi. 2020;6(2):78.
218. Mack DR, Ahrne S, Hyde L, Wei S, Hollingsworth MA. Extracellular MUC3 mucin secretion follows adherence of Lactobacillus strains to intestinal epithelial cells in vitro. Gut. 2003;52(6):827–33.
219. Morozov V, Borkowski J, Hanisch F-G. The double face of mucin-type O-glycans in lectin-mediated infection and immunity. Molecules. 2018;23(5):1151.
220. Schneider A, Streitberger K, Joos S. Acupuncture treatment in gastrointestinal diseases: a systematic review. World J Gastroenterol. 2007;13(25):3417–24.
221. Conte R, Marturano V, Peluso G, Calarco A, Cerruti P. Recent advances in nanoparticle-mediated delivery of anti-inflammatory phytocompounds. Int J Mol Sci. 2017;18(4):709.
222. Rothe G, Hachiya A, Yamada Y, Hashimoto T, Dräger B. Alkaloids in plants and root cultures of Atropa belladonna overexpressing putrescine N-methyltransferase. J Exp Bot. 2003;54(390):2065–70.
223. Davies MK, Hollman A. Atropa belladonna. Heart. 2002;88(3):215.
224. Kaye MD, Rhodes J, Sweetnam PM. Clinical evaluation of three long-acting anticholinergic compounds. Gut. 1968;9(5):590–6.
225. Malik TF, Gnanapandithan K, Singh K. Peptic ulcer disease. In: StatPearls. Treasure Island, FL: StatPearls; 2021.
226. Poonyam P, Chotivitayatarakorn P, Vilaichone R-K. High effective of 14-day high-dose PPI-bismuth-containing quadruple therapy with probiotics supplement for Helicobacter pylori eradication: a double blinded-randomized placebo-controlled study. Asian Pac J Cancer Prev. 2019;20(9):2859–64.
227. Martín-Núñez GM, Cornejo-Pareja I, Clemente-Postigo M, Tinahones FJ, Moreno-Indias I. Helicobacter pylori eradication therapy affect the gut microbiota and ghrelin levels. Front Med. 2021;8:712908.
228. Pierik M, Rutgeerts P, Vlietinck R, Vermeire S. Pharmacogenetics in inflammatory bowel disease. World J Gastroenterol. 2006;12(23):3657–67.
229. Yamamoto T, Shimoyama T, Kuriyama M. Dietary and enteral interventions for Crohn's disease. Curr Opin Biotechnol. 2017;44:69–73.
230. Lloyd-Price J, Abu-Ali G, Huttenhower C. The healthy human microbiome. Genome Med. 2016;8(1):51.

231. Spencer NJ, Hu H. Enteric nervous system: sensory transduction, neural circuits and gastrointestinal motility. Nat Rev Gastroenterol Hepatol. 2020;17(6):338–51.
232. The Rome Foundation [Internet]. https://theromefoundation.org/rome-iv/rome-iv-criteria/.
233. Bristol Stool Chart [Internet]. https://www.bladderandbowel.org/wp-content/uploads/2017/05/BBC002_Bristol-Stool-Chart-Jan-2016.pdf.
234. Arasaradnam RP, Brown S, Forbes A, Fox MR, Hungin P, Kelman L, et al. Guidelines for the investigation of chronic diarrhoea in adults: British Society of Gastroenterology, 3rd edition. Gut. 2018;67(8):1380–99.
235. Paré P, Fedorak RN. Systematic review of stimulant and nonstimulant laxatives for the treatment of functional constipation. Can J Gastroenterol Hepatol. 2014;28(10):549–57.
236. Tong Y, Tang J. Candida albicans infection and intestinal immunity. Microbiol Res. 2017;198:27–35.
237. Koboziev I, Karlsson F, Grisham MB. Gut-associated lymphoid tissue, T cell trafficking, and chronic intestinal inflammation. Ann N Y Acad Sci. 2010;1207(Suppl 1):E86–93.
238. Lord R, Burr NE, Mohammed N, Subramanian V. Colonic lesion characterization in inflammatory bowel disease: a systematic review and meta-analysis. World J Gastroenterol. 2018;24(10):1167–80.
239. Czepiel J, Dróżdż M, Pituch H, Kuijper EJ, Perucki W, Mielimonka A, et al. Clostridium difficile infection: review. Eur J Clin Microbiol Infect Dis. 2019;38(7):1211–21.
240. Alfredsson J, Wick MJ. Mechanism of fibrosis and stricture formation in Crohn's disease. Scand J Immunol. 2020;92(6):e12990.
241. Luo C, Cen S, Ding G, Wu W. Mucinous colorectal adenocarcinoma: clinical pathology and treatment options. Cancer Commun. 2019;39(1):13.
242. Guan Z-W, Yu E-Z, Feng Q. Soluble dietary fiber, one of the most important nutrients for the gut microbiota. Molecules. 2021;26(22):6802.
243. Ngoan LT, Thu NT, Lua NT, Hang LTM, Bich NN, Van HN, et al. Cooking temperature, heat-generated carcinogens, and the risk of stomach and colorectal cancers. Asian Pac J Cancer Prev. 2009;10(1):83–6.
244. Qin H-Y, Cheng C-W, Tang X-D, Bian Z-X. Impact of psychological stress on irritable bowel syndrome. World J Gastroenterol. 2014;20(39):14126–31.
245. National Institute for Health and Care Excellence (NICE). Constipation in children and young people: diagnosis and management. London: National Institute for Health and Care Excellence (NICE); 2017.
246. Kanner J. Polyphenols by generating H2O2, affect cell redox signaling, inhibit PTPs and activate Nrf2 axis for adaptation and cell surviving: in vitro, in vivo and human health. Antioxidants. 2020;9(9):797. https://pubmed.ncbi.nlm.nih.gov/32867057.
247. Calabrese EJ, Tsatsakis A, Agathokleous E, Giordano J, Calabrese V. Does Green tea induce hormesis? Dose Response. 2020;18(3):1559325820936170. https://pubmed.ncbi.nlm.nih.gov/32728352.
248. Badgujar SB, Patel VV, Bandivdekar AH. Foeniculum vulgare Mill: a review of its botany, phytochemistry, pharmacology, contemporary application, and toxicology. Biomed Res Int. 2014;2014:842674.
249. Salehi B, Zakaria ZA, Gyawali R, Ibrahim SA, Rajkovic J, Shinwari ZK, et al. Piper species: a comprehensive review on their phytochemistry, biological activities and applications. Molecules. 2019;24(7):1364.
250. Bharucha AE, Lacy BE. Mechanisms, evaluation, and management of chronic constipation. Gastroenterology. 2020;158(5):1232–1249.e3.
251. Martin CR, Osadchiy V, Kalani A, Mayer EA. The brain-gut-microbiome axis. Cell Mol Gastroenterol Hepatol. 2018;6(2):133–48.
252. Giua C, Minerba L, Piras A, Floris N, Romano F, Sifac G. The effect of sucralfate-containing ointment on quality of life in people with symptoms associated with haemorrhoidal disease and its complications: the results of the EMOCARE survey. Acta Biomed. 2021;92(1):e2021029.

253. Alammar N, Wang L, Saberi B, Nanavati J, Holtmann G, Shinohara RT, et al. The impact of peppermint oil on the irritable bowel syndrome: a meta-analysis of the pooled clinical data. BMC Complement Altern Med. 2019;19(1):21.
254. Nee J, Lembo A. Review Article: current and future treatment approaches for IBS with diarrhoea (IBS-D) and IBS mixed pattern (IBS-M). Aliment Pharmacol Ther. 2021;54(Suppl 1):S63–74.
255. Malik EM, Müller CE. Anthraquinones as pharmacological tools and drugs. Med Res Rev. 2016;36(4):705–48.
256. Gao C-C, Li G-W, Wang T-T, Gao L, Wang F-F, Shang H-W, et al. Rhubarb extract relieves constipation by stimulating mucus production in the colon and altering the intestinal flora. Biomed Pharmacother. 2021;138:111479.
257. Luo S, Wen R, Wang Q, Zhao Z, Nong F, Fu Y, et al. Rhubarb Peony Decoction ameliorates ulcerative colitis in mice by regulating gut microbiota to restoring Th17/Treg balance. J Ethnopharmacol. 2019;231:39–49.
258. Moosavi M. Bentonite clay as a natural remedy: a brief review. Iran J Public Health. 2017;46(9):1176–83. https://pubmed.ncbi.nlm.nih.gov/29026782.
259. Barberio B, Segal JP, Quraishi MN, Black CJ, Savarino EV, Ford AC. Efficacy of oral, topical, or combined oral and topical 5-aminosalicylates, in ulcerative colitis: systematic review and network meta-analysis. J Crohns Colitis. 2021;15(7):1184–96.
260. Pugliese D, Felice C, Papa A, Gasbarrini A, Rapaccini GL, Guidi L, et al. Anti TNF-α therapy for ulcerative colitis: current status and prospects for the future. Expert Rev Clin Immunol. 2017;13(3):223–33.
261. Nguyen NH, Fumery M, Dulai PS, Prokop LJ, Sandborn WJ, Murad MH, et al. Comparative efficacy and tolerability of pharmacological agents for management of mild to moderate ulcerative colitis: a systematic review and network meta-analyses. Lancet Gastroenterol Hepatol. 2018;3(11):742–53.
262. Ogobuiro I, Tuma F. Physiology, renal. In: StatPearls. Treasure Island, FL: StatPearls; 2021.
263. Dalal R, Bruss ZS, Sehdev JS. Physiology, renal blood flow and filtration. In: StatPearls. Treasure Island, FL: StatPearls; 2021.
264. Musso CG, Álvarez-Gregori J, Jauregui J, Macías-Núñez JF. Glomerular filtration rate equations: a comprehensive review. Int Urol Nephrol. 2016;48(7):1105–10.
265. Fountain JH, Lappin SL. Physiology, renin angiotensin system. In: StatPearls. Treasure Island, FL: StatPearls; 2021.
266. Zehra T, Cupples WA, Braam B. Tubuloglomerular feedback synchronization in nephrovascular networks. J Am Soc Nephrol. 2021;32(6):1293–304.
267. Osborn JW, Tyshynsky R, Vulchanova L. Function of renal nerves in kidney physiology and pathophysiology. Annu Rev Physiol. 2021;83:429–50.
268. Panicker JN. Neurogenic bladder: epidemiology, diagnosis, and management. Semin Neurol. 2020;40(5):569–79.
269. de la Taille A, Robert G, Descazeaud A. Consequences of prostatic obstruction on bladder function, impact of removal, and management of recurrence after surgery. Prog en Urol J l'Association Fr d'urologie la Soc Fr d'urologie. 2018;28(15):813–20.
270. Patel K, Batura D. An overview of hydronephrosis in adults. Br J Hosp Med (Lond). 2020;81(1):1–8.
271. Levey AS, James MT. Acute kidney injury. Ann Intern Med. 2017;167(9):ITC66–80.
272. Couser WG. Pathogenesis and treatment of glomerulonephritis-an update. J Bras Nefrol 'orgao Of Soc Bras e Latino-Americana Nefrol. 2016;38(1):107–22.
273. Rodrigues JC, Haas M, Reich HN. IgA nephropathy. Clin J Am Soc Nephrol. 2017;12(4):677–86.
274. Spivacow FR, Del Valle EE, Lores E, Rey PG. Kidney stones: Composition, frequency and relation to metabolic diagnosis. Medicina. 2016;76(6):343–8.
275. Colbert GB, Elrggal ME, Gaur L, Lerma EV. Update and review of adult polycystic kidney disease. Dis Mon. 2020;66(5):100887.

276. Samsu N. Diabetic nephropathy: challenges in pathogenesis, diagnosis, and treatment. Biomed Res Int. 2021;2021:1497449.
277. Gaitonde DY, Cook DL, Rivera IM. Chronic kidney disease: detection and evaluation. Am Fam Physician. 2017;96(12):776–83.
278. Kodner C. Diagnosis and management of nephrotic syndrome in adults. Am Fam Physician. 2016;93(6):479–85.
279. Himmelfarb J, Vanholder R, Mehrotra R, Tonelli M. The current and future landscape of dialysis. Nat Rev Nephrol. 2020;16(10):573–85.
280. Gray RE, Harris GT. Renal cell carcinoma: diagnosis and management. Am Fam Physician. 2019;99(3):179–84.
281. Aldrink JH, Heaton TE, Dasgupta R, Lautz TB, Malek MM, Abdessalam SF, et al. Update on Wilms tumor. J Pediatr Surg. 2019;54(3):390–7.
282. Chapman CL, Johnson BD, Parker MD, Hostler D, Pryor RR, Schlader Z. Kidney physiology and pathophysiology during heat stress and the modification by exercise, dehydration, heat acclimation and aging. Temp. 2021;8(2):108–59.
283. Beecroft J, Duffin J, Pierratos A, Chan CT, McFarlane P, Hanly PJ. Enhanced chemo-responsiveness in patients with sleep apnoea and end-stage renal disease. Eur Respir J. 2006;28(1):151–8.
284. Abuyassin B, Sharma K, Ayas NT, Laher I. Obstructive sleep apnea and kidney disease: a potential bidirectional relationship? J Clin Sleep Med. 2015;11(8):915–24.
285. Jean G, Souberbielle JC, Chazot C. Vitamin D in chronic kidney disease and dialysis patients. Nutrients. 2017;9(4):328.
286. Koleganova N, Piecha G, Ritz E. Prenatal causes of kidney disease. Blood Purif. 2009;27(1):48–52.
287. EGb 761. Ginkgo biloba extract, Ginkor. Drugs R D. 2003;4(3):188–93.
288. Lu Q, Zuo W-Z, Ji X-J, Zhou Y-X, Liu Y-Q, Yao X-Q, et al. Ethanolic Ginkgo biloba leaf extract prevents renal fibrosis through Akt/mTOR signaling in diabetic nephropathy. Phytomedicine. 2015;22(12):1071–8.
289. Han J, Pang X, Shi X, Zhang Y, Peng Z, Xing Y. Ginkgo biloba extract EGB761 ameliorates the extracellular matrix accumulation and mesenchymal transformation of 303. Renal tubules in diabetic kidney disease by inhibiting endoplasmic reticulum stress. Biomed Res Int. 2021;2021:6657206.
290. Coskun O, Armutcu F, Kanter M, Kuzey GM. Protection of endotoxin-induced oxidative renal tissue damage of rats by vitamin E or/and EGb 761 treatment. J Appl Toxicol. 2005;25(1):8–12. https://doi.org/10.1002/jat.1002. PMID: 15669049.
291. Sherif IO, Al-Shaalan NH, Sabry D. Ginkgo biloba extract alleviates methotrexate-induced renal injury: new impact on PI3K/Akt/mTOR signaling and MALAT1 expression. Biomolecules. 2019;9(11):691.
292. Kim SH, Lee EK, Chang JW, Min WK, Chi HS, Kim SB. Effects of Ginkgo biloba on haemostatic factors and inflammation in chronic peritoneal dialysis patients. Phytother Res. 2005 Jun;19(6):546–8.
293. Song J, Liu D, Feng L, Zhang Z, Jia X, Xiao W. Protective effect of standardized extract of Ginkgo biloba against cisplatin-induced nephrotoxicity. Evid Based Complement Alternat Med. 2013;2013:846126.
294. Chen Y-N, Wu C-G, Shi B-M, Qian K, Ding Y. The protective effect of asiatic acid on podocytes in the kidney of diabetic rats. Am J Transl Res. 2018;10(11):3733–41.
295. Guo Y-L, Gao F, Dong T-W, Bai Y, Liu Q, Li R-L, et al. Meta-analysis of clinical efficacy and safety of Tripterygium wilfordii polyglycosides tablets in the treatment of chronic kidney disease. Evid Based Complement Alternat Med. 2021;2021:6640594.
296. Tienda-Vázquez MA, Morreeuw ZP, Sosa-Hernández JE, Cardador-Martínez A, Sabath E, Melchor-Martínez EM, et al. Nephroprotective plants: a review on the use in pre-renal and post-renal diseases. Plants. 2022;11(6):818.
297. Gómez-Sierra T, Medina-Campos ON, Solano JD, Ibarra-Rubio ME, Pedraza-Chaverri J. Isoliquiritigenin pretreatment induces endoplasmic reticulum stress-mediated hormesis

and attenuates cisplatin-induced oxidative stress and damage in LLC-PK1 cells. Molecules. 2020;25(19):4442.
298. Cascella M, Palma G, Barbieri A, Bimonte S, Amruthraj NJ, Muzio MR, et al. Role of Nigella sativa and its constituent thymoquinone on chemotherapy-induced nephrotoxicity: evidences from experimental animal studies. Nutrients. 2017;9(6):625.
299. Gágyor I, Hummers E, Schmiemann G, Friede T, Pfeiffer S, Afshar K, et al. Herbal treatment with uva ursi extract versus fosfomycin in women with uncomplicated urinary tract infection in primary care: a randomized controlled trial. Clin Microbiol Infect. 2021;27(10):1441–7.
300. Brendler T, Abdel-Tawab M. Buchu (Agathosma betulina and A. crenulata): rightfully forgotten or underutilized? Front Pharmacol. 2022;13:813142.
301. Vestby LK, Grønseth T, Simm R, Nesse LL. Bacterial biofilm and its role in the pathogenesis of disease. Antibiotics. 2020;9(2):59. https://pubmed.ncbi.nlm.nih.gov/32028684.
302. Zacchino SA, Butassi E, Cordisco E, Svetaz LA. Hybrid combinations containing natural products and antimicrobial drugs that interfere with bacterial and fungal biofilms. Phytomedicine. 2017;37:14–26.
303. Melander RJ, Basak AK, Melander C. Natural products as inspiration for the development of bacterial antibiofilm agents. Nat Prod Rep. 2020;37(11):1454–77.
304. Jafri H, Ahmad I. Thymus vulgaris essential oil and thymol inhibit biofilms and interact synergistically with antifungal drugs against drug resistant strains of Candida albicans and Candida tropicalis. J Mycol Med. 2020;30(1):100911.
305. Li G, Guan C, Xu L, Wang L, Yang C, Zhao L, et al. Scutellarin ameliorates renal injury via increasing CCN1 expression and suppressing NLRP3 inflammasome activation in hyperuricemic mice. Front Pharmacol. 2020;11:584942.
306. Gomes-Neto AW, Osté MCJ, Sotomayor CG, van den Berg E, Geleijnse JM, Berger SP, et al. Mediterranean style diet and kidney function loss in kidney transplant recipients. Clin J Am Soc Nephrol. 2020;15(2):238–46.
307. Mirabelli M, Chiefari E, Arcidiacono B, Corigliano DM, Brunetti FS, Maggisano V, et al. Mediterranean diet nutrients to turn the tide against insulin resistance and related diseases. Nutrients. 2020;12(4):1066.
308. Elks CM, Reed SD, Mariappan N, Shukitt-Hale B, Joseph JA, Ingram DK, et al. A blueberry-enriched diet attenuates nephropathy in a rat model of hypertension via reduction in oxidative stress. PLoS One. 2011;6(9):e24028.
309. Siener R. Dietary treatment of metabolic acidosis in chronic kidney disease. Nutrients. 2018;10(4):512.
310. Khan SR, Pearle MS, Robertson WG, Gambaro G, Canales BK, Doizi S, et al. Kidney stones. Nat Rev Dis Primers. 2016;2:16008.
311. Nephrotoxic Medications [Internet]. https://www.ncbi.nlm.nih.gov/books/NBK553144/.
312. Gatarek P, Kaluzna-Czaplinska J. Trimethylamine N-oxide (TMAO) in human health. EXCLI J. 2021;20:301–19.
313. Pechter Ü, Raag M, Ots-Rosenberg M. Regular aquatic exercise for chronic kidney disease patients: a 10-year follow-up study. Int J Rehabil Res Int Zeitschrift fur Rehabil Rev Int Rech Readapt. 2014;37(3):251–5.
314. Kolman KB. Cystitis and pyelonephritis: diagnosis, treatment, and prevention. Prim Care. 2019;46(2):191–202.
315. Osuna-Padilla IA, Leal-Escobar G, Garza-García CA, Rodríguez-Castellanos FE. Dietary acid load: mechanisms and evidence of its health repercussions. Nefrologia. 2019;39(4):343–54.
316. Felsenfeld AJ, Levine BS. Approach to treatment of hypophosphatemia. Am J Kidney Dis. 2012;60(4):655–61.
317. Ostermann M, Liu K, Kashani K. Fluid management in acute kidney injury. Chest. 2019;156(3):594–603.
318. Xie X, Liu Y, Perkovic V, Li X, Ninomiya T, Hou W, et al. Renin-angiotensin system inhibitors and kidney and cardiovascular outcomes in patients with CKD: a Bayesian network meta-analysis of randomized clinical trials. Am J Kidney Dis. 2016;67(5):728–41.

319. Augustine J. Kidney transplant: new opportunities and challenges. Cleve Clin J Med. 2018;85(2):138–44.
320. Cuddapah VA, Zhang SL, Sehgal A. Regulation of the blood-brain barrier by circadian rhythms and sleep. Trends Neurosci. 2019;42(7):500–10.
321. Hablitz LM, Nedergaard M. The glymphatic system: a novel component of fundamental neurobiology. J Neurosci. 2021;41(37):7698–711.
322. Gulyaeva NV. Molecular mechanisms of neuroplasticity: an expanding universe. Biochemistry. 2017;82(3):237–42.
323. von Bartheld CS, Bahney J, Herculano-Houzel S. The search for true numbers of neurons and glial cells in the human brain: a review of 150 years of cell counting. J Comp Neurol. 2016;524(18):3865–95.
324. Bassett DS, Sporns O. Network neuroscience. Nat Neurosci. 2017;20(3):353–64.
325. Fan L, Li H, Zhuo J, Zhang Y, Wang J, Chen L, et al. The human brainnetome atlas: a new brain atlas based on connectional architecture. Cereb Cortex. 2016;26(8):3508–26.
326. Pöyhönen S, Er S, Domanskyi A, Airavaara M. Effects of neurotrophic factors in glial cells in the central nervous system: expression and properties in neurodegeneration and injury. Front Physiol. 2019;10:486.
327. Bach D, Brown SA, Kleim B, Tyagarajan S. Extracellular matrix: a new player in memory maintenance and psychiatric disorders. Swiss Med Wkly. 2019;149:w20060.
328. Sweeney MD, Sagare AP, Zlokovic BV. Blood-brain barrier breakdown in Alzheimer disease and other neurodegenerative disorders. Nat Rev Neurol. 2018;14(3):133–50.
329. Josselyn SA, Tonegawa S. Memory engrams: recalling the past and imagining the future. Science. 2020;367(6473):eaaw4325.
330. Mahalakshmi AM, Ray B, Tuladhar S, Bhat A, Bishir M, Bolla SR, et al. Sleep, brain vascular health and ageing. GeroScience. 2020;42(5):1257–83.
331. Acosta MT. Sleep, memory and learning. Medicina. 2019;79(Suppl 3):29–32.
332. Meeusen R, Decroix L. Nutritional supplements and the brain. Int J Sport Nutr Exerc Metab. 2018;28(2):200–11.
333. Kelly ME, Duff H, Kelly S, McHugh Power JE, Brennan S, Lawlor BA, et al. The impact of social activities, social networks, social support and social relationships on the cognitive functioning of healthy older adults: a systematic review. Syst Rev. 2017;6(1):259.
334. Hablitz LM, Plá V, Giannetto M, Vinitsky HS, Stæger FF, Metcalfe T, et al. Circadian control of brain glymphatic and lymphatic fluid flow. Nat Commun. 2020;11(1):4411.
335. Claassen JAHR, Thijssen DHJ, Panerai RB, Faraci FM. Regulation of cerebral blood flow in humans: physiology and clinical implications of autoregulation. Physiol Rev. 2021;101(4):1487–559.
336. Sweeney MD, Ayyadurai S, Zlokovic BV. Pericytes of the neurovascular unit: key functions and signaling pathways. Nat Neurosci. 2016;19(6):771–83.
337. Tripp G, Wickens JR. Neurobiology of ADHD. Neuropharmacology. 2009;57(7–8):579–89.
338. Delgado-Lobete L, Pértega-Díaz S, Santos-Del-Riego S, Montes-Montes R. Sensory processing patterns in developmental coordination disorder, attention deficit hyperactivity disorder and typical development. Res Dev Disabil. 2020;100:103608.
339. Borst K, Dumas AA, Prinz M. Microglia: immune and non-immune functions. Immunity. 2021;54(10):2194–208.
340. Hoogland ICM, Houbolt C, van Westerloo DJ, van Gool WA, van de Beek D. Systemic inflammation and microglial activation: systematic review of animal experiments. J Neuroinflammation. 2015;12:114.
341. Ali T, Rahman SU, Hao Q, Li W, Liu Z, Ali Shah F, et al. Melatonin prevents neuroinflammation and relieves depression by attenuating autophagy impairment through FOXO3a regulation. J Pineal Res. 2020;69(2):e12667.
342. Chamberlain SR, Cavanagh J, de Boer P, Mondelli V, Jones DNC, Drevets WC, et al. Treatment-resistant depression and peripheral C-reactive protein. Br J Psychiatry. 2019;214(1):11–9.
343. Mazza MG, De Lorenzo R, Conte C, Poletti S, Vai B, Bollettini I, et al. Anxiety and depression in COVID-19 survivors: Role of inflammatory and clinical predictors. Brain Behav Immun. 2020;89:594–600.

344. Obermeier B, Daneman R, Ransohoff RM. Development, maintenance and disruption of the blood-brain barrier. Nat Med. 2013;19(12):1584–96.
345. Yuan J, Amin P, Ofengeim D. Necroptosis and RIPK1-mediated neuroinflammation in CNS diseases. Nat Rev Neurosci. 2019;20(1):19–33.
346. Basil MC, Levy BD. Specialized pro-resolving mediators: endogenous regulators of infection and inflammation. Nat Rev Immunol. 2016;16(1):51–67.
347. Chen G, Zhang Y-Q, Qadri YJ, Serhan CN, Ji R-R. Microglia in pain: detrimental and protective roles in pathogenesis and resolution of pain. Neuron. 2018;100(6):1292–311.
348. Giovane RA, Lavender PD. Central nervous system infections. Prim Care. 2018;45(3):505–18.
349. Radolf JD, Strle K, Lemieux JE, Strle F. Lyme disease in humans. Curr Issues Mol Biol. 2021;42:333–84.
350. Rutsch A, Kantsjö JB, Ronchi F. The gut-brain axis: how microbiota and host inflammasome influence brain physiology and pathology. Front Immunol. 2020;11:604179.
351. Crapser JD, Spangenberg EE, Barahona RA, Arreola MA, Hohsfield LA, Green KN. Microglia facilitate loss of perineuronal nets in the Alzheimer's disease brain. EBioMedicine. 2020;58:102919.
352. Crapser JD, Arreola MA, Tsourmas KI, Green KN. Microglia as hackers of the matrix: sculpting synapses and the extracellular space. Cell Mol Immunol. 2021;18(11):2472–88.
353. van Langelaar J, Rijvers L, Smolders J, van Luijn MM. B and T cells driving multiple sclerosis: identity, mechanisms and potential triggers. Front Immunol. 2020;11:760.
354. Binvignat O, Olloquequi J. Excitotoxicity as a target against neurodegenerative processes. Curr Pharm Des. 2020;26(12):1251–62.
355. Naspolini NF, Heinz Rieg CE, Cenci VH, Cattani D, Zamoner A. Paraquat induces redox imbalance and disrupts glutamate and energy metabolism in the hippocampus of prepubertal rats. Neurotoxicology. 2021;85:121–32.
356. Cheng Y, Song Y, Chen H, Li Q, Gao Y, Lu G, et al. Ferroptosis mediated by lipid reactive oxygen species: a possible causal link of neuroinflammation to neurological disorders. Oxid Med Cell Longev. 2021;2021:5005136.
357. Gao Y, Tan L, Yu J-T, Tan L. Tau in Alzheimer's disease: mechanisms and therapeutic strategies. Curr Alzheimer Res. 2018;15(3):283–300.
358. Logsdon AF, Rhea EM, Reed M, Banks WA, Erickson MA. The neurovascular extracellular matrix in health and disease. Exp Biol Med (Maywood). 2021;246(7):835–44.
359. Dankovich TM, Rizzoli SO. The synaptic extracellular matrix: long-lived, stable, and still remarkably dynamic. Front Synap Neurosci. 2022;14:854956. https://pubmed.ncbi.nlm.nih.gov/35350469.
360. Lemus HN, Warrington AE, Rodriguez M. Multiple sclerosis: mechanisms of disease and strategies for myelin and axonal repair. Neurol Clin. 2018;36(1):1–11.
361. Freitas A, Aroso M, Rocha S, Ferreira R, Vitorino R, Gomez-Lazaro M. Bioinformatic analysis of the human brain extracellular matrix proteome in neurodegenerative disorders. Eur J Neurosci. 2021;53(12):4016–33.
362. Štěpán-Buksakowska I, Szabó N, Hořínek D, Tóth E, Hort J, Warner J, et al. Cortical and subcortical atrophy in Alzheimer disease: parallel atrophy of thalamus and hippocampus. Alzheimer Dis Assoc Disord. 2014;28(1):65–72.
363. Kleffman K, Levinson G, Rose IVL, Blumenberg LM, Shadaloey SAA, Dhabaria A, et al. Melanoma-secreted amyloid beta suppresses neuroinflammation and promotes brain metastasis. Cancer Discov. 2022;12:1314–35.
364. Woods B, Aguirre E, Spector AE, Orrell M. Cognitive stimulation to improve cognitive functioning in people with dementia. Cochrane database Syst Rev. 2012;(2):CD005562.
365. Bertholet AM, Delerue T, Millet AM, Moulis MF, David C, Daloyau M, et al. Mitochondrial fusion/fission dynamics in neurodegeneration and neuronal plasticity. Neurobiol Dis. 2016;90:3–19.
366. Quintana-Cabrera R, Bolaños JP. Glutathione and γ-glutamylcysteine in the antioxidant and survival functions of mitochondria. Biochem Soc Trans. 2013;41(1):106–10.

367. Sukumaran NP, Amalraj A, Gopi S. Neuropharmacological and cognitive effects of Bacopa monnieri (L.) Wettst—a review on its mechanistic aspects. Complement Ther Med. 2019;44:68–82.
368. Calabrese C, Gregory WL, Leo M, Kraemer D, Bone K, Oken B. Effects of a standardized Bacopa monnieri extract on cognitive performance, anxiety, and depression in the elderly: a randomized, double-blind, placebo-controlled trial. J Altern Complement Med. 2008;14(6):707–13.
369. Kongkeaw C, Dilokthornsakul P, Thanarangsarit P, Limpeanchob N, Scholfield CN. Meta-analysis of randomized controlled trials on cognitive effects of Bacopa monnieri extract. J Ethnopharmacol. 2014;151(1):528–35.
370. Lewis JE, Poles J, Shaw DP, Karhu E, Khan SA, Lyons AE, et al. The effects of twenty-one nutrients and phytonutrients on cognitive function: a narrative review. J Clin Transl Res. 2021;7(4):575–620.
371. Lopresti AL. Salvia (Sage): a review of its potential cognitive-enhancing and protective effects. Drugs R D. 2017;17(1):53–64.
372. Mitchell ES, Conus N, Kaput J. B vitamin polymorphisms and behavior: evidence of associations with neurodevelopment, depression, schizophrenia, bipolar disorder and cognitive decline. Neurosci Biobehav Rev. 2014;47:307–20.
373. Razgonova MP, Veselov VV, Zakharenko AM, Golokhvast KS, Nosyrev AE, Cravotto G, et al. Panax ginseng components and the pathogenesis of Alzheimer's disease (Review). Mol Med Rep. 2019;19(4):2975–98.
374. Choi S, Lim JW, Kim H. Korean Red Ginseng inhibits Amyloid-β-induced apoptosis and nucling expression in human neuronal cells. Pharmacology. 2020;105(9–10):586–97.
375. Rastogi V, Santiago-Moreno J, Doré S. Ginseng: a promising neuroprotective strategy in stroke. Front Cell Neurosci. 2014;8:457.
376. Jin Y, Cui R, Zhao L, Fan J, Li B. Mechanisms of Panax ginseng action as an antidepressant. Cell Prolif. 2019;52(6):e12696.
377. Lee S, Rhee D-K. Effects of ginseng on stress-related depression, anxiety, and the hypothalamic-pituitary-adrenal axis. J Ginseng Res. 2017;41(4):589–94.
378. Li X, Lu L, Chen J, Zhang C, Chen H, Huang H. New insight into the mechanisms of Ginkgo biloba extract in vascular aging prevention. Curr Vasc Pharmacol. 2020;18(4):334–45.
379. Chen Y, Yu K, Hu Y, Chang Y. Ginkgo biloba extract protects mesenteric arterioles of old rats via improving vessel elasticity through Akt/FoxO3a signaling pathway. Ann Vasc Surg. 2019;57:220–8.
380. Kandiah N, Ong PA, Yuda T, Ng L-L, Mamun K, Merchant RA, et al. Treatment of dementia and mild cognitive impairment with or without cerebrovascular disease: expert consensus on the use of Ginkgo biloba extract, EGb 761(®). CNS Neurosci Ther. 2019;25(2):288–98.
381. Choudhary D, Bhattacharyya S, Bose S. Efficacy and safety of Ashwagandha (Withania somnifera (L.) Dunal) root extract in improving memory and cognitive functions. J Diet Suppl. 2017;14(6):599–612.
382. Roda E, Priori EC, Ratto D, De Luca F, Di Iorio C, Angelone P, Locatelli CA, Desiderio A, Goppa L, Savino E, Bottone MG, Rossi P. Neuroprotective metabolites of Hericium Erinaceus promote neuro-healthy aging. Int J Mol Sci. 2021;22(12):6379. https://doi.org/10.3390/ijms22126379. PMID: 34203691; PMCID: PMC8232141.
383. Mao JJ, Xie SX, Zee J, Soeller I, Li QS, Rockwell K, et al. Rhodiola rosea versus sertraline for major depressive disorder: a randomized placebo-controlled trial. Phytomedicine. 2015;22(3):394–9.
384. Limanaqi F, Biagioni F, Busceti CL, Polzella M, Fabrizi C, Fornai F. Potential antidepressant effects of Scutellaria baicalensis, Hericium erinaceus and Rhodiola rosea. Antioxidants. 2020;9(3):234.
385. Ghasemi F, Bagheri H, Barreto GE, Read MI, Sahebkar A. Effects of Curcumin on microglial cells. Neurotox Res. 2019;36(1):12–26.

386. Benameur T, Soleti R, Panaro MA, La Torre ME, Monda V, Messina G, et al. Curcumin as prospective anti-aging natural compound: focus on brain. Molecules. 2021;26(16):4794.
387. Ganesan P, Kim B, Ramalaingam P, Karthivashan G, Revuri V, Park S, et al. Antineuroinflammatory activities and neurotoxicological assessment of curcumin loaded solid lipid nanoparticles on LPS-stimulated BV-2 microglia cell models. Molecules. 2019;24(6):1170.
388. Dolati S, Babaloo Z, Ayromlou H, Ahmadi M, Rikhtegar R, Rostamzadeh D, et al. Nanocurcumin improves regulatory T-cell frequency and function in patients with multiple sclerosis. J Neuroimmunol. 2019;327:15–21.
389. Mogharbel BF, Cardoso MA, Irioda AC, Stricker PEF, Slompo RC, Appel JM, et al. Biodegradable nanoparticles loaded with levodopa and curcumin for treatment of Parkinson's disease. Molecules. 2022;27(9):2811.
390. ElSohly MA, Radwan MM, Gul W, Chandra S, Galal A. Phytochemistry of Cannabis sativa L. Prog Chem Org Nat Prod. 2017;103:1–36.
391. Zou S, Kumar U. Cannabinoid receptors and the endocannabinoid system: signaling and function in the central nervous system. Int J Mol Sci. 2018;19(3):833. https://pubmed.ncbi.nlm.nih.gov/29533978.
392. Maroon J, Bost J. Review of the neurological benefits of phytocannabinoids. Surg Neurol Int. 2018;9:91.
393. Martín-Moreno AM, Brera B, Spuch C, Carro E, García-García L, Delgado M, et al. Prolonged oral cannabinoid administration prevents neuroinflammation, lowers β-amyloid levels and improves cognitive performance in Tg APP 2576 mice. J Neuroinflammation. 2012;9(1):8. https://doi.org/10.1186/1742-2094-9-8.
394. MacCallum CA, Russo EB. Practical considerations in medical cannabis administration and dosing. Eur J Intern Med. 2018;49:12–9.
395. Wagner H. Synergy research: approaching a new generation of phytopharmaceuticals. Fitoterapia. 2011;82(1):34–7.
396. Fragoso YD, Carra A, Macias MA. Cannabis and multiple sclerosis. Expert Rev Neurother. 2020;20(8):849–54.
397. Aviram J, Samuelly-Leichtag G. Efficacy of Cannabis-based medicines for pain management: a systematic review and meta-analysis of randomized controlled trials. Pain Physician. 2017;20(6):E755–96.
398. Bagur MJ, Murcia MA, Jiménez-Monreal AM, Tur JA, Bibiloni MM, Alonso GL, et al. Influence of diet in multiple sclerosis: a systematic review. Adv Nutr. 2017;8(3):463–72.
399. Shinto L, Quinn J, Montine T, Dodge HH, Woodward W, Baldauf-Wagner S, et al. A randomized placebo-controlled pilot trial of omega-3 fatty acids and alpha lipoic acid in Alzheimer's disease. J Alzheimers Dis. 2014;38(1):111–20.
400. Leak RK, Calabrese EJ, Kozumbo WJ, Gidday JM, Johnson TE, Mitchell JR, et al. Enhancing and extending biological performance and resilience. Dose Response. 2018;16(3):1559325818784501.
401. Calabrese EJ, Rubio-Casillas A. Biphasic effects of THC in memory and cognition. Eur J Clin Invest. 2018;48(5):e12920.
402. Mattson MP, Moehl K, Ghena N, Schmaedick M, Cheng A. Intermittent metabolic switching, neuroplasticity and brain health. Nat Rev Neurosci. 2018;19(2):63–80.
403. Mattson MP, Cheng A. Neurohormetic phytochemicals: Low-dose toxins that induce adaptive neuronal stress responses. Trends Neurosci. 2006;29(11):632–9.
404. Pallàs M, Porquet D, Vicente A, Sanfeliu C. Resveratrol: new avenues for a natural compound in neuroprotection. Curr Pharm Des. 2013;19(38):6726–31.
405. Mattson MP. Dietary factors, hormesis and health. Ageing Res Rev. 2008;7(1):43–8.
406. Trovato Salinaro A, Pennisi M, Di Paola R, Scuto M, Crupi R, Cambria MT, et al. Neuroinflammation and neurohormesis in the pathogenesis of Alzheimer's disease and Alzheimer-linked pathologies: modulation by nutritional mushrooms. Immun Ageing. 2018;15:8. https://pubmed.ncbi.nlm.nih.gov/29456585.

407. Huang J, Wang X, Zhu Y, Li Z, Zhu Y-T, Wu J-C, et al. Exercise activates lysosomal function in the brain through AMPK-SIRT1-TFEB pathway. CNS Neurosci Ther. 2019;25(6):796–807.
408. Goyal D, Ali SA, Singh RK. Emerging role of gut microbiota in modulation of neuroinflammation and neurodegeneration with emphasis on Alzheimer's disease. Prog Neuropsychopharmacol Biol Psychiatry. 2021;106:110112.
409. Wahls TL, Titcomb TJ, Bisht B, Ten EP, Rubenstein LM, Carr LJ, et al. Impact of the Swank and Wahls elimination dietary interventions on fatigue and quality of life in relapsing-remitting multiple sclerosis: The WAVES randomized parallel-arm clinical trial. Mult Scler J Exp Transl Clin. 2021;7(3):20552173211035400.
410. Wysoczański T, Sokoła-Wysoczańska E, Pękala J, Lochyński S, Czyż K, Bodkowski R, et al. Omega-3 fatty acids and their role in central nervous system—a review. Curr Med Chem. 2016;23(8):816–31.
411. An M, Shaughnessy M. The effects of exercise-based rehabilitation on balance and gait for stroke patients: a systematic review. J Neurosci Nurs J Am Assoc Neurosci Nurs. 2011;43(6):298–307.
412. Gardiner P, MacGregor L, Carson A, Stone J. Occupational therapy for functional neurological disorders: a scoping review and agenda for research. CNS Spectr. 2018;23(3):205–12.
413. Adamit T, Shames J, Rand D. Effectiveness of the Functional and Cognitive Occupational Therapy (FaC(o)T) Intervention for Improving Daily Functioning and Participation of Individuals with Mild Stroke: A Randomized Controlled Trial. Int J Environ Res Public Health. 2021;18(15).
414. Peltoniemi MA, Hagelberg NM, Olkkola KT, Saari TI. Ketamine: a review of clinical pharmacokinetics and pharmacodynamics in anesthesia and pain therapy. Clin Pharmacokinet. 2016;55(9):1059–77.
415. Goldberg SB, Pace BT, Nicholas CR, Raison CL, Hutson PR. The experimental effects of psilocybin on symptoms of anxiety and depression: a meta-analysis. Psychiatry Res. 2020;284:112749.
416. Khoy K, Mariotte D, Defer G, Petit G, Toutirais O, Le Mauff B. Natalizumab in multiple sclerosis treatment: from biological effects to immune monitoring. Front Immunol. 2020;11:549842.
417. Kueper JK, Speechley M, Montero-Odasso M. The Alzheimer's disease assessment scale-cognitive subscale (ADAS-Cog): modifications and responsiveness in pre-dementia populations. a narrative review. J Alzheimers Dis. 2018;63(2):423–44.
418. Finley CR, Chan DS, Garrison S, Korownyk C, Kolber MR, Campbell S, et al. What are the most common conditions in primary care? Systematic review. Can Fam Physician. 2018;64(11):832–40. https://pubmed.ncbi.nlm.nih.gov/30429181.
419. Zeff J, Snider P, Myers S. Naturopathic model of healing-the process of healing revisited. Integr Med (Encinitas). 2019;18(4):26–30.
420. Miernik M, Wieckiewicz M, Paradowska A, Wieckiewicz W. Massage therapy in myofascial TMD pain management. Adv Clin Exp Med. 2012;21(5):681–5.
421. Armiento AR, Alini M, Stoddart MJ. Articular fibrocartilage—why does hyaline cartilage fail to repair? Adv Drug Deliv Rev. 2019;146:289–305.
422. Longobardi L, Li T, Tagliafierro L, Temple JD, Willcockson HH, Ye P, et al. Synovial joints: from development to homeostasis. Curr Osteoporos Rep. 2015;13(1):41–51.
423. Pham S, Puckett Y. Physiology, skeletal muscle contraction. In: StatPearls [Internet]. Treasure Island, FL: StatPearls; 2022. Accessed 8 May 2022.
424. Dave HD, Shook M, Varacallo M. Anatomy, skeletal muscle. In: StatPearls. Treasure Island, FL: StatPearls; 2022. Accessed 5 Sep 2021.
425. El Sayed SA, Nezwek TA, Varacallo M. Physiology, bone. In: StatPearls [Internet]. Treasure Island, FL: StatPearls; 2022. Accessed 9 Oct 2021.
426. Elizagaray-Garcia I, Beltran-Alacreu H, Angulo-Díaz S, Garrigós-Pedrón M, Gil-Martínez A. Chronic primary headache subjects have greater forward head posture than asymptomatic and episodic primary headache sufferers: systematic review and meta-analysis. Pain Med. 2020;21(10):2465–80.

427. Jun D, Zoe M, Johnston V, O'Leary S. Physical risk factors for developing non-specific neck pain in office workers: a systematic review and meta-analysis. Int Arch Occup Environ Health. 2017;90(5):373–410.
428. Booth FW, Roberts CK, Laye MJ. Lack of exercise is a major cause of chronic diseases. Compr Physiol. 2012;2(2):1143–211.
429. Gupton M, Munjal A, Terreberry RR. Anatomy, hinge joints. In: StatPearls [Internet]. Treasure Island, FL: StatPearls; 2022. Accessed 26 Jul 2021.
430. Stephens FB, Constantin-Teodosiu D, Greenhaff PL. New insights concerning the role of carnitine in the regulation of fuel metabolism in skeletal muscle. J Physiol. 2007;581(Pt 2):431–44.
431. Selvarajah D, Kar D, Khunti K, Davies MJ, Scott AR, Walker J, et al. Diabetic peripheral neuropathy: advances in diagnosis and strategies for screening and early intervention. Lancet Diabetes Endocrinol. 2019;7(12):938–48.
432. Marmolejo VS, Arnold JF, Ponticello M, Anderson CA. Charcot foot: clinical clues, diagnostic strategies, and treatment principles. Am Fam Physician. 2018;97(9):594–9.
433. Mielgo-Ayuso J, Calleja-González J, Refoyo I, León-Guereño P, Cordova A, Del Coso J. Exercise-induced muscle damage and cardiac stress during a marathon could be associated with dietary intake during the week before the race. Nutrients. 2020;12(2):316.
434. Griffin TM, Scanzello CR. Innate inflammation and synovial macrophages in osteoarthritis pathophysiology. Clin Exp Rheumatol. 2019;37 Suppl 120(5):57–63.
435. Coskun BI. Role of inflammation in the pathogenesis and treatment of fibromyalgia. Rheumatol Int. 2019;39(5):781–91.
436. Shim H, Rose J, Halle S, Shekane P. Complex regional pain syndrome: a narrative review for the practising clinician. Br J Anaesth. 2019;123(2):e424–33.
437. Kemble S, Croft AP. Critical role of synovial tissue-resident macrophage and fibroblast subsets in the persistence of joint inflammation. Front Immunol. 2021;12:715894.
438. Sarkar S, Fox DA. Dendritic cells in rheumatoid arthritis. Front Biosci. 2005;10:656–65.
439. Ceccarelli F, Perricone C, Cipriano E, Massaro L, Natalucci F, Capalbo G, et al. Joint involvement in systemic lupus erythematosus: from pathogenesis to clinical assessment. Semin Arthritis Rheum. 2017;47(1):53–64.
440. Gupta A, Thorson P, Penmatsa KR, Gupta P. Rhabdomyolysis: revisited. Ulster Med J. 2021;90(2):61–9.
441. Pintor IA, Pereira F, Cavadas S, Lopes P. Pott's disease (tuberculous spondylitis). Int J Mycobacteriol. 2022;11:113–5.
442. Elshabrawy HA, Chen Z, Volin MV, Ravella S, Virupannavar S, Shahrara S. The pathogenic role of angiogenesis in rheumatoid arthritis. Angiogenesis. 2015;18(4):433–48. https://pubmed.ncbi.nlm.nih.gov/26198292.
443. Shi Y, Hu X, Cheng J, Zhang X, Zhao F, Shi W, et al. A small molecule promotes cartilage extracellular matrix generation and inhibits osteoarthritis development. Nat Commun. 2019;10(1):1914.
444. Rahmati M, Nalesso G, Mobasheri A, Mozafari M. Aging and osteoarthritis: central role of the extracellular matrix. Ageing Res Rev. 2017;40:20–30.
445. Mahdy MAA. Skeletal muscle fibrosis: an overview. Cell Tissue Res. 2019;375(3):575–88.
446. Bayer E, Elliott R, Bang M, Ross M, Tall M. Atlantoaxial instability in a patient with neck pain and rheumatoid arthritis. J Spinal Cord Med. 2021;44(3):433–6.
447. Ji LL, Yeo D. Mitochondrial dysregulation and muscle disuse atrophy. F1000Research. 2019;8.
448. Brown HK, Tellez-Gabriel M, Heymann D. Cancer stem cells in osteosarcoma. Cancer Lett. 2017;386:189–95.
449. CDC. Adult physical inactivity prevalence maps by race/ethnicity [Internet]. https://www.cdc.gov/physicalactivity/data/inactivity-prevalence-maps/index.html.
450. Ogino Y, Kakeda T, Nakamura K, Saito S. Dehydration enhances pain-evoked activation in the human brain compared with rehydration. Anesth Analg. 2014;118(6):1317–25.
451. Hannibal KE, Bishop MD. Chronic stress, cortisol dysfunction, and pain: a psychoneuroendocrine rationale for stress management in pain rehabilitation. Phys Ther. 2014;94(12):1816–25.

452. Tucker KL. Osteoporosis prevention and nutrition. Curr Osteoporos Rep. 2009;7(4):111–7.
453. Lubis AMT, Siagian C, Wonggokusuma E, Marsetyo AF, Setyohadi B. Comparison of glucosamine-chondroitin sulfate with and without methylsulfonylmethane in grade I-II knee osteoarthritis: a double blind randomized controlled trial. Acta Med Indones. 2017;49(2):105–11.
454. Murray M. Another positive study on glucosamine chondroitin reducing joint pain [Internet]. https://doctormurray.com/another-positive-study-on-glucosamine-chondroitin-reducing-arthritis-pain/. Accessed 31 May 2022.
455. Smith AG, Miles VN, Holmes DT, Chen X, Lei W. Clinical trials, potential mechanisms, and adverse effects of arnica as an adjunct medication for pain management. Medicine. 2021;8(10):58.
456. Schell J, Scofield RH, Barrett JR, Kurien BT, Betts N, Lyons TJ, et al. Strawberries improve pain and inflammation in obese adults with radiographic evidence of knee osteoarthritis. Nutrients. 2017;9(9):949.
457. Harrison SR, Li D, Jeffery LE, Raza K, Hewison M. Vitamin D, autoimmune disease and rheumatoid arthritis. Calcif Tissue Int. 2020;106(1):58–75.
458. Habib AM, Nagi K, Thillaiappan NB, Sukumaran V, Akhtar S. Vitamin D and its potential interplay with pain signaling pathways. Front Immunol. 2020;28(11):820. https://pubmed.ncbi.nlm.nih.gov/32547536.
459. Dimitrov V, Barbier C, Ismailova A, Wang Y, Dmowski K, Salehi-Tabar R, et al. Vitamin D-regulated gene expression profiles: species-specificity and cell-specific effects on metabolism and immunity. Endocrinology. 2021;162(2):bqaa218.
460. Uchitomi R, Oyabu M, Kamei Y. Vitamin D and sarcopenia: potential of Vitamin D supplementation in sarcopenia prevention and treatment. Nutrients. 2020;12(10):3189.
461. Majeed M, Majeed S, Narayanan NK, Nagabhushanam K. A pilot, randomized, double-blind, placebo-controlled trial to assess the safety and efficacy of a novel Boswellia serrata extract in the management of osteoarthritis of the knee. Phytother Res. 2019;33(5):1457–68.
462. Bannuru RR, Osani MC, Al-Eid F, Wang C. Efficacy of curcumin and Boswellia for knee osteoarthritis: systematic review and meta-analysis. Semin Arthritis Rheum. 2018;48(3):416–29.
463. Sarzi-Puttini P, Batticciotto A, Atzeni F, Bazzichi L, Di Franco M, Salaffi F, et al. Medical cannabis and cannabinoids in rheumatology: where are we now? Expert Rev Clin Immunol. 2019;15(10):1019–32.
464. Farpour HR, Rajabi N, Ebrahimi B. The efficacy of Harpagophytum procumbens (Teltonal) in patients with knee osteoarthritis: a randomized active-controlled clinical trial. Evid Based Complement Alternat Med. 2021;2021:5596892.
465. Menghini L, Recinella L, Leone S, Chiavaroli A, Cicala C, Brunetti L, et al. Devil's claw (Harpagophytum procumbens) and chronic inflammatory diseases: a concise overview on preclinical and clinical data. Phytother Res. 2019;33(9):2152–62.
466. Zhang Y, Mao X, Li W, Chen W, Wang X, Ma Z, et al. Tripterygium wilfordii: an inspiring resource for rheumatoid arthritis treatment. Med Res Rev. 2021;41(3):1337–74.
467. Daily JW, Yang M, Park S. Efficacy of turmeric extracts and curcumin for alleviating the symptoms of joint arthritis: a systematic review and meta-analysis of randomized clinical trials. J Med Food. 2016;19(8):717–29.
468. Charoenwoodhipong P, Harlow SD, Marder W, Hassett AL, McCune WJ, Gordon C, et al. Dietary omega polyunsaturated fatty acid intake and patient-reported outcomes in systemic lupus erythematosus: the michigan lupus epidemiology and surveillance program. Arthritis Care Res. 2020;72(7):874–81.
469. Guo R, Chen L-H, Xing C, Liu T. Pain regulation by gut microbiota: molecular mechanisms and therapeutic potential. Br J Anaesth. 2019;123(5):637–54.
470. Freidin MB, Stalteri MA, Wells PM, Lachance G, Baleanu A-F, Bowyer RCE, et al. An association between chronic widespread pain and the gut microbiome. Rheumatology (Oxford). 2021;60(8):3727–37.
471. Sánchez Romero EA, Meléndez Oliva E, Alonso Pérez JL, Martín Pérez S, Turroni S, Marchese L, et al. Relationship between the gut microbiome and osteoarthritis pain: review of the literature. Nutrients. 2021;13(3):716.

472. Minerbi A, Fitzcharles M-A. Gut microbiome: pertinence in fibromyalgia. Clin Exp Rheumatol. 2020;38 Suppl 1(1):99–104.
473. Mandel DR, Eichas K, Holmes J. Bacillus coagulans: a viable adjunct therapy for relieving symptoms of rheumatoid arthritis according to a randomized, controlled trial. BMC Complement Altern Med. 2010;10:1.
474. Ida Rolf Institute [Internet]. https://rolf.org/.
475. The Guild for Structural Integration [Internet]. https://www.rolfguild.org/.
476. Frank C, Kobesova A, Kolar P. Dynamic neuromuscular stabilization & sports rehabilitation. Int J Sports Phys Ther. 2013;8(1):62–73.
477. Vickers AJ, Vertosick EA, Lewith G, MacPherson H, Foster NE, Sherman KJ, et al. Acupuncture for chronic pain: update of an individual patient data meta-analysis. J Pain. 2018;19(5):455–74.
478. Yuan Q-L, Wang P, Liu L, Sun F, Cai Y-S, Wu W-T, et al. Acupuncture for musculoskeletal pain: a meta-analysis and meta-regression of sham-controlled randomized clinical trials. Sci Rep. 2016;6:30675.
479. Pagliai G, Giangrandi I, Dinu M, Sofi F, Colombini B. Nutritional interventions in the management of fibromyalgia syndrome. Nutrients. 2020;12(9):2525.
480. Anti-inflammatory diet in rheumatoid arthritis (ADIRA)—a randomized, controlled crossover trial indicating effects on disease activity. Am J Clin Nutr. 2020;111(6):1203–1213.
481. Schönenberger KA, Schüpfer A-C, Gloy VL, Hasler P, Stanga Z, Kaegi-Braun N, et al. Effect of anti-inflammatory diets on pain in rheumatoid arthritis: a systematic review and meta-analysis. Nutrients. 2021;13(12):4221.
482. Naumann J, Sadaghiani C. Therapeutic benefit of balneotherapy and hydrotherapy in the management of fibromyalgia syndrome: a qualitative systematic review and meta-analysis of randomized controlled trials. Arthritis Res Ther. 2014;16(4):R141.
483. Rivas Neira S, Pasqual Marques A, Pegito Pérez I, Fernández Cervantes R, Vivas CJ. Effectiveness of aquatic therapy vs land-based therapy for balance and pain in women with fibromyalgia: a study protocol for a randomised controlled trial. BMC Musculoskelet Disord. 2017;18(1):22.
484. Jordan PM, van Goethem E, Müller AM, Hemmer K, Gavioli V, Baillif V, et al. The Natural Combination Medicine Traumeel (Tr14) improves resolution of inflammation by promoting the biosynthesis of specialized pro-resolving mediators. Pharmaceuticals. 2021;14(11):1123.
485. Jacques C, Floris I, Lejeune B. Ultra-low dose cytokines in rheumatoid arthritis, three birds with one stone as the rationale of the 2LARTH(®) micro-immunotherapy treatment. Int J Mol Sci. 2021;22(13):6717.
486. Floris I, García-González V, Palomares B, Appel K, Lejeune B. The micro-immunotherapy medicine 2LARTH® reduces inflammation and symptoms of rheumatoid arthritis in vivo. Int J Rheumatol. 2020;2020:1594573.
487. Xie P, Xue W, Qi W, Li Y, Yang L, Yang Z, et al. Safety, tolerability, and pharmacokinetics of ibuprofenamine hydrochloride spray (NSAIDs), a new drug for rheumatoid arthritis and osteoarthritis, in healthy Chinese subjects. Drug Des Devel Ther. 2021;15:629–38.
488. Lawson K. A brief review of the pharmacology of amitriptyline and clinical outcomes in treating fibromyalgia. Biomedicine. 2017;5(2):24.
489. Fuggle N, Curtis E, Shaw S, Spooner L, Bruyère O, Ntani G, et al. Safety of opioids in osteoarthritis: outcomes of a systematic review and meta-analysis. Drugs Aging. 2019;36(Suppl 1):129–43.
490. Privitera R, Anand P. Capsaicin 8% patch Qutenza and other current treatments for neuropathic pain in chemotherapy-induced peripheral neuropathy (CIPN). Curr Opin Support Palliat Care. 2021;15(2):125–31.
491. Fraenkel L, Bathon JM, England BR, St Clair EW, Arayssi T, Carandang K, et al. 2021 American College of Rheumatology Guideline for the Treatment of Rheumatoid Arthritis. Arthritis Rheumatol. 2021;73(7):1108–23.

Chapter 9
Lifespan Considerations

Birth to Three Years

A developing child is like a supernova of the expression of genetic potential. The net increase in size, developmental refinement, brain cell activity, and human learning and experience is astounding. This makes requirements for nutrition, overall determinants of health, care and love, and avoidance of harmful stimuli even more important.

In screening care of a newborn, there are state requirements to fulfill, which will vary. At the very least, this include pulse oximetry (which might show a low PO_2 associated with a congenital heart defect), basic hearing test, Ortolani test for congenital hip dysplasia, and a blood test taken from a prick on the skin of the heel of the baby. This will screen for phenylketonuria and very likely maple syrup urine disease, congenital hypothyroidism, and sickle cell anemia. Other tests can be done at this time as well [1].

In well-child care, the developmental landmarks [2] of speech, fine motor control, social interaction, and gross motor skills are documented at regular visits. Height and weight are recorded and compared in percentiles to tables of aggregated data. Children fluctuate, and they vary, but long-term trends or steep changes in weight and/or height must be considered.

Office visits should *at least* be as follows: [3]

- The first week visit (3 to 5 days old).
- 1 month old.
- 2 months old.
- 4 months old.
- 6 months old.
- 9 months old.
- 12 months old.
- 15 months old.

F. Smith, *Naturopathic Medicine*, https://doi.org/10.1007/978-3-031-13388-6_9

- 18 months old.
- 2 years old (24 months).
- 3 years old (36 months).

Weight, height, head circumference, and motor/ verbal skills are documented. One hepatitis C screen is included. Autism spectrum screen or referral for analysis is possible at this stage. Naturopathic scope of practice and standards of care will vary between jurisdictions. The American Academy of Pediatrics lists Recommendations for Preventive Pediatric Health Care at www.healthychildren.org [3].

In some jurisdictions, naturopathic physicians can administer vaccines. The practice may provide complete primary care to children or may be a complementary/integrative form of care.

The current vaccine schedule from birth to 18 years is provided by the Centers for Disease Control [4].

https://www.cdc.gov/vaccines/schedules/hcp/imz/child-adolescent.html

The CDC also publishes the Appendix—Guide to Contraindications and Precautions to Commonly Used Vaccines [5].

https://www.cdc.gov/vaccines/schedules/hcp/imz/child-adolescent.html#appendix

Medical ethics, as described by the Department of Health and Human Services, for health service providers includes informed consent (as does research involving human subjects). Physicians should know when to delay or avoid a vaccine according to CDC-published guidelines, and they should provide informed consent to parents/guardians and patients.

There is sometimes a reluctance to provide information so that parents can make an informed decision because it might lead to parents being dissuaded from following an immunization schedule. Or the doctor may be concerned that they will be perceived at "talking the family out of vaccination." So the naturopathic physician should explain these schedules and immunizations as any procedure that can help someone, neither withholding information nor attempting to manipulate the family by overstating risk or by intentionally creating a vague sense of danger. Honest and forthright behavior on the part of physicians earns the trust of patients and caregivers. And this trust is conducive to people making choices that support their health and the health of their greater community.

Nutritional Requirements in Infancy

One perspective on infant nutrition relates to the first 1000 days, from the beginning of life to the second birthday. This encompasses prenatal development, perinatal and early infancy, and the rapid growth period up to the second birthday [6].

Prenatal Nutrition

Pregnancy is a time of momentous development and critical events. Folic acid is well known to prevent neural tube defects, which can lead to spina bifida. The brain and the retina require DHA (docosahexaenoic acid) and omega 3s in general, choline, protein, and carotenoids. Iron stores for the mother will be needed to ensure that hemoglobin levels are normal, which is absolutely necessary to bring oxygen to the baby. Iodine is required for thyroid function, and this mineral is transferred to the fetus and stored.

Newborns have intense energy and protein needs. Breast milk provides these and all of the other essentials. The mother needs to have adequate iron, zinc, iodine, etc., in order for breastmilk to be optimal. It has prebiotics and immune cells that have developmental benefits. In the late nineteenth century, the so-called "formula" was introduced as the industrial revolution separated mothers and infants. Sometimes this was nothing more than dehydrated milk or warm cow's milk. In the twentieth century, a popular concoction was the addition of sugar to cow's milk, in order to provide better energy. Physicians would tell parents to also give babies orange juice to prevent vitamin C deficiency. Interestingly, the go to resources for parents, the advice and care guide from Dr. Benjamin Spock, indicates in the early 1950s edition that he supported breastfeeding and that he attempted to dispel notions that it was too difficult or beyond a mother's ability (which was, it seems, a fear that some of his patients' parents had) [7]. The unusually high protein in cow's milk, and the phosphate, put a burden on the kidneys of the infants. It is possible that prior to the introduction of the feedlot, with more cattle being range fed and eating grass, that at least the omega 3 fatty acid content of this milk was higher than the milk from many of today's corn- and soy-fed cows.

The ostensible basis for this pushing of formula was that it was based on science, when in fact it was based on opinion. Starting in the 1970, a swing back to breastfeeding, very much powered by mothers, gained momentum. One example is La Leche League, which was started by a group of mothers in the Chicago area frustrated with the lack of support for breastfeeding moms [8]. Actual research into infant nutrition confirmed that the natural means of feeding infants that has developed and sustained the human race was the best. Unlike Dr. Benjamin Spock's time, many of the ways in which breast milk is beneficial are better understood, such as immune cell and compound transfer.

At the same time, formula has come a long way. Many formulations have DHA, prebiotics, probiotics, and some have somewhat denatured proteins to reduce the chance of allergy. The lutein (carotenoid) in formula is usually from synthetic chemical sources, and this underscores criticism of formula. Another is that when it is introduced to a breastfeeding baby, the ease of devouring it and its filling nature can start to displace breastmilk. The less demand from the baby, and less latching, the lower production goes.

Some babies need to be fed on formula. The reality of the situation is that some mothers work two jobs, or just have, in spite of good (or perhaps because of a lack of) coaching on best techniques, a limited supply of breastmilk. Poverty, famine, displacement due to wars, or natural disaster can upend a breastfeeding relationship between mother and child. The more formulas that can approximate breast milk, the better. Many United States infants do a stint on soy formula, which might avoid cow's milk protein but will push their genistein serum levels to about 8 to 10 times higher than that of a Japanese female adult eating a traditional diet replete with miso. Genistein has health benefits, but at these levels, it might possibly be acting like an endocrine-disrupting compound. Babies that are fed with pumped breast milk, or given formula, should be fed from glass or at the least with a BPA-free plastic.

At six months of age, babies will be depleted of their prenatal iron and zinc stores, and their growth continues to accelerate. This is a critical time for iron and zinc. Vitamin D and calcium are required for the bone growth they are experiencing. The deficiencies that occur from vitamin A can lead to corneal damage and blindness, not so common in developed countries but all too common globally. Carotenoids can be vitamin A precursors, and they have their own protective effect on the retina. Vitamin C is needed from their primary diet, although drops with supplemental C are not out of the question. B complex and the methylation critical nutrients B12 and folate must be present for both hemoglobin and neurologic development. DHA and omega 3 fats are often low in US babies and toddlers. This impacts many systems, eye, brain, immune, and respiratory.

At birth, the aerobic Enterobacteriaceae family of bacteria are the first to appear [9]. In a few days, anaerobic species *Bifidobacterium*, *Clostridium*, *Enterococcaceae*, *Streptococcaceae*, *Lactobacillaceae*, and *Bacteroides* start colonizing the gut. The milk diet of the infant particularly supports the growth of Bifidobacterium, and they come to dominance for some months. Once the baby starts eating solid food, including dietary fiber, there is a shift to increased *Bacteroides*, *Clostridium*, and *Ruminococcus*, and a decrease in *Bifidobacterium* and *Enterobacteriaceae*. In the rest of the 1000 days, the infant gut begins to develop lifelong families such as Ruminococcaceae, Lachnospiraceae, Bacteroidaceae, and Prevotellaceae.

Food Introduction

The American Academy of Pediatrics recommends exclusive breastfeeding for approximately 6 months, with continuation of breastfeeding for 1 year or longer as mutually desired by mother and infant. Solid foods should not be introduced before the 6 month mark. It was once believed that introducing protein foods at the 6- to 9-month or even the 12-month period would increase the risk for allergies. The reasoning was that the immature immune system would be overexposed to antigens from foods, particularly complex grains, meats, and eggs. This would set up the infant for a hypersensitivity to that food. In the 2000s, research into the downsides of shielding infants from a variety of foods (after 6 months of breastfeeding) became clearer. Without opportunities to become acquainted with a variety of food antigens, the tolerance mechanisms in the submucosal immune system, including regulatory T cells, didn't switch on. It now appears that there is no allergy avoidance benefit to delaying foods.

The consensus of 12 societies (i.e., American Academy of Pediatrics, American Academy of Allergy, Asthma & Immunology, American College of Allergy, Asthma & Immunology, Australasian Society of Clinical Immunology and Allergy, Canadian Society of Allergy and Clinical Immunology, European Academy of Allergy and Clinical Immunology, Israel Association of Allergy and Clinical Immunology, Japanese Society for Allergology, Society for Pediatric Dermatology, and World Allergy Organization) is that infants should be introduced to peanut between the ages of 4 and 9 months, in order to decrease the risk of peanut allergy later. This should not be whole peanut (butter or finely ground instead) to avoid choking [10].

Eggs are considered a good early protein. Other foods can be given in small quantities. In naturopathic approaches to child nutrition, these research findings are incorporated, but in the context of whole food, balanced nutrition. This means that fruits and vegetables, as well as bland (but iron fortified!) rice cereal is a better basis for the 6- to 9-month period. Other foods can rotate in and make their appearance, but the regulatory systems should be given a chance to activate. Processed and highly processed foods, as well as concentrated sweeteners (foods from NOVA categories 2,3, and 4) should be avoided in that first year [11]. Hopefully the "table food" that the older members of the family are eating is high in these whole foods. But if not, the infant should not be given pureed versions of canned, processed, adulterated foods. These are only marginally foods, and while they might be preferable to protein-calorie malnutrition (which is a stark and real choice for some families), if there is the means to keep them away from the infant, that is the correct course. Excellent cookbooks, websites, and videos are now available to help parents create good menus.

As a child moves to solid food, there is a tremendous opportunity for them to form habits and tastes that will be with them for years. Having a variety of fruits and vegetables in the diet helps normalize these natural foods. Avoiding fast food as much as possible will minimize the extreme habit forming (and palate conditioning) effects of these foods. Snacks can be whole grain crackers, fruits, milk, or beverages. Juice is a source of vitamin C, but it should be kept to 1 glass a day. It is high in sugar and can displace other foods. Likewise, milk or other calcium and D-rich beverages can provide these (and vitamin A) nutrients. But too much filling up on milk (for those who can handle the lactose and are not allergic) displaces other nutrients, including those rich in zinc, which is vital to growth. Family meals together, without screen time, is an important time for communication and reinforcement of good eating habits. Breakfasts should include a protein or very dense whole grain and fruit. Fermented foods such as natural yogurt (which should start when breastfeeding ends and solid food is introduced) is important for a healthy gut and an immune system that is interacting and growing with a diverse and commensal/symbiotic microbiome.

Urgent interventions are sometimes needed with people in their first 1000 days. (Table 9.1) While it is true that mild fever and naturally acquired infections are a part of a developing immune system, various situations can overwhelm a child. Although optimally healthy children tend to deal with these challenges with strength and emerge stronger, a few important facts have to be noted:

- The early twentieth-century naturopaths did not have the option of referring patients to a safe, evidence-based, pediatric practice or pediatric hospital. The specialty of pediatrics was just being developed in Europe, and the vast amount of research and experience in this field was yet to accrue. So while the historic writings of naturopathic doctors from 100 years ago have important things to tell us about helping children develop healthy bodies and minds, the message that medical doctors will only suppress illness and create harm is not true in today's context (and has not been true for some time and historically was only sometimes true).
- The rate of progression and severity of some illness are such that they can overwhelm an infant and cause death [12]. While not very common, something as simple as respiratory syncytial virus can lead to bronchiolitis and plummeting PO2—hypoxia. While naturopathic treatments will make this less likely, it sometimes happens.

Table 9.1 Levels of dysfunction in selected early childhood conditions The following are examples and are not an exhaustive list of pediatric conditions or treatments [14]. Although fibrotic, degenerative, and neoplastic conditions are rare in childhood, they are extremely serious and require care from a team including specialized pediatricians

Stage of dysfunction	Example	Course of action
Hypofunction	Constipation	Look at diet and fiber and water intake. Cow's milk allergy a possibility. Determine if the child is ignoring the urge to defecate (more likely at 18 to 24 months)
Impaired circulation and coordination	Developmental milestone delays in motor skills	Seek out cause and address it. Work with an occupational therapist
Inflammation	Atopic dermatitis	Consider diet, microbiome, and omega 3 intake
Deeper inflammation and immune involvement	Multisystem inflammatory syndrome in children (MIS-C) associated with COVID-19	Biochemical support to decrease inflammation; work with pediatrician; anti-inflammatory medication may be needed
Fibrosis	Neonatal acute liver failure	Will likely lead to liver transplantation
Decline of function	Acid sphingomyelinase deficiency (Niemann-pick disease type A)	Will cause sphingomyelin accumulation in viscera and organ failure
Neoplasia	Neuroblastoma	Pediatric oncologist will treat and provide integrative care, nutritional support, whole-person support

- As is mentioned in the model of naturopathic medicine, the activation of prosurvival mechanisms only goes so far. At times, maladaptive responses are so strong that they have to be reduced. In other situations, a system can collapse so rapidly (i.e., spinal meningitis, intussusception, seizure) that the only hope that person has is to induce a homeostatic state very rapidly. Some treatments in the naturopathic scope can do this, others are part of the conventional medical scope and expertise (i.e., cranial surgery, pediatric ICU, etc.)
- Health is not a level playing field. Some children are born with defects due to prenatal issues. Genetic differences can make one baby more susceptible to a pathogen than the next. Disparities in health care access, nutrition, living conditions, etc., can set a child up for far more harm from a disease challenge than a child who is better off.

All patients deserve the best care taken from the branches of medicine that help them the most at the moment. Ideology, ego, and parochialism have no place in treatment, especially in the treatment of the youngest and most vulnerable.

Many issues that infants encounter are subacute and can be managed in a nonsuppressive manner. However, the naturopathic physician must be alert to possible complications and very rapid changes of state and be willing to "err on the side of caution" at times.

Safety

Infant safety is an adaptation to any home. Public health departments and the CDC have excellent resources about this [13]. Some of the germane safety precautions include:

- A crib that meets safety standards. That means no headspace between mattress and frame. Drop-frames have a history of infant injury. Bedding should be firm to reduce risk of sudden infant death syndrome. Bedding should never be plush or soft; infants have asphyxiated this way, as they have had plush bedding or pillows in front of their face and have not had the strength to flip or move.
- Covering up electrical outlets. Using cord shortening wraps on electrical cords and cords on blinds or lamps.
- Blocking off stairways.
- Ensuring that pets are child friendly, supervised at any time they are in contact with the baby, and not allowed to co-sleep with the infant.
- Firearms are locked in a safe.
- Infants are never left in a bathtub or wash area unsupervised, even for seconds.
- Choking hazards are removed from reach.
- All household poisons, including prescription medicines, OTC medicines, and supplements, household plants, and cleaning supplies are kept away from the infant.

- Toys that meet safety standards only are used.
- Car seats and carriers meet safety standards and are properly installed. Firefighters at the local fire station are usually available to provide instruction on this. Infants, in their carriers, are only in the back seats and are rear facing as long as possible, certainly until 12 months.

  The following resources are recommended:
  Center for Disease Control resources for parents:
  https://www.cdc.gov/parents/index.html
  American Association of Poison Control Centers:
  https://www.aapcc.org/
  1-800-222-1222 to reach a local poison control center.

Examples

Examples of Typical Naturopathic Treatments in This Age Group.

Colic: Apparent pain and discomfort in the gut of an infant with crying and fussiness. No apparent serious issues beyond this discomfort. Etiology not clear.

Physician reviews formula usage or, if breastfed, mother's diet. Antibiotic use history is considered.

Treatment considerations:

Bifidobacterium: 1 billion CFU in powder added to infant food source.
Gripe water: nonalcoholic herbal extracts, based on traditional Eastern European formula.
Extracts of *Foeniculum vulgare* (fennel), *Zingiber officinale* (ginger), sodium bicarbonate, bioflavonoids, fructose, citric acid, potassium sorbate.
Homeopathic remedies: *Chamomilla, Magnesium phosphoricum, Dioscorea.*

Constipation: Decrease in frequency of stools, with difficult passage, dryness, and anal irritation (Table 9.1).

Physician reviews diet, food introduction history, child eating patterns, screen for pica or other unusual substances consumed, and history of any recent infections or trauma.

Treatment considerations: [15].

Natural yogurt or other fermented foods.
Increase dietary fiber, fruits, and vegetables.
Flax seed oil: 1 teaspoon a day.
Homeopathic medicines such as *Calcarea carbonica.*
Drink water; do not overdrink milk.
Peppermint tea with honey.
Gentle massage to the lower abdomen.

Otitis media: Pain and inflammation in the middle ear due to blockage of the eustachian tube drainage. Physician reviews temperature, examines ear, watches for signs of extension to petrous temporal bone, and educates parents about timeline.

Treatment considerations: [15].

Alcohol free *Echinacea purpurea.*
Ear oil with *Allium sativum* (Garlic), *Verbascum thapsus* (Mullein), *Rosmarinus officianlis* (Rosemary).
Zinc melts or drops.
Steam inhalation with eucalyptol and menthol—room well ventilated.
Homeopathic remedies: *Hepar sulphuricum, Chamomilla, Pulsatilla.*

Children Aged 4 to 12 Years

Although development is a continuum, children at 4 have left the toddler stage, being language proficient, and having motor skills that they previously were still working on. Most are able to attend preschool and do rudimentary sports, dance, martial arts, and other activities. Not all children develop at the same rate, and a child at 4 years who can't do these things should be evaluated. But this should be done in an appreciative way to look at how to support their development versus jumping to a conclusion that there is something wrong. There may in fact be serious issues such as celiac disease, autism spectrum disorder, or myopathy (Table 9.2). But many children who seem to lag in one area or another can, with support and time, catch up to their peers.

Table 9.2 Levels of dysfunction in childhood disorders

Level of dysfunction	Example	Course of action
Hypofunction	Difficulty with far visual acuity	Check for nutrient deficiencies, refer for complete eye examination, send child for fitting with corrective lenses
Impaired circulation and communication	Sensory processing disorder	Ensure that all nutritional requirements are met. Have child see an occupational therapist for sensory and motor integration
Inflammation	Allergy to environmental factors	Test for exact allergies, bioflavonoids, avoidance, possible desensitization therapy
Deeper inflammation and immune involvement	Asthma	Address allergies, nutritional status, omega 3 fatty acids, dietary impacts
Fibrosis	Cystic fibrosis	N acetyl cysteine, immune support, respiratory therapy
Decline of function	Muscular dystrophies	Muscle and mitochondrial support; work with physical therapist and pediatricians
Neoplasia	Leukemia	Referral to pediatric oncologist; provide supportive/integrative care

As this childhood developmental phase rolls on, learning and development continue with motor skills, language, mathematical abilities, and social skills all growing. The determinants of health, as with all people, need to be met.

This includes: [16].

Outdoor time, exposure to sunlight, natural environments.
Movement and exercise.
Limits to screen time.
Healthy diet.
Love and social support.
Sleep in a quiet space without electronics or blue light.
Hydration; water over colas, juices, sports drinks, etc.; and clean, safe drinking water.
Limits to detrimental amounts of sugars, trans fats, omega 6 fats.
Air quality at home and school.

With all minors, the parents, guardians, and all those who love and care for them have to think about harm reduction. Adverse childhood experiences can lead to long-term problems. Although children are resilient, they need to express in their own way their response to traumas. This can sometimes surprise adults who thinking that because a child has not spoken of something for a while (the passing of a family member, an accident or illness that causes suffering for the child), that it was behind them.

Abuse and neglect can take different forms, and physicians have a duty to report.

According to the Centers for Disease Control at [17]: https://www.cdc.gov/violenceprevention/childabuseandneglect/fastfact.html

Physical abuse is the intentional use of physical force that can result in physical injury. Examples include hitting, kicking, shaking, burning, or other shows of force against a child.

Sexual abuse involves pressuring or forcing a child to engage in sexual acts. It includes behaviors such as fondling, penetration, and exposing a child to other sexual activities. Please see CDC's Preventing Child Sexual Abuse webpage for more information.

Emotional abuse refers to behaviors that harm a child's self-worth or emotional well-being. Examples include name-calling, shaming, rejecting, withholding love, and threatening.

Neglect is the failure to meet a child's basic physical and emotional needs. These needs housing, food, clothing, education, access to medical care, and having feelings validated and appropriately responded to.

In practice, some signs of these forms of abuse or neglect are objectively visible, such as bruising, unkempt appearance, and failure to thrive. Children who are withdrawn or who suddenly start to exhibit strange or inexplicable behaviors should raise concern. While physicians are not investigators, they must have some basis on which to contact child and family services. Sometimes some well-placed questions to children and parents or guardians can clarify things. Sometimes it is necessary to make a report in spite of not having absolute certainty. This is one of the difficult roles of a doctor.

A well-child visit annually is indicated in this age group. Children should receive an annual visual examination and at least one audiology screen. Height and weight, motor skills, and basic language skills are documented. It should be noted if the child is receiving regular dental care [14, 16].

Examples

Examples of typical naturopathic treatments in this age group:

Upper Respiratory Infection [15]

Viral or bacterial colonization of bronchial surfaces. Physician reviews symptoms, onset, and conduct physical examinations. Determines that airways are functioning properly, and the child is not distressed, not having nuchal rigidity, tachypnea, dyspnea, etc. Viral versus bacterial etiology may be presumptive. Treatment might be empirical, but sputum culture is always a possibility. Rapid antigen tests (Streptococcus group A; SARS CoV-2, etc.) for fever, pharyngitis, family or school exposure, etc., will indicate prompt treatment if the results are positive. It is important for the physician to set a timeline for check in, so that further action can be taken if the patient has not improved.

Treatment considerations:

Alcohol-free *Echinacea purpurea* 2.5 ml bid or tid.

Also consider alcohol-free *Hydrastis canadensis* (Goldenseal), *Lentinula edodes* (Shiitake mushroom extract).

Vitamin mineral drops for small infants or dissolvable zinc and vitamin C tablet to melt in the mouth.

Vaporizer in room using modern tank vaporizer or ultrasonic vaporizer—drops of essential oil of *Eucalyptus globulus* in tank water. Room ought to have proper ventilation.

Homeopathic medicines such as *Drosera, Phosphorus (homeopathic dilution), Pulsatilla,* etc.

Insomnia: Delayed sleep, poor quality sleep, shortened sleep cycles [15].

Physician reviews any history of pain, sugar and caffeine intake, medications, neurological findings, and the presence of depression or anxiety. Ensure that room is quiet, dark, without electronic devices.

Herbal blends alcohol free: *Scutellaria lateriflora* (skullcap), *Passiflora incarnata* (passional flower).
Low-dose magnesium supplementation.
Melatonin 10 mg h.s.
Regular bed times.
Address, with input from counselor or psychologist, any anxiety or depression.

Adolescence

The span of ages from 12 to 18 years have certain common denominators. There is continued growth and maturation. Intellectual and motor skills ramp up to adult levels. Increased desire to be independent and to bond with peers is in balance, or tension, with emotional and economic dependency on parents/guardians. There are dramatic changes between 12 and 18 years. Sexual maturation takes place. The level of autonomy changes to the point that the 18 year old is able to emancipate themselves, moving out on their own, attending college, or joining the workforce. The emotional and growth aspects of this time can be confusing, disorienting, and sometimes overwhelming.

Social isolation is a great problem that in the past, with high levels of screen and social media time. Adventures with alcohol are lower, probably as a result (but certainly not out of the picture). Group parties with friends has become less frequent for this age group, but drug addiction using opioids and other drugs of abuse self-administered at home can be just as, more dangerous. Cyberstalking, online bullying, and sexual exploitation via text or social media are contemporary challenges for adolescents. The current adolescent population has endured the most prolonged period of social isolation and activity restrictions, sometimes referred to as "lockdowns," [18, 19] with effects on mental health that are still being understood. A recent systematic review indicates predictable increases in anxiety and depression, but the long-term impacts or duration, in this population, are not yet known.

Sexual health is an important aspect of caring for this population. This include contraception and protection from sexually transmitted diseases [20]. Self-acceptance of sexuality and a sense of being supported are extremely important. Peer influence and social media manipulation of body image and sexual identity are forces to be aware of, both for physicians and parents/ guardians. The issue is not one of exploration or self-education about issues of sexual identity but rather the massive amount of influence and input, even direct opinion sharing, that a modern adolescent is exposed to. This is a new phenomenon.

States differ in their laws around informed consent and informing parents and guardians about health choices. Some states do not allow any lab results to be released to parents without consent, starting at 12 years old. Some state medical boards allow treatment for children under 18 years old without parental knowledge or permission. Physicians need to be sensitive to the expectations of an adolescent patient and their obligations to parents and their duties to report and share information. At this point, they will have their own relationship with their adolescent patients that allows for conversations without parents present, and these patients will want to be included and consulted.

The major causes of death in this age group are as follows: [21].

Accidents (unintentional injuries).
Homicide.
Suicide.

Suicide prevention is an important aspect of health care in this group, including connecting families with resources for mental health and making adolescents and families aware of the warning signs [22]. Accidents, including motor vehicle deaths, are near the top, although changes to license permits and societal efforts to reduce driving under the influence have improved—the number of teens who drink and drive has decreased by 50% since 1991 (about 1 in 10 now). Teen drivers are 17 times more likely to die in a crash if the teen driver has a blood alcohol level of 0.08% or higher [23, 24]. Drug overdose and poisoning, with a longstanding risk [6] increased by 83.6% from 2019 to 2020 among children and adolescents, became the third leading cause of death in that age group [25, 26].

Violence is the leading cause of death for adolescents. Firearm deaths can be community-wide issues that pose an ever present hazard to adolescents (and children) in addition to adults. Firearm deaths and motor vehicle accidents are the leading causes of death for those under 18 years old [27].

In the United States, 21% of adolescents are obese [28].

Many others have metabolic syndrome. The precise definition of this in children adolescents is debatable [29]. What is perhaps more helpful is to examine diabetic warning signs and cardiovascular risk markers. These include the following:

- Hypertension.
- Increase waist-to-hip ratio.
- Dyslipidemia (high triglycerides, high LDL, low/dysfunctional HDL).
- Elevated hemoglobin A1C.

Annual wellness visits are needed during these years, in addition to other appointments for select needs. Adolescents, like everyone, can suffer from a range of disorders, from troublesome, but self-limiting, to extremely dangerous (Table 9.3). Education, based on a respectful and honest rapport, of patient and parents is needed around: nutrition, pregnancy, substance abuse, sexual health and identity, safety in the community and at home, emotional health and mood disorders, and safe driving. Clearly, the adolescent years are a critical time for preserving life and health, and naturopathic physicians are needed as a part of that team.

The following are examples of some clinical presentations at different levels of dysfunction [14].

Table 9.3 Levels of dysfunction in adolescent disorders

Stage of dysfunction	Example	Course of action
Hypofunction	Fatigue	Investigate causes: Lack of sleep, masked anxiety or depression, nutrition, anemia, mononucleosis, and drug use
Impaired circulation or communication	Raynaud's phenomenon	Look for other causes, such as systemic lupus erythematosus; omega 3 supplementation, proanthocyanidins, circulatory stimulant botanicals
Inflammation	Rotator cuff tear	Rehabilitative exercises, physiological therapeutics, homeopathic/arnica gel
Deeper inflammation and immune involvement	Ulcerative colitis	Dietary therapy, soluble fiber, bioflavonoids and anti-inflammatory herbs; conventional management
Fibrosis	Strictures secondary to inflammatory bowel disease, particularly Crohn's disease	Surgical referral, and overall supportive treatment with diet, anti-inflammatory botanical extracts
Decline of function	Congenital/pediatric cardiomyopathy	Surgical and cardiology management; strong naturopathic support for circulation, mitochondria, etc.
Neoplasm	Hodgkin's lymphoma	Referral for oncology treatment; integrative support

Examples

Examples of typical conditions treated by naturopathic physicians:

Attention Deficit Hyperactivity Disorder

This is a mixture of variants, some tending toward impulsivity and others, inattentiveness. Some presentations are mixed. Like any neuroatypical state, it is important to value and recognize the strengths and abilities of the individual. Although ADHD-type neurobiology can create problems of living for children and adults, overly pathologizing it is not helpful. Diagnosis should be by a neuropsychiatric consult. Problems of staying on task in school, self-care, organization, anxiety over beginning tasks, inability to complete tasks, social awkwardness, hyperfocus on certain activities, and a general pattern of inconsistency are all frequently reported [30].

Treatment

The patient should adopt strategies in daily living, such as creating visual reminders in their environment, breaking tasks down to smaller components, playing to their strengths, and recognizing their own frustration level. In addition to these organizational tactics, the patient may need support at school. A 504 Plan is indicated by federal law for students who qualify based on a qualifying assessment. The school will provide changes to the learning environment or testing situations such as the ability to move around or to take tests in a quiet environment. An individualized education plan (IEP) opens the door for specialized instruction. Both of these supportive measures are also valuable for neurotypical children who are diagnosed with being on the autistic spectrum.

Working with a counselor is valuable for many children as they can learn self-regulation strategies, how to be more aware of and communicate feelings, and to strengthen executive function.

The standard medical approach is the use of stimulant medication, such as dexmethylphenidate. These medicines, while stimulants, can activate the brain regions responsible for executive functioning. These have been used for decades and do seem to create changes and improvements.

A naturopathic physician would definitely work with the child and family to increase their exercise levels. This alone can have an impact on executive function, emotional regulation, focus, and feelings of well-being. Adding at least an hour a day of moderate to intense exercise is a good idea for an adolescent patient with ADHD.

Other helpful considerations would be:

Bacopa monnieri, 500 mg per day. An herb that helps with mental stamina and focus.
Omega 3 supplement with DHA and EPA: 2000 mg per day.
L-theanine: an amino acid that may have a calming but nonsedative effect, especially for more hyperkinetic and impulsive individuals.

There are three things to note naturopathically:

- There is nothing intrinsically wrong with the use of a low-dose stimulant for many ADHD kids. These medicines can be safe, and they can provide a useful change. Much like eyeglasses or foot orthotics can give refractive or biomechanical adjustments that someone needs, stimulant medications are also helpful. The unfortunate trend of increased prescriptions of antipsychotic medications for nonpsychotic issues is another matter. There are always cases where these can be helpful too, but they are overprescribed, in spite of low-quality evidence for this use.
- It is not a malady for a child to not feel comfortable being in a school and behind a desk for hours at a time. Most adapt fairly well. Some do not. This way of living for children is a recent development. Some children might ultimately do better with homeschooling blended with interesting sports and activities with other kids in the evenings. Others might do well at a private school with large amounts of outdoor time. Some schools have experimented with having frequent breaks for movement, even putting exercise equipment into high school math classrooms.

- Naturopathic medicine can be integratively blended with other ways of helping a child (including occupational therapy for those with sensory processing disorders and ADHD). The main thing is what will help them to live their lives happily and productively with freedom to use their talents and grow as a person.

Obesity

According to the CDC, 21.2% among 12- to 19-year-olds are obese. This is a complex problem, in spite of the fact that some of the immediate causes are simple. The incidence has disparities, and with regard to children in general, obesity prevalence was 25.6% among Hispanic children, 24.2% among non-Hispanic Black children, 16.1% among non-Hispanic White children, and 8.7% among non-Hispanic Asian children [28].

There are several factors at work. Diet is without a doubt a major one. The increases in high-carbohydrate choices, fast food, and basically ultra-processed food have deleterious effects on children and adolescents. These foods are energy rich and nutrient poor. They are often designed to encourage overeating, which is a hallmark of snack food development. Many of these foods have additive properties. While in isolation, on occasion, and within a healthy diet, these foods (like a slice of birthday cake) are all enjoyable, the reality of the situation is that they are massively overconsumed. White flour, sugar, salt, trans fat, artificial flavors, monosodium glutamate, high-fructose corn syrup, fatty meats, deep fried meats and starches, and carbonated beverages are constantly consumed by children.

With many variations, some children are not physically active enough. One third of the global population 15 years and older do not get enough exercise. The United States, in spite of a strong culture of youth sports, is no exception and adolescents in the United States have seen increases in screen time (which have adverse mental health effects at high exposures).

Disparities in health care, access to healthy food choices, socioeconomic disparities, and stressors all contribute to nutritional problems and health problems as a whole.

There are environmental aspects such as chemical obesogens, which amplify the activity and growth of adipose cells.

Treatment Approach

Work with the patient and their family to move into a nutrient-dense diet that sheds most of the nutrient-poor, high-carbohydrate, ultra-processed, and fast-food options. This may take time. Education, support, new strategies for cooking, and quite possibly a reclaiming of the family meal time around a table of healthy food choices are all part of this. The guidelines for healthy eating proposed by the USDA have greatly improved in the last several years, with more emphasis on whole foods and more warnings about health-degrading foods. The Canadian nutrition guidelines are particularly excellent, with the emphasis on plant-based foods.

There are many ways to approach this, while meeting nutritional guidelines. A Mediterranean diet is one excellent starting point, but that is not necessarily how every adolescent and their family will approach this. There are excellent cookbooks, websites, and apps that apply these guidelines to more familiar menu planning. The website and not for profit Oldways (https://oldwayspt.org/) has excellent menu choice structures and recipes [31]. Known for their Mediterranean diet tools, they have added:

- African heritage diet.
- Latin diet.
- Asian diet.
- Vegetarian/vegan diets.

These diets incorporate the principles of healthy eating but present a wider variety of foods and a connection with culinary traditions.

Other treatments:

Panax ginseng 500 mg bid—metabolic enhancement.

Momordica charantia (note: contraindicated for those with glucose 6 phosphate deficiency)—insulin sensitization, anti-inflammatory.

In general, limiting portion size; using lower glycemic index foods; adding beneficial herbs such as cinnamon, ginger, and garlic to the diet; and having a set meal time are all valuable beginnings.

Adults

Just as the journey from ages 3 to 12 or 12 to 18 years traverses great changes, the category "adult" ranges from a still developing but self-sufficient person to a mature one who is experiencing senescence. Adulthood denotes reaching a certain level of maturity, both in the body and the mind. Although the brain and body continue to refine themselves, young adults are capable of launching careers or even starting a family. Although people in their 60s are experiencing a decline of muscle mass and brain mass and increased risks of diseases such as cancer, they *can* be incredibly vital. Our contemporary society has the peculiar situation of having many adults, fortunately, living longer and not dying younger due to things like acute infections in the way that they did in the past. But the rising tide of degenerative diseases, which are enabled not only by longer lifespans, but by disturbances to health, can obscure the fact that it could be normal for people in their 60s and 70s to often be fit and unencumbered by degenerative disease. That is observable in some isolated places and in some individuals. Of course, random mutations, inescapable damage due to environmental toxins, cosmic rays, sunlight, and genetic susceptibility ensures that no matter how scrupulous someone is in their lifestyle, accidents and injuries, cancers, and chronic maladies can strike. The SARS CoV-2 pandemic certainly impacted many people who were "high risk"—having COPD, diabetes, heart disease, etc.—but it could also (with less likelihood) ravage individuals who were the picture of health.

Naturopathic physicians provide primary care health care to adults. This can include the important screening and health maintenance steps, such as regular testing of lipids and serum chemistry on an annual checkup. It can involve the treatment of acute illness, using natural and where necessary more synthetic medicines. It often involves a tandem approach, where the patient is seeing a specialist. For example, a patient with lung cancer is sent to an oncologist, and that may involve surgical approaches as well as radiation and chemotherapy. That doesn't mean that the patient ends their relationship with the naturopathic physician.

Depending on the jurisdiction, and the nature of the naturopathic practice, the patient might also be treated in tandem with a medical or osteopathic physician who does family medicine/internal medicine. Some naturopathic practices are based on working with patients who want to integrate a natural approach to their health care. Some have intractable problems that have yielded only slightly to pharmaceutical intervention. Some have been simply unhealthy for many years and have realized that illness is a progressive, feedforward situation when health begins to decline.

Some naturopathic practices provide the full-service primary care to a group of patients who elect to use them and offer naturopathic therapeutics to others, who are free to receive regular primary care from a medical or osteopathic doctor. In this sense, naturopathic physicians are capable of being part of an integrative care relationship, and they can competently (and do in many jurisdictions) provide primary care.

In working with younger adults, the issues tend to involve metabolic (obesity), autoimmune, mood, musculoskeletal, reproductive, and urologic issues. This is complemented by the common presenting complaints from most age groups: digestion, acute viral infections, headaches, sports injuries, stomach pain, irritable bowel syndrome, and nutritional advice.

In adults aged 35 to 60 years, there are stepped up efforts to screen for health issues. And processes that lead to disease have had time to further develop. Heart disease, cancers, and wear-and-tear musculoskeletal issues began to be common. In those over 60 years old, there are commonly some medical issues to manage, and often very serious ones.

At the minimum, preventive health screening [32] consists of the following:

- Cholesterol/lipid panel every 5 years from the age of 20 onwards.
- A chem-screen every 2 or 3 years for adults under 30 years, annually over 30.
- Blood pressure recorded at each wellness checkup.
- Increased frequency of lipid testing for those with cardiovascular risk factors.
- Colonoscopy for adults 45 to 75 years, every 5 years unless indicated otherwise by the surgeon.

- Skin exam by dermatologist may start at 40 but earlier depending on history (solar exposure, family history).
- Abdominal aneurysm scan for adults over 50 years old, one time.

  Based on individual risk:

Sexually transmitted disease screening based on exposure (potential).
Tuberculosis screening based on potential exposure.
Hepatitis B and C screening based on health history.

Elderly Adults

Older adults typically need more frequent screening tests, plus special examinations depending on their specific health concerns [33] (Table 9.4). For example, an 80-year-old patient with age-related macular degeneration will get ophthalmologic examinations on a regular timetable by a specialist. A 70-year-old diabetic will get more intensive examinations of the kidney, eye, nervous system, and cardiovascular systems.

The physician must check into the following:

Cognitive screen might be done if the patient and their family requests it.
Fall prevention is an important prevention measure, which involves asking the patient about their household setup, their use of a walker, and their balance.

Table 9.4 Examples of levels of dysfunction in adults [14, 15]

Level of dysfunction	Example	Course of action
Hypofunction	Dyspepsia due to mild hypochlorhydria	Bitter herbs such as *Gentiana lutea,* in small doses prior to meals
Disordered circulation and communication	Poor peripheral circulation leading to leg pain	Address atherosclerosis, *Ginkgo biloba* extra EB761, ascorbic acid, coenzyme Q10
Inflammation	Peptic ulcer with *H. pylori* involvement	Eradicate *H. pylori*, provide gastric protection, glutamine, probiotics
Deeper inflammation and immune involvement	Advanced atherosclerosis with unstable plaques and elevated inflammatory biomarkers	Adjust diet and bring in polyphenolic molecules, omega 3 fatty acids, ascorbic acid
Fibrosis and extracellular matrix degeneration	Lung parenchyma damage leading to emphysema	Increasing antioxidant status and decreased exposure to pro-oxidative forces
Decline of function	Hepatic failure secondary to fibrosis and cirrhosis	Diet with high quality but limited protein, probiotics, soluble fiber, Silymarin nanoparticle form
Neoplasm	Adenocarcinoma of colon	Referral to oncologist, supportive nutritional and herbal care

Measures for wellness checks, the presence of caregivers or relatives, and access to emergency services in the event of a fall or debilitating situation such as a stroke.

A review of their current medications.

Nutritional status in the elderly can suffer. Digestion weakens due to decline in pancreatic exocrine function, as well as atrophy of the gastric mucosa, with less hydrochloric acid and pepsin. Gallbladder disease or removal can decrease bile flow. Many seniors have dental issues such as partial plates or tooth/gum disease that makes chewing more difficult. Medicines that dry up secretions will decrease salvation. Support of digestion with enzymes and botanicals, and a review of diet to ensure that nutritional needs are being met, is necessary. Social isolation, debility, and apathy can lead to seniors falling into a more processed food/restaurant food diet. Unfortunately, this diet can lack the plant foods, antioxidants, essential fatty acids, and proteins that they need and be high in unhealthy (trans and excessive saturated) fats, sugar, and sodium.

Sample Condition in Adult Care

Hypothyroidism [15]

A 36-year-old male presents with fatigue, chills, and gradual weight gain in spite of no change to diet. A lab panel with hormones T4, T3, and TSH (thyroxine, triiodothyronine, thyroid-stimulating hormone) is taken. Results show low T4 and T3 and elevated TSH. A test for antibodies to the enzyme thyroid peroxidase is positive.

Physician discusses options of supplemental T4 (levothyroxine) or desiccated thyroid gland (USP) that has both T4 and T3. In order to decrease inflammation, the physician reviews diet and has the patient rotate some foods that are eaten too frequently, such as high-gluten grains. A multivitamin and mineral supplement that has selenium, zinc, vitamin D, and other nutrients is added.

Migraine Headache [15]

A 42-year-old female presents with migraine headache. This has been a pattern since her late teens. But lately, it has been much worse. She used to get a migraine at the beginning of the menstrual cycle, but about every 3 months. Now it is happening monthly. The headache has a pounding sensation, photophobia, vomiting, and with pain more localized to the right side of the head. It seems to be worse from eating at restaurants or drinking wine.

Physician reviews various determinants of health with the patient, finds that sleep and hydration are disturbed, and works with patient to correct these. The herb *Tanacetum parthenium* (feverfew) is started as prophylaxis, as is supplemental magnesium citrate 200 mg bid. The patient is advised to avoid red wine, canned tuna, shrimp, aged cheese, and pork, within one week of when the headaches usually start. The homeopathic remedy *Sanguinaria canadensis* is given to the patient to take for pain relief when a migraine recurs.

Women's Health

In addition to the general health screening, female patients will have a variety of goals and needs (Table 9.5). These include the following: [34].

- Breast health: Breast self-exam and physician exam are conducted throughout life. Mammograms are instituted beginning age 40 depending on family history.
- Naturopathic physicians can prescribe oral contraceptives in some jurisdictions.
- Family history of uterine and ovarian cancer is determined.

Table 9.5 Examples of typical presentations of female patients in naturopathic medicine: [14]

Level of dysfunction	Example	Course of action
Hypofunction	Oligomenorrhea	Investigate causes including lack of pituitary hormones
Disordered circulation and communication	Menopausal hot flashes	Decreased LH and vasomotor instability—Rule out other causes—Support stability with botanicals, lifestyle modification, and nutrients
Inflammation	Mastitis	Treat with topical treatments or intern antimicrobials—If breastfeeding, must consider safety of infant
Deeper inflammation and immune involvement	Cervicitis	Screen for recent antibiotic use, methods of contraception if used, and do screening tests for sexually transmitted diseases (i.e., chlamydia)
Fibrosis and extracellular matrix degeneration	Infertility due to pelvic inflammatory diseases—Blocked fallopian tube	Consult with gynecological surgeon about possibility for treatment; ensure that inciting cause of PID—Such as *Neisseria gonorrhoeae*—Is eradicated
Decline of function	Infertility after treatment for cancer—Chemotherapy and radiation have damaged the ovaries	Some patients elect to have eggs banked prior to undergoing cancer treatment
Neoplasm	Cervical cancer	Consistent lifetime screening—With cytology and DNA analysis or at the very least PAP smear Surgical treatment and integrative naturopathic care can be effective in many cases. Smoking and folic acid deficiency are often associated. New HPV vaccines are now in widespread use

- Menopausal symptoms are managed depending on the patient's experience at this time of life.
- Bone density, cardiovascular health, cognitive health, and metabolic function may change at menopause.
- Cervical dysplasia screening: Liquid cytology and human papilloma virus DNA screen. PAP smears are still accessible for screening purposes.

Breast Self-Exam [35]

Some research review committees and associations (such as breastcancer.org) discourage performing breast self-examination. Many physicians and organizations continue to support it. One criticism is that false-positive findings (a lump that creates concern) will lead to either unnecessary testing or unnecessary treatment. This is possible, and a naturopathic physician works with a patient to manage such findings. However, this strikes to the heart of what happens when a well-intentioned effort to guide all behavior by evidence, based on statistical review, goes against common sense self-care. Most naturopathic physicians would be extremely dismayed to see a patient diagnosed with breast cancer, especially a higher staging, if they had discouraged the patient from becoming familiar with their body and performing self-exam.

Abuse and Violence [36]

Primary care involves screening for safety at home and recognizing signs and symptoms of violence and abuse. This can involve additional forms of health care and reporting to the police. An additional dimension to this screening is sex trafficking, which is a global problem.

Xenoestrogens

While the absolute impact on health is still being understood, it is important to realize that synthetic compounds (and high doses of some natural ones) can bind to the estrogen receptor. These include plasticizers such as bisphenol A, B, etc., and phthalates, as well as dioxin, various agricultural and industrial compounds, and some drinking water components such as chlorinated biphenyls and excreted prescription hormones recycled into drinking water. These compounds may increase the risk for cancers of the uterus, breast, and ovary and can promote metabolic dysfunction [37].

Vaginitis and Cervicitis

Bacteria, yeast, and other organisms can cause transient infections. But in some cases, screening for *Neisseria gonorrhoeae*, *Chlamydia trachomatis*, Herpes virus, and other sexually transmitted diseases is required [14].

Fertility and Pregnancy

The general care of pregnant patients has far more visits and routine screening tests than the typical adult care.

Prenatal care guidelines are published by the National Institute of Child Health and Development. [38] Many patients will work with an obstetrician, but some work with their family doctor, who in some jurisdictions is a naturopathic doctor. The training and specifications for prenatal care and delivery and addressing complications is beyond the scope of this textbook. In general, the prenatal visit schedule is:

- Monthly in the first 27 weeks.
- Every 2 weeks from weeks 28 to 36.
- Weekly for the week 36 to birth.

To establish a baseline for the health of the mother and baby, in the first visit:

- Review prenatal plan, medical history, birthing plan (including calculated due date), and goals around prenatal testing.
- Urine sample: including HcG levels.
- Weight, height, blood pressure.
- Order ultrasound examination if not already done.
- Review need to not smoke, and not consume alcohol.
- Review need for exercise.
- Review remaining determinants of health including social support.
- Perform prenatal blood tests to do the following:
- Determine your blood type and Rh (Rhesus) factor. (Note: if mother is Rh negative and father is Rh positive, this is pertinent to pregnancy risk including immune harm to the fetus).
- Complete blood count and Chemscreen.
- Screening panel for hepatitis B, HIV, rubella, and syphilis.
- Pelvic exam and cultures for gonorrhea and chlamydia.
- If not on file recently, liquid cytology for HPV.
- Blood pressure, pulse, temperature, respiration rate, and exam of the abdomen, thorax, and extremities.

Note: Some parents elect to receive genetic screening. This can be genetic screening of mother and father to look for autosomal dominant and recessive issues. It can also involve amniocentesis to read the DNA of the infant. Genetic counselors specialize in guidance on these matters.

Subsequent visits include taking the abdominal height, weight, and blood pressure and urinalysis.

During pregnancy, adequate protein and calories, overall nutrients, and in particular folic acid are essential. Naturopathic supplements that contain vitamin A should be avoided due to its potential for teratogenic actions, but dietary vitamin A should be checked on to ensure adequacy. Exposure to smoke, lead in drinking water, and pathogens such as *Listeria monocytogenes* from deli meats and *Toxoplasma gondii* from cat feces (litter boxes) are important.

Primary Dysmenorrhea [15].

Menstrual cramping, not secondary to a pathology.

Physician ensures that dysmenorrhea is not heralding more severe issues.

Diet to introduce more plant foods, fiber, fermented foods, etc., to allow for gut health and to reduce reabsorption (enterohepatic circulation) of estrogen.

Support of hepatic detoxification including use of Diindolylmethane 100 mg bid for hormone processing in liver.

Viburnum opulus: 5 ml of tincture (hydro-ethanol extract) bid during painful periods.

Homeopathic medicines including *Magnesium phosphoricum, Cimicifuga, Lachesis,* and *Viburnum.*

Menopausal Hot Flushes [15].

Vasomotor instability during perimenopausal and menopausal phase.

Physician ensures that patients are receiving proper risk assessment and prevention for osteoporosis, cardiovascular disease, and cancer screening.

Cimicifuga racemosa: as a standardized extract 50 mg bid or tincture 5 ml bid.

Soy isoflavones: 100 mg per day.

Soy isoflavones, from *Glycine max*, may have more benefits on metabolism, cognition, and bone. *Cimicifuga racemosa* works primarily on vasomotor instability.

Evaluate determinants of health, stress level, and self-acceptance during this phase of life.

Consider supplementation with calcium, magnesium, vitamin D, and Zinc but ensure that diet is as nutritionally sound as possible prior to supplementing.

Men's Health

In addition to the adult screening and health care principles noted above, men's health includes the issues of testicular and prostate cancer and benign prostatic hyperplasia [39] (Table 9.6). Prostate cancer risk increases with age [40]. It is, after

Table 9.6 Examples of typical presentations of male patients in primary care [14]

Level of dysfunction	Example	Course of action
Hypofunction	Decreased sperm count with age	Screen for environmental factors and nutritional status
Disordered circulation and communication	Erectile dysfunction due to impaired nerve and vascular flow	Address vascular health and comorbidities such as diabetes mellitus
Inflammation	Cystitis due to impeded urinary flow	Treat prostatic hyperplasia, urinary antiseptics, biofilm disruption
Deeper inflammation and immune involvement	Urethritis due to *Neisseria gonorrhoeae*	Begin antibiotic treatment, report to health authorities
Fibrosis and extracellular matrix degeneration	Fibrosis of prostate after radiation treatment	Address any urinary incontinence or sexual dysfunction resulting from procedures
Decline of function	Low testosterone post orchitis	Consider supplemental testosterone depending on patient goals and history
Neoplasm	Prostate cancer	Screen properly and establish diagnosis—Carefully consider treatments and encourage patient to use oncology care to address the problem

nonmelanoma skin cancer, the most common cancer in men. It is not the highest cause of mortality, as it can be successfully (but not always) treated. Many men have very slow-growing adenomas and may die from some other cause before that cancer progresses to the point where it could spread. The prostate-specific antigen (PSA) test is a screening and a monitoring test. Digital rectal examination is not recommended by the United States Preventive Services Task Force because of a lack of evidence that it makes a difference. Nevertheless, many physicians perform a digital rectal exam on the premise that finding a nodule or gross asymmetry is a clue that might lead to early cancer treatment. The PSA test is somewhat controversial, because it has led to premature biopsies and treatments. Nevertheless, many physicians feel that they will not blindly overreact to positive findings on these tests, that they can properly educate their patients on how to keep these results in perspective, and they wish to avail themselves of clues that might allow for early detection.

Testicular cancer is a common cancer in males 15 to 35 years of age [39]. It is highly treatable. Self-exam and doctor exam are not universally recommended as it is not clear that it impacts long-term outcomes. However, many primary care physicians perform a testicular examination during annual wellness checks. If they were to find nodules, they could order additional testing.

Benign prostatic hyperplasia is a swelling of the prostate gland. This occurs with age in many men. It may be due to accumulation of dihydrotestosterone or an estrogen/ testosterone imbalance. This will start to impinge on the part of the urethra that travels through the prostate gland. This in turn leads to difficulty voiding, overfilling of the bladder, possible infection of bladder, nocturia, and dysuria. Sometimes, it can lead to hydronephrosis due to so much hydrostatic pressure in the bladder that it refluxes to the kidneys.

Benign Prostatic Hypertrophy [15]

Physician rules out prostate cancer and performs urinalysis.

Serenoa repens to regulate hormones in the prostate environment: 160 mg bid.

Hepatic support to encourage systemic regulation of hormones. Zinc supplementation at 50 mg per day with Copper 5 mg.

Erectile Dysfunction

Establish circulatory issues versus peripheral neuropathy.

Address atherosclerosis and add nerve-protecting agents such as alpha lipoic acid.

Address diabetes if part of the clinical picture.

Adaptogenic herbs such as *Panax ginseng* or circulatory tonics such as *Ginkgo biloba* might be helpful.

EENT

Primary Care Considerations Summary [14, 15, 41].

Actual naturopathic care involves the investigation into the real conditions and challenges that a particular patient faces. It also involves decisions about where to apply support to stimulate that person's body.

For the purposes of describing some common management considerations, examples of some keynote treatments for a range of primary care presentations are provided below.

Ocular

Eye conditions are common in primary care (Table 9.7). Many of these require referral to a specialist, an ophthalmologist in most cases (although some range of conditions can be handled by an optometrist, such as dry eye, monitoring the retina, etc.).

Table 9.7 Common ocular disorders

Condition	Diagnostic considerations	Whole-person approaches and key determining factors of health	Biochemical support and hormetic stimulation	Decreasing maladaptive responses or long-term inducement of homeostasis
Conjunctivitis	Bacterial or viral; ensure that painful extension to cornea is not occurring.	Correct for dehydration, vitamin A deficiency, medicines that dry out mucus membranes; the acupuncture approach would look at heat in the liver channel	Omega 3 fatty acids; eyedrops (sterile) with *Euphrasia officinalis*; Boric acid eye wash (pH balanced, USP)	Ocular antibiotics in solution or ointment
Uveitis	Related to autoimmune diseases or certain chronic infections; can lead to permanent visual loss rapidly	Diet and anti-inflammatory regimen for the long term Gut microbiome testing or presumptive probiotic supplementation	None	Corticosteroids as long as necessary but monitored for increase in intraocular pressure
Recurrent corneal erosions	Past injury to cornea disrupting Bowman's membrane; erosions can increase risk of corneal infection	Dehydration, dry living environment, medications that reduce tear film, food allergies	Vitamin A drops to increase mucin production; omega 3 fatty acids; sources of proanthocyanidins, such as berries, and vitamin C to provide collagen support	Artificial tears, hypertonic sodium chloride (to reduce corneal edema), excimer laser treatment or puncture treatment to strengthen corneal epithelial attachment
Cataract	Ocular exam determines extent of growth	Excessive oxidative stress, nutrient deficiency, and ultraviolet light exposure contribute. Smoking cessation if indicated. High plant food diet	A, C, and E, lutein, and zeaxanthin supplements; drops containing *N*-acetylcarnosine	Lens removal and implant

(continued)

Table 9.7 (continued)

Condition	Diagnostic considerations	Whole-person approaches and key determining factors of health	Biochemical support and hormetic stimulation	Decreasing maladaptive responses or long-term inducement of homeostasis
Macular degeneration	Degree of retinal deterioration on ocular exam	Lack of antioxidants in diet; smoking cessation if indicated; overall increase oxidative stress	A, C, and E, zinc, lutein, and zeaxanthin supplements *Ginkgo biloba*, *Vaccinium myrtillus* (bilberry)	Laser photocoagulation therapy Anti-VEGF (vegetative endothelial growth factor) treatment
Diabetic retinopathy	Extent and degree of hemorrhage and/or fibrosis	Aggressive control and reversal of diabetes; homeopathic medicines that have hemorrhage in symptom picture (i.e., *Lachesis mutans*); Mediterranean diet	*Ginkgo biloba* but not for hemorrhagic retinopathy *Vaccinium myrtillus* (Fig. 9.1), grape phenolic compounds vs. advanced glycation end products; *Crocus sativus* (Saffron); *Curcuma longa* (curcumin)	Pharmaceutical treatments for diabetes Photocoagulation; cryotherapy
Glaucoma	Measured intraocular pressure, optic nerve edema and atrophy, visual tests	Anti-inflammatory diet, ketogenic diet, acupuncture as adjunctive therapy not sole therapy	*Ginkgo biloba*	Prostaglandin analogs; beta-blockers; laser therapy to open canal drainage
Pinguecula	Assess progression rate	Hydration, vitamin A status, sunglasses, and avoid dust and wind	*Euphrasia officinalis* drops (sterile)	Eye lubricant drops; surgery for very advanced pinguecula, α-2 adrenergic agonist for temporary relief

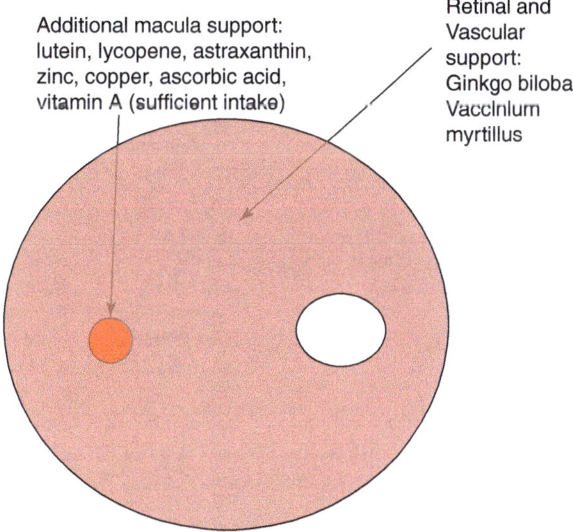

Fig. 9.1 Nutrients and the retina: Phytochemicals and carotenoids can have protective and strengthening effects on the retina

Nasal

Nasal issues can be due to allergy, infection, foreign bodies, or trauma (Table 9.8). They are often related to other issues, and diet and allergy screening is often indicated.

Ear

The ear requires treatment for both structural issues (such as an infection in the external canal) to functional ones (that ultimately have some physical change behind them), particularly hearing (Table 9.9). Changes to hearing can occur quickly after trauma or even extreme noise exposure. Some ear and hearing issues are chronic and may take a long time to heal.

Mouth

Oral pathologies of self-limiting and potential surgical natures are common in practice (Table 9.10). The mouth is an easy area to access for inspection of the tongue, gums, buccal mucosa, pharynx, and more. As resilient as these tissues are, they can break down due to infection, allergy, or physical trauma (such as burns).

Table 9.8 Common conditions of the nasal passages and sinuses

Condition	Diagnostic considerations	Whole-person approaches and key determining factors of health	Biochemical support and hormetic stimulation	Decreasing maladaptive responses or long-term inducement of homeostasis
Allergic rhinitis	Sources of allergy—Environmental or dietary	Allergy avoidance, dietary restructure, Constitutional hydrotherapy, modified fasting	Quercetin, vitamin C, nasosympatico treatment (essential oils applied nasally), (Fig. 9.2) nasal irrigation with saline	Nasal corticosteroids, nasal decongestants (very short-term use), allergy desensitization injections
Rhinitis medicamentosa	Determine that the patient has other solutions to nasal congestion—Discontinue decongestants and steroids	Steam inhalation, modified fasting, dietary triggers for congestion (dairy, gluten containing grains, sucrose), Homeopathic *Allium cepa*, *Mercurius solubilis*, etc	Dilute therapies in sterile nasal mist to provoke drainage reactions (3× dilutions, sterile of *Euphorbium*, *Hepar sulphuricum*, etc.)	Patient may return to using decongestants that caused the mucosal atrophy if they cannot find relief—Not advisable
Sinusitis	Determine extent of sinus filling with fluid— CT scan	Steam inhalation, hot foot bath; wet sheet pack; Homeopathic medicines such as Mercurius corrosivus, Kali bichromium	Nasal irrigation with or with herbal extracts such as *Hydrastis canadensis*; essential oil applications; oral *Lomatium dissectum*, *Echinacea purpurea*	Antibiotic therapy

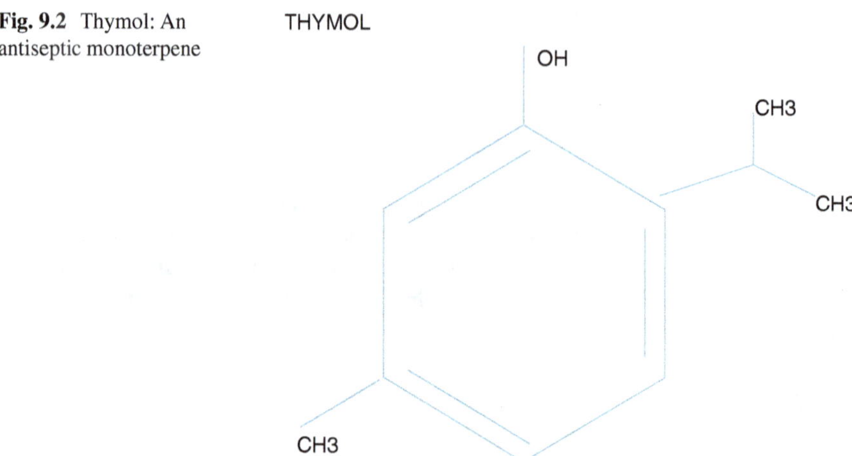

Fig. 9.2 Thymol: An antiseptic monoterpene

Table 9.9 Selected otic/auditory conditions

Condition	Diagnostic considerations	Whole-person approaches and key determining factors of health	Biochemical support and hormetic stimulation	Decreasing maladaptive responses or long-term inducement of homeostasis
Acute sensorineural hearing loss	Auditory testing: Degree of bone and air conduction, frequency ranges, avoid sources of hearing damage	Acupuncture/ electro-acupuncture, homeopathic remedies such as (arnica or Hypericum if due to physical trauma), replace ear buds with ambient speakers at lower decibel	Vitamin A and D supplementation	Hyperbaric oxygen therapy, short-term corticosteroid injection
Meinniere's disease	Ear and neurologic examination: Idiopathic or secondary to lesion	Epley maneuver, acupuncture, Chinese herbal medicines for kidney qi deficiency or liver yang rising	*Ginkgo biloba* extract GBE761 or other standardized extracts, neuro hormesis via Coriolus versicolor and *Hericium erinaceus*	Antihistamines, steroids
Otitis externa	Determine etiology (bacterial, fungal)	Reduce sugar consumption and increase omega 3 fatty acids	Drops or washes with *Hydrastis canadensis*, *Allium sativum*, *Eucalyptus globulus*, *Thymus vulgaris*, *Rosmarinus officinalis*	Antibiotic or antifungal drops or internally
Otitis media	Rule out mastoiditis	Homeopathic medicines such as Chamomila, Pulsatila, silica; Address environmental and food allergy; microbiome repair and gut repair in children with food hypersensitivities or history of repeated antibiotic use; steam inhalation with vaporizer in a ventilated room with essential oils such as *Eucalyptus globulus* oil	Ear oil with *Hypericum perforatum*, *Hydrastis canadensis*, *Verbasum thapsus*, *Allium sativum*; vitamin C, zinc, *Echinacea purpurea*	Prescription antibiotics, myringotomy tubes (Fig. 9.3)

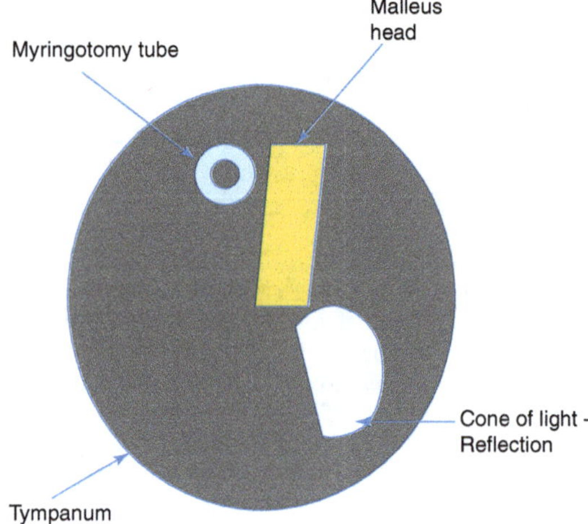

Fig. 9.3 Examining the tympanum: Dullness where the normal reflection of the otoscope should be suggests fluid buildup

Table 9.10 Selected conditions of the oral cavity and pharynx

Condition	Diagnostic considerations	Whole-person approaches and key determining factors of health	Biochemical support and hormetic stimulation	Decreasing maladaptive responses or long-term inducement of homeostasis
Aphthous ulceration	Determine cause: Allergy, acidic food, side effect of drug, infection; associated with inflammatory bowel disease, Bechet's disease, and neoplasm (squamous cell	Consider dietary allergies and mast cell activation	Deglycerinated licorice tablets to chew *Calendula officinalis* tea—Swish Zinc lozenges	Tetracycline, benzocaine application
Gingivitis	Review oral hygiene regimen, date of last dental visit	Dietary vitamin C and bioflavonoids, smoking cessation	Folic acid, coenzyme Q 10, mouthwash with *Thymus vulgaris* and *Hydrastis canadensis*, toothpaste with *Commiphora myrrha*	Antibiotic rinse, dental irrigation with peroxide
Pharyngitis	Diagnosis agent (viral, bacterial, fungal), screen for neoplasm (HPV-associated cancer - requires different treatment protocol than this table indicates for infectious pharyngitis)	*Homeopathic medicines such as Hepar sulphuricum, Mercurius corrosivus, and Atropa belladonna, constitutional hydrotherapy, Microcurrent stimulation to acupoints LI 4 and LU7*	*Gargle of Hydrastis canadensis extract and water, Verbascum thapsus tea and Ulmus fulva gruel or tea for soothing effect, zinc, Astragalus membranaceus, Panax ginseng*	Antibiotics if nonresolving

Diabetes

Diabetes is a health concern of such magnitude, it deserves special consideration. It is estimated that 37.3 million people in the United States have diabetes. Prediabetes, with higher than normal glucose readings and hemoglobin A1c, and metabolic abnormalities, is found in 96 million people aged 18 years and up. That number is 38% of the adult United States population. Looking at the population of adults 65 years and older, the prediabetic numbers rise to 48.8%. The Centers for Disease Control and Prevention estimates that by 2050, 1 in 3 American adults will be diabetic [42].

Diabetes mellitus impacts multiple organ systems [43].The pancreas is of course involved, due to the insulin secretion cells there. Adipose tissue, muscle, the cardiovascular system, nerves, kidneys, and the eye are all strongly impacted.

Obesity is the strongest risk factor for diabetes. The higher someone's body mass index, the younger they are likely to be diagnosed with it.

Testing for glucose in the bloodstream is one way to diagnose diabetes. The other is to measure levels of hemoglobin A1C (Table 9.11) [44]. It is the protein hemoglobin that has been glycated—it has glucose attached to it. It reflects blood glucose levels over time. It used to be used to monitor treatment efficacy but is not an acceptable diagnostic criterion.

Glucose testing in the bloodstream is done in three ways. The most common is fasting glucose, where patients have had nothing to eat or any liquid besides water for the last 12 to 14 h (Table 9.12). A special way of testing blood glucose is to have a patient drink a glucose beverage with a known amount of sugar in it and then measure their serum glucose at certain intervals. This is done with pregnant women to measure gestational diabetes (Table 9.13). Some patients cannot get this test because they have reactive hypoglycemia. Their insulin surge after this type of challenge is so intense that their blood sugar levels. This can lead to palpitations,

Table 9.11 Hemoglobin A1C

Test result	Significance
6.5% or higher	Diabetes
5.7%–6.4%	Prediabetes
Lower than 5.7%	Normal Nondiabetic

Table 9.12 Fasting serum glucose

Test result	Significance
126 mg/dL or higher	Diabetes
100 to 125 mg/dL	Prediabetes
99 mg/dL or lower	Normal—Nondiabetic

Table 9.13 Glucose tolerance test

Test result	Significance
200 mg/dL or higher	Diabetes
140—199 mg/dL	Prediabetes
99 mg/dL or lower	Normal—Nondiabetic

dizziness, confusion, or even losing consciousness. Random glucose readings in a nonfasting patient are not typically used to diagnose, although any reading over 200 mg/dL probably indicates a diabetic result for that person.

Diabetes mellitus takes its name from a bygone era when physicians would taste their patient's urine. The name literally means "sweet" or "honey-like" urine. When glucose levels become very high, glucose will start to spill out into the urine. It can't be reabsorbed fast enough, and it doesn't return from kidney tubules very well when the blood is already saturated with it. Very high levels of glucose will start to increase the osmotic pressure of the bloodstream. This can become so powerful that it can pull water out of the brain, leading to diabetic coma (a form of encephalopathy).

There are two forms of diabetes: insulin-dependent diabetes mellitus (IDDM) and non-insulin-dependent diabetes mellitus (NIDDM) [14, 15, 43]. These are sometimes called types I and II. The form IDDM (type I) used to be called juvenile diabetes. It is more common in children but can strike adults. In IDDM, an autoimmune event begins to cause attrition of the beta cells of the pancreas. The beta cells are a population of endocrine cells in the pancreas containing a sensor protein known as GLUT2. When blood glucose levels go high, more glucose binds to GLUT2, and this leads to influx of calcium into the beta cell. This in turn causes vesicles containing the hormone insulin to migrate to the cell membrane, fuse with it, and release insulin into the bloodstream. Insulin binds with receptors on muscle and other cells and leads to more presence and activity of the glucose transport protein GLUT4, which pulls glucose into the cell.

In IDDM, the damage to the beta cell population, over weeks or months, leads to a sharp decrease in the total amount of insulin that the patient is capable of secreting. This leads to blood glucose levels rising. The brain can run itself on ketone bodies, such as hydroxybutyrate and acetoacetate, which are made from fatty acids. IDDM patients will have a fruity smelling breath due to these ketones, including acetone, a byproduct of acetoacetate. Muscles will begin to waste due to lack of glucose uptake. And IDDM patients are at risk of encephalopathy.

NIDDM patients can develop alarming levels of glucose. They are different, in that they can make insulin, although the output of insulin is less than what is needed. Their muscles and their GLUT4 receptors become resistant to insulin. Some variants of this illness actually have high insulin levels. Over years, the insulin levels of these patients decline, and many of them actually end up needing insulin in order to control their disease. But unlike IDDM, they don't start off with an absolute need for injected insulin in order to stay alive.

NIDDM used to be called adult-onset diabetes. Sadly, according to the CDC, the rate of new cases (or incidence) of diabetes in youths younger than 20 years increased in the United States between 2002 and 2015, with a 4.8% increase per year for type 2 diabetes in the period 2008 to 2015. Prediabetes rates indicate that many adolescents will soon be diagnosed as well—18% of adolescents in the United States are prediabetic.

Ground Causes

The dysfunctions that precede diabetes are some of the common ground states that lead to illness of other systems. Certainly, obesity sets the stage for this progression, but so do genetic predispositions, diet, and changes to microbiome [45].

Experimental evidence shows that insulin resistance and NIDDM can be related to dysbiosis, a maladaptive change to the gut microbiome [46]. A high-fat diet can cause lipopolysaccharide to increase. This is a product of gram-negative bacteria. The reduction in short-chain fatty acid synthesis that can occur with some shifts in microbiome can decrease insulin production. Intensive research is underway to identify links between gut microbiome and NIDDM. This requires extensive analysis, using DNA (of gut bacteria) analysis. One contender for possible risk increase is *Clostridia citroniae* (now reclassified as *Enterocloster* genus). Microbiome changes can lead to an increase in the production of amino acids that are absorbed into the circulation such as branched chain amino acids (BCAA) and aromatic amino acids. Although the BCAA are helpful in other conditions, such as liver failure, elevations of plasma levels of these amino acids have been associated with a fivefold future risk of NIDDM.

MicroRNAs (miRNAs) are small non-coding RNA sequences. They are formed in both the nucleus and cytoplasm. They act as activators or suppressors of messenger RNA. Dysfunctional miRNA are implicated in suppressing beta cell function and insulin production. These miRNAs are a form of what is now called "metabolic memory." They can persist even when someone's glucose levels have been normalized. This is why early childhood dysglycemia and obesity are so dangerous; they create a "normal-abnormal" that creates a holding pattern that is difficult to break free from. It is not surprising at all that diet fads have often failed these patients, nor is it at all surprising that bariatric surgery has increased in popularity. There are many reasons why patients have bariatric procedures, but one is to break the hold of metabolic memory and reverse morbid obesity [47, 48].

Hypofunction [14, 15]

Physical deconditioning and lack of exercise will decrease glucose flow into the muscles and decrease the utilization of glucose that might occur during work done by the muscles.

Insulin secretion can be impaired in some patients who develop NIDDM (Table 9.14). This is not always the case. Other patients develop insulin resistance first. Dimas et al. found through genetic analysis risk loci into four major categories with glycemic changes related to what have been identified as glycemic phenotypes.

- The first cluster had genetic predisposition to effects on insulin sensitivity.

Table 9.14 Levels of dysfunction in diabetes mellitus

Level of dysfunction	Example
Hypofunction	Mild decrease in insulin secretion
Impaired coordination and circulation	Insulin resistance
Inflammation	Advanced glycation end products initiated inflammation
Deeper inflammation and immune involvement	Cyclic reinforcement of adipose tissue growth, inflammation, insulin resistance, and mitochondrial damage
Fibrosis and extracellular matrix degeneration	Polyol pathway, AGE, fibrotic changes to kidney
Decline of function	Diabetic complications in cardiovascular system, kidney, eye, nerves, and the pancreas itself
Neoplasm	Pancreatic cancer (associated higher incidence but not necessarily caused by diabetes)

- The second cluster had risk alleles associated with reduced insulin secretion and fasting hyperglycemia.
- The third cluster had defects in insulin processing.
- The fourth cluster had secretion of insulin changes but not to the degree that they had hypoglycemia when fasting.

Decrease in insulin secretion tends to happen earlier and to a greater degree than insulin resistance (which is going to happen earlier in those who have mutations of GLUT4). Some patients have both and will progress to higher serum glucose levels quickly.

Disordered Circulation and Communication

Insulin resistance is a hallmark of NIDDM (Table 9.14). In normal circumstances, GLUT2 acts as a sensor for the beta cells. When glucose is taken up by GLUT2 into pancreatic beta cells, it is metabolized, and the intracellular ATP levels rises and certain ATP-dependent potassium channels close. This leads to a depolarization and an opening of calcium channels. The influx of calcium sets off the completion and transfer of granules packed with insulin to the beta cell membrane. Insulin is then released into the bloodstream.

Obesity is a driver of insulin resistance-breakdown of communication in the above process. Adipose tissue can develop resistance to insulin and not only let glucose remain in the plasma, it leads to the release of free fatty acids (FFA). These FFA can trigger hepatic gluconeogenesis.

Blood sugar levels rise. In adipose tissue in an obese individual, there is less ability to receive glucose and more likely to release free fatty acids [44].

Beta cells that are exposed to high free fatty acid levels have depressed insulin secretion in response to glucose levels, less genetic expression of insulin-producing genes, and more apoptosis. Excessive free fatty acids appear to harm the mitochondria and endoplasmic reticulum.

Inflammation

Mitochondria are damaged in diabetes. High free fatty acid levels due to adipose insulin resistance can lead to mitochondrial stress. More ATP production than is needed due to the "force feeding" of mitochondria leads to reactive oxygen species. This leads to oxidized proteins, increasing cell death. This also leads to more advanced glycemic end products (AGE). [49] These AGEs have specific receptors, and when bound with AGE, this drastically increases inflammation. In diabetes, the mitochondria are more likely to fuse which can impair their functions. Some amount of fused mitochondria are always present, but continued damage will increase the percentage. Defective autophagy in the oxidative stress mitochondria leads to a failure of mitochondrial fission. This means that more poorly functioning mitochondria, which also leak more reactive oxygen, are left in place, instead of being sent to the proteasome for degradation.

Deeper Inflammation and Immune Involvement

The cycle of lowered insulin secretion, muscle and adipose insulin resistance, and gluco- and lipotoxicities causes an intensification of inflammation. Excessive glucose in the blood will have two effects on the liver. It might lead to triglyceride accumulation and lipotoxicity in the liver, resulting in inflammatory changes and fatty liver disease. Alternately, the liver may succeed in exporting more of these fats created from excess glucose uptake to the liver, with VLDL and triglyceride released into the bloodstream. This creates a dyslipidemia. The triglyceride-rich lipoproteins in this case are extra atherogenic. This process also lowers protective HDL. And there are more small dense LDLs, which are easily oxidized and very atherogenic. As the vascular endothelium is damaged, the inflammation and atherosclerosis that result enter a positive feedback loop.

Fibrosis and Extracellular Matrix Degeneration

Extreme oxidative stress and inflammation lead to the following issues in diabetes:

Increased activity of the polyol pathway. This leads to the accumulation of sorbitol. Flooding cells with glucose overwhelms the hexokinase pathway. A secondary enzyme aldose reductase converts the glucose to sorbitol. Some of that sorbitol will end up as fructose, but it can also accumulate. This is an energy-dependent reaction that uses up NADPH—which has effects such as lowering of glutathione levels. Sorbitol will draw water into the cells, causing them to swell, via simple osmosis. This causes generation of the lens of the eye, the retina, the kidney, and the Schwann cells that support peripheral nerves. These tissues do not convert much sorbitol to fructose, and under sustained hyperglycemia, they have buildups of sorbitol and then permanent structural damage [44].

Formation of advanced glycation end products. As mentioned above, AGEs are deleterious to the body. Sorbitol can damage proteins and create AGEs as well. More AGE receptors seem to occur under these conditions as well, which reinforces inflammation.

Protein kinase C is activated by these factors of AGE and oxidative stress. Protein kinases change the activity of proteins by phosphorylating serine residues. The upregulation of protein kinase C in diabetes has an accelerating effect on atherosclerosis via increased cytokine activity in the endothelium. PKC activation also results in endothelium-dependent vasodilator dysfunction by altering the bioavailability of nitric oxide (NO). It also lowers protective prostacylin but raises thromboxanes, endothelin-1, and vascular endothelial growth factor (VEGF). VEGF will thicken the vessel walls. Macrophages, which attempt to engulf oxidized lipids but simply add to the inflammatory process, are more destructive in the presence of high PKC activation [49].

Diabetics sustain kidney damage by sorbitol accumulation, but there are other pathways. The extracellular matrix thickens and, along with glomerular basement membrane thickening, decreases the flow rate into the glomeruli—decreasing filtration rate and kidney function. In patients with nephropathy from diabetes, the kidney mesangium fills up with types IV and VI collagen, fibronectin, and laminin.

Decline of Function

The above inflammatory, fibrotic, and extracellular matrix disrupting factors are self-reinforcing. Increased mitochondrial damage creates leakage of the mitochondrial membranes and more reactive oxygen species. More protein damage, AGE, and very importantly protein kinase C lead to increasing levels of inflammation and vascular, kidney, and nerve damage (Table 9.14). Even in NIDDM, the continual cell turnover, inflammation, ongoing lipo- and glucotoxicity, and free radical activity will wipe out much of the pancreatic beta cells. Many type 2 diabetics eventually require some measure of insulin [44].

Some of the key complications of diabetes include the following: [44].

Vascular disease. Mortality from cardiovascular disease is increased in diabetics. This is not only the serious issues of cardiac and cerebrovascular disease but also peripheral circulation. Loss of blood flow to the extremities, erectile dysfunction, and retinal deterioration are all found in diabetes.

Diabetic neuropathy or nerve deterioration due to the above factors has a number of consequences. Diabetics can lose sensory input from their feet, and this, combined with poor arterial flow and degenerated microcirculation, can lead to serious foot infections. Diabetic wound management is a major concern. Healing can be slow or nonexistent. Debridement of necrotic tissue and even amputations of toes, foot, or legs are frequent surgical events.

Nerve damage can lead to erectile dysfunction, with or without vascular issues. The diabetic nerve damage can strike in the bowel leading to motility issues and to the stomach and pyloric valve, resulting in gastroparesis. In this condition, the stomach does not release its contents after eating, resulting in nausea, bloating, and difficulty eating.

Autonomic neuropathy does not only impact the gastrointestinal tract. The heart has extensive connections to the central nervous system via the autonomic nervous system. In the case of neuropathy, imbalances in sympathetic and parasympathetic input into the heart occur. This can make any kind of heart failure resulting from atherosclerosis much worse. Sympathetic activation of the heart can serve as a short-term compensation to address reduced output. Sympathetic overactivation or poor parasympathetic offsetting of sympathetic input can cause increased risk of sudden cardiac death.

Renal failure is common in diabetes, and in addition to the decreased glomerular filtration rate, destruction of the kidney endothelium can lead to permanent loss of functional renal tissue.

Eye damage and visual impairment is common in diabetes. The lens will age quickly, and the blood supply to the retina becomes compromised. The oxidative stress, mitochondrial dysfunction, and glycation damage can destroy the retina. Hemorrhages and retinal detachment are ultimate consequences.

Treatment

Address Determinants

Diet is of course a high priority for prevention. Some examples of diets likely to be therapeutic are given below under whole-person approaches.

In terms of avoiding the disturbances to health determinants, limiting the amount of refined sugars and refined flours in the diet is important (Table 9.15). A small amount of excess refined carbohydrates is generally not harmful. The average child in the United States consumes about 18 teaspoons of sugar per day. A full-grown adult eating a 2000-calorie diet, at 10% of their calories from sugars, would only consume 12 teaspoons (which in itself is too much). For children, 18 teaspoons of sugar per day (rendering 4 g of sugar per teaspoon) adds up to 26 kg of sugar per year. Depending on the age of that child, they may be eating their own weight in sugar (added) per year. No amount of vaguery, obfuscation, or statistical shenanigans could paint this as an acceptable situation in terms of health. Adults, as well as children, need to limit these sugars [50].

Table 9.15 Treatment considerations in diabetes mellitus

Level of treatment	Treatment	Comments
Address determinants	Dietary liabilities	Excessive refined sugars, trans and damaged fats have to be reduced
Address determinants	Exercise	Needed to maintain insulin sensitivity, expend caloric energy, and condition cardiovascular system
Address determinants	Sleep	Poor sleep quality and sleep apnea will increase inflammation and risk of NIDDM
Address determinants	Infants: Breastfeeding as long as possible—First year at least	Reduces risk of autoimmune events that lead to beta cell attrition and IDDM
Biochemical support	White tea extract	Protect against advanced glycation end products
Biochemical support	*Momordica charantia*	Decrease insulin resistance, vascular inflammation
Biochemical support	Quercetin	Increase insulin production via MAPK pathway, protect tissues from inflammation, lower NFkB
Biochemical support	*Cinnamomum verum/islandica*	Improve glucose uptake
Biochemical support	*Curcuma longa*	Nanoparticle curcumin, reduced inflammation, reduction in lipid peroxidation which is toxic to mitochondria
Biochemical support	*Ginkgo biloba*	Improve vascular health, endothelial function, pretreatment against ischemia
Biochemical support	Magnesium	Insulin receptor efficacy; deficiency leads to impairment, more inflammation
Hormetic stimulation	Exercise	Sirtuin 1, 2 production and protection of mitochondria
Hormetic stimulation	Caloric restriction	Sirtuin activation, mitochondrial protection
Hormetic stimulation	Very low dose metformin	Mitochondrial support
Whole-person support	Mediterranean diet	Glycemic balance, protective plant molecules, antioxidants, omega 3s, high fiber
Whole-person support	Low-carbohydrate diets	Plant foods provide many benefits in this diet, but emphasis on controlled (not eliminating) carbohydrates as energy source helps the patient escape the trap of insulin resistance
Whole-person support	Acupuncture	Reduce neuropathic pain
Whole-person support	Hydrotherapy	Improved circulation, better glycemic control (must take causation with warm treatments due to thermal damage and sensory deficits in diabetes, caution with hypoglycemia)

(continued)

Table 9.15 (continued)

Level of treatment	Treatment	Comments
Dampen maladaptive resources	Pharmacotherapy	Increasing insulin secretion, decreasing insulin resistance, increasing renal glucose excretion, decreasing gut glucose absorption
Dampen maladaptive responses	Alpha-lipoic acid	Address neuropathy
Induce homeostasis	Insulin	Usually long acting and rapid acting for background, nighttime, and postprandial coverage

Although saturated fats, from sources such as butter, have benefits for cooking, overconsumption can tilt the microbiome toward species that might increase diabetes risk.

Exercise is necessary to burn off calories and create an energy balance (Table 9.15). Exercise also helps maintain insulin sensitivity. If caloric intake is kept in balance, exercise can help control levels of intra-abdominal fat, which increase the risk of diabetes and cardiovascular disease. The glucose uptake and improved insulin sensitivity are going to decrease inflammation and oxidative stress. These injurious responses are part of the deadly feed-forward phenomena that diabetes unleashes [51].

Sleep deprivation and sleep apnea appear to increase inflammation and diabetes risk. To what degree sleep correction is an intervention for diabetes is not clear, but poor sleep quality or deprivation is likely having an undermining effect on all those prediabetic and diabetic patients who already have the metabolic imbalances [52, 53].

Biochemical Support

White Tea

This is made from nonoxidized/nonfermented *Camellia sinensis* leaves. It has long been known that (−)-epigallocatechin-O-gallate (EGCG), a polyphenol, has antioxidant, cancer preventive, and anti-inflammatory effects. There are also flavoalkaloids (a molecule with a flavonoid and a nitrogen group) in the plant:

- (−)-6-(5‴-S)-*N*-ethyl-2-pyrrolidinone-epigallocatechin-*O*-gallate (ester-type catechin pyrrolidinone A, etc-pyrrolidinone A, 1)
- (−)-6-(5‴-R)-*N*-ethyl-2-pyrrolidinone-epigallocatechin-*O*-gallate (etc-pyrrolidinone B, 2),
- (−)-8-*N*-ethyl-2-pyrrolidinone-epigallocatechin-*O*-gallate (etc-pyrrolidinone C, 3a, and etc- pyrrolidinone D, 3b)

These flavoalkaloids and the EGCG can work to neutralize advanced glycation end products [54].

Quercetin

This bioflavonoid is widely used for its cell protective and anti-allergy effects, including in the gut. Quercetin has some blocking ability of the pro-inflammatory compounds in diabetes, including NFkB. Quercetin appears to be able to stimulate glucose uptake through an MAPK insulin-dependent mechanism. This leads to more presence of GLUT4. Quercetin, in animal model experiments, has been protective to the retina in diabetic animals [55].

Momordica charantia

This is a versatile anti-inflammatory herb that has several mechanisms of benefit for diabetic (Table 9.15). It is worth noting that while generally safe, it is contraindicated for people with inherited glucose-6-phosphate dehydrogenase (G6PD) deficiency. It can cause severe anemia in people who have G6PD deficiency due to hemolysis. It appears to have anti-inflammatory effects on blood vessels and some decrease in insulin resistance. It has been observed to lower glucose levels postprandial. Based on its vascular effects alone, bitter melon is a serious consideration in biochemical support in diabetes. Its evidence profile does not support it as a mainstay treatment. That doesn't diminish its usefulness as part of a larger ensemble of treatments [56].

C. verum or *C. zeylanicum*

Ceylon cinnamon is not the same as the more common cassia cinnamon found in supermarkets. That form has some health benefits, but for more intense biochemical support, the Ceylon variety is better studied. *C. verum* and *C. zeylanicum* are also better tolerated as *C. cassia* can cause gastric upset. The bark contains cinnamaldehyde, and the leaves have eugenol and other phenolics such as rutin, catechins, quercetin, kaempferol, and isorhamnetin. Eugenol is a hypoglycemic agent, and the polyphenols activate insulin receptor kinase leading to better glucose uptake. Cinnamaldehyde is also hypoglycemic. Cinnamon does not drive down cytokines or C-reactive protein as much as some herbs too, but given its low cost and ease of consumption, it is something that diabetic patients can use frequently [57].

Vaccinium myrtillus

Bilberry, and for that matter, other berries, are recommended for diabetes to support the retina. They have proanthocyanidins that protect the retina from oxidative stress and strengthen the retina which is important for its integrity and stromal grounding. *Vaccinium myrtillus* also has been shown, in human clinical trials, to lower blood glucose levels and insulin levels by about 18% [58–60].

Curcuma longa

Turmeric contains curcumin, a substance that has been studied for many health benefits. Because it is poorly absorbed and distributed throughout the body, it may not arrive at molecular targets with sufficient force. Nanoparticles containing curcumin are presently being studied and appear to be one of the best delivery forms to date. Curcumin blocks lipid peroxidation through the preservation of levels of superoxide dismutase, catalase, and glutathione peroxidase. This is important as lipid peroxidation leads to mitochondrial dysfunction and the creation of AGEs. It may also lower IL-6, TNF-α, and NF-κB, but the degree to which it can do this in humans versus animals exposed to massive amounts is unclear. Improved beta cell function, lower glucose levels, and improvement in lipid profile have been seen in human trials with *Curcuma longa* [61].

Magnesium

Patients with deficiencies or borderline deficiencies of these minerals should be given foods that are good sources and supplemented especially with magnesium, which is a widely deficient mineral. Magnesium helps to regulate electrical activity and, via potassium channel operation and calcium influx, ultimately impacts insulin secretion in pancreatic beta cells. Intracellular magnesium concentrations are critical for the phosphorylation of the insulin receptor. If magnesium in the cell is low, the insulin receptor does not signal the cellular effects (postreceptor effects) properly. Glucose transport into the cell is impacted. Magnesium deficiency in general can increase systemic inflammation, which is double harmful to the diabetic. That does not mean that providing extra magnesium to those with good status will have additional anti-inflammatory effects, but it does underscore the need to address deficiency in diabetic patients [62].

Chromium

Chromium is best obtained from foods, but supplementation with safe levels can improve glucose tolerance and lower LDL [63].

Gingko biloba

This plant is usually used in a concentrated form. Due to its flavone glycosides and terpenes, it has protective effects on the vascular system. *Ginkgo biloba*, although a mild blood thinner, is generally a very safe herb. EGB761 is one powerful extract that has been widely studied. It would seem to be appropriate as a long-term prophylactic treatment for vascular inflammation. It has shown benefit to reducing cognitive decline in diabetics [64] as well as improving cardiovascular health [65].

Hormetic Effects

Caloric restriction and exercise are important for improving sirtuins, which are protective of the mitochondria. This is beneficial to all tissues, including the kidneys. These practices (fasting and exercise) may also protect mitochondria via the AMP-activated protein kinase pathway. Diabetic patients might not be able to fast, especially on an insulin regimen. The mild cell stresses that come from exercise can lead to expression of protective proteins [66]. *Panax ginseng* and *Ginkgo biloba* are reported by Calabrese to show hormetic responses. *Panax ginseng* in the low-dose zone is neuroprotective and reduces inflammasome activity [67, 68].

Whole-Person Support

Mediterranean diets and similarly structured diets can benefit diabetics (Table 9.15). The use of healthy fats, polyphenols, and nutrient-dense foods in general, as well as the limitation of refined carbohydrates, lead to benefits [69].

Low-carbohydrate diets are excellent options for many patients. Given the amount of refined grains and sugars many patients have consumed for their entire lives, it is not surprising that many are ultrasensitized to carbohydrates [70]. The unsurpassed work of the naturopathic physician Dr. Mona Morstein has brought to light how low-carbohydrate diets are beneficial and how they fit into the overall plan of diabetic patient care [71]. These diets have less than 30% of calories coming from carbohydrates, with fats or proteins providing the rest of daily energy. This type of diet has been shown to reduce body mass index, stabilize blood sugar, and, in one study, reduce the needed insulin dose for patients that had type 2 diabetes but needed insulin for control. A low-carbohydrate diet is not the same as a ketogenic diet, which pushes the carbohydrate intake to low levels and induces ketosis.

Hydrotherapy that uses contrast warmth and cold to increase circulation and metabolism might be helpful. Any warm application for a diabetic must always be checked to ensure that it is not too hot—some diabetics cannot tell if it will burn them due to neuropathy and loss of sensation. A 2018 study using acupuncture and hydrotherapy for diabetics with peripheral arterial disease found that blood flow to the leg and physical performance improved on a number of exercise and movement tests [72]. While these two therapies did not lower blood sugar per se, at the end of the 6-week follow-up, acupuncture plus hydrotherapy appeared to reduce inflammatory response by decreasing IL 6, TNF α, malondialdehyde, and SOD and increasing glutathione. A 2020 study found that nerve growth factor and patients' balance improved with hydrotherapy and massage [73].

Dampen Maladaptive Responses

Pharmacotherapy for diabetes is widely used, and metformin, a biguanide, is probably the most versatile of these drugs (Table 9.15). It decreases insulin resistance and lowers blood sugar between meals by blocking glucose release from the liver. It seems to have some interesting life extension capabilities that are under investigation. Metformin may stress the mitochondria at usual doses, but some evidence suggests that at microdoses, metformin has a hormetic effect and stimulates the mitochondria [74].

Some common pharmaceuticals to control glucose levels in diabetes are the following: [74, 14].

Meglitinides:

Example: Nateglinide.
Function: Stimulate the release of insulin.
Side effect: Hypoglycemia, gastric upset.

Sulfonylureas:

Example: Glyburide (DiaBeta, Glynase).
Function: Gets the pancreas to pump out more insulin.
Side effect: Hypoglycemia.

Dipeptidyl Peptidase-IV Inhibitors:

Example: Saxagliptin (Onglyza).
Function: Stimulates the release of insulin when blood glucose is rising/blocks gluconeogenesis.
Side effects: Upper respiratory tract infection, sore throat, headache.

Biguanides:

Example: Metformin (Glumetza, Riomet, Fortamet).
Function: Inhibits the release of glucose from the liver, improve sensitivity to insulin.
Side effect: Nausea, diarrhea, lactic acidosis (rare, a caution in renal or hepatic failure).

Thiazolidinediones:

Example: Rosiglitazone (Avandia).

Function: Improves sensitivity to insulin, inhibits the release of glucose from the liver.
Side effect: Weight gain, myocardial infarction, contraindicated in renal or cardiac disease.

Alpha-glucosidase inhibitors:

Example: Acarbose.
Function: Slows the breakdown of starches and some sugars (a malabsorptive effect).
Side effect: Nausea, bloating, diarrhea.

Medications:

Canagliflozin (Invokana).
Dapagliflozin (Farxiga).
Empagliflozin (Jardiance).
Function: Blocks glucose from being reabsorbed by the kidneys.
Possible side effects: Urinary tract infections, yeast infections, medications.

Alpha-Lipoic Acid

In terms of reducing nerve inflammation, one useful supplement is α-lipoic acid (1,2-dithiolane-3-pentanoic acid or thioctic acid). In humans, it is found in the mitochondria.

It is an enzymatic cofactor in some glucose and lipid metabolic pathways and has a role in gene transcription. For example, in the mitochondria, it can act as a cofactor for both pyruvate dehydrogenase and α-ketoglutarate dehydrogenase. Alpha-lipoic acid is both fat and water soluble and supports antioxidant systems of the body. It was studied in the 1950s as part of aerobic metabolism, particularly with German and some Italian and other European research. It was referred to as thioctic acid [75]. Early clinical investigations look at its role in protecting liver tissue from the toxin of *Amanita phalloides* (toxic death cap mushroom). Research in the 1960s showed it had some ability to protect the mitochondria from arsenic damage [76]. Research in the next several decades looked at its use for heart mitochondrial damage and nerve damage associated with some seizure disorders. In the 1990s, alpha-lipoic acid supplementation grew in patient use and research for reducing the pain of diabetic peripheral neuropathy. [77] Interestingly, it had been used by physicians in Germany back to the 1950s for this purpose. Recent and legacy clinical trials support its use for neuropathy, diabetic and toxin induced.

It is found in nature as enantiomers and R and S form. Supplements have both, but the R form is found in nature. Humans can synthesize it in small amounts, enough it seems to support function, but plant foods are a very important source. In addition to reducing inflammation and pain in the peripheral nerves, it turns out that alpha-lipoic acid has some benefits on glycemic control, probably due to supporting metabolism. Since mitochondrial function can generate oxygen free radicals, the fact that alpha-lipoic acid is protective of the mitochondria makes it particularly useful [78].

Homeostatic Control

Insulin is a form of homeostatic control, and it has saved many lives. It is necessary for IDDM (type 1) and often eventually necessary for NIDDM (type 2) diabetics [79].

Studies in the later twentieth century confirmed that tight control reduced complications. From that point on, it was no longer sufficient to prescribe a long-acting insulin only. Patients might use a background insulin for nighttime control, but shorter-acting varieties for meal time/post prandial control.

Some frequently used types of insulin: (Table 9.16).

(Note, this list is not exhaustive, consult manufacturer guidelines and the American Diabetes Association *Standards of Care*). This does not mean that a naturopathic physician cannot be beyond these standards with safe methods that support the body's intrinsic ability to adapt. But when using potent hormones like insulin, or pharmacologic intervention, it's vital to use aggregated best evidence based on the work of thousands of researchers and clinicians.

(https://diabetesjournals.org/clinical/article/40/1/10/139035/Standards-of-Medical-Care-in-Diabetes-2022)

Table 9.16 Below is a summary of insulin types, based on information from the CDC [80]

Type of insulin	Onset time	Time to maximum efficacy	Duration of action	Directions
Rapid-acting insulin	15 min	1 h	3 h	Taken immediately before a meal Delays in eating may cause hypoglycemic symptoms Usually used in conjunction with a daily longer-acting insulin
Regular/short acting	30 min	3 h	3 to 6 h	Taken 30 to 60 min before a meal May not achieve as precise a post prandial control as rapid, but allows patients more time to eat before onset of action
Intermediate	2 to 4 h	4 to 12 h	12 to 18 h	Insulin coverage for half of a day May be used as an overnight insulin to regulate glucose and suppress hepatic gluconeogenesis Often combined with a short or rapid acting which is then used right before meals
Long acting	2 h	No particular peak—a steady release	Up to 24 h	Insulin coverage for an entire day Often combined with a short or rapid acting which is then used right before meals

References

1. Dubay KS, Zach TL. Newborn Screening. [Updated 2022 May 8]. Treasure Island (FL): StatPearls Publishing; 2022.
2. Misirliyan SS, Huynh AP. Development Milestones. Treasure Island (FL): StatPearls Publishing; 2022.
3. The American Academy of Pediatrics. The AAP Parenting Website [Internet]. [cited 2022 Jun 1]. Available from: https://www.healthychildren.org/English/Pages/default.aspx
4. Center for Disease Control and Prevention. Child and Adolescent Immunization Schedule [Internet]. [cited 2022 Jun 1]. Available from: https://www.cdc.gov/vaccines/schedules/hcp/imz/child-adolescent.html
5. Center for Disease Control and Prevention. Appendix - Guide to Contraindications and Precautions to Commonly Used Vaccines [Internet]. [cited 2022 Jun 1]. Available from: https://www.cdc.gov/vaccines/schedules/hcp/imz/child-adolescent.html#appendix
6. Beluska-Turkan K, Korczak R, Hartell B, Moskal K, Maukonen J, Alexander DE, et al. Nutritional gaps and supplementation in the first 1000 days. Nutrients. 2019;11(12):2891.
7. Spock B. The pocket book of baby and child care. New York: Pocket Books; 1953.
8. Marinelli K. An Interview With La Leche League Founders Marian Tompson and Mary Ann Kerwin, JD. J Hum Lact. 2018;34:14–9.
9. Dominguez-Bello MG, Godoy-Vitorino F, Knight R, Blaser MJ. Role of the microbiome in human development. Gut. 2019;68(6):1108–14.
10. Fleischer DM, Sicherer S, Greenhawt M, Campbell D, Chan E, Muraro A, et al. Consensus communication on early Peanut introduction and prevention of Peanut allergy in high-risk infants. Pediatr Dermatol. 2016;33(1):103–6.
11. EduChange. NOVA Food Classification System [Internet]. Available from: https://educhange.com/wp-content/uploads/2018/09/NOVA-Classification-Reference-Sheet.pdf
12. Center for Disease Control and Prevention. Infant Mortality [Internet]. [cited 2022 Jun 1]. Available from: https://www.cdc.gov/reproductivehealth/maternalinfanthealth/infantmortality.htm
13. Center for Disease Control and Prevention. Information on Safety in the Home & Community for Parents with Infants & Toddlers (Ages 0-3) [Internet]. [cited 2022 Jun 1]. Available from: https://www.cdc.gov/parents/infants/safety.html
14. Papdakis M, McPhee S, Rabow M. Current medical diagnosis & treatment. New York: McGraw Hill; 2020.
15. Smith F. Introduction to principles and practices of naturopathic medicine. Vancouver: CCNM Press; 2008.
16. Child and Adolescent Health and Development. 3rd edition. Bundy DAP, Silva Nd, Horton S, et al., editors. Washington (DC): The International Bank for Reconstruction and Development/The World Bank; 2017.
17. Center for Disease Control and Prevention. Fast Facts: Preventing Child Abuse & Neglect [Internet]. [cited 2022 Jun 1]. Available from: https://www.cdc.gov/violenceprevention/childabuseandneglect/fastfact.html
18. Singh S, Roy D, Sinha K, Parveen S, Sharma G, Joshi G. Impact of COVID-19 and lockdown on mental health of children and adolescents: a narrative review with recommendations. Psychiatry Res. 2020;293:113429.
19. Panchal U, Salazar de Pablo G, Franco M, Moreno C, Parellada M, Arango C. et al, The impact of COVID-19 lockdown on child and adolescent mental health: systematic review. Eur Child Adolesc Psychiatry. 2021:1–27.
20. Center for Disease Control and Prevention. Sexually Transmitted Diseases. Adolescents and Young Adults [Internet]. [cited 2022 Jun 1]. Available from: https://www.cdc.gov/std/life-stages-populations/adolescents-youngadults.htm
21. Cunningham RM, Walton MA, Carter PM. The major causes of death in children and adolescents in the united states. N Engl J Med. 2018;379(25):2468–75.

22. Patra KP, Kumar R. Screening For Depression and Suicide in Children. [Updated 2022 Feb 19]. In: StatPearls [Internet]. Treasure Island (FL): StatPearls Publishing; 2022.
23. Goldstick JE, Cunningham RM, Carter PM. Current causes of death in children and adolescents in the United States. N Engl J Med. 2022;386(20):1955–6. https://doi.org/10.1056/NEJMc2201761.
24. CDC. Teen drinking and Driving [Internet]. Available from: https://www.cdc.gov/vitalsigns/teendrinkinganddriving/index.html
25. Volkow ND. Principles of adolescent substance use disorder treatment: A research-based guide. Bethesda: National Institutes of Health; 2014. p. 1–42. Available from: http://www.drugabuse.gov
26. Center for Disease Control and Prevention. Drug Overdose Deaths in the U.S. Up 30% in 2020 [Internet]. [cited 2022 Jun 1]. Available from: https://www.cdc.gov/nchs/pressroom/nchs_press_releases/2021/20210714.htm
27. Theodorou CM, Beyer CA, Vanover MA, Brown IE, Salcedo ES, Farmer DL, et al. The hidden mortality of pediatric firearm violence. J Pediatr Surg. 2022;57(5):897–902.
28. Center for Disease Control and Prevention. Childhood Obesity Facts [Internet]. Available from: https://www.cdc.gov/obesity/data/childhood.html
29. DeBoer MD. Assessing and managing the metabolic syndrome in children and adolescents. Nutrients. 2019;11(8):1788.
30. Drechsler R, Brem S, Brandeis D, Grünblatt E, Berger G, Walitza S. ADHD: current concepts and treatments in children and adolescents. Neuropediatrics. 2020;51(5):315–35.
31. Oldways. Traditional Diets [Internet]. [cited 2022 Jun 1]. Available from: https://oldwayspt.org/traditional-diets
32. Givler DN, Givler A. Health Screening. [Updated 2022 May 1]. Treasure Island (FL): StatPearls Publishing; 2022.
33. Center for Disease Control and Prevention. Promoting Health For Older Adults [Internet]. Available from: https://www.cdc.gov/chronicdisease/resources/publications/factsheets/promoting-health-for-older-adults.htm
34. Center for Disease Control and Prevention. Women's Health [Internet]. Available from: https://www.cdc.gov/women/index.htm
35. Pippin MM, Boyd R. Breast Self-Examination. [Updated 2022 Feb 17]. Treasure Island (FL): StatPearls Publishing; 2022.
36. Walker-Descartes I, Mineo M, Condado LV, Agrawal N. Domestic violence and its effects on women, children, and families. Pediatr Clin N Am. 2021;68(2):455–64.
37. Rattan S, Zhou C, Chiang C, Mahalingam S, Brehm E, Flaws JA. Exposure to endocrine disruptors during adulthood: consequences for female fertility. J Endocrinol. 2017;233(3):R109–29.
38. Development NI of CH and. What Happens During a Prenatal Visit [Internet]. [cited 2022 Jun 1]. Available from: https://www.nichd.nih.gov/health/topics/preconceptioncare/conditioninfo/prenatal-visits%0A
39. Center. Men's Health [Internet]. Available from: https://www.cdc.gov/nchs/fastats/mens health.htm
40. Jain MA, Sapra A. Prostate Cancer Screening. [Updated 2021 Oct 9]. Treasure Island (FL): StatPearls Publishing; 2022.
41. Golden MI, Meyer JJ, Patel BC. Dry Eye Syndrome. [Updated 2021 Nov 2]. Treasure Island (FL): StatPearls Publishing; 2022.
42. Zimmet P, Alberti KG, Magliano DJ, Bennett PH. Diabetes mellitus statistics on prevalence and mortality: facts and fallacies. Nat Rev Endocrinol. 2016;12(10):616–22. https://doi.org/10.1038/nrendo.2016.105.
43. Center for Disease Control and Prevention. Diabetes Tests [Internet]. Available from: https://www.cdc.gov/diabetes/basics/getting-tested.html
44. Galicia-Garcia U, Benito-Vicente A, Jebari S, Larrea-Sebal A, Siddiqi H, Uribe KB, et al. Pathophysiology of type 2 diabetes mellitus. Int J Mol Sci. 2020;21(17):6275.

45. Muñoz-Garach A, Diaz-Perdigones C, Tinahones FJ. Gut microbiota and type 2 diabetes mellitus. Endocrinol Nutr. 2016;63(10):560–8.
46. Brown AE, Walker M. Genetics of insulin resistance and the metabolic syndrome. Curr Cardiol Rep. 2016;18(8):75. Available from: https://pubmed.ncbi.nlm.nih.gov/27312935
47. Hathaway QA, Pinti MV, Durr AJ, Waris S, Shepherd DL, Hollander JM. Regulating microRNA expression: at the heart of diabetes mellitus and the mitochondrion. Am J Physiol Heart Circ Physiol. 2018;314(2):H293–310.
48. Berezin A. Metabolic memory phenomenon in diabetes mellitus: achieving and perspectives. Diabetes Metab Syndr. 2016;10(2 Suppl 1):S176–83.
49. Giacco F, Brownlee M. Oxidative stress and diabetic complications. Circ Res. 2010;107(9):1058–70. Available from: https://pubmed.ncbi.nlm.nih.gov/21030723
50. The Diabetes Council 45 Alarming Statistics on American's Sugar Consumption and the Effects of Sugar on Americans' Health [Internet]. Available from: https://www.thediabetescouncil.com/45-alarming-statistics-on-americans-sugar-consumption-and-the-effects-of-sugar-on-americans-health/
51. Carbone S, Del Buono MG, Ozemek C, Lavie CJ. Obesity, risk of diabetes and role of physical activity, exercise training and cardiorespiratory fitness. Prog Cardiovasc Dis. 2019;62(4):327–33.
52. Ogilvie RP, Patel SR. The epidemiology of sleep and diabetes. Curr Diab Rep. 2018;18(10):82.
53. Zimmet P, Alberti KGMM, Stern N, Bilu C, El-Osta A, Einat H, et al. The circadian syndrome: is the metabolic syndrome and much more! J Intern Med. 2019;286(2):181–91.
54. Li X, Liu G-J, Zhang W, Zhou Y-L, Ling T-J, Wan X-C, et al. Novel Flavoalkaloids from white tea with inhibitory activity against the formation of advanced glycation end products. J Agric Food Chem. 2018;66(18):4621–9.
55. Chen S, Jiang H, Wu X, Fang J. Therapeutic effects of quercetin on inflammation, obesity, and type 2 diabetes. Mediat Inflamm. 2016;2016:9340637.
56. Yin RV, Lee NC, Hirpara H, Phung OJ. The effect of bitter melon (Momordica charantia) in patients with diabetes mellitus: a systematic review and meta-analysis. Nutr Diabetes. 2014;4(12):e145. Available from: https://pubmed.ncbi.nlm.nih.gov/25504465
57. Singh N, Rao AS, Nandal A, Kumar S, Yadav SS, Ganaie SA, et al. Phytochemical and pharmacological review of Cinnamomum verum J. Presl-a versatile spice used in food and nutrition. Food Chem. 2021;338(127773)
58. Singh N, Rao AS, Nandal A, Kumar S, Yadav SS, Ganaie SA, et al. Phytochemical and pharmacological review of Cinnamomum verum J. Presl-a versatile spice used in food and nutrition. Food Chem. 2021;338(127773)
59. Ma H, Johnson SL, Liu W, DaSilva NA, Meschwitz S, Dain JA, et al. Evaluation of polyphenol anthocyanin-enriched extracts of blackberry, black raspberry, blueberry, cranberry, red raspberry, and strawberry for free radical scavenging, reactive carbonyl species trapping, anti-glycation, anti-β-amyloid aggregation, and mic. Int J Mol Sci. 2018;19(2):461. Available from: https://pubmed.ncbi.nlm.nih.gov/29401686
60. Pires TCSP, Caleja C, Santos-Buelga C, Barros L, Ferreira ICFR. Vaccinium myrtillus L. fruits as a novel source of phenolic compounds with health benefits and industrial applications - a review. Curr Pharm Des. 2020;26(16):1917–28.
61. Yavarpour-Bali H, Ghasemi-Kasman M, Pirzadeh M. Curcumin-loaded nanoparticles: a novel therapeutic strategy in treatment of central nervous system disorders. Int J Nanomedicine. 2019;14:4449–60.
62. Feng J, Wang H, Jing Z, Wang Y, Cheng Y, Wang W, et al. Role of magnesium in type 2 diabetes mellitus. Biol Trace Elem Res. 2020;196(1):74–85.
63. Suksomboon N, Poolsup N, Yuwanakorn A. Systematic review and meta-analysis of the efficacy and safety of chromium supplementation in diabetes. J Clin Pharm Ther. 2014;39(3):292–306.
64. Palta P, Carlson MC, Crum RM, Colantuoni E, Sharrett AR, Yasar S, et al. Diabetes and cognitive decline in older adults: the ginkgo evaluation of memory study. J Gerontol A Biol Sci Med Sci. 2017;73(1):123–30.

65. Tabrizi R, Nowrouzi-Sohrabi P, Hessami K, Rezaei S, Jalali M, Savardashtaki A, et al. Effects of Ginkgo biloba intake on cardiometabolic parameters in patients with type 2 diabetes mellitus: A systematic review and meta-analysis of clinical trials. Phytother Res. 2020;8. https://doi.org/10.1002/ptr.6822.
66. Winnik S, Auwerx J, Sinclair DA, Matter CM. Protective effects of sirtuins in cardiovascular diseases: from bench to bedside. Eur Heart J. 2015;36(48):3404–12.
67. Sharma K. Mitochondrial hormesis and diabetic complications. Diabetes. 2015;64(3):663–72. Available from: https://pubmed.ncbi.nlm.nih.gov/25713188
68. Calabrese EJ. Hormesis and ginseng: ginseng mixtures and individual constituents commonly display Hormesis dose responses, especially for neuroprotective effects. Molecules. 2020;25(11):2719.
69. Mirabelli M, Chiefari E, Arcidiacono B, Corigliano DM, Brunetti FS, Maggisano V, et al. Mediterranean diet nutrients to turn the tide against insulin resistance and related diseases. Nutrients. 2020;12(4):1066.
70. Bolla AM, Caretto A, Laurenzi A, Scavini M, Piemonti L. Low-carb and ketogenic diets in type 1 and type 2 diabetes. Nutrients. 2019;11(5):962.
71. Morstein M. Master your diabetes: a comprehensive integrative approach for both type 1 and type 2 diabetes. White River Junction, VT: Chelsea Green; 2017.
72. Qi Z, Pang Y, Lin L, Zhang B, Shao J, Liu X, et al. Acupuncture combined with hydrotherapy in diabetes patients with mild lower-extremity arterial disease: a prospective, randomized, nonblinded clinical study. Med Sci Monit. 2018;24:2887–900.
73. Shourabi P, Bagheri R, Ashtary-Larky D, Wong A, Motevalli MS, Hedayati A, et al. Effects of hydrotherapy with massage on serum nerve growth factor concentrations and balance in middle aged diabetic neuropathy patients. Complement Ther Clin Pract. 2020;39:101141.
74. Padhi S, Nayak AK, Behera A. Type II diabetes mellitus: a review on recent drug based therapeutics. Biomed Pharmacother. 2020;131:110708.
75. Rausch F. Clinical observations on thioctic acid (lipoic acid); preliminary report. Arzneimittelforschung. 1955;5(1):32–4.
76. Facchini G, Cenacchi GC, Di Paolo E. Activity of prothrombin and of factor V and factor VII in experimental poisoning by sodium arsenite; protective effect of thioctic acid. Arch Patol Clin Med. 1959;36(2):135–43.
77. Sachse G, Willms B. Efficacy of thioctic acid in the therapy of peripheral diabetic neuropathy. Horm Metab Res Suppl. 1980;9:105–7.
78. Salehi B, Berkay Yılmaz Y, Antika G, Boyunegmez Tumer T, Fawzi Mahomoodally M, Lobine D, et al. Insights on the use of α-lipoic acid for therapeutic purposes. Biomol Ther. 2019;9(8):356.
79. Wilson LM, Castle JR. Recent advances in insulin therapy. Diabetes Technol Ther. 2020;22(12):929–36.
80. Center for Disease Control and Prevention. Types of Insulin [Internet]. [cited 2022 Jun 2]. Available from: https://www.cdc.gov/diabetes/basics/type 1 types of insulin.html

Further Reading

Brown JC, Gerhardt TE, Kwon E. Risk Factors For Coronary Artery Disease. [Updated 2021 Jun 5]. Treasure Island (FL): StatPearls Publishing; 2022.

Calcaterra V, Verduci E, Cena H, Magenes VC, Todisco CF, Tenuta E, et al. Polycystic ovary syndrome in insulin-resistant adolescents with obesity: the role of nutrition therapy and food supplements as a strategy to protect fertility. Nutrients. 2021;13(6):1848.

CDC. Infant Mortality [Internet]. Available from: https://www.cdc.gov/reproductivehealth/maternalinfanthealth/infantmortality.htm

Center for Disease Control and Prevention. Adolescent Health [Internet]. Available from: https://www.cdc.gov/nchs/fastats/adolescent-health.htm

Goldstein DS. Concepts of scientific integrative medicine applied to the physiology and pathophysiology of catecholamine systems. Compr Physiol. 2013;3(4):1569–610.

Kesari A, Noel JY. Nutritional Assessment. [Updated 2022 Apr 16]. Treasure Island (FL): StatPearls Publishing; 2022.

Lindner B, Thomas PJ, Fellous J-M, Tiesinga P. Biological cybernetics: 60 years and more to come. Biol Cybern. 2021;115(1):5–6. Available from: https://pubmed.ncbi.nlm.nih.gov/33620520

Malleshaiah M, Gunawardena J. Cybernetics, redux: An outside-in strategy for unraveling cellular function. Dev Cell. 2016;36(1):2–4.

O'Rourke MC, Jamil RT, Siddiqui W. Suicide Screening and Prevention. [Updated 2022 Mar 9]. Treasure Island (FL): StatPearls Publishing; 2022.

Chapter 10
Roles in Health Care

Naturopathic medicine is a professionalized form of health care. Naturopathic physicians are trained to see patients with undefined health issues. That means, the naturopathic doctor can be the first health-care practitioner that a patient sees. They are also trained to make decisions about what other health-care providers the patient needs to see and with what urgency. For example, a patient that has bloodwork that reveals a very distorted pattern of white blood cell changes, with fever and fatigue, will be sent to a hematologist for further diagnostic workup. A child who presents with high fever, vomiting, and neck rigidity will be sent to the pediatric ER for diagnosis of possible meningococcal infection. Even if that naturopathic physician uses a rapid diagnostic test to diagnose meningococcal infection, if it were positive, they would still send that patient to the hospital for lumbar puncture and intensive antibiotic therapy (There are some circumstances, including afebrile patients, where this condition can be treated outpatient, and that is essentially for adults.). That is not to say that naturopathic physicians simply refer to the ED for any serious issue. But like any first-line practitioner, they are alert to situations which go beyond their scope of practice. This is not only common-sense doctoring, it is a condition of being a licensed health-care practitioner.

Naturopathic physicians in the United States, at the time of this writing, are licensed in 26 jurisdictions (23 states plus the District of Columbia, Puerto Rico, and the United States Virgin Islands) that have licensing or registration laws for naturopathic doctors (NDs/NMDs) [1]. In Canada, there are five provinces that regulate the practice of naturopathic doctors: British Columbia, Alberta, Saskatchewan, Manitoba, and Ontario. The Naturopathic Doctors Act of 2008 grants title protection for naturopathic doctors in the province of Nova Scotia [2].

The naturopathic doctors in the United States and Canada have similarities in training and practice. In any jurisdiction that regulates the practice of naturopathic medicine, the applicant for licensure or registration must have attended a naturopathic medicine program that is recognized by the Council on Naturopathic Medical Education (CNME) [3]. The CNME is an accreditation agency that is a member of

F. Smith, *Naturopathic Medicine*, https://doi.org/10.1007/978-3-031-13388-6_10

the Association of Specialized and Professional Accreditors (ASPA) and abides by the ASPA's Code of Good Practice. CNME is recognized by the United States Department of Education. It is also a member of the Association of Accrediting Agencies of Canada.

Graduates who seek a license or registration from any of these jurisdictions must pass licensing examinations, as with any health-care profession. In the United States, regulated jurisdictions accept the Naturopathic Physicians Licensing Examinations (NPLEX) [4].

The licensing of naturopathic physicians allows for varying scopes of practice. In some jurisdictions, they can prescribe a very broad formulary of pharmaceutical medications, administer vaccinations, and perform in-office procedures such as suturing of lacerations or skin biopsy.

In other jurisdictions, there is a more limited formulary that still includes various hormones and medicines that are needed to have on hand during intravenous therapies, such as epinephrine and diphenhydramine. Intravenous therapeutics are used by about a third of naturopathic physicians in their practice to deliver antioxidants, magnesium, and other natural products.

Some jurisdictions have a more limited scope that includes dietary supplements, herbal medicines, various manual therapies, and the diagnostic ability to collect blood, urine, and sputum specimens in office and to order laboratory tests. This might also extend to performing male- and female-sensitive examinations.

What these various settings have in common are the unifying principles and concepts of naturopathic medicine. This includes looking at the causes of disease and creating the conditions for health. The use of natural therapeutics is meant to support and stimulate the ability of the body to heal. Sometimes these natural therapies are used to palliative or reduce suffering. The choice of tool is not what defines a naturopathic physician, it is their commitment to working with the self-healing mechanisms.

Prior to 1989, there was no published definition of naturopathic medicine by the profession. A narrow, modality-centered definition was on file with the United States Department of Labor. This definition described the profession in terms of its treatment methods–by the tools it used. The profession came together, and in an effort commissioned by the American Association of Naturopathic Physicians (AANP), a definition was created and adopted by AANP's House of Delegates (HOD) at the annual AANP convention held at Rippling River, OR [5].

These principles are as follows:

1. The healing power of nature
2. Identify and treat the cause
3. First do no harm
4. Doctor as teacher
5. Treat the whole person
6. Prevention

There are approximately 8000 naturopathic physicians with this type of training in North America. New jurisdictions are being added, such as the passage of a licensing law in the midwestern state of Wisconsin in 2022.

Types of Roles

General Practitioner of Naturopathic Medicine

Generalist works in tandem with more conventionally oriented primary health-care providers.

In this scenario, the naturopathic doctor sees patients who most always have a family medicine or internal medicine MD or DO. The naturopathic doctor provides some services in terms of screening tests, advanced lipid testing perhaps. The patient uses this care to improve their own health and to repair or rehabilitate themselves for any chronic issue, and many acute. This improvement would be to the level that pharmaceutical or surgical intervention is not needed. Conversely, the naturopathic physician recognizes that due to the severity or rapid progressive nature of some conditions and that the patient should follow conventional care regimens at times. Other reasons for that can be difficulty adhering to a change in behavior, at least temporarily, or some susceptibility that cannot be completely overcome. For example, a patient with PARK2 gene in an autosomal recessive sense develops neurologic symptoms. Overall better health and specific support for the neurological system helps with tremor, but they see a neurologist and do use L-Dopa and a small dose of anticholinergic medicine.

This role for the naturopathic physician is not necessarily adjunctive. They may see many acute presentations and work with patients with some very serious chronic diseases. There are many practices like these. Practically speaking, the naturopathic physician in this situation is like any doctor—they have to know their limitations, and they need to keep the patient's needs foremost.

Complete Primary Care

There are naturopathic physicians who provide comprehensive primary care. This is going to be found in jurisdictions with a broader scope of practice. It could be in a densely populated urban area or a town in a more remote location, or a rural area. This would include care for all ages, including the milestone evaluations for children. It will mean depending on the skill of the doctor but certainly at some point the use of medications, when necessary (such as antibiotics, antihypertensive drugs, pain control, etc.) for situations that need rapid reversal. Many of these naturopathic physicians provide immunizations. This is done with informed consent to families and following the CDC and manufacturer guidelines, so as not to administer a vaccine at a time when a child is suffering from a febrile illness or some other contraindication. Some naturopathic physicians in this role will work with parents to create an alternate vaccine schedule, and others would prefer not to deviate from the CDC immunization schedule.

Part of this kind of role includes arranging for the screening tests that patients ought to have, such as lipid testing and a colonoscopy after age 50 (some authorities prefer a younger start). It also means arranging for referrals for specialist care and admitting patients to the hospital. There are naturopathic medical clinics that are certified medical homes, meeting the various criteria for these. This role also includes the continuing education to stay abreast of certain issues.

The issue is not that other naturopathic physicians are not acting in a primary care role. But the comprehensiveness of this kind of practice and the extent of coordination with other providers and agencies make this more like the general practitioner-gatekeeper role that MD or DO family physicians or internists often fill.

Specialty by System or Health Condition

Some naturopathic doctors develop a practice focus in a certain area. For instance, they will spend much of their day working with patients that have gastrointestinal issues. Or they will develop an expertise in helping patients diagnosed with Lyme disease and who suffer from a variety of long-term debilitating issues (and in many cases, getting that patient an accurate diagnosis is the first step).

This idea of practice focus is looked upon in different ways by licensing authorities. Some jurisdictions do not allow the use of the word "specialize," or the doctor must meet certain criteria. There are a number of specialty associations in naturopathic medicine that include postgraduate training and credentialing beyond the ND degree.

Specialty by Treatment Modality

Although naturopathic medicine is not defined by the tools or modalities, some naturopathic physicians delve into one therapy. For instance, some acquire advanced standing in acupuncture and traditional Chinese medicine and make that a practice focus. Others make homeopathic medicine their primary tool. If someone applies these different methods according to naturopathic medicine principles, they have much common ground with others and are still practicing naturopathic medicine.

Member of an Integrative Team

Much has been made of integrative medicine as an evolution, and it can be a productive arrangement. This is where several or more doctors practice in a unit or coherent network and see the same patients. As Orr 2019 pointed out, there are various levels of integration for naturopathic physicians. Using nomenclature from Boone et al., Orr draws a distinction between "parallel practice" where nonantagonistic practitioners essentially share real estate or coordinated practice where patients might be sent to different types of doctors for different complaints. Truly integrative practice involves communication and collaboration among members of a healthcare team, and it elevates the patient needs and preferences to the superordinate function. That is, the group will come together to discuss what a patient wants and needs and what selection, and order, of approaches within the group are best suited to *this patient*. As in coordinated care, a case manager or practice manager might be on hand to ensure that the patient is getting that care and not merely being passed from doctor to doctor. But the intent in the truly integrative practice is for practitioners to make joint decisions and to keep learning from each other.

In some cases of naturopathic practice focus, naturopathic doctors who specialize have trained with, or currently work with, medical and osteopathic doctors in that field. In others, they are not associated directly with these doctors. For example, there are a small number of naturopathic physicians who specialize in cardiology, who have done much training with MD cardiologists.

The profession has a number of specialty associations. Membership in these require evidence of advanced training, via postgraduate coursework and in many cases completion of a residency. There is also ongoing education and attendance at special conferences.

According to the American Association of Naturopathic Physicians [6], the following are the current specialty associations:

- Endocrinology Association of Naturopathic Physicians (AANP Affiliate)
- American Association of Naturopathic Midwives
- Gastroenterology Association of Naturopathic Physicians
- Homeopathic Academy of Naturopathic Physicians (AANP Affiliate)
- Institute of Naturopathic Generative Medicine
- Naturopathic Association of Environmental Medicine (AANP Affiliate)
- Oncology Association of Naturopathic Physicians (AANP Affiliate)
- Pediatric Association of Naturopathic Physicians (AANP Affiliate)
- Psychiatric Association of Naturopathic Physicians (AANP Affiliate)

Residencies

Most naturopathic medicine jurisdictions do not require a residency. This is the same as chiropractic, dentistry, or physical therapy. Many naturopathic graduates pursue a residency of 1 or 2 years. Residencies are supervised by certain participating accredited naturopathic medical schools. The standards that the schools are expected to hold the various sites to are published by the Council on Naturopathic Medical Education (CNME). According to the CNME, the Council, through its Committee on Postdoctoral Naturopathic Medical Education (CPNME), periodically reviews naturopathic residency training programs and school sponsors to make sure that residencies meet CNME requirements.

Naturopathic Physicians and Conventional Therapies

It may seem odd that a profession that originated from practitioners in the late nineteenth and early twentieth century, who eschewed conventional care, would be inclined to make use of it. There are a number of reasons for this. One is that the practice of medicine in the 2020s is very different than in the early 1900s. At that time, there were no antibiotics, no steroids, and no modern intensive care units. Imaging was confined to radiography which came to include fluoroscopy and contrast imaging. There were some medical doctors who were excellent diagnosticians. But the tools of the trade often included what were essential purified extracts from herbal sources.

Conventional medicine has undergone major transformations. Many childhood infections and surgical emergencies have a very high survival rate under standard care. Trauma care and intensive care are extremely advanced. Imaging and other diagnostic technologies are very precise. There are many pharmaceutical treatments that act powerfully and rapidly to stabilize potentially fatal shutdowns of the body.

When a naturopathic physician prescribes these types of therapies or refers a patient to someone who can, it is due to a recognition of the scientific basis of these measures. They have strong proof of efficacy in many cases.

If that is true, it can also be asked why then naturopathic physicians don't just use the same approaches that medical and osteopathic doctors use? The reason is that naturopathic physicians are working to recreate the basis of health and to facilitate the healing process. As Zeff, Snider, and others have described, healing follows an order. Naturopathic doctors work with patients to create the conditions for health and to support the patient's progression through an orderly healing process.

In this textbook, a model of progressive dysfunction and rational intervention is presented. Aside from very virulent infectious disease or trauma, many illnesses progress from hypofunction to disordered communication and circulation, increasingly inflammation, and then fibrosis and the breakdown of the extracellular matrix.

Inevitable decline of function, and sometimes total breakdown or even neoplasm, follows.

In healing, there is a balance to be achieved between promoting and strengthening the adaptive responses of the human being and reducing the intensity of maladaptive resources. These adaptive responses include cell regeneration, removal of toxins from tissues and excretion from the body, and the resynchronization of circadian and bioregulatory control systems, to name a few. The means to do so involve biochemical support, hormetic stimulation, and whole-person therapies that stimulate global healing responses. Maladaptive responses include excessive inflammation and immune engagement, rapid or extreme oscillation of bioregulatory systems, and extreme remodeling of tissues. In some cases, the immediate severity or long-term deficits of a condition require medication or surgery to extrinsically establish a type of homeostasis. Without those drastic means, the person can die.

Naturopathic physicians exert the most leverage in a patient's health care when they use their skills to enhance adaptive responses and always to address those deficiencies in factors required for health (Fig. 10.1). But they also recognize that

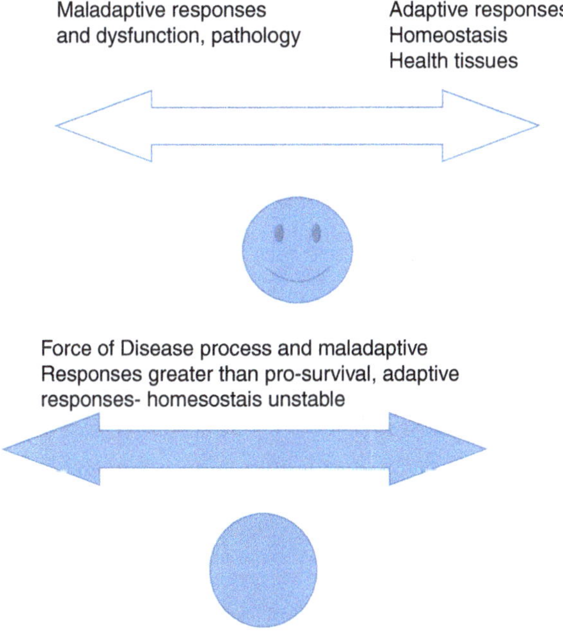

Fig. 10.1 Ascendency of maladaptive responses: When adaptive responses can, with assistance, restore homeostasis, naturopathic medicine is highly indicated. When maladaptive responses and the forces of disease (which can become self-perpetuating) are on the ascendancy, patients often need assistance to reduce those responses and to quell the forces of disease. This doesn't preclude naturopathic therapies, and it definitely does not mean that ignoring deficient or disturbed determinants of health is wise, even if temporary relief is given by medical therapies

sometimes relieving the patient of the constraints of overwhelming symptoms can permit healing. That actual healing may yet need more direct support. For example, a patient has a substantial injury to the glenohumeral joint, and it becomes massively inflamed, in spite of some natural therapies to support it. One single cortisol injection put excessive inflammation in check and prevented a degree of damage that might have led to permanent damage.

Symptom-based treatment, used judiciously, can lead to healing. Medical and osteopathic doctors do many things that are reasonable, and they see improvements in their patient's lives. Naturopathic physicians are attempting to assist patients who are past the point where they can rebalance themselves with simple interventions. Their level of dysfunction has become profound enough that even with symptomatic therapy, their system does not self-correct. Naturopathic doctors are not eager to interfere with the process of healing but recognize that it is sometimes necessary and that medical interventions used intelligently can create benefits far beyond temporary relief. Conventional treatments are based on a deep foundation of scientific understanding of how the body works. They create stability and can often eliminate inciting causes. That is their proper use. But in our modern health-care milieu, millions of people are using standard medical treatments to buttress what is in effect a crumbling physiology and a weakened body. These therapies, as great as they are, can too often become only palliative. To create balance in the provision of health care, it's necessary for more emphasis to be placed on maximizing self-healing and adaptation, instead of so many patients bypassing these measures and lapsing into a lifetime on multiple prescriptions and several chronic disease diagnoses.

If a person lives without addressing disturbed determinants of health, and they are progressing through stages of dysfunction, in time it will become very difficult and resource intensive to keep their body functioning. This is particularly true after about the age of 50 (Fig. 10.2).

So the tendency of the modern naturopathic physician to use and incorporate the broadest range of options for patients is practical and scientific. It can be said that in terms of turning around the current health situation, with its rampant obesity, cardiovascular disease, diabetes, cancer, mood disorders, and addiction, it takes all available means and that there is plenty of work to do for physicians of all types.

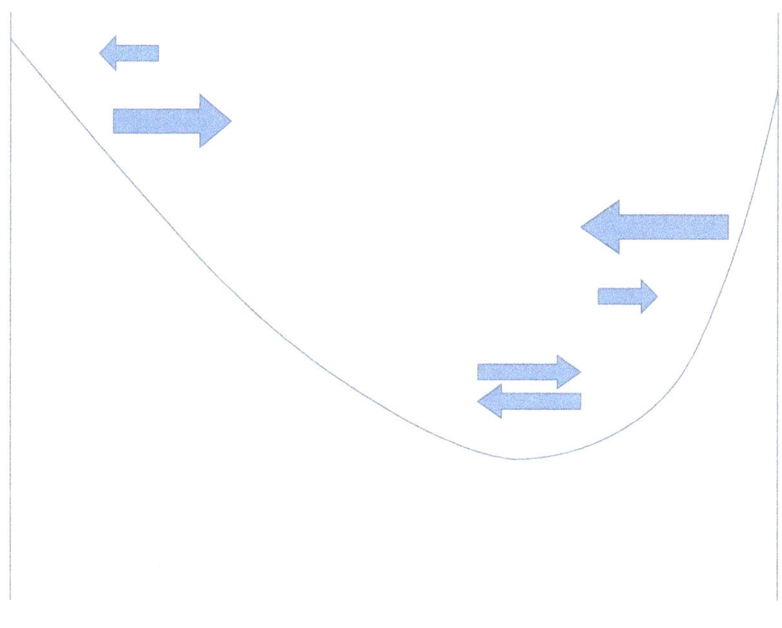

Fig. 10.2 The effects of time across the lifespan: As people age, they still can mount adaptive responses, but their cellular reserves and biological plasticity have decreased. If they have not addressed many of their health requirements, then it is not uncommon to require some form of medical intervention to preserve life even by the age of 50

References

1. American Association of Naturopathic Physicians. Regulatory states and regulatory authorities. https://naturopathic.org/page/RegulatedStates.

2. Canadian Association of Naturopathic Doctors. Naturopathic medicine today. https://www.cand.ca/naturopathic-medicine-today/.
3. Council on Naturopathic Medical Education. About CNME. https://cnme.org/about-cnme/#about.
4. North American Board of Naturopathic Examiners. https://nabne.org.
5. Snider P, Zeff J. Unifying principles of naturopathic medicine origins and definitions. Integr Med. 2019;18(4):36–9.
6. American Association of Naturopathic Physicians. Specialty affiliates. https://naturopathic.org/page/SpecialtyAffiliates.

Chapter 11
Science and Naturopathic Medicine

Science is an enterprise that produces knowledge about the world. A key component in science is the experimental method, which is the testing of hypotheses under controlled conditions. For example, if we had an experimental model where we added nitric acid of different concentrations to magnesium, we'd find that diluted nitric acid formed magnesium nitrate and hydrogen gas. If we used a very concentrated nitric acid with magnesium, it produced magnesium nitrate and nitrogen dioxide (instead of hydrogen). This would occur every time we did the same experiment under the same conditions with the same reagents in the same amounts and concentrations. Others would precisely replicate what we did and would get the same results.

A hypothesis to the effect that the low concentration nitric acid will produce hydrogen gas, which will combust easily, is something that could be tested. Science philosopher Sir Karl Popper described a scientific proposition as consisting of a "falsifiable" hypothesis. It can be tested and proven false. If it is never proven false, it stands and is considered true until proven otherwise. This excludes hypotheses that don't meet Popper's criterion, if they are nonfalsifiable. Even though scientists might not think in terms of falsification in each experiment they run, the criterion of falsifiability is useful. The proposition that "the psyche remains the same in the afterlife" is not a scientifically testable hypothesis, although it might have interest to us in other ways.

Theories are essentially models, as Thomas Kuhn pointed out [1]. Theories are models that explain the world, and they allow us to not only understand nature but also to make predictions. They also provide a scaffolding for creating experiments. A strongly supported theory, such as one that says "increased catecholamine activity in the brain has an inverse association with depressive symptoms" is something that is useful. Some theories are useful for a while and, then as knowledge accumulates or better instrumentation to conduct experiments (more sensitive data capture, more refined probing of material), are replaced by better theories.

F. Smith, *Naturopathic Medicine*, https://doi.org/10.1007/978-3-031-13388-6_11

A group of theories usually are tied in with what Kuhn called a "paradigm." This is a large and stable model of nature that doesn't change, at least not very often. Normal science works within a stable paradigm. Newtonian physicians, thermodynamics, etc., was the dominant paradigm in physics until relativity and quantum mechanics came along. While these did not negate Newtonian physics, they delimited that paradigm of nature as an explanation for many phenomena. According to Kuhn, paradigms change when the prevailing paradigm has failed for some time to adequately explain and provide a framework for studying various phenomena. A new paradigm slowly takes hold as it does a better job. Often, scientists trained in the old paradigm simply work to refine it until the end of their career, with younger scientists picking up the new one. The use of the word paradigm as a twenty-first-century colloquialism is more akin to the idea of a worldview or a smaller-scale model (i.e., our sales force is operating with a whole new paradigm since the pandemic) and is not what Kuhn was referring to.

The scientific method as we know it began to take shape in the sixteenth century in Europe, with important inputs from people such as Sir Francis Bacon, Sir Isaac Newton, Galilee Galileo, Nicolas Copernicus, and many others. Slowly, the fields of physics, chemistry, and then biology began to emerge. By the early twentieth century, the basic chemistry and some physiology of the body were known, but much of what went on in a cell and between organs was a mystery. By the mid-twentieth century, basic physiology and a good deal of biochemistry was sorted out. At that point, the discovery of DNA and, within just a few decades, the ability to identify chromosomes and then sequence genetic code were made. Molecular cell biology advanced to the point that by the end of the twentieth century, the basic operations of the genome and of cells were understood and could even be manipulated to some extent. The mapping of the human genome and the increased power of microprocessors and software they ran to process genetic and proteomic information began to fill in the gaps of knowledge of specific interactions in nature, such as how a foreign protein elicits a chain reaction of immune responses.

In the late nineteenth century, some important fundamentals of biological sciences were discovered that are simple by early twenty-first-century standards but were transformative of medicine. Virchow coined the term "cellular pathology," and the relationship between clinically apparent disease states and observable changes to the cell was demonstrated. This led to a deep probing into the pathological basis of disease and a whole new way to establish a diagnosis. Every time that a biopsy is interpreted today, this harkens back to the work of Virchow and others. Louis Pasteur set much of the foundation for microbiology, as did Robert Koch. The ability to culture a sample of sputum or pus from a patient, and identify a microorganism, not only created a new diagnostic method but also opened the door for future chemotherapeutics. Roentology, or "X-ray" diagnosis, discovered by Wilhelm Roentgen, leads to an ability to see into the body. Henri Becquerel, Marie Curie, and Pierre Curie won the Nobel Prize for discovering so much about where this energy came from and its nature.

This advance in science and technology derived from it started to reshape medicine. Physicians began to trust the data from laboratory or imaging methods.

Therapies could be created or at least evaluated in light of their action on cell and organ pathology. The real shift, however, was the admitting of new information into the body of knowledge of medicine based on its derivation by scientific activity. This led over the years to a narrowing of therapeutics but also an increase in their precision and the depth of the diagnosis that supported their use. An example is the synthesis of cortisol. Prior to that discovery, those with hypoadrenal states such as Addison's disease had little hope of completely regaining their health. Or the discovery of insulin, and it's purification, which gave new hope and life to type I/ juvenile diabetics. Insulin, derived from animal pancreases, remained a precious substance until another technology that developed from scientific inquiry, DNA recombination, created a bacterial source of this hormone that could then be created on an industrial scale.

The advent of the scientific method does not negate the intelligence and industry of human beings in the past or in the present using nonscientific endeavors. In ancient Rome, engineers constructed aqueducts to bring fresh water to the city, which still stand in some parts of Italy. Metallurgists in what are now Tanzania, Rwanda, and Uganda were able to forge incredible metals using smelts that were reaching 1800 °C according to modern calculations based on the materials they left. There are countless examples of the intelligent application of human reasoning to experience: gunpowder creation in ancient China, astronomy in Mesoamerica, and forest management and ecology of native North and South Americans were discovered prior to the modern scientific methods.

Nevertheless, the use of the scientific method has undoubtedly propelled medicine forward. This method has allowed knowledge to build upon itself. It also allows for competition among models of understanding and changes to those models as evidence accumulates. For example, physicians 200 years ago knew that the kidneys were connected to the bladder and were involved in urination. Physicians 100 years ago could diagnose some problems such as proteinuria and nephritis, or kidney infection, based on laboratory methods, physical examination, and patient history. Now, we have a thorough understanding of the physiology of the kidney and a great deal of its molecular cell biology. For example, the processes that lead to fibrosis of the kidney in an autoimmune disease are explainable in terms of each step, each enzyme, and signaling pathways that control the entire process.

Naturopathic medicine and other forms of healing that focus on supporting the body's intrinsic healing abilities are certainly able to draw on the scientific enterprise. For example, the type of diet to prescribe for a patient with celiac disease or giving a B12 injection for a patient with pernicious anemia is something that is obvious to a naturopathic doctor. The changes to physiology that occur when some requirement for health, such as hydration, is not adequately met can be understood using knowledge of physiology, anatomy, and biochemistry. The entire concept of an organism repairing itself is amenable to scientific study.

This leads to the areas where naturopathic medicine has struggled with a scientific footing. One is the general nature of some of its concepts.

Scientific Realism

What is testable and empirically provable is knowable. While models of science are imperfect, there is an underlying assumption that they represent reality [2]. The problem is, of course, that patients are complex and far outside of a controlled experiment. Even stacking experiments and statistically combining their data, and attempting to eliminate bias, only informs practice. This is not only because our knowledge is incomplete. It is because a human being is an open system and a vastly complex network of interacting systems. While it is quite possible to make predictions about consistent responses in this complex entity we call a patient, this is not the totality of that entity. For example, it's extremely likely that injecting any person with epinephrine will accelerate their heart rate. It's somewhat predictable that boosting norepinephrine in the brain in someone with depressive disorder will help them. But the way that multiple treatments interact in a person in a situation of chronic illness is less predictable. To put it another way, much of the reasoning and techniques of conventional medicine emerged from the root sciences of the early twentieth century, but also the battlefields of World War 2. Things work, or they do not. An antibiotic has to reduce bacteria replication, or it is ineffective. A surgical repair of a torn artery is successful, or it is unsuccessful.

When we apply this logic to therapy, it is useful, to a point. Lowering lipid levels in highly inflamed 50-year-olds who have already had a coronary event seems to help. Lowering lipids in those with high LDL and triglycerides seems to lower the likelihood of future events. But does preemptive suppression of LDL in, say, a 30-year-old lead to dementia in the future due to the fact that a biosynthetic pathway for cholesterol was suppressed, and the central nervous system needed it? Will lowering LDL not work because the underlying disturbances that were not addressed led to degenerative changes through other mechanisms? That is not to disparage statins or the value of LDL as a predictor of future morbidity, but to point out that even with an enormous amount of research, it is harder to answer questions about chronic disease and health maintenance than to address acute illness.

Another way to consider this seeming lack of comparison between short and long term effects, is to compare reliability versus validity. Reliability, in a test or a measurement, tells us that the same measurement, or on a test, the same question, will perform in a similar manner. A perfectly calibrated blood pressure cuff in the hands of a very experienced nurse is rather reliable. A lower end use at home blood pressure monitor, less so. It might tell you that your BP is 140/90 mmHG when it's 137/86 mmHg, or it may tell you that your blood pressure is 120/75 mmHg when in fact it's higher. It may be reliable enough over many BP readings to get the job done, or perhaps for someone with still uncontrolled hypertension, it's not reliable enough at all. A molecular test to diagnose HIV must be supremely reliable.

Validity is about the relevance of a test or measurement to the thing one is trying to find out. A very reliable BP cuff might not have much validity for measuring serum cholesterol or how much iron someone has in their blood.

The test of an antibiotic to inhibit the growth of a bacteria in a culture medium is a pretty valid test as far as in vitro goes. Testing a tolerable (to the patient) dose of this antibiotic to see if it cleared the bacteria from, say, the urine, would be a little less valid but still valid enough to mean something. Patients have immuno systems of different competence, they have different diets, and the total census of their microbiome is different. So how a bacteria behave in their body is a bit unique. And what antibiotics might work to suppress a certain bacterium in *that.*

To cause a biochemical change, such as lowering cholesterol, to prevent a state of disease 20 years into the future has rendered the observed pre- and posttreatment effects that might be measured not so valid. This is not because the drug did not cause the actions it was meant to. It is due to the fact that there are dozens of intervening factors.

Medical research takes the problems of reliability and validity into account. For instance, researchers, and those who review the experiments of others, seek to eliminate bias from the experiment or clinical trial. Bias can creep into an experiment in many ways. Sometimes it is a product of good intentions. A doctor treating a patient *wants* them to get well. That intentionality contributes to the healing process on some level. But reliability suffers if personal likes and dislikes and blind spots of the caregivers can warp what is being recorded as, ostensibly, facts. In nonclinical research, one way this is overcome is by having researchers precisely describe their methods and materials, and for other, impartial, or even highly skeptical, research groups to *replicate the experiment.*

To overcome the validity issues of many variables, medical research introduces certain practices and certain statistical instruments. Randomization is an important method. If a study has 1000 participants, and there is a treatment group, and non -treatment group (500 people each), the researchers attempt to randomize these groups. Neither group should be more homogenous than the other. There are limits to randomization–patient sex and age enrolled in the study. This can yield shortcomings, such as medicines tested only on males, and then prescribed to females. Randomization disperses effects to very different individuals, so that a general but verifiable effect of the treatment might emerge.

Statistical instruments, in biology and in medical research, eliminate effects due to chance. They clarify the true magnitude of effects. Human reasoning is powerful, but it has blind spots. Sometimes, what seems like an impressive effect from a treatment cannot be differentiated from random chance. In other words, if you did not treat a group of people and just kept measuring a symptom or physiological parameter, you might see, on certain days or certain subjects, an improvement. If we superimpose a treatment on this group, and we see an improvement, we might be inclined to credit the treatment with the good turn of events. Perhaps, the treatment does cause improvements, but the use of biostatistics is necessary to discern that the treatment added an effect.

One common practice is to attempt to disprove the "null hypothesis," which is that the observed changes are due to chance alone. Statistical inference can be done according to a number of methodologies, but they all look at a distribution of probability. A cause-and-effect relationship between intervention and outcome for instance (or risk factor and disease) can have a very strong probability, or a very weak one that is perhaps more than random chance but insufficient for making recommendations.

A modern randomized controlled trial makes use of these methods (including sufficient participant size, length of follow-up, and many details about how the trial was conducted). In the late twentieth century, the shortcomings of one RCT were made evident. So multiple RCTs were combined using systematic reviews. These reviews use an explicit search of the scientific literature using a set of terms. Kept results are justified, and various markers of quality are used to filter the studies. A risk of bias checklist is included. Some studies may end up being discarded due to multiple issues. The overall strength and conclusions of the research are summarized. If there is enough quantitative data in this set of studies, a meta-analysis is conducted. This uses statistical reasoning to extract and combine data from a set of individual studies. This requires the use of more advanced statistical reasoning than basic biological science level statistics. Standardized reviews and meta-analyses will yield conclusions to the effect that the current evidence is strong, moderate, weak, or insufficient to support a conclusion. The studies in question might all ask the same question. Usually, when creating searches for these studies, a "PICO" is formed. This acronym stands for "patient, intervention, condition, and outcomes." An example of a question formulated in a PICO query is: "Crestor to lower C-reactive protein in middle-aged males with established cardiovascular disease."

Why did systematic reviews come into being? Partly, it is to acknowledge the fact that no physician can read all the studies on a broad range of questions, unless they are in a very narrow subspecialty. Systematic reviews (SR) also came about because looking at just one study might be misleading. Looking at a group of studies that were filtered through an SR process created more certainty.

This was hastened by the explosion of medical publications and, importantly, the ability to retrieve them using computerized searching of the indexed medical literature. Medline, a bibliographic database of the National Library of Medicine (NLM), Bethesda, Maryland (on the campus of the National Institutes of Health), is searchable online. For some years it was published on CD-ROM, and with the advent of widely available internet access, it is now searchable through PubMed, which is hosted by the National Center for Biotechnology Information (NCBI), a part of the NLM. Before computerization, the librarians at the NLM created indexes of the medical literature, published in large volumes. Some indexes were by subject and were permuted (branched) based on levels of specificity the researcher sought. For example, a researcher might want to see what had been published in 1979 under pulmonary infections, and then under specific types of bacteria. These grew up into the MESH headings, which according to the NLM are:

> The Medical Subject Headings (MeSH) thesaurus is a controlled and -organized vocabulary produced by the National Library of Medicine. It is used for indexing, cataloging, and searching of biomedical and health-related information. MeSH includes the subject headings appearing in MEDLINE/PubMed, the NLM Catalog, and other NLM databases [3].

This is important to note. Because the PubMed interface is very easy to use, and because natural language queries via "Google Scholar" are easy for anyone to execute, it's easy to overlook the fact that this information is structured in a logical manner.

Because the amount of knowledge accrued (and accruing rapidly) is vast, and retrieval is very easy (compared to the intriguing but fatiguing walking of the journal stacks of 40 years ago), it is natural to think that a database can simply whip up an answer to any question. In a way it can, but these results are really carefully constructed questions, answered through a precise methodology, documented in a standardized manner, and indexed according to some very long-standing conventions.

All of this progress in managing information is excellent. There are, however, some critiques to keep in mind. These include:

(a) Overall quality or lack thereof of systematic reviews.
(b) The assumption that the randomized controlled trial is *always* the superior method.
(c) The ability of the highly successful RCT/SR complex to limit the advancement of other models of creating valid and reliable research results.
(d) The potential for error due to the isomorphism of the RCT to the state of scientific knowledge of the 1960s, at a time when system theory, proteomics, etc., are stretching the boundaries of what we believe to be cause and effect, signal, and feedback.

As it was presented its earlier development in the 1990s, evidence-based medicine was supposed to include biomedical research and clinical judgment. It has had its successes, but an overreliance upon it, partly due to the fallacy of thinking that systematic reviews and RCT are synonymous with science in some total fashion, has turned it into an authoritarian model that can encourage groupthink. Ioannadis [4] and others have critiqued the SR in general by saying that it *could* be a better guide, but most SR are so poorly done that they are meaningless.

In Defense of the Phenomenon

Observable phenomena are considered inferior evidence because of bias, subjectivity, etc., but there are severe limitations to discarding the reasoning emerging from information from our senses.

If people from 200 or 300 years ago were overly deterministic in their thinking, to the point of being trapped by fallacies of reasoning that looked for cause and effect all the time, then it would seem that the twenty-first century is an age of seeking randomness in medical research. Phenomena arise from studying data, and theories, such as they can come and go, arise from these phenomena. Theories can help generate more tests. Scientists work with nature, and create data that they can abductively apply to reasoning about these theories. The RCT/SR, while useful for deducing probabilities of a drug having a certain effect within a defined group of randomized subjects, lacks external validity to the wide variety of nonrandomized individual patients who flow through a practice. It is not without usefulness, and the

RCT/SR can pull the veil from biased thinking about treatments that are not useful, but it was never a tool that was good enough to be the last word on all of medicine.

Experiments

There would be no validation of theories without experiments. Babies experiment. Craftspeople experiment. The original scientific method was based on experimentation. Theory, of course, allows for a set of assumptions and construction of models based on the hypothesis testing from numerous experiments. It networks knowledge and generates new hypotheses. It allows for predictions. Theory allows for streamlining the thoughts and conclusions of many who have come before.

Medicine is the ultimate set of experiments, using a treatment on a given individual, under a certain set of present circumstances, when their health, physiology, and microbiome are at the precise state they are on that day. What becomes of medicine if the value of the $n = 1$ clinical experiment in the treatment room becomes worthless—a phantasm? Then the ability of physicians to observe and reason abductively becomes downgraded, and of course, will atrophy from disuse. In this new scenario, the physician collects data and applies a diagnostic algorithm to it. The result is that the treatment that has risen to the highest probability, or a large group of individuals with a similar condition (but dissimilar health, physiology, and microbiome), is selected. If it doesn't work, there is no runner up in this contest. The reason is that the supreme treatment that arose from the RCT/SR process is the only acceptable one. The others are not evidence based.

Individual Observations and Science

Lyme Disease Example

Certainly, a bandwagon and good reasons not to overprescribe antibiotics.

The fact that the medical literature will categorize a large group of people as "anti-science" because they present a phenomenon that is not explainable in current opinion and research shows the problem with the current model. Certainly, in the population of patients who have chronic Lyme symptoms, there are those who have been misdiagnosed, self-diagnosed, or sold on an expensive treatment regimen. There are others who have chronic symptoms (sequelae) or even chronic infection. Some infectious disease specialists in the scientific literature have attempted to address this and the reality of chronic issues for some patients. Others scoff and dismiss any unresolvable issue as hysteria, naivete, or just a defiant and oppositional attitude to "science." Of course, science as an enterprise must constantly reconcile data, phenomena that are constructed from data, models, calculations, and theory.

The fact that some in the industry decry stubborn or confounding or disconfirming data in the form of patients who won't go away belies the fact that they are confusing the greater scientific enterprise, with their own personal work. Even though there are patients and members of the general public who cling to ideas that are mostly disproven, there are many who are providing the outlying information, and through their daily suffering, a reminder that models and understanding of health phenomena don't progress without real-world input. The problem here is not the calling out of a mindset of those who might lack the education in rigorous scientific method who are convinced of a point of view without good evidence. The problem is a certain arrogance that the scientific enterprise can operate in a self-contained manner to a greater extent than it can. It was patients and physician reports who identified that thalidomide caused teratogenicity, reserpine caused depression, statin induced neuromuscular issues, and the suicidal effects of antidepressants in children. Even in a time of proliferating pet theories that are easy to propagate on social media, some physicians and scientists still need to keep a more open mind and do more listening and less scoffing.

Consensus is difficult to communicate to the public or nonscientists, and in fairness to clinicians who see patients seize upon a convenient but flawed theory that explains their problems, it's not always possible to impart everything an expert knows.

Treating the Individual

A system of medicine that does not have a theory of healing, or a cogent theory of disease, has very little in the way of navigational tools through therapies. Some have a clear physiological rationale, but for the most part, if drug X truly benefits condition (generalized) Y, is an unknown and unpredictable outcome. The only solution is to look for increasingly refined correlations. There are exceptions with antimicrobial therapy, where the ability of a drug to inhibit a bacteria can be benchmarked in vitro, or some emergency medicine therapies, whose effects and benefits are expected to and observed to take effect in the span of minutes. But the vast majority of treatments are for chronic or potentially chronic situations. For reasons discussed above, to assign a person to a disease category is often fallacious. Some disease categories, such as "poor FEV1 due to pulmonary fibrosis," are so localized, measurable, and similar that they can be standardized for the purposes of making a "PICO" question. For many other situations, the individual variability makes this less, and less, valid.

Moreover, the human being contains a group of serial and intermeshed systems that are open to the environment. This is purportedly what statistical analysis without individual data is meant to overcome. But the premises, or in this case, the patients do not provide the relevant or adequately true data to this enterprise, because they are *not* the homogenous group they may appear to be on paper.

Still, given how conventional medicine is delivered, the brute force of highly powered randomized clinical trials aggregated by meta-analyses can yield probabilities about therapies given on a nonindividualized basis for generalized disease categories. This is in fact what the majority of patients have known as the only approach to medicine throughout their lives, and are naturally seeking as medical treatment. A diabetic patient who has had a myocardial infarction and has peripheral vascular disease is placed on intensive statin therapy. This is known to probably improve their lot.

For a system of medicine that is seeking improvements in physiological function, systems integration, and a long-term de-dependance on extrinsic biochemical support, such as naturopathic medicine, this kind of logic is insufficient. It lacks navigational tools to see a particular patient through that process.

This presents a conundrum, simply because the RCT/SR methodology is a powerful one, and it introduces levels of certainty about what interventions can lead to desired outcomes and which fall short. It was inevitable that conventional medical therapy would come to devolve upon statistical analysis, in this drawn-out manner. Conventional practice bases its premise on the knowledge of the human body that comes from anatomy, pathology, molecular cell biology, biochemistry, immunology, etc. These disciplines all interrelate at the cellular and molecular level. These disciplines are necessary to describe a *state of affairs* that underlies the disease presentation. This knowledge also suggests what a therapeutic approach might target, in that point of breakdown can be more accurately described. That is why many pharmaceutical therapies can yield reliable results. For example, a child with a seizure disorder is put on medication that changes the threshold for depolarization in the central nervous system, and their seizure events become much less frequent.

What is lacking in conventional approaches is a science of therapeutics. This is somewhat present in rehabilitative medicine and, actually, surgery, which may be invasive but is a type of procedure that works closely with the repair processes of the body. The surgeon counts on the adaptive responses of the body asserting themselves, so that the time comes where they can remove the sutures and close out that case. But in the by and by of everyday medical practice—the millions of prescriptions given—it is based on probabilities of creating the desired result rather than a whole-system approach to healing.

An analogous situation would be that of an engineer building a suspension bridge. If that bridge was starting to swing or oscillate a bit too much in high winds, the engineer would use physics, engineering science, plenty of mathematical computations, and their own tests, to determine what was causing this. But whatever they end up doing, they would consider the impact on the different components of the bridge, because the forces that travel through them all interact—the suspension cables, the vertical suspenders, stiffening girders/trusses, the main towers, anchorages for the main cables, the connection between the main cables and towers, and the connections between the main cables, the vertical suspending cables, and the bridge deck (the things we walk or drive across). No engineer would keep their license if they did not consider these factors. Bridge engineering science, of course, has plenty of real-world tests and model-based experimentation to make excellent calculations. They work amazingly well—the ambassador bridge between Detroit, Michigan and Windsor, Ontario, carries over 200 million dollars of truck-based commerce per day, and it was built in the 1920s (and maintained constantly).

Medicine is different. Scientists certainly think about the impact of treatments if there is toxicity to other organs. But the science of that interaction, the science of what it means to introduce a strongly stimulating treatment into a complex open system like a human being, is underdeveloped. Conversely, naturopathic medicines' therapies, for a variety of reasons, extrinsic and intrinsic, are underdeveloped in terms of statistical information based on RCT/SR.

This is why any drug treatment, with some emergency treatment exceptions (in a very narrow time frame for a very specific purpose), is an event that is governed by randomness. And the probability sciences, that act as navigation through randomness, are the best tool that conventional medicine currently has.

An unfortunate consequence of this dominance of conventional medicine by the RCT/SR process is that physicians are less likely to engage in the kind of abductive reasoning which the human brain excels at.

Naturopathic medicine is undertheorized. But the theories it needs (those that go beyond the useful and applicable theories of biological science) in order to expand scientific activity of naturopathic therapeutics have an important prerequisite. These are theories that must be very inferential from facts, from clinic phenomena. This is opposed to theories that would tell us *not to see obvious clinical states of affairs that are in front of us*.

Professor Nancy Cartwright, of the London School of Economics, published an important paper in 2007 entitled *Are RCTs the Gold Standard*? [5] Cartwright differentiates between what she calls "clinchers," which are forms of deductive reasoning that more or less prove something to be the case, and "vouchers," which are often adductive forms of reasoning that suggest that something is the best explanation at the moment or that something is probably the case. The clinchers tend to have high internal validity and high reliability. The vouchers have much higher external validity but are less reliable. RCTs have high internal validity but poor external validity—even randomized, the constellation of variables involved in a group of people at one point in time is not easily replicated elsewhere. That is hypothetically important because the claim is that randomization increases significance and internal validity and eliminates selection bias. That is true, but it does not mean that the RCT necessarily translates to practice, unless the cross section of people being treated is very similar to those within the study group. For some conditions, this is easier to achieve, and "ideal RCT" has a high level of external validity. A study of the diagnosis of bacterial meningitis, for instance, might reach this, because this condition is so overwhelming and it produces such drastic symptoms and signs that the sameness between a large-enough study group and patients in the real world is enough to make it a good assessment of the facts.

Cartwright notes the many non-RCT deductive methods used in science including the following:

- Econometric methods.
- Galilean experiments.
- Probabilistic/Granger causality.
- Derivation from established theory.

- Tracing the causal process.

She furthermore proposes that the power of **statistical sameness,** the power of accrued specific observations, is achievable with sufficiently rigorous repetition in medical science. This swings the pendulum from utter faith in randomization to a more balanced view that for many aspects of practice, a type of research that is more akin to other scientific fields, are more productive.

Some standards in research become that way by rote. For instance, a study with a confidence internal of $p > 0.05$ is not necessarily false, and the "significance" standard of 0.05, adopted by Fisher is subject to appraisal based on the specifics of the experiment [6].

Lack of Theory

Refinements to models for testing pharmaceuticals are insufficient, although still useful. In terms of truly understanding the benefits of the naturopathic approach, the following principles could be studied with regard to naturopathic medicine.

Proposition I

Creating the conditions for health will lead to rectification of disordered systems and resolution of problems. By subjective and objective means, the symptoms, signs, and disruptions to bioregulatory systems will often improve when the conditions for health are met. This is constrained by the degree to which permanent structural pathological changes to cells and extracellular matrix have set in.

Proposition II

Supporting prosurvival mechanisms will lead to rectification of disordered systems and resolution of problems. This is constrained by the degree to which conditions for health are met and the degree to which permanent structural pathological changes to cells and extracellular matrix have set in.

Proposition III

Reduction in the magnitude of maladaptive responses can lead to rectification of disordered systems and resolution of problems. This is constrained by the extent to which prosurvival responses are robust enough to assert themselves, the conditions for health are met, and the degree to which permanent structural pathological changes to cells and extracellular matrix have set in.

The fact that homeostatic balance can be induced by the external means, such as a synthetic pharmaceutical, is beyond question and is the subject of massive research. It is also not questionable that this does great good and in many cases is the best starting point for patients.

Homeostatic maintenance with external agents will become either intolerable or will be unsustainable if:

(a) Started without addressing the conditions for health.
(b) Begun in a patient with unrealized or defective prosurvival mechanisms.
(c) Carried on for a long period of time.
(d) Is too disruptive or carries too high of a toxic burden.

It might be prolonged with adjustments in dose and the addition of more agents. This might be an acceptable trade-off for the elderly. For the young or middle aged, this can lead to very few options for maintaining function and a level of health that is functioning but not optimal and is tenuous.

Below is a proposed model of studying naturopathic treatments that aim to address determining factors of health, stimulate the healing process, and support the expression of adaptive responses (Fig. 11.1). In this model, the pinnacles are observational studies with replication. A plausible mechanism and careful documentation about the specific nature of patients by their clinicians are necessary here. In some cases, overlapping confidence intervals between observational studies would be one

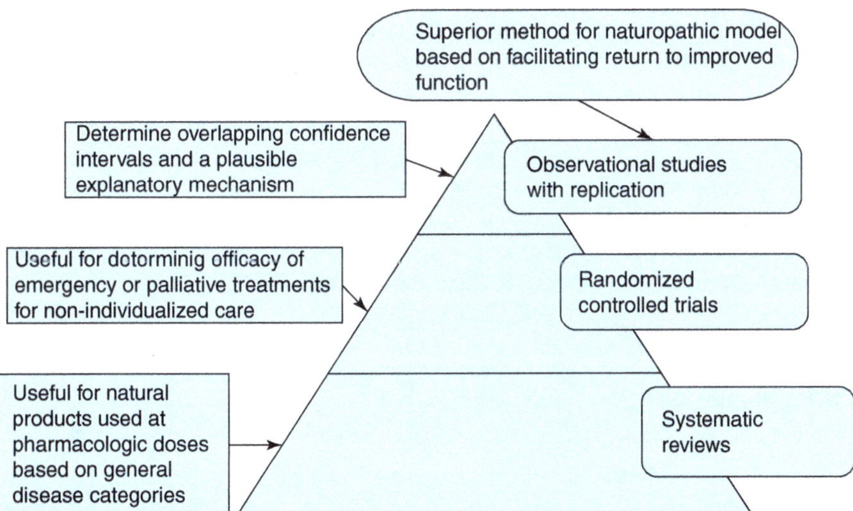

Fig. 11.1 A prioritizing model for naturopathic medical research: All types of studies and analyses have their place. Rigorous replication of treatment effects, with very close observation and documentation of specific patient traits, is essential to building the knowledge base that supports naturopathic therapeutics

way to create replication rigor. Experience becomes more powerful as it accumulates. The fact that fallacy can persist is not a reason to discount replicable outcomes. If that were true, science would not have developed as it has. A vacuum of nihilism about the value of physician observation and the power of replication and sameness over a fixation on randomization has brought us to where we now are. By the narrowest of margins, some drugs pass muster of being statistically significant ($p < 0.05$), and unlike other sciences where intense experimentation can grow practical knowledge, medicine has slowed down.

There is definitely applicability of RCT and SR to naturopathic medicine. But this becomes more valid when the topic at hand is a very standardized treatment, such as herbs used at pharmaceutically high doses, for disease states that tend to produce a very similar clinical picture.

In other eras, as a model of medicine reached maturity, a certain stagnation set in. This happened with Galenic medicine in the Middle Ages in Europe. Some innovation, often injected by Arab physicians, helped float this model along well past its expiration date. The lack of the modern scientific method allowed for authoritarianism. But when a medical system is too invested in dogma, when it values methods over the sometime murky amalgam of observation, bedside experimentation, biomedical sciences plausibility, and the study of similar (versus random) patients compared together in valid ways, it can become therapeutically sterile. Such systems begin to have increasing difficulty dealing with the new diseases of the time. This intensifies, until a crisis occurs. Such a crisis occurred in Europe in the 1600s as syphilis became epidemic, and the theories of the time, and the legacy of Galenic medicine, had no answers. What kept the answers out? It was the adherence to a worldview based on what worked for the diseases of the past. The diseases of today are many, and there are still awesomely effective treatments for them, and new treatments all the time. But the frustrating situations are those related to a collapse of health itself. Diabetes climbs with a projection to 1/3 of the population by 2050. Cardiovascular disease, in spite of some victories in vulnerable groups with statin therapy, marches on. And it will roar as the many, many obese American children and prediabetic teenagers reach the age of 40 years and up. These disorders are being studied in great detail, which are all useful information. But these maladies will not yield solely to an approach that seeks to reduce them to lesions or one-degree cause-and-effect entities, because they are not.

Biocybernetics

Naturopathic medicine suffers from a certain hypocognition in research. This is the linguistic phenomenon whereby it becomes difficult to discuss or express something because of a lack of words for it. This is not to say that there is no linguistic apparatus to discuss naturopathic medicine. The processes of biology and healing are plain to see. What can be undertheorized and in some ways limited is the distinct therapeutic model of naturopathic medicine. The work by Zeff, Snider, and many others to articulate the healing order in naturopathic medicine (one that approximates the healing order of the human body and mind) has brought with it a great deal of codified language which has moved the profession forward.

Cybernetics as a scientific system has been described since the mid-twentieth century [7]. Ross Ashby contributed much to a general theory of cybernetics. The concept of homeostasis arises from cybernetic concepts. These have been applied to natural neural networks in understanding how complex neurological systems function through interaction of components. Biocybernetics is the application of these principles of how enmeshed whole systems work [8]. Systems biology makes use of this. It is likely that one area of testable and theorizable science in the therapeutics and practice of naturopathic medicine will use biocybernetic principles to understand how small stimulations and soft guidance from natural therapy inputs can permit complex systems to move from a state of disorder or chaotic oscillations back into one of balance.

References

1. Ridgway E, Baker P, Woods J, Lawrence M. Historical developments and paradigm shifts in public health nutrition science, guidance and policy actions: a narrative review. Nutrients. 2019;11(3):531.
2. Allzén S. Scientific realism and empirical confirmation: a puzzle. Stud Hist Phil Sci. 2021;90:153–9.
3. Medicine NL of. Preface. [cited 2022 Jun 2]. Available from: https://www.nlm.nih.gov/mesh/intro_preface.html
4. Ioannidis JPA. The mass production of redundant, misleading, and conflicted systematic reviews and meta-analyses. Milbank Q. 2016;94(3):485–514.
5. Cartwrjight N. Are RCTs the gold standard? BioSocieties. 2007;2(1):11–20.
6. Wasserstein RL, Schirm AL, Lazar NA. Moving to a World Beyond "p < 0.05.". Am Stat. 2019;73(sup1):1–19. https://doi.org/10.1080/00031305.2019.1583913.
7. Lindner B, Thomas PJ, Fellous J-M, Tiesinga P. Biological cybernetics: 60 years and more to come. Biol Cybern. 2021;115(1):5–6. Available from: https://pubmed.ncbi.nlm.nih.gov/33620520
8. Goldstein DS. Concepts of scientific integrative medicine applied to the physiology and pathophysiology of catecholamine systems. Compr Physiol. 2013;3(4):1569–610.

Chapter 12
Artificial Intelligence

Artificial intelligence (AI) is predicted to have a major impact on medicine as the twenty-first century unfolds [1]. AI is the programming and initiation of computer-based systems that can make choices based on a type of rule application. In the concept of AI versus that of a simple computer program, there is a certain implied plasticity, a reinvention or reapplication of the rules, so that the AI system can confront a variety of situations. Machine learning is a subset of AI and is the type of information accumulation by a programmed system that can adapt its models and algorithms as it accrues more information. For example, machine learning is being used to review medical records from large hospital EHR databases to detect trends about diagnoses, patient statistics, treatments, and outcomes.

Machine learning and, more robustly, artificial neural nets that can function autonomously are already here. With increased sophistication and increased computing power, they will grow in efficacy. What sort of functions are they predicted to play in medicine.

Diagnosis

AI is capable of amassing a large amount of information and filtering it. Physicians will one day have an AI assist utility that will access millions of citations and thousands of biological facts. This doesn't mean that the AI system will have the last word but rather will search and refine, not just aggregate information.

F. Smith, *Naturopathic Medicine*, https://doi.org/10.1007/978-3-031-13388-6_12

Treatments

As data about treatments accumulates, so does the need to have a comprehensive overview of it. The AI scan of treatments will also be able to factor in biological facts such as pharmacokinetics, pharmacodynamics, statistical predictions, and actions of similar agents. Another dimension to this tool is to factor in the patient's specific information including results of many lab tests.

Genomic Analysis

Genes, and the proteins they code for, create an order of complexity that is too high to predict the impact of many genes. Some mutations or autosomal dominant and recessive genes are so striking in their actions that they are predictable. The cystic fibrosis gene is an example. But there is much more than this. DNA is a code that contains information. There is also a high degree of complexity in how genes activate and repress each other. The influences of the environment and the microbiome add even more variables and possible pathways. This is an area where the ability of an AI system to navigate incredible amounts of data will be useful.

What Will Be the Containers, the Queries of These Powerful Algorithms?

Much like Kant connected reason to the pre-existing categories of the human mind, when we assemble an automated system to process data, we need to provide categories that are, abstractly, going to allow that machine to support sense-making. Humans are sense-making creatures, and to the degree that these machines are more useful to us beyond speed of calculations or the automated control of other machines, they must process and apprehend the patterns in data that are supportive of us in our sense-making.

Naturopathic medicine might fear that an infinitely vast and fast set of computations might allow a one-side approach to health care to prevail. Through sheer processing power and brute force analysis of data points, it will empower physicians to simply treat symptoms as they emerge. Or perhaps, the actions to take will be so far over our heads, that we'll just do what the program tells us to do, being unable to make the connections and casualties for ourselves. Much like a tourist driving through a strange city just following GPS directions without understanding the terrain, we'll accept the fact that the medical AI knows best, and we'll cooperate, so the story goes. There are discussions now about the fact that the sheer computational power of AI will leave our scientific method behind. That causation as we are capable of comprehending it might be superceded by a machine's ability to assemble patterns and associations from terabytes of data and make predictions that are more accurate than those derived by a logical/deductive method arising from scientific knowledge [2].

This may be true to some extent; the selection of certain drugs, or nutrients, based on health status and genome, might be aided by lightning speed software based on machine learning. But this is to fail to imagine what might be possible using these tools that was not possible before.

The current state of the extracellular matrix, its communications, and its impact on cells is something we can study in specific ways for tissues and in certain illnesses. To be able to aggregate biochemical and matrix function information about a patient and discern where disruptions due to communication, toxin deposition, inflammation, and other extracellular matrix activities could be remedied.

The feature engineering of these systems could be imbued with categories—features—that enable us to better understand the patient as a whole person and a vastly complex system and being.

The muscular aspect of computing power can help in the following ways:

1. Aggregating cases and small trials to establish a replication effect—this is knowable to actual human doctors but the retrieval and assembling of these cases, observations, and small trials can become challenging as medical research grows by millions of indexed entries.
2. Interpolation and extrapolation, of a sort, might be aided by such software. To some extent, the pattern recognition and insight of the human mind is superior. But the apprehension of shared traits within a group or between a group and the rest of the population can be aided by computer and various electronic networks that can carry out tasks that will superceded what we currently think of as computing power.
3. To the degree that is valid, present statistical analysis, but without a tyrannical model of conflating any statistical computation with "the truth." Going beyond the idea of statistical sameness is a discernible but rigorous replication, and the AI assistance may make a highly individualized system of medicine much more reliable in its assumptions.
4. Executing queries regarding genes and DNA sequences, which is in its vast amount of coded data, occurring naturally.

Aside from aiding us in these abductive reasoning processes, this computing power can help us with the evaluation of functional states of whole systems and also with predictive tasks in medicine.

Functional States: Biocybernetics

Applying biocybernetic principles to understand whole systems, and how they are operating based on inputs and outputs, requires a massive amount of real-time data. AI tools may bring this to life in a case-by-case manner. Rather than erase the individuality and artfulness of a patient-centered medicine, AI may actually empower it [3].

Humans First

These tools will arise, but they need not dominate us. One of the ethical and societal challenges of the twenty-first century will be to establish the primacy of the human and not to let the tools of our technology become the main value that supercedes other considerations. That is to say, that part of the expression of human life and its value is to realize one's abilities and to express oneself in time and in action. The highest good is not necessarily to be found by cleverly replacing all human activity. There are already many powers in the universe that exceed ours and could swallow up the earth, such as black holes. The ability to build a machine that can compare images faster than a human brain doesn't mean that it should have all the fun. The question is not even what humans can do better, which is in fact, at this moment, a lot. The human brain literally changes with experience, with life. It doesn't emulate something else, it is a part of us, as living, thinking, and feeling beings.

And at the root of that truth is the fact that patients suffer, and the role of the physician is to be there with them. Certainly, the work of physicians in saving livings, and resources, with the power of data sciences and AI is a good thing and, for those who receive the benefit, makes all the difference in the world. But no mountain of machine learning can ever replace what we mean to each other. The day may come when some patients are content with whatever treatment a supercomputer will dispense from a vending machine of sorts. But whenever a person suffers, seeks to realize that they can heal, and takes the steps to allow that healing to proceed, many will want a physician as their guide and their doctor. This need and this practice is as old as the human race, and to be human is to need other humans.

References

1. Noorbakhsh-Sabet N, Zand R, Zhang Y, Abedi V. Artificial intelligence transforms the future of health care. Am J Med. 2019;132(7):795–801.
2. Voit EO. Perspective: dimensions of the scientific method. PLoS Comput Biol. 2019;15(9):e1007279.
3. Lindner B, Thomas PJ, Fellous J-M, Tiesinga P. Biological cybernetics: 60 years and more to come. Biol Cybern. 2021;115(1):5–6. https://pubmed.ncbi.nlm.nih.gov/33620520.

Chapter 13
The Broader Mission of Naturopathic Medicine

Mission

Naturopathic medicine has a lot to offer individual patients. But the people we aim to serve live in a world that influences their health and welfare, and which they in turn influence. If we truly address causes and treat the whole person, we must consider community, societal, and global issues [1]. There are many, some being widely recognized, and others more personal or known to a smaller or local group. The impact of human activities on climate and the impact of heat, drought, and rising oceans on human life and food production are issues that matter now and will in all likelihood loom over life as the twenty-first century unfolds. A naturopathic physician cannot act on all of these issues every day, but being aware opens the door to making choices (such as sustainable health-care practice) and choosing what specific issues they want to put (time, money, and energy) into.

Food Access

As discussed earlier in this textbook, food access is a problem for many people, including access to healthy foods. At the same time, the average patient is confronted with a vast array of edible choices that carry health risks. So called food "swamps" are places where there is a preponderance of vendors of processed and fast foods. At least one third of the United States adults eat fast food each day [2]. Many people cannot drive to work or to recreational activities without passing through a gauntlet of fast-food choices. In Canada, there are older statistics indicating that about a third of Canadians visit a fast-food outlet per day, but newer information indicates that fast food contributes to about 6% of the total energy intake of Canadians [3].

F. Smith, *Naturopathic Medicine*, https://doi.org/10.1007/978-3-031-13388-6_13

Disparities in Health Care

Health-care disparities take many forms. Simple lack of access to care due to being unable to afford it is one. The problems of access in more private insurance and market orientation systems versus government single-payer systems differ. But at the end of the day, there are finite resources. In the United States, Medicare and Medicaid provide funding for millions of people. But not all health providers opt into these systems, or rather, they opt out because they are not happy with the administrative time and cost nor the remuneration.

The health-care system in the United States and those who study it are taking a closer look at racial disparities in terms of how care is delivered [4–8]. This goes beyond looking at outcomes and relates to the experience that patients have, and how this differs based on self-identified racial category. For instance, does one group get a less serious approach to the physician obtaining informed consent? African Americans are more likely to be misdiagnosed with mental illness. To what degree is that a function of physician behavior, or to training (which impacts behavior in practice), or to the way that diagnostic standards for mental illness are constructed? If someone has food insecurity and work insecurity, and their neighborhood has had a recent episode of violence, does that constitute an anxiety disorder if they are feeling overwrought? The placing of patient symptoms and signs into categories is a necessary function of diagnosis, but is that diagnosis done blindly in some instances?

During the COVID 19 pandemic, treatment for some Black and Latino patients was delayed or not ordered due to faulty pulse oximeters that overestimated their blood PO2. It appears that these devices do not work as well on pigmented skin and are not correctly calibrated for these patients [9].

There are many other kinds of disparities, by age, gender, sexual orientation, gender identity, and economic. Combined, these make delivery of limited resources for health very uneven and have ripple effects through the society in terms of mortality, morbidity, and distress.

These are necessary studies and conversations, and naturopathic physicians will need to be a part of them, as they are part of health care and, as with any doctor, are not above falling into the errors of bias or discrimination.

Leadership

In a doctor-and-patient relationship, a naturopathic physician will educate patients about meeting their own requirements for health and perhaps provide resources about how to shop, cook, and live in a way that is more sustainable. But what kind of leadership can a naturopathic physician provide?

Leadership has many definitions. There are academic fields that study it, including Leadership Studies, and Organizational Development and Effectiveness. This field came to maturity, in terms of theory and research, in the twentieth century. As an example of breadth, the Encyclopedia of Leadership is a 4-volume set [10], and this simply provides an overview of many topics for graduate students in this field. One way of characterizing leadership is that it is a process of influence that allows an organization and its members to direct their activities in a way that moves toward a goal. There are leadership settings and styles where leadership is authority based—command and control.

What Are Ways of Influencing These Issues?

Understanding that leadership is not so much about titles, but about influence, helps to see that a naturopathic physician in a community can be a leader. They can lead their patient into clear thinking about good health choices and behaviors. They can participate in community, national, or global groups that have a stated purpose that aligns with their values. They can conduct research and publish the results. They can use public forms of communication, such as social media (always with professionalism and restraint), and broadcast to reach a wider audience. They can volunteer for professional association work or give their time to a worthy not-for-profit organization.

Lessons from Indigenous Peoples

Naturopathic medicine has its distinct genealogy and a specific history. It has its roots in Hippocratic medicine and is something of a prodigy of European nature cure and hydrotherapy medicine. It is very much a product of the American milieu of natural medicine of the early twentieth century, which has its parallel with Canadian wellness movements. But its principles are easily seen in parallel with traditional medicine systems. The idea of the body healing itself and the primacy of being in harmony with nature is integral to indigenous medicine systems. These traditional practices have their own context and those who bear the expertise and experience with them.

Studying them should not be a way to co-opt aspects of their linguistic categories of nature, without acknowledging that these are very rooted, traditional systems that precede naturopathic medicine. But with an open mind and humility, there are lessons that can make naturopathic medicine better. Influence by these systems can help to keep naturopathic medicine from sliding into a more reductionistic and less relevant stance. This has been a trend in Hippocratic-whole system schools of medicine that, having reached their apogee, tend to formalize or systematize their work and lose their distinct framework and value system. As these indigenous systems developed many of the herbs and practices that naturopathic medicine inherited, there is also a duty to help to protect and sustain these systems. Not only are many of these traditional systems of indigenous medicine less prominent in some countries because of patient movement to more conventional systems of care. Many of these systems are threatened, and the knowledge passed down for centuries is at risk of being lost.

This is not only tragic for the loss it would mean to those indigenous communities. It is at this very time that the knowledge, the wisdom, the approach to problem-solving, and the connection with nature, and the whole-person integration that many indigenous systems practice, are needed. Our societal progress in using the scientific method and technologies that arise from it has brought us incredible good. For example, babies born with congenital heart defects have them repaired every day. Infections that can overwhelm the defenses of even a hearty individual can often be nullified with antimicrobials. But our one-sided pursuit of dominance of nature is in a sense consuming our world. The declining health of Americans doesn't appear to yield to more elaborate and precise treatments (although those treatments can treat the end stages of that declining health). The world itself, in the sense of a biosphere, is buckling under the demands of an industrial world.

Dr. Nicole Redvers is a naturopathic physician and an assistant professor in both the Department of Family and Community Medicine and the Department of Indigenous Health at the University of North Dakota. Dr. Redvers' recent publications outline the need for sustainable healthcare and the education of physicians who are able to create and deliver it [11]. Her recent review on the research of indigenous healing systems reveals that there has been progress in creating research and some co-education models [12]. But there is also a long history of dismissive or disrespectful attitudes of physicians to indigenous healing. This arises not only from a sense of superiority but also from a true ignorance of what these healing systems really are. It would be ironic and regrettable if naturopathic medicine, a field with great promise in modeling an integrative approach (and which has in many ways), was unable to hear the voices of indigenous medicine and cultures during a time in history that is a turning point.

The world is at a level of nonsustainability. Industrial economies, science, technology, etc., have given the human race new tools and new gifts that created the world we live in. But the twenty-first century will require new ways to live, new ways to treat each other, and a recalibrated sense of how to treat the planet. As exciting as the concept of creating human colonies on near-to-Earth places like Mars or the Moon may be, the 7 and ¾ billion people who live on Earth are needing this biosphere to be whole and healing. We won't be able to simply exploit the planet for much longer. That doesn't mean a return to a patheolithic lifestyle for just a few millions of people. But it will mean a new approach to respecting the health of the planet and realizing that our health is bound up with it.

Naturopathic physicians can teach patients in their clinic, or impart to them, a sense of what that means. They can also be involved in efforts to help our world, be it creating economic alternatives to deforestation in countries such as Borneo or seeing that agriculture moves to a sustainable model that doesn't waste resources but doesn't create food scarcity.

The ethos that naturopathic physicians can often impart, through their actions, is this: technology and energy-intensive methods to solve health problems are wonderful and can save lives. But to flaunt the laws of nature and then expect that these technologies can erase the consequences is foolish.

That is not a judgment of any person who suffers from a disease. But it is a call to help awaken patients to their own healing abilities and to see that being a modern, twenty-first-century member of the human race can include older ways of living and thinking, as well as our contemporary technologies.

Naturopathic medicine is one profession among many that seeks to alleviate suffering and help people rebuild their health. Because it is based on sound principles that ring true in each generation, it has survived the vicissitudes of the technological era in medicine and remade itself into a viable, contemporary profession. With every day that passes, naturopathic physicians and their patients come together to learn, to work, and to create the conditions that allow healing to take place. For it is ultimately the systems, forces, and instincts that pull all living things toward survival and growth, that creates health. The healing power of nature, or vis medicatrix naturae, as Hippocrates termed it, is the central idea that can bring order and wholeness out of chaos and disharmony. No matter what new tools and technologies the naturopathic physicians of tomorrow adopt, they will still exert their efforts to work with that force for health, which is the birthright of every single person in this world.

References

1. Smith F. Remedium Mundi. Naturopathic Doct News Rev. 2022;6
2. CDC. 2018. https://www.cdc.gov/nchs/products/databriefs/db322.htm. Accessed 30 Apr 2022.
3. Black JL, Billette JM. Fast food intake in Canada: differences among Canadians with diverse demographic, socio-economic and lifestyle characteristics. Can J Public Health. 2015;106(2):e52–8. https://doi.org/10.17269/cjph.106.4658. PMID: 25955672, PMCID: PMC6972105.
4. Wheeler SM, Bryant AS. Racial and ethnic disparities in health and health care. Obstet Gynecol Clin N Am. 2017;44(1):1–11.
5. Sutton MY, Anachebe NF, Lee R, Skanes H. Racial and ethnic disparities in reproductive health services and outcomes, 2020. Obstet Gynecol. 2021;137(2):225–33.
6. Center for Disease Control and Prevention. Health disparities. https://www.cdc.gov/healthyyouth/disparities/. Accessed 20 May 2022.
7. Thornton RLJ, Glover CM, Cené CW, Glik DC, Henderson JA, Williams DR. Evaluating strategies for reducing health disparities by addressing the social determinants of health. Health Aff. 2016;35(8):1416–23.
8. Saeed SA, Masters RM. Disparities in health care and the digital divide. Curr Psychiatry Rep. 2021;23(9):61.
9. Fawzy A, Wu TD, Wang K, Robinson ML, Farha J, Bradke A, et al. Racial and ethnic discrepancy in pulse oximetry and delayed identification of treatment eligibility among patients with COVID-19. JAMA Intern Med. 2022;182:730. https://doi.org/10.1001/jamainternmed.2022.1906.
10. SAGE. https://us.sagepub.com/en-us/nam/encyclopedia-of-leadership/book220818. Accessed 30 Apr 2022.

11. Redvers N, Schultz C, Vera Prince M, Cunningham M, Jones R, Blondin B. Indigenous perspectives on education for sustainable healthcare. Med Teach. 2020;42(10):1085–90. https://doi.org/10.1080/0142159X.2020.1791320.
12. Redvers N, Blondin B. Traditional Indigenous medicine in North America: a scoping review. PLoS One. 2020;15(8):e0237531. https://doi.org/10.1371/journal.pone.0237531. PMID: 32790714; PMCID: PMC7425891.

Appendix A: Resources

The following are a list of resources for those who wish to learn more about naturopathic medicine. This is merely a sample, and there are many excellent books, articles, websites, databases, and conferences to choose from.

- Books

  Murray M, Pizzorno J. Editors. A Textbook of Natural Medicine. St. Louis, Churchill Livingstone, 2020.

  Saunders P, Barlow K. Principles and Practices of Naturopathic Botanical Medicine. Toronto, CCNM Press, 2022.
- Databases

  Natural Medicines [database on the Internet]. Somerville (MA): Therapeutic Research Center; publication year [July 1, 2022]. Available from: https://naturalmedicines.therapeuticresearch.com. Subscription required to view.
- Journals

  Natural Medicine Journal. Portland (ME): American Association of Naturopathic Physicians. Available from: https://www.naturalmedicinejournal.com/
- Trade Publications

  Naturopathic Doctors News and Review. Scottsdale (AZ). Available from: https://www.ndnr.com

F. Smith, *Naturopathic Medicine*, https://doi.org/10.1007/978-3-031-13388-6

Appendix B: Professional Organizations

The following are professional organizations in Naturopathic Medicine.

- United States
  American Association of Naturopathic Physicians
  300 New Jersey Ave NW, Suite 900
  Washington, DC 20001
  P: 202-237-8150
  http://www.naturopathic.org
- Canada
  Canadian Association of Naturopathic Doctors
  20 Holly St., Ste. 200
  Toronto, Ontario, Canada M4S 3B1
  Tel: 416-496-8633
  Toll-free: 1-800-551-4381
  http://www.cand.ca
- Accreditation
  The Council on Naturopathic Medical Education
  PO Box 178
  Great Barrington, MA 01230
  413-528-8877
  http://www.cnme.org
- Licensing Examinations (multi-jurisdiction)
  North American Board of Naturopathic Examiners
  Suite 119, #321
  9220 S.W. Barbur Blvd.
  Portland, OR 97219
  503-246-0694
  http://www.nabne.org

F. Smith, *Naturopathic Medicine*, https://doi.org/10.1007/978-3-031-13388-6

- Accredited Naturopathic Programs
  Association of Accredited Naturopathic Medical Colleges
  1717 K Street NW, Suite 900
  Washington, DC 20006
  800-345-7454
  http://www.aanmc.org
- Globally
  World Naturopathic Federation
  20 Holly Street, Suite 200
  Toronto, Ontario
  M4S 3B1
  905-940-2727
  http://www.worldnaturoapthicfederation.org

Index

F. Smith, *Naturopathic Medicine*, https://doi.org/10.1007/978-3-031-13388-6

N

GPSR Compliance
The European Union's (EU) General Product Safety Regulation (GPSR) is a set of rules that requires consumer products to be safe and our obligations to ensure this.

If you have any concerns about our products, you can contact us on

ProductSafety@springernature.com

In case Publisher is established outside the EU, the EU authorized representative is:

Springer Nature Customer Service Center GmbH
Europaplatz 3
69115 Heidelberg, Germany

www.ingramcontent.com/pod-product-compliance
Lightning Source LLC
LaVergne TN
LVHW022122110326
833723LV00022B/818

* 9 7 8 3 0 3 1 1 3 3 9 0 9 *